Improving the fat content of foods

Related titles:

Food, diet and obesity
(ISBN-13: 978-1-85573-958-1; ISBN-10: 1-85573-958-5)
Obesity is a global epidemic affecting both developed and developing countries. There has been a wealth of research on the complex interactions between genetic susceptibility, diet and lifestyle in determining individual risk of obesity. With its distinguished editor and international team of contributors, this important collection sums up the key findings in weight control research and its implications for the food industry.

Functional foods, ageing and degenerative disease
(ISBN-13: 978-1-85573-725-9; ISBN-10: 1-85573-725-6)
As the proportion of the elderly increases in many developed countries, there is an increasing emphasis on preventing some of the chronic diseases particularly associated with ageing. This important collection reviews the role of functional foods in preventing a number of degenerative conditions from osteoporosis and cancer to immune function and gut health.

Functional foods, cardiovascular disease and diabetes
(ISBN-13: 978-1-85573-735-8; ISBN-10: 1-85573-735-3)
Cardiovascular disease and diabetes pose a serious and growing health risk to populations in the developed world. This authoritative collection reviews dietary factors affecting disease risk and the ways individual functional foods can help prevent them.

Details of these books and a complete list of Woodhead titles can be obtained by:

- visiting our web site at www.woodheadpublishing.com
- contacting Customer Services (email: sales@woodhead-publishing.com; fax: +44 (0) 1223 893694; tel.: +44 (0) 1223 891358 ext. 30; address: Woodhead Publishing Limited, Abington Hall, Abington, Cambridge CB1 6AH, England)

Improving the fat content of foods

Edited by
Christine Williams and Judith Buttriss

CRC Press
Boca Raton Boston New York Washington, DC

WOODHEAD PUBLISHING LIMITED
Cambridge England

Published by Woodhead Publishing Limited
Abington Hall, Abington
Cambridge CB1 6AH
England
www.woodheadpublishing.com

Published in North America by CRC Press LLC
6000 Broken Sound Parkway, NW
Suite 300
Boca Raton, FL 33487
USA

First published 2006, Woodhead Publishing Limited and CRC Press LLC

British Library Cataloguing in Publication Data
A catalogue record for this book is available from the British Library.

Library of Congress Cataloging-in-Publication Data
A catalog record for this book is available from the Library of Congress.

Woodhead Publishing Limited ISBN-13: 978-1-85573-965-9 (book)
Woodhead Publishing Limited ISBN-10: 1-85573-965-8 (book)
Woodhead Publishing Limited ISBN-13: 978-1-84569-107-3 (e-book)
Woodhead Publishing Limited ISBN-10: 1-84569-107-5 (e-book)
CRC Press ISBN-10: 0-8493-9208-X
CRC Press order number: WP9208

The publishers' policy is to use permanent paper from mills that operate a sustainable forestry policy, and which has been manufactured from pulp which is processed using acid-free and elementary chlorine-free practices. Furthermore, the publishers ensure that the text paper and cover board used have met acceptable environmental accreditation standards.

Project managed by Macfarlane Production Services, Dunstable, Bedfordshire
(e-mail: macfarl@aol.com)
Typeset by Godiva Publishing Services Ltd, West Midlands
Printed by TJ International Limited, Padstow, Cornwall, England

Contents

Part II Reducing saturated fatty acids in food

Contributor contact details

(* = main contact)

Editors

Professor Christine M. Williams
School of Food Biosciences
University of Reading
Reading RG6 6AP
UK

E-mail: c.m.williams@reading.ac.uk

Professor Judith Buttriss
British Nutrition Foundation
52–54 High Holborn
London WC1V 6RQ
UK

E-mail: j.buttriss@nutrition.org.uk

Chapter 1

Dr Peter L. Zock
Unilever Research and Development Vlaardingen
Olivier van Noortlaan 120
3133 AT Vlaardingen
Netherlands

E-mail: peter.zock@unilever.com

Chapter 2

Dr Danielle I. Shaw and Professor Christine M. Williams
Hugh Sinclair Unit of Human Nutrition
School of Food Biosciences
The University of Reading
PO Box 226
Whiteknights
Reading RG6 6AP
UK

Dr Wendy L. Hall*
Department of Nutrition and Dietetics
School of Biomedical and Health Sciences
King's College London
Franklin Wilkins Building

150 Stamford Street
London SE1 9NH
UK

E-mail: wendy.hall@kcl.ac.uk

Chapter 3

Professor Denis Lairon* and Richard Planells
INSERM
Faculté de Médecine
Université de Marseille
27 Bd Jean Moulin
13385 Marseille 5
France

E-mail: denis.lairon@medecine.univ-mrs.fr
richard.planells@medecine.univ-mrs.fr

Chapter 4

Dr José López-Miranda*, Dr Pablo Pérez-Martínez and Dr Francisco Pérez-Jiménez
Unidad de Lípidos y Arteriosclerosis
Hospital Universitario Reina Sofia
Facultad de Medicina
Universidad de Córdoba
Avda. Menéndez Pidal s/n
14004 Cordoba
Spain

E-mail: jlopezmir@uco.es

Chapter 5

Dr Anne M. Minihane* and Dr Julie A. Lovegrove
Hugh Sinclair Unit of Human Nutrition
School of Food Biosciences
University of Reading
Reading RG6 6AP
UK

E-mail: j.a.lovegrove@reading.ac.uk
a.m.minihane@reading.ac.uk

Chapter 6

Dr Patrick Schrauwen* and Professor Wim H. M. Saris
Nutrition and Toxicology Research Institute Maastricht (NUTRIM)
Department of Human Biology
Maastricht University
PO Box 616
6200 MD Maastricht
The Netherlands

E-mail: p.schrauwen@hb.unimaas.nl

Chapter 7

Dr Margriet S. Westerterp-Plantenga
Department of Human Biology
Maastricht University
PO Box 616
6200 MD Maastricht
The Netherlands

E-mail: M.Westerterp@HB.unimaas.nl

Chapter 8

Dr Parveen Yaqoob* and Dr Sabine Tricon
Hugh Sinclair Unit of Human Nutrition
School of Food Biosciences
PO Box 226
University of Reading
Whiteknights
Reading RG6 6AP
UK
E-mail: P.Yaqoob@reading.ac.uk

Dr Graham C. Burdge and
Professor Philip C. Calder
Institute of Human Nutrition
School of Medicine
University of Southampton
Bassett Crescent East
Southampton SO16 7PX
UK

Chapter 9

Professor Zdzisław E. Sikorski
Gdańsk University of Technology
Department of Food Chemistry,
Technology and Biotechnology
Gabriela Narutowicza 11/12
80952 Gdańsk-Wrzeszcz
Poland

E-mail: sikorski@chem.pg.gda.pl

Dr Grażyna Sikorska-Wiśniewska
Medical Academy of Gdańsk
Clinic of Pediatrics, Gastroenterology
and Pediatric Oncology
Nowe ogrody 1–7
80-803 Gdańsk
Poland

E-mail: graszkasikorska@op.pl

Chapter 10

Dr Liisa Lähteenmäki
Chief Scientist: Consumer Studies
VTT
PO Box 1000
FI-02044 VTT
Finland

E-mail: Liisa.Lahteenmaki@vtt.fi

Chapter 11

Professor D. I. Givens*
School of Agriculture
The University of Reading
Whiteknights
Reading RG6 6AR
UK

E-mail: d.i.givens@reading.ac.uk

Dr K. J. Shingfield
MTT AgriFood Research Finland
Finland

E-mail: kevin.shingfield@mtt.fi

Chapter 12

Dr Y. Chilliard
Unité de Recherches sur les
Herbivores
INRA Theix
63122- St-Genès-Champanelle
France

E-mail:
yves.chilliard@clermont.inra.fr

Chapter 13

Dr Aidan P. Moloney
Teagasc
Grange Research Centre
Dunsany
Co. Meath
Ireland

E-mail: amoloney@grange.teagasc.ie

Chapter 14

Dr John F. Kerry and Dr Joe P. Kerry*
Department of Food and Nutritional
Sciences
University College Cork

Cork City
Co. Cork
Ireland

E-mail: Joe.Kerry@ucc.ie

Chapter 15

Professor Julie M. Jones*
Department of Nutrition and Food Science
College of St. Catherine
4030 Valentine Ct
Arden Hills, MN 55112
USA

E-mail: juliemjones@comcast.net

Dr Satya S. Jonnalagadda
Senior Medical Affairs Specialist
Novartis Medical Nutrition
1541 Park Place Blvd
St. Louis Park, MN 55416
USA

E-mail:
satya.jonnalagadda@novartis.com

Chapter 16

C. M. Logan, J. M. W. Wallace, P. J. Robson and Professor M. B. E. Livingstone
Northern Ireland Centre for Food and Health (NIHCE)
Room W2022
Centre for Molecular Biosciences
University of Ulster
Cromore Road
Coleraine, BT55 ISA
UK

E-mail:
mbe.livingstone@ulster.ac.uk
cm.logan@ulster.ac.uk

Chapter 17

Dr Eckhard Flöter* and Dr Arjen Bot
Unilever Research and Development Vlaardingen
Olivier van Noortlaan 120
3133 AT Vlaardingen
Netherlands

E-mail:
eckhard.floter@unilever.com
Arjen.Bot@unilever.com

Chapter 18

Dr Charlotte Jacobsen* and Ms Mette Bruni Let
Department of Seafood Research
Danish Institute for Fisheries Research
Building 221, Søltofts Plads
Technical University of Denmark
DK-2800 Kgs, Lyngby
Denmark

E-mail: cja@dfu.min.dk
mbl@dfu.min.dk

Chapter 19

Professor Tom A. B. Sanders*
Nutritional Sciences Research Division
King's College London
Franklin-Wilkins Building
150 Stamford Street
London SE1 9NH
UK

E-mail: Tom.Sanders@kcl.ac.uk

Chapter 20

Professor Johnathan A. Napier
Rothamsted Research
Harpenden
Herts AL5 2JQ
UK

E-mail:
Johnathan.napier@bbsrc.ac.uk

Chapter 21

Dr Gerrit van Duijn, Dr Erich E. Dumelin* and Dr Elke A. Trautwein
Unilever Research and Development Vlaardingen
Olivier van Noortlaan 120
3133 AT Vlaardingen
Netherlands

E-mail: erich.dumelin@unilever.com
Gerrit-van.Duijn@unilever.com

Chapter 22

Dr Jon Skorve, Dr Karl Johan Tronstad, Dr Hege Vaagenes Wergedahl, Dr Kjetil Berge, and Dr Rolf Kristian Berge*
Institute of Medicine
Section of Clinical Biochemistry
Haukeland University Hospital
Jonas Lievsei 65
N-5021 Bergen
Norway

E-mail: rolf.berge@med.uib.no

Dr Jon Songstad
Department of Chemistry
University of Bergen
N-5021 Bergen
Norway

Part I

Dietary fats and health

1

Health problems associated with saturated and *trans* fatty acids intake

P. L. Zock, Unilever Research and Development Vlaardingen

1.1 Introduction

Saturated fatty acids occur in the diet in different chain lengths, with lauric, myristic, palmitic, and stearic acids as the major ones. *Trans* fatty acids predominantly occur as monounsaturated fatty acids with the *trans* double bond at different positions in the carbon chain. Dietary saturated and *trans* fatty acids have important effects on health. In particular, epidemiological studies and randomised controlled trials on hard clinical end-points indicate that reducing the intake of saturated and *trans* fatty acids will reduce the risk of coronary heart disease (CHD).

The most important metabolic effect by which saturated and *trans* fatty acids increase CHD risk is through an adverse influence on blood lipid levels. High levels of total blood cholesterol and of cholesterol in low-density lipoproteins (LDL) raise the risk for CHD, whereas a high level of cholesterol in high-density lipoproteins (HDL) lowers it. Dietary saturated fatty acids strongly raise total and LDL cholesterol levels in blood. *Trans* fatty acids not only raise LDL cholesterol, but also lower HDL cholesterol. Different saturated fatty acids can have different effects on lipoprotein cholesterol levels, but it is unclear if this translates to different effects on CHD risk. Different positional isomers of *trans* fatty acids probably have similar adverse effects on CHD risk.

Together, the evidence from epidemiological, clinical, and metabolic studies convincingly shows that replacing saturated and *trans* fatty acids in the diet with *cis*-monounsaturated and polyunsaturated fatty acids is an effective way to reduce the risk of CHD. Reducing the total fat content of the diet, i.e. replacing saturated and *trans* fatty acids with carbohydrates, seems less effective.

1.2 Saturated and *trans* fatty acids in the diet

Dietary fats largely consist of triglycerides, molecules with three fatty acids esterified to a glycerol backbone. Fatty acids are classified on the basis of their chain length, the number of double bonds in the molecule, the position of the first double bond from the methyl end and the configuration of the double bonds (*trans* or *cis*). Accordingly, fatty acids are categorised as saturated, (*cis*)-monounsaturated, *trans* and polyunsaturated (Fig. 1.1).

Saturated fatty acids (SAFAs) have no double bonds. They primarily come from animal products such as meat and dairy products, and from tropical oils such as palm oil, palm kernel oil, and coconut fat. In general, such fats are solid at room temperature. Stearic acid is a saturated fatty acid that may have different biological effects from other saturated fatty acids. Important food sources of stearic acid are beef, hydrogenated vegetable oils and chocolate. Monounsaturated fatty acids (MUFAs) have one double bond. Plant sources that are rich in MUFAs are liquid vegetable oils, such as rapeseed oil, olive oil, high-oleic sunflower oil, and nuts. Polyunsaturated fatty acids (PUFAs) have two or more double bonds. The large majority of PUFA in the diet (90% or more) is linoleic acid, an n-6 (or omega-6) fatty acid. Vegetable oils such as soybean, rapeseed and sunflower oils are important sources. PUFAs also occur as the n-3 (or omega-3) fatty acid alpha-linolenic acid in some vegetable oils and nuts, and as the very long chain n-3 fatty acids in fish and other seafood. *Trans* fatty acids (TFAs) are unsaturated fatty acids that contain at least one double bond in the *trans* configuration. TFAs are formed during partial hydrogenation of vegetable oils, and also by natural bio-hydrogenation of fats in the rumen of cattle and sheep. The partial hydrogenation of polyunsaturated oils with *cis* double bonds causes isomerisation of some of the remaining double bonds and migration of others, resulting in an increase in the *trans* fatty acid content and the hardening of the oil. Most TFAs are monounsaturated, with the *trans* double bond at different positions in the carbon chain. Processed fats thus contain a range of *trans* positional isomers (*trans*-C18:1n-6 to *trans*-C18:1n-14), with elaidic acid (*trans*-C18:1-n-9; Fig. 1.1) often in the largest amount. Dietary sources of *trans* fatty acids are foods made with partially hydrogenated vegetable oils, such as shortenings, commercially prepared baked goods, snack foods, fried foods and margarine. *Trans* fatty acids also are present in foods that come from ruminant animals (cattle and sheep); these include dairy products, beef and lamb. The predominant naturally occurring TFA is vaccenic acid (*trans*-C18:1n-7; Fig. 1.1).

The descriptors 'hydrogenated' and 'partially hydrogenated' on food labels are often used interchangeably but both indicate the presence of TFA in the processed vegetable oil used to prepare the food. For the sake of accuracy, in oil that is fully hydrogenated (i.e. the unsaturated fatty acids have all been converted to stearic acid), there are no *trans* unsaturated fatty acids. Thus, fats that are partially hydrogenated have variable amounts of TFA depending on the extent of hydrogenation.

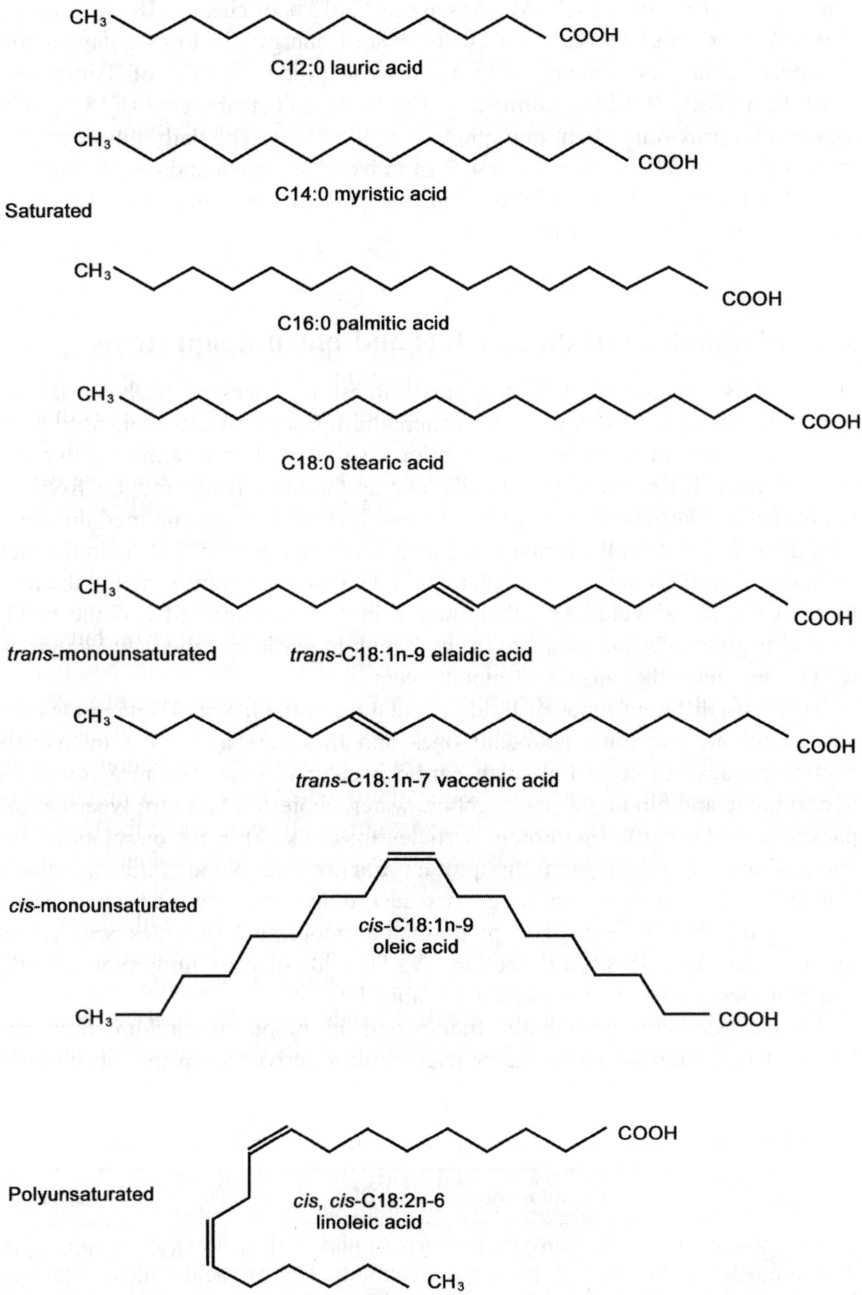

Fig. 1.1 Chemical structures and nomenclature of major dietary fatty acids.

Intakes of SAFAs are on average 5 to 10-fold higher than intakes of TFA. The average daily intake of SAFAs is about 11–13% of energy (18–32 g/day) in North America and ranges from 10 to 19% of energy (24 to 60 g/day) across European countries. Dietary SAFAs consist predominantly of lauric acid (C12:0), myristic (C14:0), palmitic acid (C16:0), and stearic acid (C18:0), with stearic acid providing about one-quarter of all SAFAs. The daily intake of total TFA is about 2–3% of energy (*ca* 4–7 g) in North America and ranges from 0.5 to 2.1% of energy (1.2 to 6.7 g/day) in Europe (Allison *et al.*, 1999; Briefel & Johnson, 2004; Hulshof *et al.*, 1999).

1.3 Metabolism of dietary fats and blood lipoproteins

Dietary fats are absorbed in the small intestine. Ingested triglycerides (or triacylglycerols) are hydrolysed by pancreatic lipases into glycerol, fatty acids and some mono-acylglycerol. Absorption of dietary fats is almost complete; 98% or more. Intestinal mucosal cells take up the hydrolysis products from the gut lumen and largely re-esterify these to triglycerides. Short and medium chain fatty acids (C4:0–C10:0), which make up a very small part of SAFAs in the diet, are not re-esterified but directly taken up in the blood and transported to the liver through the portal vein. All other fatty acids are re-esterified and the newly formed triglycerides are excreted in the lymph in particles called chylomicrons, which then enter the peripheral bloodstream.

There are different types of lipids circulating in the blood. Triglycerides and cholesterol are the most abundant ones and these are also most intensively studied because of their link with cardiovascular disease. Because lipids are hydrophobic and blood plasma largely is water, cholesterol and triglycerides are packaged into specific lipoprotein particles for transport in the circulation. The composition of the different lipoprotein fractions in blood varies markedly (Table 1.1). Lipoproteins are categorised according to their density, which varies between 0.9 and 1.1 kg/l. The predominant lipoprotein particles are: chylomicrons, very low-density lipoproteins (VLDL), low-density lipoproteins (LDL) and high-density lipoproteins (HDL) (Table 1.1).

Triglycerides are principally transported in blood in chylomicrons and VLDL. Chylomicrons mainly carry triglycerides derived from the diet through

Table 1.1 Composition and physical characteristics of plasma lipoproteins

	Chylomicrons	VLDL	LDL	HDL
Density (g/ml)	<0.95	0.95–1.006	1.019–1.063	1.063–1.210
Protein (mass %)	2	7	20	50
Phospholipids (mass %)	7	20	22	22
Triglycerides (mass%)	83	50	10	8
Cholesterol (mass %)	8	22	48	20

intestinal absorption, whereas VLDL mainly carries triglycerides that are endogenously synthesised in the liver. Total serum cholesterol is the sum amount of cholesterol found in different lipoproteins in the blood. Chylomicrons do transport dietary cholesterol after absorption from the intestine, but most cholesterol in blood is transported by LDL, HDL and VLDL. LDL contains about 60–70% of total serum cholesterol, and HDL carries approximately 20–30% of total serum cholesterol (Table 1.1).

A high total cholesterol concentration is a risk factor for CHD. Total cholesterol consists mainly of LDL cholesterol, and an increase in LDL cholesterol increases the risk of CHD. Lowering levels of LDL cholesterol reduces the risk for CHD. A high level of HDL cholesterol is inversely associated with risk for CHD, and a high level of blood triglycerides in the fasting state is positively associated with CHD. A causal relationship between LDL cholesterol and CHD is clearly established, but there is also strong evidence for a causal role of low HDL cholesterol and high triglyceride levels. A high triglyceride level and low HDL cholesterol level are also important diagnostic criteria for metabolic syndrome, a condition that increases risk of cardiovascular disease.

The relationship between the change in level of some lipid parameters and the resulting risk for heart disease has been quantified in several large population studies and meta-analyses. Generally accepted estimates at the population level predict that a decrease of 1% in total cholesterol will reduce risk by 1–2% (Expert Panel, 2001) or even more at younger age (Law *et al.*, 1994), and that an increase of 1% in HDL decreases risk by approximately 2 to 3% (Boden, 2000). The total to HDL cholesterol (TC/HDL) ratio combines the two opposite effects of LDL and HDL cholesterol on CHD risk, and in this way provides a single, powerful predictor of the effects of dietary fatty acids on CHD risk (Stampfer *et al.*, 1991; Kinosian *et al.*, 1995; Pedersen *et al.*, 1998; Natarjan *et al.*, 2003). In fact, the ratio of total to HDL cholesterol is increasingly considered superior to total or lipoprotein cholesterol concentrations regarding its predictive value for risk for CHD. A decrease of 1% in the TC/HDL ratio decreased risk by 1.3% based in one study population (Pedersen *et al.*, 1998) and a decrease of 1 unit (e.g. from 5 to 4) decreased risk by 50% based on another study population (Stampfer *et al.*, 1991). The latter implies that for a starting TC/HDL ratio of 5, a decrease of 1% in the ratio (0.05 unit) would give a 2.5% decrease in risk. For a starting ratio of 8, a decrease of 1% in the ratio (0.08 unit) would give a 4% decrease in risk.

1.4 Dietary fats and the risk of coronary heart disease

1.4.1 Epidemiological studies and clinical trials

Cardiovascular diseases comprise many different disorders related to impaired blood flow, including disease of the heart (mostly coronary heart disease), the brain (ischaemic and haemorrhagic stroke) and peripheral blood vessels (e.g.

deep vein thrombosis). Effects of dietary fats on the risk of coronary heart disease have been most widely studied and are established by both epidemiological studies and randomised controlled clinical trials.

Of all cardiovascular diseases, a causal relationship with blood lipid levels is most clear for coronary heart disease. Although cholesterol lowering by drug treatment (HMG-CoA-reductase inhibitors, statins) lowers both the risk of coronary heart disease and that of stroke, the epidemiological data on dietary fats and stroke are very limited and show no clear associations with the amount or type of dietary fats (He *et al.*, 2003). In contrast, for CHD there are several epidemiological studies that addressed the associations with dietary fats as well as randomised clinical trials that studied the effects of changing the intake of specific fatty acids (Hu & Willett, 2002) on disease outcome. This section therefore focuses on the relations between intake of saturated and *trans* fatty acids and the risk of coronary heart disease.

Epidemiological studies on associations with dietary fats

A higher intake of fat and in particular of saturated fat is already long believed to contribute to the development of CHD. This belief originates in geographical and migration studies comparing the intake of fats and rates of CHD between countries (Keys, 1980) or in population groups moving from one country to another (Kato *et al.*, 1973). In the Seven Countries Study (Keys, 1980), the percentage of energy as saturated fat in the diet was strongly correlated ($r = 0.86$) with coronary death rates across 16 different populations. Notably, the correlation between percentage energy from total fat and CHD rate was much weaker ($r = 0.39$). CHD rates were highest in Finland and lowest in Crete, but both regions had the same high amount of total fat intake (40% of energy). Because the high fat intake in Finland was mainly due to a high dairy fat intake (SAFA-rich diet) and that in Crete mainly due to high olive oil intake (MUFA-rich diet), Keys proposed that in particular the type of dietary fat is important. In a more recent analysis of the Seven Countries Study, Kromhout *et al.* (1995) found strong positive correlations between CHD death rates during 25-year of follow-up and initial intakes of SAFA ($r > 0.80$) and of TFA ($r = 0.78$).

Data from international comparisons and migration studies show the importance of diet, lifestyle and other environmental factors for developing CHD. However, such data do not provide strong evidence for the causal role of individual dietary components, because relations with CHD are easily confounded by other dietary aspects, physical activity, smoking habits, obesity and socio-economic status. Prospective cohort studies of individuals within a population, in which diet is assessed before the onset of disease and in which confounding factors can to a certain extent be controlled for, are considered as the strongest type of epidemiological evidence. Surprisingly, despite the long history of dietary fat and CHD research, the number of earlier cohort studies that have directly investigated associations between dietary fat intake and risk of CHD is relatively small and the results are not consistent. A statistically significant positive association between saturated fat intake and risk of CHD was found in two studies (McGee *et al.*, 1984; Kushi *et al.*, 1985), but not in several others (e.g. Gordon, 1981; Shekelle *et al.*, 1981; Ascherio *et al.*, 1996). Possible explanations for these inconsistent findings are that most of these earlier studies were limited by small study size, inadequate dietary assessment, or insufficient adjustment for confounding factors.

The largest prospective epidemiological analysis of dietary fatty acids and risk of CHD is from the Nurses' Health Study cohort (Hu *et al.*, 1997) in more than 80 000 women over 14 years of follow-up. This study found a weak relation between saturated fat intake and increased CHD risk; 5% of energy from saturated fatty acids as compared with the same amount of energy from carbohydrates was associated with a 17% higher risk of CHD. *Trans* fatty acid intake was much more strongly associated with CHD; it was estimated that 2% of energy as *trans* fatty acid as compared with carbohydrates was associated with a 93% higher CHD risk. Higher intakes of non-hydrogenated polyunsaturated fats and monounsaturated fat were associated with decreased risk. Total fat intake was not significantly related to risk, probably because of the opposing effects of different fat types.

In addition to the Nurses' Health Study (Hu *et al.*, 1997), three other large prospective studies consistently found increased risks of CHD with higher intakes of *trans* fatty acids (Ascherio *et al.*, 1996; Pietinen *et al.*, 1997; Oomen *et al.*, 2001). When the results of these four studies were combined (Oomen *et al.*, 2001), the pooled relative risk of CHD with a difference of 2% of energy as *trans* fatty acids was 1.25 (a 25% increase in risk). Results from other types of epidemiological studies, such as case-control studies using biochemical markers of TFA intake, are less consistent (Ascherio *et al.*, 1999). In a more recent case-control study, higher red-cell membrane levels of TFA were associated with significantly increased risk of primary cardiac arrest (Lemaitre *et al.*, 2002). One study found no association between adipose tissue TFA and sudden death (Roberts *et al.*, 1995), but another found a positive association between adipose TFA and myocardial infarction (Clifton *et al.*, 2004). Because intake of SAFA is, unlike intake of TFA, not reliably reflected in body tissue, there are no epidemiological data on SAFA and heart disease using such biochemical markers of intake.

Randomised clinical trials of changes in dietary fats

The strongest type of evidence for a causal role of diet in the development of CHD is provided by long-term randomised trials on clinical end-points. If a randomised trial is successfully conducted with high compliance of subjects and few patients are lost to end-point ascertainment, then results can be fully ascribed to effects of the dietary intervention, without confounding by other lifestyle factors or the subjects' own choices. Important drawbacks of clinical trials are their practical limitations, required large sample sizes, long duration and high costs. Therefore, there are only a few trials that specifically tested the effects of changing dietary fat intake, without involving other treatments, such as blood pressure or plasma lipid lowering medication or combined lifestyle and

Table 1.2 Randomised clinical trials aimed at changing dietary (saturated) fat and CHD outcome (adapted from Hu & Willett, 2002)

Trial	Subjects in the intervention group	Energy of dietary fat in intervention group (%)	Energy from polyunsaturated (P) and saturated fat (S) in intervention group (%)	Duration of intervention (years)	Change in serum cholesterol (%)*	Change in incidence of CHD (%)*
Low-fat, high-carbohydrate approach						
MRC low-fat (Research Committee, 1965)	123 men with CHD	22 (41 in control)	Not reported	3	−5	+4
DART (Burr *et al.*, 1989)	1015 men with CHD	32 (35 in control)	P:S ratio = 0.8	2	−4	−9
High-polyunsaturated fat approach						
Finnish Mental Hospital Study (Turpeinen *et al.*, 1979)	676 men without CHD	35	P =13; S = 9	6	−15	−43**
Oslo Diet-Heart Study (Leren, 1966, 1970)	206 men with CHD	39	P =21; S = 9	5	−14**	−25**
MRC soy oil (Morris *et al.*, 1968)	199 men with CHD	46	P: S ratio = 2	4	−16**	−12
Los Angeles Veteran Study (Dayton *et al.*, 1969)	424 men, most without evidence of CHD	40	P = 16; S = 19	8	−13**	−20 for CHD −31** for CVD
Minnesota Coronary Survey (Frantz *et al.*, 1989)	4393 men and 4664 women	38	P = 15; S = 9	1	−14**	No change

* Changes refer to the percentage difference or change in the treatment group compared with the control group.
** $P < 0.05$.

diet combinations. These trials were conducted a few decades ago, mostly in patients with or at high risk of CHD (see Sacks & Katan, 2002 for review) (Table 1.2).

Only two clinical trials tested the effect on CHD end-points of a low-fat, high-carbohydrate diet (Research Committee, 1965; Burr *et al.*, 1989). Both trials included patients with a recent myocardial infarction. Reduction in saturated fat was planned to reduce total fat intake, and therefore carbohydrate-rich foods were advised. Neither of these low-fat trials showed significant benefits (Table 1.2). It could be argued that the two or three years' duration of intervention was too short to produce a reduction in CHD by lipid-lowering, or that the sample sizes were too small. In addition, dietary adherence could have been low in both trials, because the serum cholesterol reduction expected with lower saturated fat intake was not observed (Table 1.2). Nevertheless, these trials do not support the contention that advice to replace saturated fat by carbohydrates is in the long term an effective way to reduce cholesterol and CHD risk.

In five trials, saturated fat intake was reduced by prescribing unhydrogenated soybean oil and other vegetable oils to hypercholesterolaemic patients, and thus tested the effect on CHD end-points of a high-polyunsaturated fat diet. Three of these were primary prevention trials in subjects with no evidence of existing CHD at baseline (Dayton *et al.*, 1969; Turpeinen *et al.*, 1979; Frantz *et al.*, 1989). These trials were conducted among institutionalised subjects so as to increase control over the diets. In all three trials, serum cholesterol was substantially reduced. In the Los Angeles Veteran Study (Dayton *et al.*, 1969), the trial with the most rigorous methodology, CHD rate was reduced by 31% during eight years of follow-up, while in the Finnish Mental Hospital study (Turpeinen *et al.*, 1979) CHD rate was reduced by 43% over 6 years. In both these trials, the substantial increase of linoleic acid in adipose tissue of subjects confirmed compliance with the high-polyunsaturated fat, low-saturated fat diets. In the Finnish study, subjects in the intervention group also replaced hard stick margarine for soft tub margarine, so that the reduction in cholesterol and CHD was probably in part also due to a reduction in TFA intake (Turpeinen *et al.*, 1979). In the third primary prevention trial (Frantz *et al.*, 1989), CHD rate was not affected despite a 14% reduction in cholesterol. However, this study was relatively short in duration, and the achieved changes in intakes of saturated and polyunsaturated fat (P:S ratio = 1.6) was much lower than the goals (P:S ratio = 2.5).

The effect of a high-polyunsaturated fat diet was also tested in two secondary prevention trials (Leren, 1970; Morris *et al.*, 1968). The Oslo Diet Heart study, which provided as much as 21% of energy as polyunsaturated fat, found significant reductions in both serum cholesterol and CHD after 5 years of follow-up (Leren, 1970). Trends towards lower cardiovascular mortality were also seen after an additional 6 years of follow-up (Leren, 1970). Another secondary prevention trial prescribed a high amount of soybean oil. In this trial, serum cholesterol was also effectively reduced by 16%, but the reduction in CHD rate of 12% after 4 years was not statistically significant (Morris *et al.*, 1968).

Other clinical trials on diet and risk of CVD tested either total dietary pattern approaches (De Lorgeril *et al.*, 1999; Singh *et al.*, 2002), investigated effects on intermediary end-points of CHD such as coronary atherosclerosis measured by angiography (Arntzenius *et al.*, 1985; Watts *et al.*, 1992), or applied a broad multifactorial intervention approach also including other lifestyle elements such as physical exercise, stopping smoking and drug treatment. Both the Lyon Diet Heart Study (De Lorgeril *et al.*, 1999) and the Indo-Mediterranean Diet Study (Singh *et al.*, 2002) tested effects on clinical end-points of a total dietary approach, including more grains, fruit, vegetables and fish, and less meat, dairy products and hydrogenated oils. These interventions effectively lowered the risk of mortality from heart diseases in patients with CHD. Although it is impossible to determine which of the dietary changes was responsible for reduced risk, it is notable that total amount of fat in these trials did not change much. Thus, they support the contention that the right types of fatty acids and other dietary components are more important than total fat intake. Two trials measuring atherosclerosis in coronary arteries focused on dietary interventions. The Leiden Intervention trial (Arntzenius *et al.*, 1985) tested a vegetarian diet with a high ratio of polyunsaturated to saturated fatty acids (P:S = 2) and found a significantly slower progression of atherosclerotic lesions in patients. The St. Thomas' Atherosclerosis Regression Study (Watts *et al.*, 1992) tested a moderate-fat diet with a relatively high amount of polyunsaturated fat, and also found less progression of coronary atherosclerosis.

Together, the randomised clinical trials on the quality of dietary fat provide strong support that dietary intervention can be an effective way to reduce CHD risk. In these trials, fats from meats, dairy products and hydrogenated fats were replaced with soybean, corn, sunflower and safflower oils. In terms of fatty acids, this shows beneficial effects of replacing mainly SAFA and some TFA by mainly linoleic acid (C18:2n-6) and some alpha-linolenic acid (C18:3n-3), with similar intakes of total fat and MUFA. The randomised trials of lowering the amount of total fat in the diet are limited in number and methodology, but they do not support a major benefit of replacing saturated fat with carbohydrates. There are no randomised trials conducted that directly addressed effects of MUFA on CHD end-points.

1.4.2 Effects on risk factors in humans

Blood lipids

The effect of dietary fats on the risk of coronary heart disease (CHD) has traditionally been estimated by their effects on serum total cholesterol (Keys *et al.*, 1965). However, as described above, there is now abundant evidence that effects on different types of lipoprotein cholesterol are important. In particular, specific effects of fatty acids of LDL and HDL cholesterol should be considered.

Mensink *et al.* (2003) recently performed a meta-analysis of 60 selected metabolic dietary studies in humans on the amount and type of fatty acids on blood lipids. The studies that were included had to meet strict criteria, including a thorough control over food intake, dietary fatty acids as the single variable with constant cholesterol intake, study designs that included direct comparisons with a control group, feeding periods that were long enough (at least 2 weeks), and stable body weights of subjects during the study period. The 60 studies investigated effects of 159 experimental diets with different fatty acid compositions in a total of 1672 subjects. Most studies were from North America and Europe, and included both men and women in the age range between 21 and 72 years, without gross disturbances of lipid metabolism or diabetes. Therefore, the results from this meta-analysis apply to the general population in Western societies.

The Mensink *et al.* (2003) meta-analysis provides predictive equations for the effects of SAFAs, MUFAs, PUFAs and TFAs on blood lipids and lipoproteins. Figure 1.2 shows what happens with total, LDL and HDL cholesterol if 1% of energy as carbohydrates in the diet is replaced by 1% of a particular fatty acid. The figure depicts effects of the different specific SAFAs, and it must be noted that these effects were derived from a smaller set of studies than the effect of all SAFAs together as a class. Nevertheless, palmitic acid is the most abundant dietary SAFA, and the effects of SAFAs together were comparable to those of palmitic acid alone (for C12–C18 SAFAs together: +0.036 mmol/l for total cholesterol, +0.032 mmol/l for LDL cholesterol, and +0.010 mmol/l for HDL cholesterol). These data show that SAFA and TFA powerfully raise total and LDL cholesterol, while *cis*-MUFA and *cis*-PUFA lower it. All classes of fatty acids except TFAs raise HDL cholesterol when they replace carbohydrates;

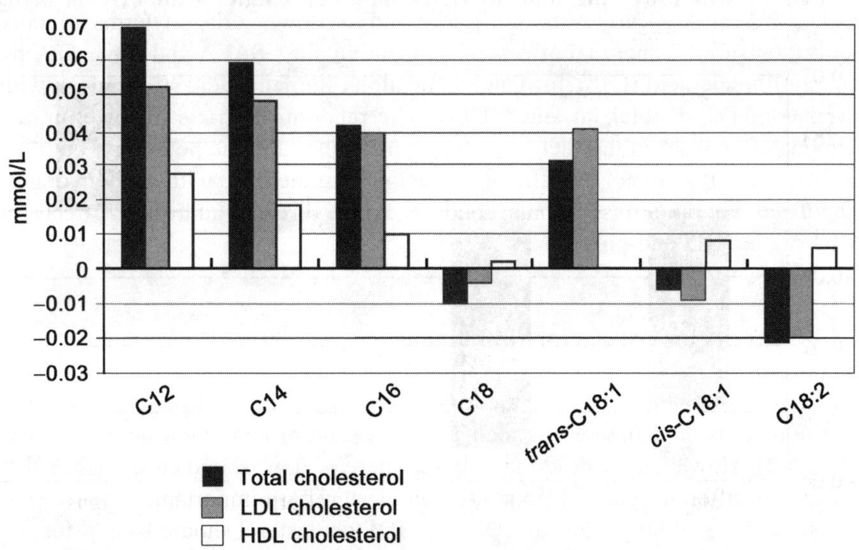

Fig. 1.2 Effects of different dietary fatty acids on plasma total, LDL and HDL cholesterol levels (mmol/l) when they replace 1% of energy as carbohydrates (data from Mensink *et al.*, 2003).

TFAs have the same effect as carbohydrates. Effects on triglycerides are not shown, but these are opposite to HDL cholesterol: all classes of fatty acids except TFA lower fasting triglycerides levels by about 0.02 mmol/l per 1% of energy when they replace carbohydrates. The effect of PUFA on triglycerides is slightly, but not significantly, larger than that of other fatty acids. This contrasts with the powerful triglyceride-lowering effect of larger doses n-3 PUFA from fish (Harris, 1997) (see elsewhere in this book), which is evidently not shared by n-6 fatty acids.

Figure 1.2 expresses the effects on blood lipids relative to 1% of energy as carbohydrates as a reference. In fact, the choice of the reference is arbitrary. However, some reference for comparison is needed, because there is no such thing as a placebo for energy-yielding nutrients. Also, the amount of energy for comparison is flexible, because the effects of the fatty acids fit well in linear relationships. Thus, the effects per 1% of energy shown in Fig. 1.2 can be used as coefficients to predict the effects of exchanging variable amounts of different fatty acids and carbohydrates in the diet. For example, the effects (coefficients) predict that replacing 2% of energy as *trans* fatty acids with 2% of polyunsaturated fatty acids will lower LDL cholesterol by ~ -0.12 mmol/l.

The total to HDL cholesterol ratio combines the two distinctive effects of LDL and HDL cholesterol and in this way provides a single, powerful predictor of the effects of dietary fatty acids on CHD risk (Stampfer *et al.*, 1991; Kinosian *et al.*, 1995; Natarjan *et al.*, 2003). Figure 1.3 shows the predicted effect on the total to HDL cholesterol ratio when 1% of energy as saturated fat is replaced by another class of fatty acids or by carbohydrates. Replacing SAFAs with MUFAs or PUFAs will lower the total to HDL cholesterol ratio, with PUFAs being

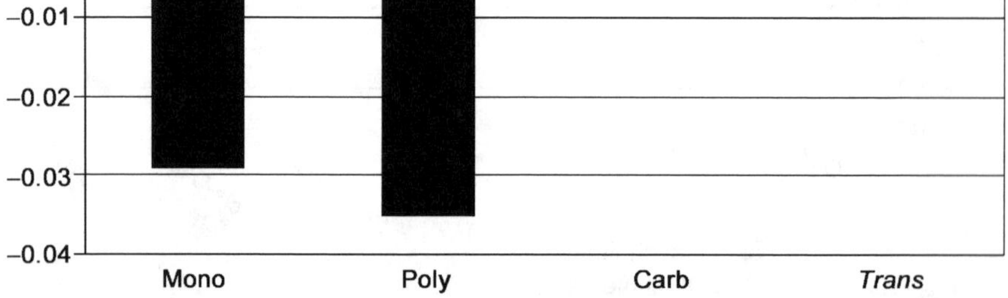

Fig. 1.3 Change in the total to HDL cholesterol ratio when 1% of energy as saturated fatty acid is replaced with other fatty acids or carbohydrates (data from Mensink *et al.*, 2003).

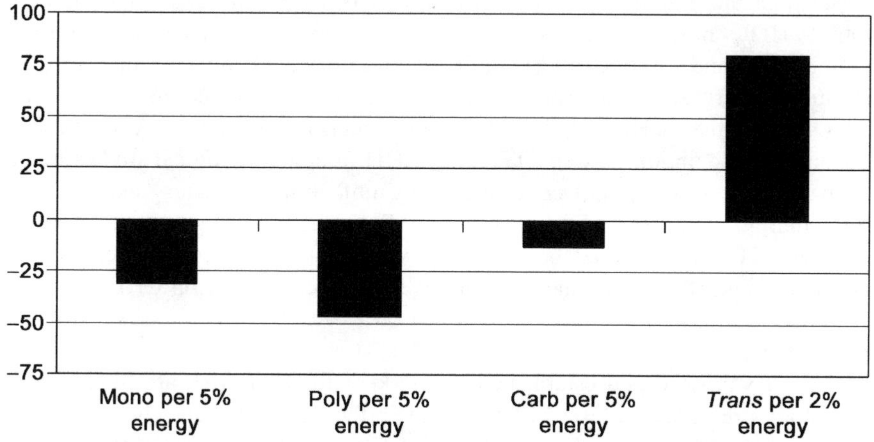

Fig. 1.4 Difference in observed risk for coronary heart disease when saturated fatty acids are iso-energetically replaced with monounsaturated fatty acids (Mono), polyunsaturated fatty acids (Poly), carbohydrates (Carb) or *trans* fatty acids (*Trans*). Data from the Nurses' Health Study (Hu *et al.*, 1997).

slightly superior. Replacing SAFAs with carbohydrates, i.e. lowering the total fat content of the diet, does not improve the total to HDL cholesterol ratio, and replacing saturated fatty acids with TFA raises the total to HDL cholesterol ratio.

Thus, metabolic studies on blood lipids suggest that for reducing CHD risk, the type of fat is more important than the total amount. The effects of SAFAs versus PUFAs and carbohydrates on blood lipids are well in line with the effects on disease outcome as seen in randomised clinical trials (Sacks & Katan, 2002). The metabolic studies also suggest that the effects of TFAs on blood lipids are even more unfavourable than those of SAFAs. There are no clinical trial data on TFAs, but the metabolic effects can be compared with epidemiological data on disease end-points. Figure 1.4 shows differences in risk as observed in women in the Nurses' Health Study (Hu *et al.*, 1997), expressed as replacement of SAFAs with either MUFAs, PUFAs, or carbohydrates (each as 5% of energy), or with TFAs (2% of energy). The direction of the differences in risk is very well in line with the different effects on blood lipids measured in the metabolic studies (Fig. 1.3). The size of the difference in risk with *trans* fatty acids, however, is much larger than predicted by blood lipid effects from metabolic studies. Note that the risk difference between TFAs and SAFAs in Fig. 1.4 is expressed for a smaller amount of energy than the risk difference between SAFAs and other fatty acids and carbohydrates, whereas the effects in Fig. 1.3 on the total to HDL cholesterol ratio are expressed in equal energy amounts.

Other epidemiological studies found smaller increases in risk with TFAs (Oomen *et al.*, 2001) than observed by Hu *et al.* (1997), but still considerably larger than one might predict from the effects of TFAs on LDL, HDL, and the total to HDL cholesterol levels alone. Increases in fasting triglycerides (Mensink *et al.*, 2003) and Lipoprotein(a) (Lp(a)) with TFA can account for only a small additional increase in risk. Therefore, it is conceivable that other mechanisms by which TFA raises CHD may be involved (Ascherio *et al.*, 1999). Alternatively, the strong association between TFA and CHD in epidemiological studies could be partly due to (residual) confounding by unfavourable dietary and lifestyle traits that go along with TFA consumption. Regardless the apparent discrepancy in sizes of effects, the metabolic and epidemiological studies together provide consistent and strong evidence for an adverse effect of TFA on CHD risk.

Other risk factors

The most validated and established biomarkers for CVD risk are blood lipids and blood pressure. As described above, the effects of fatty acids on blood lipids have been widely and intensively studied. Different comprehensive reviews and meta-analyses of well-controlled metabolic studies consistently report adverse effects of SAFA and TFA on blood lipids. For blood pressure, however, there is no convincing evidence for any physiologically significant effects of SAFA and TFA. Other potential modes of action of fatty acids by which CVD risk could be affected include effects on thrombosis and haemostasis, the vascular endothelial wall and inflammation.

Thrombosis clearly plays a role in many aspects of coronary disease. Dietary fatty acids may influence blood platelets and proteins that regulate thrombosis tendency and blood coagulation, and consequently affect the risk for heart disease. However, effects on this system cannot be measured directly, and there is no clear consensus on the functionality and relevance of different markers. The effects of dietary fatty acids on markers of thrombosis in humans are sometimes suggestive, but inconclusive (Lefevre *et al.*, 2004). On the whole, these studies may suggest a beneficial effect when SAFA is replaced with MUFA or PUFA, but the clinical meaning is unclear (Kris-Etherton *et al.*, 2001).

The evidence for effects of dietary fats on endothelial wall function is also not consistent (Sanderson *et al.*, 2004). It is established that a fatty meal has acute effects on endothelial reactivity directly after intake, but longer-term effects are not clear. Some studies show that replacing SAFAs with a high-fat MUFA diet, but not with a low-fat, high-carbohydrate diet, improves endothelial function (Sanderson *et al.*, 2004). One study specifically addressed the effects of SAFAs and TFAs (de Roos *et al.*, 2002) on endothelial function in humans. Acute effects after ingestion of TFAs and SAFAs were not different, but in the longer-term TFAs resulted in impaired endothelial function as compared with SAFAs. This could contribute to the higher risk with TFAs than with SAFAs seen in epidemiological studies (Ascherio *et al.*, 1999).

There is emerging evidence that markers of low-grade, subclinical inflammation play an important role in cardiovascular disease, or at least may be relevant indicators of CVD risk. These markers include pro-inflammatory cytokines such as interleukin 6 (IL-6) and acute phase proteins such as C-reactive protein (CRP). There are as yet few data on the effects of diet on subclinical inflammation. Most studies have focused on polyunsaturated fatty acids, and in particular on relative effects of omega-3 versus omega-6 polyunsaturated fatty acids (see other chapters in this book). One metabolic study found that TFA increased CRP and other markers of inflammation (Baer *et al.*, 2004). A cross-sectional epidemiological analysis also found positive associations between *trans* fatty acid intake and markers of systemic inflammation (Mozaffarian *et al.*, 2004). An effect of TFA on subclinical inflammation could also contribute to the higher risk with TFA than with SAFA seen in epidemiological studies (Ascherio *et al.*, 1999) However, these effects and their clinical relevance need to be confirmed by further studies.

1.4.3 Specific saturated and *trans* fatty acids and CHD risk

Specific saturates

Different specific saturated fatty acids may have different effects on CHD risk. In particular, there is a growing interest in stearic acid as a substitute for TFA to give texture and solidity to foods. Metabolic studies show that lauric acid most markedly increases total and LDL cholesterol, whereas stearic acid somewhat lowers total and LDL cholesterol when it replaces carbohydrates (Fig. 1.2) (Mensink *et al.*, 2003). However, lauric acid also has the strongest HDL raising effect, whereas stearic acid raises HDL cholesterol less than other saturated or *cis*-unsaturated fatty acids. The net effect is that lauric and stearic acid have less unfavourable effects on the total to HDL cholesterol ratio than myristic and palmitic acids. However, consequences of these differences for CHD risk are unclear. Saturated fatty acids tend to occur together in diets due to shared food sources, there are therefore hardly any epidemiological data for specific saturated fatty acids. Only one published study provides evidence about the effects of stearic acid and other specific saturates on CVD end-points (Hu *et al.*, 1999). In this study, the relative risk for a 1% increase in intake of stearic acid was 1.19, which was not substantially different from the relative risks for other saturated fatty acids (Hu *et al.*, 1999). Effects of stearic acid on risk factors other than blood lipids, such as blood clotting tendency, also do not provide a conclusive answer on whether stearic acid may have different effects on CHD risk.

As mentioned, the available studies on effects of SAFA on these risk factors are not consistent, and the clinical meaning of these effects is unclear. For example, one recent study suggests that stearic acid has less unfavourable effects on haemostatic factors than other saturates (Tholstrup *et al.*, 2003), but others found the opposite (Baer *et al.*, 2004; Lefevre *et al.*, 2004). Baer *et al.* found that a diet with 8% of energy as stearic acid increased fibrinogen concentration, which would theoretically translate to an increased risk of CHD. This study also compared the haemostatic effects of a diet with 4% of energy as stearic acid plus 4% of energy as TFA with those of a high-carbohydrate, low-fat control diet. In this comparison, there was no effect on fibrinogen concentration. Thus, at this realistic level of intake of stearic acid, no adverse effects on fibrinogen levels would be expected. Another study in 105 healthy subjects found no differences between stearic and palmitic acids in their effects on vascular function (Sanderson *et al.*, 2004).

Thus, metabolic studies show that different saturated fatty acids can have different effects on lipoprotein cholesterol levels. However, data on CHD risk beyond blood lipids are limited. There is no clear evidence that supports making a distinction between stearic acid and other saturated fatty acids.

Specific trans *fatty acids*

The two major dietary sources of TFA are ruminant dairy and meat fat, mainly providing vaccenic acid (*trans*-C18:1n-7), and industrial hydrogenated vegetable oils, providing a broad range of positional *trans* isomers with elaidic acid (*trans*-C18:1n-9) being the most abundant. It has been suggested that TFA from ruminant sources may be less detrimental for health than TFA from industrial sources. The few epidemiological comparisons of ruminant and industrial TFA have investigated associations of CHD risk with *relative* intakes of TFA (i.e. the highest *vs* the lowest categories of intake), without taking differences in absolute intake in the population between ruminant and industrial TFA into account. A recent review describes the epidemiological associations of CHD risk with *absolute* TFA intakes (i.e. grams eaten per day) (Weggemans *et al.*, 2004). This analysis reveals that there are no differences in CHD risk between total, ruminant, and industrial TFA for intakes up to 2.5 g/day. At higher intakes (more than 3 g/day), total and industrial TFA were associated with CHD, but at these levels of intake there are insufficient data on ruminant TFA.

There are no human data comparing effects of ruminant versus industrial TFA on blood lipids. The metabolic studies on industrial TFA show that different mixtures of *trans* isomers obtained by slightly different hydrogenation procedures of different types of vegetable oils have similar adverse effects on blood lipids (Ascherio *et al.*, 1999). This would suggest that the position of the *trans* double bond in the carbon chain is not an important determinant. Thus, the scarce data that are available do not support discriminating between ruminant and industrial TFA.

1.5 Dietary fats, obesity, diabetes and cancer

This chapter focuses on the effects of SAFA and TFA on CHD risk, because the evidence is most extensive and strong for this relationship. However, SAFA and TFA may also have other health effects. Next to CVD, the most important chronic diseases in Western societies for which a role of dietary fats has been suggested are obesity (and the resulting diabetes) and cancer.

There has long been and still is debate about the role of the total amount of fat in the diet in the aetiology of obesity (Katan *et al.*, 1997). If the total amount of dietary fat would in the long term increase body weight (Astrup *et al.*, 2000), this would increase CHD risk through adverse changes in blood lipids (Leenen *et al.*, 1993) and higher risk of diabetes. However, data supporting a major role of dietary fat per se in determining body weight are not strong, with long-term clinical trials being scarce and conflicting (Willett & Lebel, 2002). This seems counter-intuitive given the high energy content of dietary fat, but it is often forgotten that dietary fat forms only part of the equation determining energy balance. In the United States, the prevalence of obesity has rapidly increased despite a decline in the relative amount of fat in the diet over the past decades (Willett & Lebel, 2002). Apparently, other factors play an important role in caloric overconsumption. Indeed, many foods high in carbohydrates are also energy-dense (e.g. refined foods, soft drinks), and energy expenditure (physical activity) is a major determinant of energy imbalance and weight gain.

It has also been suggested that the type of dietary fat, in particular reducing SAFA and TFA intake and increasing MUFA intake, could directly improve insulin sensitivity and reduce the risk of type 2 diabetes (Hu & Willett, 2002). This would be an additional mechanism to reduce CHD risk. However, most experts and food and health authorities agree that the predominant way in which dietary fat quality can reduce CHD risk is through improving blood lipids.

A high consumption of fat, and in particular of animal fat and saturated fatty acids, has been associated with higher risks of breast, colorectal and prostatic cancers (Zock, 2001). However, there is no convincing evidence for a role of dietary fats. The idea derives from geographical comparisons, showing that cancer is more frequent in countries where fat consumption is high. These findings were supported by animal studies, showing that saturated fats promoted growth of artificially induced tumours. However, comparisons between countries do not provide strong evidence for causal relationships, and for animal studies it remains uncertain to what extent results can be extrapolated to humans. Moreover, well-conducted, prospective cohort studies show no or only weak relations between cancer incidence and dietary fats (Zock, 2001). One recent meta-analysis of 23 case-control studies and 12 cohort studies on dietary fat and breast cancer risk found a summary relative risk for saturated fat of 1.19 (Boyd *et al.*, 2003). Taken together, there is some evidence that intake of SAFA may somewhat increase the risk of cancer, but the evidence is not strong. There are no clear indications that TFA increases the risk of cancer.

1.6 Implications: controlling fat intake

During the past several decades, reduction in fat intake has been the main focus of dietary recommendations to decrease the risk of chronic diseases, including coronary heart disease. However, several lines of evidence indicate that the quality of dietary fat has a more important role in reducing risk than the total amount of dietary fat. Metabolic studies have clearly established that replacing saturated and *trans* fatty acids with *cis*-unsaturated fatty acids has the most favourable effect on plasma total and LDL cholesterol levels, and that reducing the total amount of fat can reduce HDL cholesterol and increase fasting TG levels. Results from epidemiological studies and controlled clinical trials show that replacing saturated and *trans* fatty acids with *cis*-unsaturated fatty acids is more effective in lowering risk of CHD than reducing total fat consumption. There is still no consensus on whether the total amount of dietary fat increases body weight in the long term and in this way offsets favourable effects of high unsaturated fat diets. In any case, the evidence favouring low-fat diets to prevent CHD is not convincing. Nevertheless, diets high in fat are often also high in energy. Therefore, it seems prudent to limit the total intake of fat, in particular for people who are not physically active and for those who experience weight gain.

The different specific saturated fatty acids can differ in their effect on blood lipid levels. In particular, stearic acid does not raise cholesterol levels as much as other saturated fatty acids. However, the implications for the risk of coronary heart disease are unclear. Because of the growing interest in stearic acid as a substitute for *trans* fatty acids to add texture and solidity in foods, there is a need to assess the effects of this fatty acid on cardiovascular disease end-points and risk factors beyond blood lipids and lipoproteins. Different types of TFA in the diet probably have similar detrimental effects on health, and there do not seem to be compelling reasons to discriminate between these.

Modern dietary recommendations agree on the need to set limits for the intake of total fat, saturated fatty acids, and *trans* fatty acids. In setting the limits for total fat, the optimal intakes rather than the maximal intakes to prevent chronic diseases are increasingly taken into account. There is good agreement on the limits set. Most recommendations for Europe and North America advise that total fat intakes should be in the range of 20–35 energy %. In addition, all recommendations stress the importance of maintaining energy balance to prevent weight gain. Saturated fat intake should be less than 10 energy % (*ca* 20 g/day)), and TFA intake should be less than 1 or 2 energy % (2–4 g/day). Although intakes of saturated fat and *trans* fat should both be decreased, saturated fat should be the primary focus of dietary modification, because saturated fat consumption is proportionately much larger than that of TFA.

1.7 Future trends

Current dietary recommendations to keep saturated fat and *trans* fat as low as possible are increasingly recognised by consumers and food regulatory agencies. This will be a driving force for the edible oil industry and food manufacturers to develop fats and foods with nutritionally improved fatty acid compositions. New processing technologies will have to create dietary fats and oils that are compatible with CHD health.

In Europe, food producers have responded rapidly to emerging evidence that *trans* fatty acids have adverse health effects by developing margarines very low in *trans* fatty acids without a concomitant increase in saturated fatty acids

(Katan, 1995). Responses in the United States have been much slower, but will also take place now that labelling of TFA on foods is mandatory as of January 2006. It can be expected that research on alternatives for *trans* fatty acid to add texture and solidity to foods will grow. Processing technologies such as interesterification, aiming at hard fats with lower TFA and SAFA contents, will become more standard and replace partial hydrogenation techniques. Research on dietary fats and health will increasingly extend beyond the classical CHD risk factors such as blood cholesterol. In particular the role of subclinical inflammation markers and their influence on vascular function and CHD risk will receive more attention. Nutrition research will also focus more on differentiating the health effects of specific saturated fatty acids, such as stearic acid. For future dietary recommendations, it can be expected that more emphasis will be put on reaching the optimal intakes of different types of fatty acids and less on decreasing the total amount of fat in the diet.

1.8 Sources of further information

A comprehensive scientific review that addresses the health effects of saturated and *trans* fatty acids in the context of a broader healthy diet is provided by Hu and Willett (2002). Several internet sites provide easily accessible information on dietary sources, health effects, and practical guidelines for fatty acids. For example, the sites of the American Heart Association, http://www.americanheart.org/presenter.jhtml?identifier=532, the British Nutrition Foundation, http://www.nutrition.org.uk/home.asp?siteId=43&sectionId=s, and OMNI http://omni.ac.uk/browse/mesh/D004041.html. The most recent dietary recommendations in the USA, with useful links are found on http://www.healthierus.gov/dietaryguidelines/

1.9 References

ALLISON DB, EGAN SK, BARRAJ LM, CAUGHMAN C, INFANTE M, HEIMBACH JT (1999). 'Estimated intakes of *trans* fatty and other fatty acids in the US population', *J Am Diet Assoc*, **99**, 166–74.

ARNTZENIUS AC, KROMHOUT D, BARTH JD, *et al.* (1985). 'Diet, lipoproteins, and the progression of coronary atherosclerosis. The Leiden Intervention Trial', *N Engl J Med*, **312**, 805–12.

ASCHERIO A, RIMM EB, GIOVANNUCCI EL, *et al.* (1996). 'Dietary fat and risk of coronary heart disease in men: cohort follow-up study in the United States', *BMJ*, **313**, 84–90.

ASCHERIO A, KATAN MB, ZOCK PL, STAMPFER MJ, WILLETT WC (1999). 'Trans fatty acids and coronary heart disease', *N Engl J Med*, **340**, 1994–8.

ASTRUP A, GRUNWALD GK, MELANSON EL, SARIS WH, HILL JO (2000). 'The role of low-fat diets in body weight control: a meta-analysis of ad libitum dietary intervention studies', *Int J Obes Relat Metab Disord*, **24**, 1545–52.

BAER DJ, JUDD JT, CLEVIDENCE BA, TRACY RP (2004). 'Dietary fatty acids affect plasma markers of inflammation in healthy men fed controlled diets: a randomized crossover study', *Am J Clin Nutr*, **79**, 969–73.

BODEN WE (2000). 'HDL-cholesterol as an independent risk factor in CVD: assessing the data from Framingham to the Veterans Affairs HDL intervention trial', *Am J Cardiol*, **86**, 19.

BOYD NF, STONE J *et al.* (2003). 'Dietary fat and breast cancer risk revisited: a meta-analysis of the published literature', *Br J Cancer*, **89**, 1672–85.

BRIEFEL RR, JOHNSON CL (2004). 'Secular trends in dietary intake in the United States', *Annu Rev Nutr*, **24**, 401–31.

BURR NIL, FEHILY AM, GILBERT JF *et al.* (1989). 'Effects of changes in fat, fish and fibre intakes on death and myocardial reinfarction: diet and reinfarction trial (DART)', *Lancet*, **2**, 757–61.

CLIFTON PM, KEOGH JB, NOAKES M (2004). '*Trans* fatty acids in adipose tissue and the food supply are associated with myocardial infarction', *J Nutr*, **134**, 874–9.

DAYTON S, PEARCE ML, HASHIMOTO S *et al.* (1969). 'A controlled clinical trial of a diet high in unsaturated fat in preventing complications of atherosclerosis', *Circulation*, **40**, Suppl 1SI–S63.

DE LORGERIL M, SALEN P, MARTIN J-L *et al.* (1999). 'Mediterranean diet, traditional risk factors, and the rate of cardiovascular complications after myocardial infarction: final report of the Lyon Diet Heart Study', *Circulation*, **99**, 779–85.

DE ROOS NM, SIEBELINK E, BOTS ML, VAN TOL A, SCHOUTEN EG, KATAN MB (2002). '*Trans* monounsaturated fatty acids and saturated fatty acids have similar effects on postprandial flow-mediated vasodilation', *Eur J Clin Nutr*, **56**, 674–9.

EXPERT PANEL ON DETECTION, EVALUATION AND TREATMENT OF HIGH BLOOD CHOLESTEROL IN ADULTS (2001). 'Executive summary of the third report of the national cholesterol education program (NCEP) expert panel on detection, evaluation and treatment of high blood cholesterol in adults (Adult treatment panel III)', *JAMA*, **285**, 2486–97.

FRANTZ ID JR, DAWSON EA, ASHMAN PL *et al.* (1989). 'Test of effect of lipid lowering by diet on cardiovascular risk: the Minnesota Coronary Survey', *Arteriosclerosis*, **9**, 129–35.

GORDON T, KAGAN A, GARCIA-PALMIERI M, KANNEL WB, ZUKEL WJ, TILLOTSON J, SORLIE P, HJORTLAND M (1981). 'Diet and its relation to coronary heart disease and death in three populations', *Circulation*, **63**, 500–15.

HARRIS WS (1997). 'n-3 Fatty acids and serum lipoproteins: human studies', *Am J Clin Nutr*, **65** (Suppl.), 1645S–54S.

HE K, MERCHANT A, RIMM EB *et al.* (2003). 'Dietary fat intake and risk of stroke in male US healthcare professionals: 14 year prospective cohort study', *BMJ*, 327, 777–82.

HU FB, WILLETT WC (2002). 'Optimal diets for prevention of coronary heart disease', *JAMA*, **288**, 2569–78.

HU FB, STAMPFER MJ, MANSON JE *et al.* (1997). 'Dietary fat intake and risk of coronary heart disease in women', *N Engl J Med*, **337**, 1491–9.

HU FB, STAMPFER MJ, MANSON JE *et al.* (1999). 'Dietary saturated fats and their food sources in relation to the risk of coronary heart disease in women', *Am J Clin Nutr*, **70**, 1001–8.

HULSHOF KFAM, VAN ERP-BAART MA, ANNTOLAINEN M *et al.* (1999). Intake of fatty acids in Western Europe with emphasis on *trans* fatty acids: The TRANSFAIR study', *Eur J Clin Nutr*, **53**, 157.

KATAN MB (1995). 'Exit *trans* fatty acids', *Lancet*, **346**, 1245–6.

KATAN MB, GRUNDY SM, WILLETT WC (1997), 'Beyond low-fat diets', *N Engl J Med*, **337**, 563–6.

KATO H, TILLOTSON J, NICHAMEN MZ *et al.* (1973). 'Epidemiological studies of coronary heart disease and stroke in Japanese men living in Japan, Hawaii and California: serum lipids and diet', *Am J Epidemiol*, **97**, 372–85.

KEYS A (1980). *Seven Countries: A Multivariate Analysis of Death and Coronary Heart Disease*, Cambridge, Massachusetts: Harvard University Press.

KEYS A, ANDERSON JT, GRANDE F (1965). 'Serum cholesterol response to changes in the diet: IV. Particular saturated fatty acids in the diet', *Metabolism*, **14**, 776–86.

KINOSIAN B, GLICK H, PREISS L, PUDER KL (1995). 'Cholesterol and coronary heart disease: predicting risks in men by changes in levels and ratios', *J Invest Med*, **43**, 443–50.

KRIS-ETHERTON P, DANIELS SR, ECKEL RH *et al.* (2001). 'Summary of the scientific conference on dietary fatty acids and cardiovascular health', *Circulation*, **103**, 1034–9.

KROMHOUT D, MENOTTI A, BLOEMBERG B *et al.* (1995). 'Dietary saturated and *trans* fatty acids and cholesterol and 25-year mortality from coronary heart disease: the Seven Countries Study', *Prev Med*, **24**, 308–15.

KUSHI LH, LEW RA, STARE FJ *et al.* (1985). 'Diet and 20-year mortality from coronary heart disease: the Ireland–Boston Diet–Heart Study', *N Engl J Med*, **312**, 811–18.

LAW MR, WALD NJ, THOMPSON SG (1994). 'By how much and how quickly does reduction in serum cholesterol concentration lower risk of ischaemic heart disease', *BMJ*, **308**, 367–73.

LEENEN R, VAN DER KOOY K, MEYBOOM S, SEIDELL JC, DEURENBERG P, WESTSTRATE JA (1993). 'Relative effects of weight loss and dietary fat modification on serum lipid levels in the dietary treatment of obesity', *J Lipid Res*, **34**, 2183–91.

LEFEVRE M, KRIS-ETHERTON PM, ZHAO G, TRACY RP (2004). 'Dietary fatty acids, hemostasis and cardiovascular disease risk', *J Am Diet Assoc*, **104**, 410–19.

LEMAITRE RN, KING IB, RAGHUNATHAN TE *et al.* (2002). 'Cell membrane *trans*-fatty acids and the risk of primary cardiac arrest', *Circulation*, **105**, 697–701.

LEREN P (1966). 'The Oslo diet-heart study: eleven-year report', *Circulation*, **42**(5), 935–42.

McGEE DL, REED DM, YANO K *et al.* (1984). 'Ten-year incidence of coronary heart disease in the Honolulu Heart Program: relationship to nutrient intake', *Am J Epidemiol*, **119**, 667–76.

MENSINK RP, ZOCK PL, KESTER ADM, KATAN MB (2003). 'Effects of dietary fatty acids and carbohydrates on the ratio of serum total to HDL cholesterol and on serum lipids and apolipoproteins; a meta-analysis of 60 controlled trials', *Am J Clin Nutr*, **77**, 1146–55.

MORRIS JN, BALL KP, ANTONIS A *et al.* (1968). 'Report of a Research Committee to the Medical Research Council. Controlled trial of soya-bean oil in myocardial infarction', *Lancet*, **2**, 693–700.

MOZAFFARIAN D, PISCHON T, HANKINSON SE *et al.* (2004). 'Dietary intake of *trans* fatty acids and systemic inflammation in women', *Am J Clin Nutr*, **79**, 606–12.

NATARJAN S, GLICK H, CRIQUI M *et al.* (2003). 'Cholesterol measures to identify and treat individuals at risk for coronary heart disease', *Am J Prev Med*, **25**, 50–57.

OOMEN CM, OCKE MC, FESKENS EJ, ERP-BAART MA, KOK FJ, KROMHOUT D (2001). 'Association between *trans* fatty acid intake and 10-year risk of coronary heart disease in the Zutphen Elderly Study: a prospective population-based study', *Lancet*, **357**, 746–51.

PEDERSEN TR, OLSSON AG, FAERGEMAN O *et al.* (1998). 'Lipoprotein changes and reduction in the incidence of major CHD events in the 4S study', *Circulation*, **97**, 1453–60.

PIETINEN P, ASCHERIO A, KORHONEN P *et al.* (1997). 'Intake of fatty acids and risk of coronary heart disease in a cohort of Finnish men. The Alpha-Tocopherol, Beta-Carotene Cancer Prevention Study', *Am J Epidemiol*, **145**, 876–87.

RESEARCH COMMITTEE (1965). 'Low-fat diet in myocardial infarction: a controlled trial' *Lancet*, **2**, 501–4.

ROBERTS TL, WOOD DA, RIEMERSMA RA *et al.* (1995). 'Trans isomers of oleic and linoleic acids in adipose tissue and sudden cardiac death', *Lancet*, 345, 278–82.

SACKS FM, KATAN MB (2002). 'Randomized clinical trials on the effects of dietary fat and carbohydrate on plasma lipoproteins and cardiovascular disease', *Am J Med*, 113, Suppl 9B, 13S–24S.

SANDERSON P, OLTHOF M, GRIMBLE RF *et al.* (2004). 'Dietary lipids and vascular function: UK Foods Standards Agency workshop report', *Brit J Nutr*, 91, 491–500.

SHEKELLE RB, SHRYOCK AM, PAUL O *et al.* (1981). 'Diet, serum cholesterol, and death from coronary heart disease: the Western Electric Study', *N Engl J Med* 304, 65–70.

SINGH RB, DUBNOV G, NIAZ MA *et al.* (2002). 'Effect of an Indo-Mediterranean diet on progression of coronary artery disease in high risk patients (Indo-Mediterranean Diet Heart Study): a randomised single-blind trial', *Lancet* 360, 1455–61.

STAMPFER MJ, SACKS FM, SALVINI S, WILLETT WC, HENNEKENS CH (1991). 'A prospective study of cholesterol, apolipoproteins, and the risk of myocardial infarction', *N Engl J Med* 325, 373–81.

THOLSTRUP T, MILLER GJ, BYSTED A, SANDSTROM B (2003). 'Effect of individual dietary fatty acids on postprandial activation of blood coagulation factor VII and fibrinolysis in healthy young men', *Am J Clin Nutr* 77, 1125–32.

TURPEINEN O, KARVONEN MJ, PEKKARINEN M *et al.* (1979). 'Dietary prevention of coronary heart disease: the Finnish Mental Hospital Study' *Int J Epidemiol* 8, 99–118.

WATTS GF, LEWIS B, BRUNT JNH *et al.* (1992). 'Effects of coronary artery disease of lipid-lowering diet, or diet plus cholestyramine, in the St. Thomas' Atherosclerosis Regression Study (STARS)', *Lancet*, 339, 563–69.

WEGGEMANS RM, RUDRUM M, TRAUTWEIN ET (2004), 'Intake of ruminant versus industrial *trans* fatty acids and risk of coronary heart disease – what is the evidence?', *Eur J Lipid Sci Technol*, **106**, 390–7.

WILLETT WC, LEBEL R (2002), 'Dietary fat is not a major determinant of body fat', *Am J Med*, **113**, Suppl 9B, 47S–59S.

ZOCK PL (2001), 'Dietary fats and cancer', *Curr Opin Lipidol*, **12**, 5–10.

2

Dietary fatty acids, insulin resistance and diabetes

D. I. Shaw, University of Reading, UK, W. L. Hall, King's College London, UK and C. M. Williams, University of Reading, UK

2.1 Introduction

Insulin is an important hormone produced and secreted from pancreatic beta cells. It plays a central role in the coordinated metabolism of the major sources of energy for the body; glucose and fat. Variation in insulin secretion during the fed and fasted states ensures optimal oxidation of glucose and storage of fat (lipid) during the fed state, and oxidation of fat and conservation of glucose during the fasted state. If this system is disturbed, adverse effects on energy supply to tissues and on circulating blood glucose and lipid levels can occur.

Insulin resistance is described as the clinical state in which a normal or increased insulin level produces a reduced/impaired biological response. In the early stages, development of insulin resistance results in compensatory hyper-insulinaemia. As secretion of insulin from the pancreatic beta cell becomes increasingly impaired, compensatory increased insulin secretion cannot be maintained and hyperglycaemia (raised blood glucose) results. At this stage subjects may have impaired glucose tolerance but no symptoms of diabetes. When insulin secretion is severely reduced, symptoms of type 2 diabetes are present and subjects can be diagnosed according to clinical criteria. Insulin resistance can be present long before the onset of hyperglycaemia and type 2 diabetes (Cefalu, 2001) and this can be referred to as the pre-diabetic state. The term 'metabolic syndrome' has also come into general use to describe a condition of insulin resistance, usually associated with overweight, impaired glucose tolerance, dyslipidaemia and hypertension. In many, but not all, individuals, the metabolic syndrome may precede the development of frank diabetes. Recent estimates suggest the prevalence of this syndrome may be as high as 25% and 10–15% of the adult populations of the USA and Europe, respectively (Shaw *et al.*, 2005) There is increasing concern about the increased prevalence of the metabolic syndrome in Westernised countries because of its strong link with risk of type 2 diabetes and cardiovascular disease, both major causes of mortality and morbidity (Laaksonen *et al.*, 2002a; Wilson, 2004; Shaw *et al.*, 2005).

The cellular mechanisms involved in the development of insulin resistance and the role of diet are yet to be fully elucidated (Cefalu, 2001). Recent research has identified effects of fatty acids on both insulin signalling and on insulin secretion, as well as on transcription factors involved in the regulation of cellular lipid and energy homeostasis, which provide new insight into the mechanisms by which high-fat diets, and disturbances in fatty acid metabolism in obesity, could impair insulin sensitivity. These are considered as part of this review which summarises the evidence for a possible role of dietary fat in the development of insulin resistance and type 2 diabetes. Evidence is considered from a number of sources including cell and tissue studies, experimental studies in animals and from observational epidemiology and dietary intervention studies in humans.

2.2 Adverse effects of fatty acids on glucose and insulin

An increased supply of free fatty acids (FFAs) has been identified as a possible factor in the development of insulin resistance. Although elevated FFA levels are considered to be typical of the fasted state, in the case of subjects consuming high-fat diets, overspill of fatty acids into the circulation, following the breakdown of circulating fat, results in elevated FFA levels within the fed/postprandial state also. Since most subjects on Westernised diets are in an almost continuous postprandial state, it follows that circulating FFA are likely to be elevated for the greater part of the day (Frayn *et al.*, 1996). This 'FFA overspill' may be exacerbated in overweight and obese subjects, in whom fasted FFA levels are also raised due to greater fat mass (Boden, 1997). These disturbances in circulating FFA are considered by some as the essential link between obesity, insulin resistance and the development of type 2 diabetes (Boden, 1997). This metabolically disturbed situation, in which both FFA and glucose are elevated simultaneously, imposes limits on the normal coordination of glucose and lipid metabolism at cellular level. Cellular disturbances in insulin action may be further exacerbated by adverse effects of FFAs on insulin secretion and on the normal regulation of beta cell function which, in extreme situations, may lead to impaired insulin action.

2.2.1 Pathways in the coordination of cellular glucose and fat metabolism

The metabolism of fat and carbohydrate are closely linked; optimal oxidation of fat and conservation of glucose occur in the fed state and the opposite in the fasted state. Current theory identifies two major biochemical pathways as central components of this integrated coordination of energy metabolism. These are the glucose–fatty acid cycle first described in 1963 (Randle *et al.*, 1963) and the malonyl CoA/carnitine palmitoyl transferase (CPT)-1 pathway which was suggested by the studies of McGarry and coworkers in the late 1970s (McGarry *et al.*, 1977). Importantly, these two pathways complement each other (Fig. 2.1).

The glucose–fatty acid cycle links carbohydrate and fat metabolism and was one of the first theories to describe how fatty acids influence glucose metabolism. It centres on the proposition that increased beta-oxidation (utilisation) of fatty acids in skeletal muscle results in a reduced uptake and oxidation of glucose (Fig. 2.1), offering additional fine-tuning to the 'coarse' control of glucose and fat utilisation that is enforced at whole body level, by insulin (Frayn, 2003). Although recent advances in the study of whole body glucose metabolism in humans using nuclear magnetic resonance (NMR) spectroscopy, have challenged details of the glucose fatty acid cycle theory, they do confirm that fatty acids can antagonise glucose metabolism and insulin action at cellular level (Shulman, 2000).

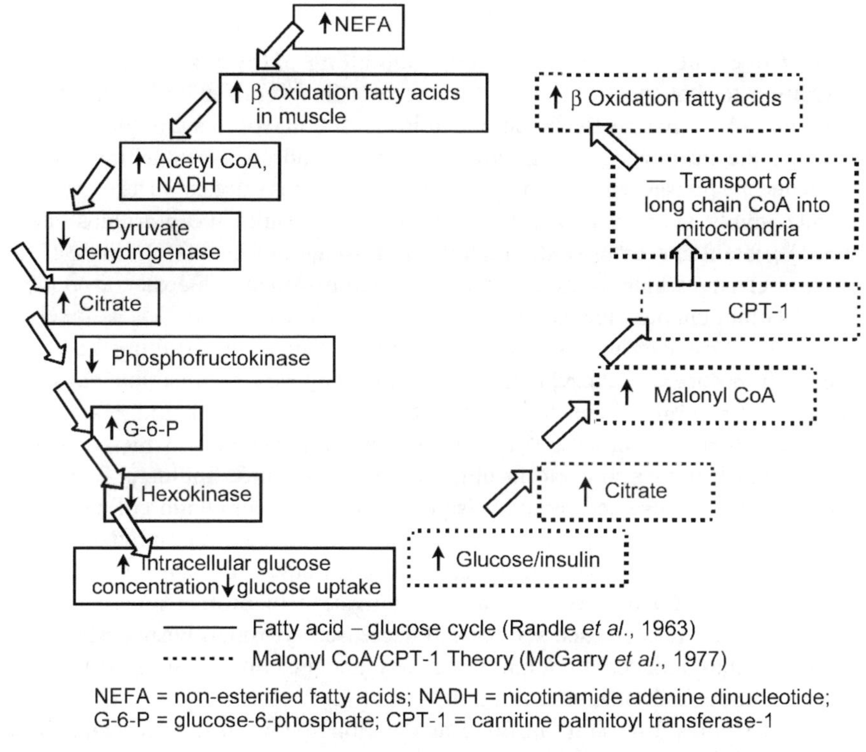

Fig. 2.1 Schematic diagram representing the fatty acid/glucose cycle and the malonyl CoA/CPT-1 system involved in coordination of glucose and lipid metabolism.

The malonyl CoA/CPT-1 pathway operates in a reverse manner to the glucose fatty acid cycle (Fig. 2.1), in restraining the rate of fatty acid oxidation under situations of high glucose provision. Increased levels of intracellular malonyl CoA (which accumulate under conditions of high glucose and insulin) inhibit the activity of CPT-1, essential for the transport of long chain (LC) acyl CoA (intermediate fatty acid metabolite) into the mitochondria for oxidation. The effects of increased glucose provision on fatty acid utilisation have been shown in a study using a pancreatic beta cell line. This study demonstrated that increased provision of glucose caused a 31% reduction in palmitate oxidation, but not under conditions where the rise in malonyl CoA was prevented, emphasising the regulatory role of malonyl CoA in intracellular glucose and lipid homeostasis (Mulder *et al.*, 2001). Importantly, this control of lipid and carbohydrate partitioning by malonyl CoA is fatty acid specific, owing to differences in the transport of long and medium chain fatty acids into the mitochondria (Sidossis *et al.*, 1996). Therefore the metabolism of long chain fatty acids (e.g. palmitate, oleate, linoleate), but not medium chain fatty acids (e.g. octanoate), can be attenuated by increased cellular glucose and insulin levels.

2.2.2 Effects of fatty acids on insulin signalling pathways

In addition to their possible effects on the coordination of energy metabolism, FFAs may also have effects on the critical actions of insulin through, for example, the insulin signalling cascade. This cascade is essential for insulin-stimulated responses such as insulin-stimulated glucose uptake. The signalling cascade involves tyrosine phosphorylation of the insulin receptor substrate 1 (IRS-1) protein and thereby stimulation of phosphatidyl inositol 3 kinase (PI-3 kinase) activity which is essential for the expression of glucose transporters (GLUT4) that enable glucose uptake.

Elevated FFA can adversely affect insulin-stimulated glucose uptake at the glucose transport/phosphorylation stage. This may occur either due to direct effects of FFA on the glucose transporter, GLUT4, or via indirect effects through upstream modification of the insulin signalling cascade, which regulates GLUT4 density in response to insulin secretion (Boden & Shulman, 2002).

Impaired insulin signalling may also be caused by accumulation of metabolic intermediaries (e.g. malonyl CoA, LC acyl CoA) and end-products (e.g. triacylglycerol, TAG) of fatty acid metabolism. LC acyl CoA can be esterified to diacylglycerides (DAG), which via their activation of protein kinase C theta (PKCθ) may cause increased serine- and decreased tyrosine-phosphorylation of IRS-1 and thus reduced PI-3 kinase activity and insulin signalling (Shulman, 2000; Le Marchand-Brustel *et al.*, 2003).

Recent studies also show positive associations between intramuscular lipid content (IMLC) and insulin resistance and suggest accumulation of TAG in non-adipose tissue cells may be important in the pathogenesis of insulin resistance (Manco *et al.*, 2004). In experiments with fatless mice and with non-obese males, accumulation of intramuscular lipid has been shown to cause a reduction in PI-3 kinase activity and intracellular insulin signalling (Yki-Jarvinen, 2002). This over-accumulation of TAG may result from excess fatty acid supply or a reduction in fatty acid utilisation within tissue (Kraegen *et al.*, 2002). As well as adverse effects on insulin signalling, TAG accumulation in pancreatic islets has been associated with beta cell apoptosis and reduced insulin secretion and has been referred to as pancreatic lipotoxicity (Manco *et al.*, 2004).

In addition to these effects of fatty acids on sites downstream of the insulin receptor, it has also been suggested that fatty acids may affect insulin receptor accessibility via changes in membrane fluidity following incorporation into membrane phospholipids (Boden, 1997). Clearly this mechanism may be subject to variability according to dietary fatty acid type.

2.2.3 Effects of fatty acids on gene expression

A large number of genes have been identified that may be associated with increased risk of diabetes (Mir *et al.*, 2003). These 'candidate' or 'susceptibility' genes have either been chosen because of their known function in insulin secretion, synthesis or cellular action or have been identified from genome-wide scans and linkage analysis of affected families. Their relevance in the context of this review is because fatty acids may have a direct or indirect effect on the level of expression of these regulatory genes, either through modification of transcription, translation or post-translational events. In this way, fatty acids may enhance or antagonise the action of insulin on key genes. For example, it is well established that dietary polyunsaturated fatty acids (PUFA) inhibit lipogenic enzymes such as fatty acid synthase and acetyl CoA carboxylase and stimulate lipid oxidation genes such as fatty acid binding proteins (see review by Clarke, 2001). Interest in the role of fatty acids in gene expression has increased since the identification of specific fatty acid-activated transcription factors such as the peroxisome proliferator-activated receptor (PPAR) and its main sub-types (PPARα, PPARβ/δ and PPARγ) which have fatty acids as their natural ligands. These transcription factors bind as heterodimers with a retinoid X receptor to response elements in the promoter region of genes involved in fatty acid oxidation, glucose homeostasis and adipogenesis. It is believed that PPARs act as fatty acid sensors, with binding affinity to PPARs increasing with the length and degree of unsaturation of the fatty acid. However, the relative binding affinities of different fatty acids to each of the PPAR subtypes has not yet been fully elucidated (Kersten, 2002). Activation of PPARα by ligands such as PUFA induces the transcription of fatty acid oxidation genes, whereas activation of PPARγ leads to altered expression of genes involved in adipocyte differentiation, lipid storage and insulin sensitisation.

Dietary fatty acids are also capable of regulating other transcription factors such as sterol-regulatory-element-binding protein-1c (SREBP-1c). SREBP-1c is expressed mainly in adipose tissue, the liver and in pancreatic β cells (Kakuma *et al.*, 2000) and has been shown to be over-expressed in animal models of insulin resistance (Kakuma *et al.*, 2000; Shimomura *et al.*, 2000; Tobe *et al.*, 2001). SREBP-1c binds to sterol regulatory elements in the promoter regions of genes that regulate lipogenesis (e.g. fatty acid synthase, acetyl CoA carboxylase and stearoyl-CoA desaturase), cholesterol transport (e.g. HMG-CoA reductase) and glucose metabolism (e.g. glucose kinase, glucose-6-phosphate dehydrogenase) (Fouelle & Ferre, 2002). Expression of SREBP-1c is increased by insulin and inhibited by glucagon, and the SREBP-1c promoter region also contains regulatory elements that respond to PUFAs. The main effect of PUFAs is to down-regulate SREBP-1c mRNA and inhibit post-translational processing of SREBP-1c (Kim *et al.*, 1999; Xu *et al.*, 1999; Yahagi *et al.*, 1999). Consequently there is a down-regulation of lipogenic and glycolytic enzymes following exposure to elevated PUFA, an effect that could counteract the actions of insulin. As knowledge of the effects of different fatty acids on gene transcriptional regulation increases, this is likely to lead to a better understanding of the molecular basis of fatty acid-dependent insulin resistance.

2.2.4 Effects of fatty acids on insulin secretion

As well as evidence for FFA modulation of energy metabolism and insulin action at cellular level, there is also increasing evidence to support the view that the amount and type of fatty acids influence the secretion of insulin, and in particular, modulate glucose-stimulated insulin secretion (GSIS). This appears to be an important physiological response which ensures insulin secretion is enhanced in situations where glucose uptake and oxidation could otherwise be compromised owing to inhibitory effects of high circulating FFA levels (via the glucose fatty acid cycle). There may also be fatty acid specific effects since in both human and rat islets, saturated fats (SFA) cause greater potentiation of GSIS compared with unsaturated fatty acids, as do long chain fatty acids compared with medium chain fatty acids (Gravena *et al.*, 2002). However, this specificity is not confirmed as relevant human studies that could demonstrate this *in vivo* have not been carried out. It is important to note that this ability of fatty acids to stimulate insulin secretion, and thereby control blood glucose levels when fatty acid and glucose levels are simultaneously raised is limited. Indeed as described later, there is evidence that following chronic exposure fatty acids may also reduce insulin secretion.

The mechanism by which fatty acids cause stimulation of insulin secretion appears to be via increased intracellular LC acyl CoA (Yaney & Corkey, 2003; Roduit *et al.*, 2004). LC acyl CoA are thought to act as lipid signalling factors for cellular processes such as exocytosis in the beta-cell and manipulation of beta-cell LC acyl CoA or malonyl CoA levels has been shown to promote insulin secretion (Chen *et al.*, 1994; Zhang & Kim, 1998). Some fatty acids may also alter insulin secretion via direct modulation of ion channel activity, with myristic acid shown to increase both K^+ and Ca^{2+} channel activity, while arachidonic acid may increase Ca^{2+} entry through indirect effects, following conversion to prostaglandins PGI_2 or PGE_2 (Haber *et al.*, 2002). Palmitate also appears to enhance insulin secretion via acylation of membrane proteins which promote Ca^{2+} dependent insulin secretion (Yajima *et al.*, 2000; Haber *et al.*, 2002).

2.2.5 Effects of fatty acids on insulinotrophic gut hormones

One of the limitations of the isolated beta cell islet studies is that, largely, they fail to take account of other factors that modulate insulin secretion *in vivo*. Such factors include the incretin hormones glucagon-like-peptide-1 (GLP-1) and glucose-dependent insulinotrophic peptide. It has been reported in both healthy humans (Thomsen *et al.*, 1999) and those with type 2 diabetes (Thomsen *et al.*, 2003) that olive oil intake caused increased GLP-1 response compared with butter intake. Furthermore, postprandial plasma GLP-1 concentrations were increased more after an oral fat test containing MUFAs compared to PUFAs and SFAs (Beysen *et al.*, 2002). Recent work has suggested that fatty acids may modulate the effects of GIP on GLP-1 and thereby insulin secretion. Experiments using an isolated ileal L cell model suggest that improvements in glycaemic response seen in MUFA compared with SFA fed rats may be due to increased GLP-1 receptor activation in response to increased GIP secretion (Rocca *et al.*, 2001).

2.2.6 Relevance of fatty acid modulation of GSIS in the pathogenesis of insulin resistance and type 2 diabetes

While on the one hand fatty acid-mediated increases in insulin secretion may be important in ensuring adequate insulin release in situations where both FFA and glucose are elevated, on the other hand chronic over-exposure to fatty acids could lead to hypersecretion of insulin and hyperinsulinaemia. Boden (1997) propose that in non-diabetic and moderately insulin-resistant subjects, FFA stimulation of gluconeogenesis is counteracted by the FFA stimulation of insulin secretion, and is thereby an important counter-regulatory mechanism for maintaining circulating glucose concentration. However, in the development of type 2 diabetes in obese subjects, FFAs fail to stimulate the required compensatory insulin response, resulting in peripheral under-utilisation and hepatic over-production of glucose, with resultant hyperglycaemia.

It has been proposed that chronic over-exposure to FFA and LC acyl CoA results in the accumulation of lipid components within the beta-cell, with lipotoxicity and apoptosis leading to possible failure in insulin biosynthesis and secretion (Roduit *et al.*, 2004). This beta cell failure typifies severe type 2 diabetes and explains the fact that many of these subjects ultimately require insulin treatment to bring their glucose intolerance under control. A model of beta-cell lipotoxicity based on over-expression of SREBP-1c in INS-1 cells has been developed (Yamashita *et al.*, 2004). This model showed lipotoxicity was associated with enhanced expression of lipogenic genes, e.g. acetyl CoA carboxylase, TAG accumulation, and a reduction in the ATP : ADP ratio. Such investigations provide evidence for possible mechanisms involved in the chronic effects of over-provision of dietary lipid on insulin resistance, although studies are required to elucidate the mechanisms involved when this stage of insulin resistance is reached.

2.2.7 Summary – cellular mechanisms involved in fatty acid-dependent effects on insulin sensitivity

In summary, there are various mechanisms proposed to explain the biochemical pathways involved in the progressive development of dietary fat-induced insulin resistance (Fig. 2.2). Fatty acids seem able to modulate the intracellular metabolism of glucose either directly (e.g. glucose fatty acid cycle), or indirectly via their effects on the insulin signalling cascade and on insulin secretion. This cross-talk between glucose (and insulin) and fatty acids plays a vital role in the coordination of whole body and cellular energy metabolism. Fatty acid stimulation of insulin secretion ensures a heightened insulin response under conditions where the adverse effects of the glucose–fatty acid cycle would otherwise result in impaired glucose uptake and hyperglycaemia. However, under conditions of chronic over-provision (either via the diet or through excessive release into the circulation from adipose tissues stores as in obesity), excess fatty acids may lead to intracellular accumulation of LC acyl CoA, with adverse effects on insulin signalling leading to cellular insulin resistance. In the beta cell, LC acyl CoA-mediated insulin secretion may break down, with consequent inability to mount an adequate insulin response to carbohydrate ingestion. Eventually over-exposure of the beta cell to excess fatty acids may lead to the abolishment of insulin secretion in the beta cell through apoptosis.

FFA and/or metabolites may:

- have direct effects on insulin stimulated glucose uptake via GLUT4
- have indirect effects on insulin signalling cascade, influencing phosphorylation of IRS-1
- affect membrane fluidity and thereby insulin receptor accessibility
- have direct or indirect effects on GSIS via modulation of ion channels
- affect GSIS differently dependent on chain length and degree of saturation
- regulate insulin secretion through protein acylation
- lead to hyperinsulinaemia through LC acyl CoA accumulation
- affect gene expression

FFA: free fatty acids, IRS-1: insulin receptor substrate-1 protein, GSIS: glucose stimulate insulin secretion, LC: long chain.

Fig. 2.2 Summary of proposed mechanisms that may be involved in fatty acid induced insulin resistance.

2.3 Evidence from animal studies

Animal studies have shown that high-fat diets reduce insulin sensitivity (Huang *et al.*, 2004; Marotta *et al.*, 2004), and that they may lead to damage of the pancreas and impaired insulin secretion (Huang *et al.*, 2004). There are also data from animal studies that suggest that dietary fat quality may influence insulin action. Table 2.1 shows a summary of a selection of studies that have investigated the effects of different dietary fatty acids on markers of insulin action in animal models.

High-fat diets caused a marked increase (2–5-fold) in fasting and postprandial plasma insulin compared with a high-carbohydrate diet in rats (Marotta *et al.*, 2004). Further investigation revealed that fasting glucose levels also increased following SFA and MUFA diets, but not an *n*-6 PUFA diet. Interestingly the greatest increment of fasting plasma insulin was noted in the *n*-6 PUFA group. This shows that the *n*-6 diet resulted in compensatory hyperinsulinaemia which maintained glucose levels, preventing the rise that occurred with SFA and MUFA feeding (Marotta *et al.*, 2004). Insulin sensitivity was significantly decreased in all high-fat groups compared with the high carbohydrate group. Further research has demonstrated that fat quality may influence insulin action even when the level of fat intake is low. For example, a low-fat MUFA diet (5% fat), compared to a low-fat SFA diet, improved glucose tolerance in lean Zucker rats (Rocca *et al.*, 2001). In contrast to these results, Lardinois and Starich (1991) demonstrated that fasting insulin concentrations were lower in rats following a PUFA diet compared with a SFA or MUFA diet, with no differences in fasting glucose among the diets. Thus, the reported effects of fat quality on insulin action and glycaemic response in animals are conflicting. Overall, the data from these studies are consistent with the hypothesis that high-fat diets compromise glucose utilisation and lead to reduced insulin sensitivity, and suggest that dietary fat quality could modulate this effect.

Recently the role of LC n-3 PUFA in insulin action has been of considerable interest. Replacing 7% of energy as SFA with fish oil (24 h), reduced insulin hypersecretion caused by high SFA feeding in rats (Holness *et al.*, 2004). However, impaired glucose tolerance was observed, suggesting the reduced insulin secretion in the LC n-3 group was an unfavourable outcome since it prevented the hypersecretion of insulin necessary to maintain normal glucose levels under situations of high SFA feeding. Similar findings were obtained when GSIS was also measured *ex vivo* on perfused beta cells obtained from treated rats. Thus, in the short term, high levels of LC n-3 PUFA could have an adverse diabetogenic effect, causing insulin secretion to be lowered but with no beneficial impact on insulin sensitivity (Holness *et al.*, 2004). In another study, replacement of 3% of dietary energy from SFA with LC n-3 PUFA over a longer period (10 weeks) was shown to have no beneficial effect on insulin-resistant mice (Muurling *et al.*, 2003). However, a further study showed replacement of 10% of dietary energy from SFA for n-3 PUFA (5 weeks) significantly reduced the impairment of glucose tolerance in male Wistar rats (Alsaif, 2004). Thus, in

Table 2.1 Summary of animal studies investigating the impact of dietary fat on markers of insulin action

			Composition of diets				
Study	Animal	Diet duration	High fat	MUFA	*n*-3 PUFA	*n*-6 PUFA	SFA
Huang *et al.* (2004)	Sprague Dawley	7 weeks	✗ S_I				
Marotta *et al.* (2004)	Male Wistar	4 weeks	✗ S_I	✗ f. glucose		✗ insulin hypersecretion ✗ S_I	✗ f. glucose
Holness *et al.* (2004)	Female Wistar	SFA 4 weeks *n*-3 24 h	✗ S_I		✓ insulin hypersecretion ✗ glucose tolerance		✓ insulin hypersecretion
Alsaif (2004)	Male Wistar	5 weeks		↔ glucose tolerance ↔ S_I	✓ glucose tolerance ✓ S_I		✗ glucose tolerance ✗ S_I
Muurling *et al.* (2003)	Apo E leiden mice	SFA 20 wks *n*-3 10 wks	✗ S_I		C		C
Rocca *et al.* (2001)	Lean Zucker rats	2 weeks		✓ glucose tolerance			✗ glucose tolerance
Jucker *et al.* (1999)	Sprague-Dawley	4–5 weeks			✓ insulin resistance	✗ insulin resistance	
Fickova *et al.* (1998)	Wister males	1 week			✓ f. insulin ✗ S_I	✗ f. insulin	
Lardinois & Starich (1991)	Rats	8 weeks		✗ f. insulin	✓ glucose clearance ✓ f. insulin		✗ f. insulin

MUFA, monounsaturated fatty acids; PUFA, polyunsaturated fatty acids; SFA, saturated fatty acids; ✓ associated with beneficial changes in identified parameter; ✗ associated with non-beneficial changes in identified parameter; C, comparable effects; S_I, insulin sensitivity; f. fasting.

the diet of animals, the effects of LC n-3 PUFA on insulin sensitivity are yet to be confirmed as beneficial, harmful or neutral.

In addition, studies have shown PUFA subtype to have variable effects on markers of insulin action in animals. Rats fed diets rich in LC n-3 PUFA compared with n-6 PUFA for 1 week had significantly lower serum concentrations of insulin but there was no difference in serum glucose, suggesting greater insulin sensitivity in the LC n-3 PUFA-fed animals (Fickova *et al.*, 1998). In another study, rats fed safflower oil (78% n-6 PUFA), were found to be more insulin resistant compared with those fed fish oil (Jucker *et al.*, 1999). This study also found the insulin-stimulated glucose disposal rate was lower in the n-6 PUFA group than in the fish oil group (Jucker *et al.*, 1999). Care needs to be taken in extrapolating many of the animal studies to the human situation because, in many cases, unphysiological levels of fatty acids have been employed; this is particularly the case with studies that have used intakes of fish oils in excess of 1–2% of the total diet.

In vivo studies in animals reinforce the importance of fatty acids in GSIS that was illustrated in the *in vitro* studies described in section 2.2, and confirm that there are varying insulinotrophic potencies of the different fatty acid classes. Fatty acid type influences the degree of insulin secretion in rats, and also insulin secretion from the perfused rat pancreas, which is potentiated with increasing chain length and decreased with degree of unsaturation (Stein *et al.* 1997).

This brief review of the animal data reveals the inconsistencies of current findings for the effects of different dietary fats on insulin sensitivity in the literature. Variability in study design, e.g. age, sex, insulin sensitivity measurement protocol, state of animal (diabetic, obese, healthy), dietary composition, fatty acid class (MUFA, SFA, etc.) or specific fatty acids investigated, may underlie the differences in outcome. Overall, the evidence appears to indicate that SFAs have a detrimental effect on insulin sensitivity. There may be beneficial effects of LC n-3 PUFA but these depend upon the overall level of fat intake and the proportion of LC n-3 PUFA of total fat intake. Both detrimental and beneficial effects of LC n-3 PUFA on glucose tolerance and insulin secretion have been observed.

2.4 Evidence from human studies

There is now good evidence from large-scale controlled intervention trials to show that diet and exercise regimes reduce the risk of type 2 diabetes in individuals with impaired glucose tolerance (Pan *et al.*, 1997; Tuomilehto *et al.*, 2001; Knowler *et al.*, 2002) and improve insulin sensitivity in normal, healthy individuals (McAuley *et al.*, 2002). The diets in these studies were generally low fat, high fibre or high in complex carbohydrates, and in most of the studies, the subjects also engaged in regular high level aerobic exercise (two to four times per week). It is, however, impossible from these studies alone to answer the question of whether fat quality, per se, is an important determinant of insulin sensitivity. There are data available from observational epidemiology, as well as from a small number of controlled dietary fatty acid intervention trials, that suggest that high-fat diets with a high percentage of SFAs may be detrimental to insulin sensitivity in humans.

2.4.1 Epidemiological studies of dietary fatty acids, insulin sensitivity and diabetes

Although many epidemiological and human experimental studies have investigated the role of dietary fatty acids in coronary heart disease (CHD), and on cardiovascular risk biomarkers such as cholesterol, there are only a limited number of human studies that have investigated the role of dietary fat, specifically, in the development of insulin resistance.

A number of prospective studies have focused on associations between dietary fatty acid intakes or plasma and tissue fatty acid compositions in relation to either insulin action or risk of type 2 diabetes. In the Nurses' Study, intakes of dietary SFA or MUFA were neutral, but intakes of PUFA were negatively, and *trans* fatty acids were positively, related to increased risk of type 2 diabetes (Salmeron *et al.*, 2001). Other prospective studies have shown that risk of type 2 diabetes is greatest in subjects showing relatively high proportions of SFA and low proportions of unsaturated fatty acids in blood lipids at baseline (Vessby *et al.*, 1994), and that increased serum levels of linoleic acid (18:2), linolenic acid (18:3), total PUFA and PUFA : SFA were associated with a more favourable insulin outcome (Laaksonen *et al.*, 2002b). In addition Pelikanova *et al.* (2001) demonstrated that serum phospholipid SFA and PUFA were negatively and positively associated with insulin sensitivity, respectively. Furthermore, higher proportions of oleic and linoleic acids and lower SFA in plasma phospholipids were associated with increased insulin sensitivity at baseline (Louheranta *et al.*, 2002).

In general these studies support the hypothesis that unsaturated fats are protective and saturated fats are harmful with respect to risk of type 2 diabetes. This is supported by a recent review of the epidemiological evidence by Parillo & Riccardi (2004), which concluded that saturated fat from animal sources results in adverse effects on risk of type 2 diabetes, compared with unsaturated fat from vegetable sources. It was surmised that total dietary fat intake did not seem to predict the development of type 2 diabetes, although it was recognised that total fat intake may influence the development of type 2 diabetes indirectly, via excess body weight. However, it must be recognised that observational studies that measure associations between dietary intakes (or biomarkers such as serum fatty acids) and disease risk are limited in the extent to which they can provide evidence of causal relationships between measured variables, even when confounding factors are considered. Controlled intervention studies provide firmer evidence for causal associations but such studies are limited in number.

2.4.2 Evidence from human intervention studies saturated versus unsaturated fatty acids

Dietary intervention studies investigating effects of dietary fatty acids on insulin sensitivity have produced inconclusive results (Table 2.2). Many studies have been of short duration and have used small subject numbers (Popp-Snijders *et al.*, 1987; Heine *et al.*, 1989; Fasching *et al.*, 1991; Garg *et al.*, 1992; Christiansen *et al.*, 1997; Brynes *et al.*, 2000; Ryan *et al.*, 2000; Lauszus *et al.*, 2001; Louheranta *et al.*, 2002; Summers *et al.*, 2002; Gerhard *et al.*, 2004). However, the KANWU study, which used a larger sample size ($n = 162$) for a longer duration (2 diets $\times$ 12 weeks), showed that a diet high in SFA resulted in a significant reduction in insulin sensitivity, measured by the intravenous glucose tolerance test (IVGTT), the gold standard method. This was in contrast to a diet rich in MUFA, which reduced fasting insulin. Importantly, favourable effects of the MUFA diet were only seen when total fat intake was below 37% energy from fat. When the total fat intake was above 40.2% energy from fat, there were no longer significant differences in the effects of SFA and MUFA diets on insulin action (Vessby *et al.*, 2001).

In contrast, another study found that SFA, MUFA and *trans* fatty acids (TFA) (28% energy from fat) had no significant effects on insulin sensitivity (IVGTT) in a study lasting 4 weeks ($n = 25$) (Lovejoy *et al.*, 2002). Interestingly, when subjects were divided into lean and overweight subgroups, insulin sensitivity was reduced by 24% in the overweight subgroup on the SFA diet and by 11% on the TFA diet compared with the MUFA diet, with no differences within the lean subgroup (Lovejoy *et al.*, 2002).

It seems that dietary fat quantity and body weight (a possible indicator of background diet) may affect insulin action in healthy humans. Current dietary reference values recommend an average population fat intake of no more than 35% fat energy intake daily, largely based on maintenance of normal circulating cholesterol levels (Henderson *et al.*, 2003). Results from the KANWU study (Vessby *et al.*, 2001) suggest intake levels slightly above this recommendation could have beneficial effects on insulin sensitivity, as long as SFA intake remains low.

It is critical to note these effects were found in healthy human subjects and optimum dietary fat intake may be different in those carrying risk factors for disease or for those already with disease. Some studies demonstrated no marked effect of feeding either low-fat or high SFA, PUFA or MUFA diets on insulin sensitivity in type 2 diabetics (Garg *et al.*, 1992). In addition, a high MUFA, compared with a low-fat, high-carbohydrate diet, had no effect on insulin sensitivity, fasting insulin or glucose levels in subjects with gestational diabetes (Lauszus *et al.*, 2001).

There are studies, however, that have found differing effects of fatty acids in obese or diabetic subjects and that support beneficial effects of unsaturated compared with saturated fat diets on insulin sensitivity. Reductions in post-prandial insulin and glucose levels, and increased insulin stimulated glucose transport, were observed in obese diabetic patients following 6 weeks of a high

Table 2.2 Summary of human intervention studies investigating the impact of dietary fat on markers of insulin action

Study	Subject (n)	Diet duration (weeks)	Diets compared	Reported effect on insulin/glucose outcome
Healthy subjects				
Vessby *et al.* (2001)	H (162)	12	MUFA *vs* SFA	SFA: ✗ S_I MUFA: ✓ Fasting insulin*
Lovejoy *et al.* (2002)	H (25)	4	SFA *vs* MUFA *vs* TFA	All diets: ↔ S_I SFA, TFA: ✗ S_I**
Subjects with various conditions				
MUFA studies				
Christiansen *et al.* (1996)	O,D (16)	6	SFA *vs* MUFA *vs* TFA	SFA, TFA: postprandial insulinaemia
Gerhard *et al.* (2004)	D (11)	6	Low-fat *vs* high-fat MUFA	All diets: ↔ glycaemic control or lipid profile
Lauszus *et al.* (2001)	GD (27)	5	High CHO *vs* high MUFA	All diets: ↔ S_I, fasting glucose/insulin
Garg *et al.* (1992)	D (8)	3	Low-fat *vs* high-fat MUFA	All diets: ↔ S_I
SFA vs PUFA studies				
Summers *et al.* (2002)	D, nonO, O (17)	5	SFA *vs* PUFA	PUFA: ✓ S_I***
Heine *et al.* (1989)	D (14)	30	SFA *vs* PUFA	All diets: ↔ S_I

MUFA vs PUFA studies				
Louheranta *et al.* (2002)	IGT (31)	8	MUFA *vs* PUFA	MUFA: ✓ Fasting glucose
Brynes *et al.* (2000)	D (9)	3	MUFA *vs* PUFA	All diets: ↔ S_I
Ryan *et al.* (2000)	D (11)	8	MUFA *vs* PUFA	MUFA: ✓ Fasting glucose/insulin
n-3 PUFA studies				
Woodman *et al.* (2002)	D (59)	6	EPA *vs* DHA *vs* MUFA	EPA, DHA: ✗ fasting glucose All diets: ↔ S_I, insulin release
Sirtori *et al.* (1997)	HT, w, w/o IGT, w, w/o D (935)	24	n-3	↔ S_I
Annuzzi *et al.* (1991)	D (8)	2	n-3	↔ S_I
Fasching *et al.* (1991)	OIGT (8)	2	n-3	✓ S_I
Popp-Snijders *et al.* (1987)	D (6)	8	n-3	✓ S_I

MUFA, monounsaturated fatty acids; PUFA, polyunsaturated fatty acids; SFA, saturated fatty acid; TFA, *trans* fatty acids; H, healthy; D, type 2 diabetes; GD, women with gestational diabetes; O, obese; ✓ associated with beneficial changes in insulin/glucose outcome; ✗ associated with non-beneficial changes in insulin/glucose outcome; ↔ no changes to insulin/glucose outcome; S_I, insulin sensitivity; HT, hypertriglyceridaemia; * Only when energy from fat <37%; ** In overweight subgroup only; *** did not improve when groups were analysed individually.

MUFA diet compared with a high SFA or high TFA diet (Christiansen *et al.*, 1997). SFA-rich diets have been reported to have adverse effects on insulin sensitivity compared with PUFA-based diets in a group of subjects including those with diabetes, obesity or neither of these conditions (Summers *et al.*, 2002). A MUFA-based diet reduced fasting glucose and/or insulin compared with a PUFA diet in type 2 diabetics and those with impaired glucose tolerance (Ryan *et al.*, 2000; Louheranta *et al.*, 2002). It was suggested these findings may relate to the increased oleic and alpha-linolenic acid concentrations of the serum phospholipids found in the MUFA group compared with the PUFA group (Louheranta *et al.*, 2002). However, although these findings are supportive of the view that increased levels of these fatty acids in serum phospholipids are associated with beneficial changes in insulin sensitivity, it should be noted that the diets within the same study not only differed in fatty acid composition but also with respect to percentage total fat so that definitive conclusions cannot be drawn.

2.4.3 Evidence from human intervention studies – LC n-3 PUFA

There is mounting evidence for protective effects of LC n-3 fatty acids in the prevention of heart disease (Ruxton *et al.*, 2004); however their influence on insulin action and glucose metabolism is not as clear. Popp-Snijders *et al.* (1987) found 3 g/day LC n-3 PUFA (8 weeks) increased insulin-stimulated glucose uptake significantly in subjects with type 2 diabetes. Similar improvements after LC n-3 supplementation were reported by Fasching *et al.* (1991) in subjects with impaired glucose tolerance. Furthermore, n-3 supplementation on subjects with hypertriglyceridaemia both with and without IGT or diabetes significantly reduced TAG but did not worsen glucose intolerance (Sirtori *et al.*, 1997). Similarly, Annuzzi *et al.* (1991) found no adverse effect of fish oil (10 g/day) on glycaemic control in type 2 diabetics ($n = 8$). It has been hypothesised that the fatty acid composition of phospholipids in skeletal muscle is closely related to insulin action, and that LC n-3 PUFA, especially, play a beneficial role in insulin action with a higher n-6/n-3 ratio worsening insulin action (Storlien *et al.*, 1997).

Once again, however, there exists contrasting evidence in the literature. For example, following eicosapentaenoic acid (EPA), docosahexaenoic acid (DHA) (both LC n-3 PUFA) and olive oil (MUFA) supplementation in type 2 diabetics, fasting glucose was observed to be significantly higher in both LC n-3 PUFA supplementation groups compared with MUFA; indicative of impaired glucose tolerance, with no significant differences in fasting insulin, insulin sensitivity or insulin release (Woodman *et al.*, 2002). Many authors have found no improvement in glucose tolerance in type 2 diabetics following LC n-3 PUFA supplementation (see review by Vessby, 2000) and this was confirmed by a recent meta-analysis (Montori *et al.*, 2000).

A recent review of the role of LC n-3 PUFA in type 2 diabetes concluded that LC n-3 PUFA (1–2 g/day) could have cardioprotective effects in those with this condition without adversely affecting glucose control and insulin sensitivity, and that supplementation could prevent the conversion from IGT to diabetes in overweight individuals (Nettleton & Katz, 2005). The authors concluded that studies in the late 1980s to early 1990s which found adverse effects on glycaemia and insulin action were the result of the high doses of LC n-3 PUFA used and this conclusion would also be consistent with some of the findings from animal studies.

2.4.4 Summary of evidence from human studies

Findings from human studies are contradictory and it is yet to be confirmed whether, and to what extent, dietary fat quantity and/or quality may affect insulin action in humans. There is a paucity of studies that have measured insulin sensitivity using direct, rather than indirect or surrogate, measures. Where direct measurements have been made, comparisons are complicated by differences in methods of measurement of insulin sensitivity, study duration and dietary composition. Critically there have been no reported studies in which the effects of dietary fat substitution (SFA/MUFA or SFA/PUFA) on insulin sensitivity have been studied in subjects with the metabolic syndrome. Lipgene is a multicentre, 5-year pan-European project that will address this gap in our knowledge. This study will investigate the impact of dietary fat quality, and diet-sensitive genotypes, on insulin sensitivity and risk markers for the metabolic syndrome. RISCK is another ongoing multicentre, 4-year, UK-based study. The impact of the quantity and quality of dietary fat and carbohydrate on those with the metabolic syndrome will be investigated. In conclusion, current available data from human studies show that dietary SFAs, compared with MUFAs and PUFAs, have an adverse effect on insulin action, but more controlled intervention studies are required to substantiate such a conclusion.

2.5 Conclusions: fatty acids and insulin sensitivity

There are plausible biological mechanisms by which excessive provision, cellular uptake and metabolism of fatty acids may lead to impaired peripheral uptake and metabolism of glucose. These include direct attenuation of glucose-metabolising pathways and/or antagonism of the action of insulin at receptor or post-receptor level, or activation/inhibition of transcription factors involved in the regulation of glucose and lipid homeostasis at cellular level. Fatty acid-induced enhancement of glucose-stimulated insulin secretion (GSIS) appears to be a normal part of the whole body response to excessive fatty acid provision which ensures a compensatory increase in secretion of insulin under such circumstances. However in the long term this compensatory response can lead to hyper-insulinaemia and, ultimately, failure in beta cell secretion of insulin, leading to diabetes. There is some evidence, from cell and animal studies, that SFA are more likely than other fatty acids to promote an inappropriate hypersecretion of insulin. Although animal data and data from controlled human studies are contradictory in some cases, there does appear to be consistent evidence to support an adverse role for SFA in maintenance of normal insulin sensitivity. Less consistent, though suggestive, is the evidence that unsaturated fatty acids may have beneficial effects on insulin sensitivity. This latter question is one which is important to answer to enable policy makers to draw conclusions regarding the relative benefits of low-fat versus fat-substituted diets in the prevention of insulin resistance, metabolic syndrome and type 2 diabetes. Until this question is adequately addressed through controlled human studies, it is not possible to provide adequate guidance to agriculturalists and food manufacturers concerning the optimal compositions of oils to be produced and used in food manufacturing and processing.

2.6 Future trends

Adequately powered human intervention studies using n-3 and n-6 PUFA and MUFA are required to firmly establish the relative benefits of different types of dietary fat compared with SFA on glucose homeostasis. In addition, the effectiveness of different fatty acids on insulin action may be modulated by variation in an individual's genes. Dietary intervention studies require large subject numbers to show a significant effect, as there is such a large variation in individual response to any given dietary modification. Single nucleotide polymorphisms (SNPs) in candidate genes for insulin resistance/type II diabetes, e.g. the Pro12Ala SNP in the PPARγ gene (Luan *et al.*, 2001), provide us with a way to investigate further the interaction between genetic variation in susceptibility to disease and response to dietary change, and perhaps to determine why some individuals will show an improvement in health following fatty acid supplementation whereas others will not. Studies that investigate gene polymorphisms, insulin sensitivity and response to dietary fatty acids are scarce as this area of research is still in its infancy.

2.7 Sources of further information

Websites

http://www.lipgene.tcd.ie
http://www.risck.org.uk
http://www.diabetes.org.uk

Books

Encyclopaedia of Human Nutrition, edited by MJ Sadler, JJ Strain and B Caballero. Academic Press, 2004.

Frayn KN (2003), *Metabolic Regulation: a Human Perspective*, 2nd edn, Oxford, UK: Blackwell Publishing.

Review articles

Cefalu WT (2001), 'Insulin resistance: cellular and clinical concepts', *Expl Bio Med*, **226**, 13–26.

Manco M, Calvani M & Mingrone G (2004), 'Effects of dietary fatty acids in insulin sensitivity and secretion', *Diabetes Obes Metab*, **6**, 402–413.

Nettleton JA & Katz R (2005), 'n-3 long chain polyunsaturated fatty acids in type 2 diabetes: a review', *J Am Diet Assoc*, **105**, 428–440.

Parillo M & Riccardi G (2004), 'Diet composition and the risk of type 2 diabetes: epidemiological and clinical evidence', *Br J Nutr*, **92**, 7–19.

Boden G & Shulman GI (2002), 'Free fatty acids in obesity and type 2 diabetes: defining their role in the development of insulin resistance and beta-cell function', *Eur J Clin Invest*, **32**, 14–23.

2.8 References

ALSAIF A (2004), 'Effect of dietary fatty acids on glucose tolerance, insulin sensitivity and membrane free fatty acids in rats', *Pakistan J Nutr*, **3**, 56–63.

ANNUZZI G, RIVELLESE A, CAPALDO B, DI MARINO L, IOVINE C, MAROTTA M & RICCARDI G (1991), 'A controlled study on the effects of n-3 fatty acids on lipid and glucose metabolism in non-insulin-dependent diabetic patients', *Atherosclerosis*, **87**, 65–73.

BEYSEN C, KARPE F, FIELDING B, CLARK A, LEVY J & FRAYN K (2002), 'Interaction between specific fatty acids, GLP-1 and insulin secretion in humans', *Diabetalogia*, **45**, 1533–1541.

BODEN G (1997), 'Role of fatty acids in the pathogenesis of insulin resistance and NIDDM', *Diabetes*, **45**, 3–10.

BODEN G & SHULMAN G (2002), 'Free fatty acids in obesity and type 2 diabetes: defining their role in the development of insulin resistance and beta-cell function', *Eur J Clin Invest*, **32**, 14–23.

BRYNES A, EDWARDS C, JADHAV A, GHATEI M, BLOOM S & FROST G (2000), 'Diet induced change in fatty acid composition of plasma triacylglycerols is not associated with change in glucagon-like peptide 1 or insulin sensitivity in people with type 2 diabetes', *Am J Clin Nutr*, **72**, 1111–1118.

CEFALU W (2001), 'Insulin resistance: cellular and clinical concepts', *Expl Bio Med*, **226**, 13–26.

CHEN S, OGAWA A, OHNEDA M, UNGER R, FOSTER D & McGARRY J (1994), 'More direct evidence for a malonyl-CoA-carnitine palmitoyltransferase I interaction as a key event in pancreatic beta-cell signaling', *Diabetes*, **43**, 878–883.

CHRISTIANSEN E, SCHNIDER S, PALMVIG B, TAUBER-LASSEN E & PEDERSEN O (1997), 'Intake of a diet high in trans monounsaturated fatty acids or saturated fatty acids. Effects on postprandial insulinaemia and glycaemia in obese patients with NIDDM', *Diabetes Care*, **20**, 881–887.

CLARKE SD (2001), 'Polyunsaturated fatty acid regulation of gene transcription: a molecular mechanism to improve the metabolic syndrome', *J Nutr*, **131**, 1129–1132.

FASCHING P, RATHEISER K, WALDHAUSAL W, ROHAC M, OSTERRODE W, NOWOTNY P &

VIERHAPPER H (1991), 'Metabolic effects of fish-oil supplementation in patients with impaired glucose tolerance', *Diabetes*, **40**, 583–589.

FICKOVA M, HUBERT P, CREMEL G & LERAY C (1998), 'Dietary (n-3) and (n-6) polyunsaturated fatty acids rapidly modify fatty acid composition and insulin effects in rat adipocytes', *J Nutr*, **128**, 512–519.

FOUELLE F & FERRE P (2002), 'New perspectives in the regulation of hepatic glycolytic and lipogenic genes by insulin and glucose: a role for the transcription factor and sterol refulatory element binding protein 1-c', *Biochem J*, **366**, 377–391.

FRAYN K (2003), 'The glucose/fatty acid cycle 1963–2003: a tribute to Sir Philip Randle', *Biochem Soc Trans*, **31**, 1115–1119.

FRAYNE KN, WILLIAMS CM & ARNER P (1996), 'Are increased plasma non-esterified fatty acid concentrations a risk marker for coronary heart disease and other chronic diseases?', *Clin Sci*, **90**, 243–253.

GARG A, GRUNDY S & UNGER R (1992), 'Comparison of effects of high and low carbohydrate diets on plasma lipoproteins and insulin sensitvity in patients with mild NIDDM', *Diabetes*, **41**, 1278–1285.

GERHARD G, AHMANN A, MEEUWS K, MCMURRY M, DUELL P & CONNOR W (2004), 'Effects of a low fat diet compared with those of a high monounsaturated fat diet on body weight, plasma lipids and lipoproteins, and glycemic control in type 2 diabetes', *Am J Clin Nutr*, **80**, 668–673.

GRAVENA C, MATHIAS P & ASHCROFT S (2002), 'Acute effects of fatty acids on insulin secretion from rat and human islets of Langerhans', *J Endocrinol*, **173**, 73–80.

HABER E, XIMENES H, PROCOPIO J, CARVALHO C, CURI R & CARPINELLI A (2002), 'Pleiotropic effects of fatty acids on pancreatic beta cells', *J Cell Physiol*, **194**, 1–12.

HEINE R, MULDER C, POPP-SNIJDERS C, VAN DER MEER J & VAN DER VEEN E (1989), 'Linoleic-acid-enriched diet: long-term effects on serum lipoprotein and apolipoprotein concentrations and insulin sensitivity in noninsulin-dependent diabetic patients', *Am J Clin Nutr*, **49**, 448–456.

HENDERSON L, GREGORY J, IRVING K & SWAN G (2003) *The National Diet and Nutrition Survey: adults aged 19–64 years, Vol. 2 Energy, Protein, Carbohydrate, Fat and Alcohol Intake*, London: HMSO.

HOLNESS M, SMITH N, GREENWOOD G & SUGDEN M (2004), 'Acute omega-3 fatty acid enrichment selectively reverses high saturated fat feeding induced insulin hypersecretion but does not improve insulin resistance', *Diabetes*, **53**, S166–S171.

HUANG B, CHIANG H, YAO H & CHIANG W (2004), 'The effect of high-fat and high-fructose diets on glucose tolerance and plasma lipid and leptin levels', *Diabetes Metab*, **6**, 120–126.

JUCKER B, CLINE G, BARUCCI N & SHULMAN G (1999), 'Differential effects of safflower oil versus fish oil feeding on insulin stimulated glycogen synthesis, glycolysis, and pyruvate dehydrogenase flux in skeletal muscle', *Diabetes*, **48**, 134–140.

KAKUMA T, LEE Y, HIGA M, WANG Z-W, PAN W, SHIMOMURA I & UNGER R (2000), 'Leptin, troglitazone, and the expression of sterol regulatory element binding proteins in liver and pancreatic islets', *Proc Natl Acad Sci USA*, **97**, 8536–8541.

KERSTEN S (2002), 'Effects of fatty acids on gene expression: role of peroxisome proliferator-activated receptor alpha, liver X receptor alpha and sterol regulatory element-binding protein-1c', *Proc Nutr Soc*, **61**, 371–374.

KIM H-J, TAKAHASHI M & EZAKI O (1999), 'Fish oil feeding decreases mature sterol regulatory element binding protein 1 (SREBP-1) by down regulation of SREBP-1c mRNA in mouse liver', *J Biol Chem*, **274**, 25892–25898.

KNOWLER WC, BARRETT-CONNOR E, FOWLER SE, HAMMAN RF, LACHIN JM, WALKER EA, NATHAN DM; DIABETES PREVENTION PROGRAM RESEARCH GROUP (2002), 'Reduction in the incidence of type 2 diabetes with lifestyle intervention or metformin', *N Engl J Med*, **346**, 393–403.

KRAEGEN E, COONEY G, YE J & FULER S (2002), 'Peroxisome proliferator activated receptors, fatty acids and muscle insulin resistance', *J R Soc Med*, **95**, 14–22.

LAAKSONEN D, LAKKA H, NISKANEN L, KAPLAN G, SALONEN J & LAKKA T (2002a), 'Metabolic Syndrome and development of diabetes mellitus: application and validation of recently suggested definitions of the metabolic syndrome in a prospective cohort study', *Am J Epidemiol*, **156**, 1070–1077.

LAAKSONEN D, LAKKA T, LAKKA H, NYYSSONEN K, RISSANEN T, NISKANEN L & SALONEN J (2002b), 'Serum fatty acid composition predicts development of impaired fasting glycaemia and diabetes in middle-aged men', *Diabetic Med*, **19**, 456–464.

LARDINOIS C & STARICH G (1991), 'Polyunsaturated fats enhance peripheral glucose utilization in rats', *J Am Coll Nutr*, **10**, 340–345.

LAUSZUS F, RASMUSSEN O, HENRIKSEN J, KLEBE J, JENSEN L, LAUSZUS K & HERMANSEN K (2001), 'Effect of a high monounsaturated fatty acid diet on blood pressure and glucose metabolism in women with gestational diabetes mellitus', *Eur J Clin Nutr*, **55**, 436–443.

LE MARCHAND-BRUSTEL Y, GUAL P, GREMEAUX T, GONALEZ T, BARRES R & TANTI J-T (2003), 'Fatty acid induced insulin resistance: role of insulin receptor substrate 1 serine phosphorylation in the retroregulation of insulin signalling', *Biochem Soc Trans*, **31**, 1152–1156.

LOUHERANTA A, SARKKINEN E, VIDGREN H, SCHWAB U & UUSITUPA M (2002), 'Association of the fatty acid profile of serum lipids with glucose and insulin metabolism during 2 fat-modified diets in subjects with impaired glucose tolerance', *Am J Clin Nutr*, **76**, 331–337.

LOVEJOY J, SMITH S, CHAMPAGNE C, MOST M, LEFEVRE M, DELANY J, DENKINS Y, ROOD J, VELDHUIS J & BRAY G (2002), 'Effects of diets enriched in saturated (palmitic), monounsaturated (oleic), or trans (elaidic) fattyacids on insulin sensitivity and substrate oxidation in healthy adults', *Diabetes Care*, **25**, 1283–1288.

LUAN J, BROWNE PO, HARDING AH, HALSALL DJ, O'RAHILLY S, CHATTERGEE VK, WAREHAM NJ (2001), 'Evidence for gene-nutrient interaction at the PPARgamma locus', *Diabetes*, **50**(3), 686–689.

MANCO M, CALVANI M & MINGRONE G (2004), 'Effects of dietary fatty acids in insulin sensitivity and secretion', *Diabetes Metab*, **6**, 402–413.

MAROTTA M, FERRER-MARTINEZ A, PARNAU J, TURINI M, MACE K & GOMEZ FOIX A (2004), 'Fiber type and fatty acid composition dependent effects of high fat diets on rat muscle triacylglyceride and fatty acid transporter protein-1 content', *Metabolism*, **53**, 1032–1036.

McAULEY KA, WILLIAMS SM, MANN JI, GOULDING A, CHISHOLM A, WILSON N, STORY G, McLAY RT, HARPER MJ & JONES IE (2002), 'Intensive lifestyle changes are necessary to improve insulin sensitivity: a randomized controlled trial', *Diabetes Care*, **25**, 445–52.

McGARRY J, MANNAERTS G & FOSTER D (1977), 'A possible role for malonyl-CoA in the regulation of hepatic fatty acid oxidation and ketogenesis', *J Clin Invest*, **60**, 265–270.

MIR AA, MYAKISHEV MV, POLESSKAYA OO, MOITRA J, PETERSEN D, MILLER L, OROSZ A & VINSON C (2003), 'A search for candidate genes for lipodystrophy, obesity and diabetes via gene expression analysis of A-ZIP/F-1 mice', *Genomics*, **81**, 378–390.

MONTORI V, FARMER A, WOLLAN P & DINNEEN S (2000), 'Fish oil supplementation in type 2 diabetes', *Diabetes Care*, **23**, 1407–1415.

MULDER H, LU D, FINLEY J, AN J, COHEN J, ANTINOZZI P, MCGARRY J & NEWGARD C (2001), 'Overexpression of a modified human malonyl-CoA decarboxylase blocks the glucose-induced increase in malonyl-CoA level but has no impact on insulin secretion in INS-1 derived (832/13) beta cells', *J Biol Med*, **276**, 6479–6484.

MUURLING M, MENSINK R, PIJI H, ROMIJN J, HAVEKES L & VOSHOL P (2003), 'A fish oil diet does not reverse insulin resistance despite decreased adipose tissue TNF alpha protein concentration in ApoE-3 leiden mice', *J Nutr*, **133**, 3350–3355.

NETTLETON J & KATZ R (2005), 'n-3 long chain polyunsaturated fatty acids in type 2 diabetes: a review', *J Am Diet Assoc*, **105**, 428–440.

PAN XR, LI GW, HU YH, WANG JX, YANG WY, AN ZX, HU ZX, LIN J, XIAO JZ, CAO HB, LIU PA, JIANG XG, JIANG YY, WANG JP, ZHENG H, ZHANG H, BENNETT PH & HOWARD BV (1997), 'Effects of diet and exercise in preventing NIDDM in people with impaired glucose tolerance. The Da Qing IGT and Diabetes Study', *Diabetes Care*, **20**, 537–544.

PARILLO M & RICCARDI G (2004), 'Diet composition and the risk of type 2 diabetes: epidemiological and clinical evidence', *Br J Nutr*, **92**, 7–19.

PELIKANOVA T, KAZDOVA L, CHVOJKOVA S & BASE J (2001), 'Serum phospholipid fatty acid composition and insulin action in type 2 diabetes', *Metabolism*, **50**, 1472–1478.

POPP-SNIJDERS C, SCHOUTEN J, HEINE R, VAN DER MEER J & VAN DER VEEN E (1987), 'Dietary supplementation of omega-3 polyunsaturated fatty acids improves insulin sensitivity in non insulin dependent diabetes', *Diabetes Res*, **4**, 141–147.

RANDLE P, GARLAND P, HALES C & NEWSHOLME E (1963), 'The glucose fatty-acid cycle its role in insulin sensitivity and the metabolic disturbances of diabetes mellitus', *Lancet*, **1**, 785–789.

ROCCA A, LAGRECA J, KALITSKY J & BRUBAKER P (2001), 'Monounsaturated fatty acid diets improve glycemic tolerance through increased secretion of glucagon-like peptide-1', *Endocrinology*, **142**, 1148–1155.

RODUIT R, NOLAN C, ALARCON C, MOORE P, BARBEAU A, DELGHINGARO-AUGUSTO V, PRZYBYKOWSKI E, MORIN J, MASSE F, MASSIE B, RUDERMAN N, RHODES C, POITOUT V & PRENTKI M (2004), 'A role for the malonyl CoA/long chain acyl CoA pathway of lipid signaling in the regulation of insulin secretion in response to both fuel and non fuel stimuli', *Diabetes*, **53**, 1007–1019.

RUXTON C, REED S, SIMPSON M & MILLINGTON K (2004), 'The health benefits of omega-3 polyunsaturated fatty acids: a review of the evidence', *J Hum Nutr Diet*, **17**, 449–459.

RYAN M, MCINERNEY D, OWENS D, COLLINS P, JOHNSON A & TOMKIN G (2000), 'Diabetes and the Mediterranean diet: a beneficial effect of oleic acid on insulin sensitivity, adipocyte glucose transport and endothelium-dependent vasoreactivity', *Q J Med*, **93**, 85–91.

SALMERON J, HU F, MANSON J, STAMPFER M, COLDITZ G, RIMM E & WILLET W (2001), 'Dietary fat intake and risk of type 2 diabetes in women', *Am J Clin Nutr*, **73**, 1019–1026.

SHAW D, HALL W & WILLIAMS C (2005), 'Metabolic Syndrome: What is it and what are the implications', *Proc Nutr Soc*, **64**(3), 349–357.

SHIMOMURA I, MATSUDA M, HAMMER RE, BASHMAKOV Y, BROWN MS & GOLDSTEIN JL (2000), 'Decreased IRS-2 and increased SREBP-1c lead to mixed insulin resistance and sensitivity in livers of lipodystrophic and ob/ob mice', *Mol Cell*, **6**, 77–86.

SHULMAN G (2000), 'Cellular mechanisms of insulin resistance', *J Clin Invest*, **106**, 171–176.

SIDOSSIS L, STUART C, SHULMAN G, LOPASCHUK G & WOLFE R (1996), 'Glucose plus insulin regulate fat oxidation by controlling the rate of fatty acid entry into the mitochondria', *J Clin Invest*, **98**, 2244–2250.

SIRTORI C, PAOLETTI R, MANCINI M, CREPALDI G, MANZATO E, RIVELLESE A, PAMPARANA F & STRAGLIOTTO E (1997), 'n-3 fatty acids do not lead to an increased diabetic risk in patients with hyperlipidemia and abnormal glucose tolerance. Italian fish oil multicenter study', *Am J Clin Nutr*, **65**, 1874–1881.

STEIN D, STEVENSON B, CHESTER M, BASIT M, DANIELS M, TURLEY S & McGARRY J (1997), 'The insulinotrophic potency of fatty acids is influenced profoundly by their chain length and degree of saturation', *J Clin Invest*, **100**, 398–403.

STORLIEN L, KRIKETOS A, CALVERT G, BAUR L & JENKINS A (1997), 'Fatty acids, triglycerides and syndromes of insulin resistance', *Prostaglandins, Leukot Essent Fatty Acids*, **57**, 379–385.

SUMMERS L, FIELDING B, BRADSHAW H, ILIC V, BEYSEN C, CLARK M, MOORE N & FRAYN K (2002), 'Substituting dietary saturated fat with polyunsaturated fat changes abdominal fat distribution and improves insulin sensitivity', *Diabetologia*, **45**, 369–377.

THOMSEN C, RASMUSSEN O, LOUSEN T, HOLST J, FENSELAU S, SCHREZENMEIR J & HERMANSEN K (1999), 'Differential effects of saturated and monounsaturated fatty acids on postprandial lipemia and incretin responses in healthy subjects', *Am J Clin Nutr*, **69**, 1135–1143.

THOMSEN C, STORM H, HOLST J & HERMANSEN K (2003), 'Differential effects of saturated and monounsaturated fats on postprandial lipemia and glucagon-like peptide 1 responses in patients with type 2 diabetes', *Am J Clin Nutr*, **77**, 605–611.

TOBE K, SUZUKI R, AOYAMA M, YAMAUCHI T, KAMON J, KUBOTA N, TERAUCHI Y, MATSUI J, AKANUMA Y, KIMURA S, TANAKA J, ABE M, OHSUMI J, NAGAI R & KADOWAKI T (2001), 'Increased expression of the sterol regulatory element-binding protein-1 gene in insulin receptor substrate-2(−/−) mouse liver', *J Biol Chem*, **276**, 38337–38340.

TUOMILEHTO J, LINDSTROM J, ERIKSSON JG, VALLE TT, HAMALAINEN H, ILANNE-PARIKKA P, KEINANEN-KIUKAANNIEMI S, LAAKSO M, LOUHERANTA A, RASTAS M, SALMINEN V, UUSITUPA M; FINNISH DIABETES PREVENTION STUDY GROUP (2001), 'Prevention of type 2 diabetes mellitus by changes in lifestyle among subjects with impaired glucose tolerance', *N Engl J Med*, **344**, 1343–1350.

VESSBY B (2000), 'Dietary fat and insulin action in human', *Br J Nutr*, **83**, S91–S96.

VESSBY B, ARO A, SKARFORS E, BERGLUND L, SALMINEN I & LITHELL H (1994), 'The risk to develop NIDDM is related to the fatty acid composition of the serum cholesterol esters', *Diabetes*, **43**, 1353–1357.

VESSBY B, UUSITUPA M, HERMANSEN K, RICCARDI G, RIVELLESE A, TAPSELL L, NALSEN C, BERGLUND L, LOUHERANTA A, RASMUSSEN B, CALVERT G, MAFFETONE A, PEDERSEN E, GUSTAFSSON I & STORLIEN L (2001), 'Substituting dietary saturated for monounsaturated fat impairs insulin sensitivity in healthy men and women: the KANWU study', *Diabetologia*, **44**, 312–319.

WILSON P (2004), 'Estimating cardiovascular disease risk and the metabolic syndrome: a Framingham view', *Endocrinol Metab Clin N Am*, **33**, 467–481.

WOODMAN R, MORI T, BURKE V, PUDDEY I, WATTS G & BEILIN L (2002), 'Effects of purified eicosapentaenoic and docosahexaenoic acids on glycemic control, blood pressure, and serum lipids in type 2 diabetic patients with treated hypertension', *Am J Clin Nutr*, **76**, 1007–1015.

XU J, NAKAMURA M, CHO H & CLARKE D (1999), 'Sterol regulatory element binding protein-

1 expression is suppressed by dietary polyunsaturated fatty acids', *J Biol Chem*, **274**, 23577–23583.

YAHAGI N, SHIMANO H, HASTY A, AMEMIYA-KUDO M, OKAZAKI H, TAMURA Y, IIZUKA Y, SHIONORI F, OHASHI K, OSUGA J, HARADA K, GOTODA T, NAGAI R, ISHIBASHI S & YAMADA N (1999), 'A crucial role of sterol regulatory element binding protein-1 in the regulation of lipogenic gene expression by polyunsaturated fatty acids', *J Biol Chem*, **274**, 35840–35844.

YAJIMA H, KOMATSU M, YAMADA S, STRAUB S, KANEKO T, SATO Y, YAMAUCHI K, HASHIZUME K, SHARP G & AIZAWA T (2000), 'Cerulenin, an inhibitor of protein acylation, selectively attenuates nutrient stimulation of insulin release. A study in rat pancreatic islets', *Diabetes*, **49**, 712–717.

YAMASHITA T, ETO K, OKAZAKI Y, YAMASHITA S, YAMAUCHI T, SEKINE N, NAGAI R, MITSUHIKO N & KADOWAKI T (2004), 'Role of uncoupling protein-2 up-regulation and triglyceride accumulation in impaired glucose stimulated insulin secretion in beta cell lipotoxicity model overexpressing sterol regulatory element binding protein 1-c', *Endocrinology*, **145**, 3566.

YANEY G & CORKEY B (2003), 'Fatty acid metabolism and insulin secretion in pancreatic beta cells', *Diabetologia*, **46**, 1297–1312.

YKI-JARVINEN H (2002), 'Ectopic fat accumulation: an important cause of insulin resistance in humans', *J R Soc Med*, **95**, 39–45.

ZHANG S & KIM K (1998), 'Essential role of acetyl CoA carboxylase in the glucose-induced insulin secretion in pancreatic beta cell line', *Cell Signal*, **10**, 35–42.

3

Lipid–gene interactions, diet and health

D. Lairon and R. P. Planells, INSERM, France

3.1 Introduction

Dietary patterns, for about 150 000 years, have reflected a hunter-gatherer way of life that merely sustained scarce human populations of *Homo sapiens*. Depending on the seasons, there might be predominance of either animal or plant foods, with consequently large seasonal variations in nutrient intakes (Cordain *et al.*, 2000). Although it is difficult to get exact figures, it is estimated that fat intake was low, while carbohydrate and protein intakes were high in the Palaeolithic stone age. This primitive lifestyle has been significantly modified by the intensification of agriculture that progressively spread out over the world and permitted a huge increase in population. From 10 000 BC to the last century, nutrient intakes changed and worldwide figures currently estimate ranges of intakes to be 10–17% of energy for protein, 40–60% of energy for carbohydrate and 20–50% of energy for fat.

During the last century, new techniques for the production of food facilitated an exponential increase in population and the lengthening of average lifespan. However, this improvement in food availability, along with changes in lifestyles toward less physical activity, but perhaps with more 'stress', was also accompanied by substantial changes in dietary patterns. Indeed, at least in industrialized countries, energy intake increased, and the contribution of dietary fat (40–50% energy), especially saturated fatty acids, became more and more important. At the same time, the prevalence of metabolic diseases (obesity, metabolic syndrome, diabetes and subsequently cardiovascular diseases) dramatically increased. Because of the economic costs of these conditions, we have been driven to ask whether changes in diets, and dietary fat more particularly, could, at least in part, be responsible for this significant rise in metabolic diseases.

Almost all metabolic diseases involve serious disturbances in lipid metabolism, and a wealth of epidemiologic studies have identified alterations in plasma lipid levels as major risk markers for cardiovascular diseases (CVD) as well as type 2 diabetes or obesity. This observed correlation between plasma lipid alterations and chronic diseases has raised the question of the role played by dietary fat in their genesis, and it is now usual to recommend dietary measures to reduce the prevalence of such diseases. Nevertheless, the use of diet to reduce risk of chronic disease raises a number of important questions, since most studies have shown that the responsiveness to diets is a complex process, dependent on both individual (genetic) features and interactions between nutrients.

Responsiveness to a change in dietary pattern depends on the activity of several proteins, all intricately involved in complex metabolic pathways. We know that, though all human beings belong to the same species, *Homo sapiens sapiens*, minor alterations in gene structures could be responsible for determining differences between subjects. Indeed, every gene encoding a protein involved in response to diets can be polymorphic, the product of a given allele acting differently from the product of another allele. The overall response resulting from the addition of these slight differences may lead to an important variability from subject to subject, which is particularly well demonstrated during intervention studies. In such studies, for an identical change in diet, a majority of subjects (the responders) display a large modification of a parameter, while a minority of subjects (the non-responders) do not exhibit any marked change or may even modify this parameter in the opposite direction. However, the same modification of the diet would lead to a different response pattern when another parameter is studied.

To date gene–diet interaction studies are aimed at associating with each of these groups, responders or non-responders, a significant distribution of allelic variants in candidate gene locus. In most cases these candidate genes will be those encoding apolipoproteins and enzymes involved in lipid metabolism, those involved in lipid signalling and those coding for the transcriptional factors controlling the expression of enzymes, receptors, apolipoproteins, etc., involved in regulating lipid metabolism. Over time, several single nucleotide polymorphisms (SNPs) have been identified and associated with particular responses to changes in nutrients or in dietary patterns.

Nowadays, in light of the Human Genome Project, a wealth of genetic data is being generated, thanks to new methodological tools allowing easy and cost-sensitive determination of a large number of gene polymorphisms. In addition, owing to the development of informatics tools, these data can be more and more easily connected to physiological information. This opens a new era where studies dedicated to interactions between diets; metabolic parameters, disease risk factors and gene polymorphisms can be carried out on small or large groups of healthy subjects or patients.

In this chapter, we will first review the available literature data discussing some polymorphisms of selected key proteins involved in lipid and lipoprotein metabolism. We will describe successively their responsiveness to dietary fatty acids, then to dietary cholesterol and finally the metabolic syndrome. We shall then focus on the mechanisms of regulation of gene expression by fat, a process that involves, for a large part, nuclear receptors. This extensively studied gene family of transcription factors provides a heuristic paradigm of regulation of gene expression. Finally, we will suggest what can be deduced currently from these studies in terms of 'optimal' dietary fat and possible ways toward a better knowledge of diet–genetic background interactions.

3.2 Genetic influences on lipid metabolism

Two main pathways are involved in the intravascular transport of lipids in the form of lipid–apoprotein complexes called lipoproteins (Ye and Kwiterovich, 2000). The first endogenous pathway controls parameters that can be measured at fasting: the liver produces and secretes very low-density lipoproteins (VLDL) bearing apoproteins apoB-100, apoE, apoCII and apoCIII. Triglycerides, then phospholipids, are hydrolysed by endovascular lipoprotein lipase and hepatic lipase, to large intermediate density lipoproteins (IDL), then to small remnants known as low-density lipoproteins (LDL), which are enriched in cholesterol and which, owing to their longer half-life, tend to accumulate in the circulation.

The second pathway can be referred to as 'exogenous' and originates from the digestion and absorption in the gut of dietary fat provided by meals. The absorptive enterocyte secretes into the bloodstream large triglyceride-rich lipoproteins, which contain apoB-48, apoA1, apoA-IV, then apoE, apoCII and apoCIII. This results in the transient accumulation of postprandial chylomicrons, from which triglycerides and phospholipids are progressively withdrawn by the combined activity of lipoprotein and hepatic lipases. This generates smaller chylomicron remnants in a few hours. Endogenous and exogenous remnants are then cleared from the circulation thanks to receptor-driven mechanisms, i.e. liver apoB,E and remnant receptors or peripheral tissue apoB,E receptor and scavenger receptor.

Circulating high-density lipoproteins (HDL) bearing apoA1 and apoAII can exchange lipids with VLDL. Chylomicrons, through the transfer activity of cholesterol esters, transfer protein (CETP) or phospholipid transfer protein (PLTP) and ensure the reverse cholesterol transport to the liver through the scavenger receptor type I (SR-BI). Within liver and intestine cells, the production of VLDL or chylomicrons is controlled by the action of specific proteins such as fatty acid binding proteins (FABPs) and the microsomal transfer protein (MTP).

Two major genetic defects are known to dramatically affect lipoprotein metabolism. The most famous is the defect in apoB,E-receptor that induces familial hypercholesterolaemia and elevated LDL levels (Brown and Goldstein, 1974). The second one is the defect in MTP that almost completely abolishes triglyceride-rich lipoprotein (TRL) production by the liver and small intestine resulting in abetalipoproteinaemia (Gregg and Wetterau, 1994). Such marked and rare genetic defects are not within the scope of the present review, the aim of which is to provide some examples of common gene polymorphisms that may have implications for large proportions of the population, especially in determining variation in response to dietary fat.

3.2.1 ApoE and lipoprotein metabolism

ApoE is a key apoprotein involved in triglyceride-rich lipoprotein (IDL and chylomicron remnants) uptake by the liver and peripheral tissues through interaction with apoB,E and remnant receptors. Two common variations exist through C to T transition, leading to variations in the amino acids p.Cys112Arg* and p.Arg158Cys. This results in three major alleles (E2, E3, E4) with relative frequencies of 0.1, 0.8 and 0.15, respectively. The apoE-E2 allelic product binds poorly to the remnant receptor, leading to accumulation of triglyceride-rich lipoproteins in the circulation. Conversely, the apoE-E4 allelic product has high affinity and increases TRL uptake by the liver, thus inducing a down-regulation of the apoB,E receptor level, reduced LDL uptake and increased LDL accumulation (Sing and Davignon, 1985). It is noteworthy that such apoE polymorphisms account for about 8–10% of total plasma cholesterol-rich variation (Schaefer *et al.*, 1994).

Several studies have investigated the relationship between apoE polymorphisms and responses to diets. Healthy men ingesting a low-fat diet *vs* their usual high-fat, cholesterol diet showed extents of reduction in LDL cholesterol in the following order E4/E4 = E4/E3 > E3/E3 > E3/E2 (Dreon *et al.*, 1995). In a cohort of men and women with coronary heart disease, a high sucrose intake resulted in higher plasma triglyceride concentration only in patients with the apoE-E2 allele. In these patients too, saturated fat or fibre intake predicted serum cholesterol levels (Erkkila *et al.*, 2001). The response to a fat-rich test-meal was also investigated in normolipidaemic patients with type 2 diabetes (Reznik *et al.*, 1996). In this study the accumulation of TRL remnants (retinyl palmitate) was postprandially exacerbated in patients with E2/E3 or E3/E4 genotypes. Finally, the response to alcohol drinking was evaluated in a cohort of healthy men and women (Corella *et al.*, 2001). In this study men and women with the apoE-E2 allele had lower LDL cholesterol levels, while men with the E4 allele had the highest LDL cholesterol levels. We have also investigated the influence of the combination of apoE-E2 and a rare apoE-E3 'Christchurch' mutant p.Arg136Ser (Vialettes *et al.*, 2000). This genotype was associated with type V hyperlipoproteinaemia and it exacerbated postprandial lipaemia and TRL-remnant accumulation. Taken together, information available on apoE polymorphisms clearly indicate that apoE-E2 or E4 variants are associated with disturbed lipid metabolism and altered lipoprotein response to dietary challenge.

* Genetic variations are described according to the recommendations of the Human Genome Variation Society (http://www.genomic.unimelb.edu.au/mbi/dblist/dblist.html).

3.2.2 ApoB and lipoprotein metabolism

Apolipoprotein B is the main apolipoprotein of chylomicrons and low-density lipoproteins (LDL). It occurs in the plasma in two main forms, apoB48 and apoB100. The first is synthesized exclusively by the intestine, the second by the liver. ApoB is thus essential for lipoprotein assembly and apoB-100 serves as the principal ligand ensuring interaction between LDL and the apoB,E receptor.

Several common mutations have been found in the human *apoB* gene. Owing to the protein's dual role as a transport protein and a peripheral recognition signal for LDL clearance, these mutations have been shown to result either in reduced VLDL secretion or in hypercholesterolaemia (LDL accumulation). Several studies have investigated the influence of some of the *apoB* polymorphisms on responses to change from high-fat to low-fat diets (or the opposite). Three polymorphisms have been mostly associated with diet-induced LDL cholesterol changes: a XbaI restriction site located in exon 26, an EcoRI site in exon 29 and a MspI site. Lopez-Miranda *et al.* (1997) reported that subjects with the homozygous absence of the XbaI site have a greater postprandial response (retinyl palmitate and apoB48 levels) to a fat-rich meal than the subjects with the presence of the XbaI site. More recently, it has been shown that a high-fat diet also induced a larger increase in plasma LDL cholesterol in subjects presenting the homozygous absence of the EcoRI restriction site. Subjects displaying the homozygous presence of the MspI restriction site were also more responsive to such a diet than heterozygous subjects (Rantala *et al.*, 2000).

3.2.3 ApoA-IV and lipoprotein metabolism

ApoA-IV is an apoprotein secreted by the small intestine and specifically associated to chylomicron and chylomicron remnants. Among possible roles are interactions between chylomicrons and HDL particles. A common SNP has been identified on the *apoA-IV* gene as a G to T substitution resulting in an allelic variation, p.Gln360His. The absence or presence of the restriction site (Fnu4HI) gives *apoA-IV-1* or *apoA-IV-2* variants with three genotypes (1/1, 1/2 and 2/2). The frequency of the *apoA-IV-2* form is 7–9% in the USA and France. The *apoA-IV-2* form has increased affinity for lipid particles and displays more competition towards apoE and apoCII binding. In homozygous women, higher fasting triglycerides and lower HDL cholesterol concentrations have been reported.

Several recent studies have reported interaction between *apoAIV* genotypes and metabolic responses. The postprandial response to a fat-rich meal has been shown to be higher in apoAIV-1/2 carriers compared with apoAIV-1/1 ones for plasma, chylomicron and VLDL triglyceride concentrations (Hockey *et al.*, 2001). This is in line with other data showing that apoAIV-1/2 carriers have somewhat lower intestinal cholesterol absorption rates than 1/1 carriers (Weinberg *et al.*, 2000) or that carriers of the H allele produced a higher increase in HDL cholesterol in response to substitution of carbohydrates for monounsaturated fatty acids (Jansen *et al.*, 1997).

The effects of this polymorphism on LDL cholesterol change in response to high- *vs* low-fat diets have been recently reviewed (Weggemans *et al.*, 2000). It appears that carriers of the allele number 2 have a smaller increase or a smaller decrease in LDL-cholesterol level in response to a high-fat/high-cholesterol diet or a low-fat/low-cholesterol diet, respectively. However, some studies show different responses: in response to a low-fat diet, hypercholesterolaemic subjects presented a significant decrease in apo B but not in LDL cholesterol for example (Carmena-Ramon *et al.*, 1998).

3.2.4 Intestinal FABP and lipoprotein metabolism

Intestinal fatty acid binding protein (I-FABP or FABP2) is a cytosolic intracellular protein capable of binding free fatty acids and delivering them to membranes. A common SNP in the I-FABP gene has been found at exon 2, with a G to A substitution resulting in a p.Ala54AThr substitution (Baier *et al.*, 1995). The frequency of the T allele has been evaluated as 0.29 in Pima Indians and 0.27 in European students. Subjects presenting the T allelic variant show higher fatty acid binding and transport as well as higher triglyceride secretion into plasma from the intestine. In addition, clinical traits associated with the T allelic variant are higher insulinaemia and insulin-resistance, higher fasting LDL cholesterol and apoB levels, higher BMI and fasting triglycerides (Hegele, 1998; Agren *et al.*, 1998). Moreover, the LDL cholesterol and apoB-lowering effects of diets rich in high-soluble fibre were more pronounced in subjects with the T variant (Hegele *et al.*, 1997). In addition, subjects homozygous for the T variant have been shown to display increased postprandial insulin (Baier *et al.*, 1995) or triglyceride responses (Agren *et al.*, 1998), although in another study (Pratley *et al.*, 2000) no marked difference was evidenced for glucose, non-esterified fatty acids or triglycerides.

3.2.5 Lipoprotein lipase and lipoprotein metabolism

Lipoprotein lipase (LPL) is the key enzyme responsible for TRL triglyceride lipolysis within blood vessels; from VLDL or chylomicrons it generates TRL remnants that can be taken up by the liver or peripheral tissues and thus cleared from the circulation. Among more than 50 known polymorphisms, several common and important ones have been found in *LPL* gene, such as p.Asp9Asn or p.Asn291Ser, which both present a 4–6% frequency in Western populations, and SNP8393 in intron 8 (restriction site HindIII).

LPL activity can be somewhat reduced in subjects bearing the p.291S or the p.9N allele and these variants are associated with higher fasting triglycerides and lower HDL cholesterol levels (Gerdes *et al.*, 1997; Senti *et al.*, 2000). In heterozygote carriers of the p.291S variant, postprandial levels of large VLDL apoB48, triglycerides and retinyl palmitate were higher than in non-carriers (Mero *et al.*, 1999). Regarding long-term dietary interventions, it has been reported that homologous carriers of the HindIII site had a significantly smaller change in mean total plasma cholesterol in response to diet than others (Humphries *et al.*, 1996).

3.2.6 Lipid transfer proteins

In humans, cholesteryl ester, triglycerides and phospholipids can be exchanged between circulating lipoprotein particles thanks to proteins that are active in the plasma. The plasma also displays a cholesterol esterification activity associated with lecithin acyl cholesterol transferase (LCAT), a glycoprotein thought to play a role in the HDL-mediated transport of cholesterol. Interestingly, the activation of LCAT needs the apolipoprotein AI, which is associated with the HDL particles (Frank and Marcel, 2000). Three arginine residues on apoA1 have been shown to be critical for LCAT activation by apoAI and conversely, mutations in the *apoAI* gene induced a severe decrease in LCAT activity (Roosbeek *et al.*, 2001). LCAT deficiency is usually associated with low plasma HDL levels, which thus addresses the potential role of this enzyme in the development of coronary heart disease (Peelman *et al.*, 1999). For example, a p.Pro143Leu mutation has been identified in 5.79% of Chinese patients suffering from coronary heart disease (Zhang *et al.*, 2004).

A lipotransfer protein, the cholesterol ester transfer protein (CETP) promotes the exchange of cholesterol from HDL particles to triglyceride-rich particles (TRL) and of triacylglycerol from TRL to HDL. Since HDL can be roughly considered as responsible for transferring to the liver endogenously synthesized cholesterol, the CETP activity would modify the ratio between LDL cholesterol and HDL cholesterol. For example, in a recent study undertaken in a population from diverse origins, an association was demonstrated between the g.−629>C allele and a 30% decrease in CETP mass (Thompson *et al.*, 2003). In another study, such a decrease in mass has been shown to result in changes in the size of HDL particles with a marked increase in the large alpha-1 HDL particles and decrease in the small pre-beta-1 particles, features that have been clearly associated with lower risk for coronary heart disease (Asztalos *et al.*, 2000, 2002). Interestingly, in a recent study on a large cohort of German patients, the patients bearing the g.−629>C allele were significantly more sensitive to statin therapy and those homozygous for this allele displayed a cardiovascular mortality reduced by half (Blankenberg *et al.*, 2003). The Taq1B polymorphism in the *CETP* gene has also been extensively studied. This polymorphism generates three genotypes, namely B1/B1 (frequency about 0.33), B1/B2 (approx. 0.5) and B2/B2 (approx 0.17). This latter genotype seems to be associated with a lower CETP activity and therefore a reduction in CVD risk, an effect certainly due to a significantly higher plasma HDL (Brousseau *et al.*, 2002). Nevertheless, other recent studies do not support this finding and conclude that the Taq1 B polymorphism does not predict cardiovascular events and does not discriminate those who will and those who will not benefit from statin treatment (de Grooth *et al.*, 2004).

3.2.7 Miscellaneous

The reader can refer to recent reviews to obtain literature data on the effects of other gene polymorphisms studied – such as those encoding for apoA1, apoCIII, hepatic lipase or SR-BI (Ye and Kwiterovich, 2000; Ordovas, 2001; Masson *et al.*, 2003; Masson and McNeill, 2005). To summarize, most studied polymorphisms of genes encoding for key proteins involved in lipid and lipoprotein metabolism have been associated with some documented effects on fasting and/or postprandial metabolic markers in humans. This consistently supports the concept that interaction between genetic susceptibility and inappropriate diet is a key determinant of CVD risk.

3.3 Genetic influences on the uptake and absorption of cholesterol

Cholesterol is essential for all mammalian cells, and nearly all tissues of the body have the ability to produce cholesterol necessary for the formation of cell membranes. Cellular cholesterol requirements are met through *de novo* synthesis and uptake of plasma lipoproteins. In humans, plasma lipoproteins transport two sources of cholesterol: cholesterol derived from diets and that endogenously synthesized by the liver and other tissues. While LDL seems to transport both dietary or neo-synthesized cholesterol from liver to tissues, HDL has been consistently shown to be responsible for the transport of cholesterol from peripheral tissues to the liver, in order for it to be eliminated from the body. To achieve this aim, cholesterol has to be excreted into bile, either directly or after conversion into bile acids. However, cholesterol excreted into bile can be reabsorbed from the gut into the bloodstream and thus contributes to the exogenous source of cholesterol. Therefore, cholesterol homeostasis is maintained by balancing dietary absorption and endogenous synthesis of cholesterol with its biliary excretion, but through complex interacting molecular mechanisms that still remain poorly understood.

These complex interactions certainly explain why, in humans, responses to diet vary considerably between subjects: for example, a low-fat, low-cholesterol diet resulted in a 30% reduction in plasma cholesterol in some subjects while others could elicit no response to such a diet (Beynen *et al.*, 1987). Similarly, when the intake of dietary cholesterol increases, some studies have shown that this elicits a modest elevation in plasma cholesterol concentration (Ginsberg *et al.*, 1994, 1995), while other studies have shown that dietary cholesterol has no effect (Kestin *et al.*, 1989; Vorster *et al.*, 1992). It is thus logical to wonder to what extent genetic variations could explain these discrepancies (Gylling and Miettinen, 2002).

There is an important limitation to the extent of cholesterol absorption, as only 40–60% of dietary cholesterol is absorbed on average (with a broad interindividual variation) (McNamara, 1987; Sehayek *et al.*, 1998; Bosner *et al.*, 1999; Ostlund *et al.*, 1999). In addition, cholesterol absorption has been shown to be largely dependent on several factors, particularly the presence of other nutrients (Beynen and Katan, 1985; Ginsberg *et al.*, 1994, 1995; Mekki *et al.*, 1997). In fact, although the relationship between dietary fat and cholesterol absorption has been one of the most extensively studied issues in lipid nutrition, many of the studies have led to contradictory conclusions. For example, a meta-analysis of several cholesterol feeding studies in humans concluded that dietary factors play an insignificant role in the blood cholesterol response to dietary cholesterol (McNamara, 1995). However, in a more recent study, it has been shown that a dietary cholesterol challenge of 100 mg resulted in a higher increase in LDL cholesterol on a high versus a low saturated fat diet (Weggemans *et al.*, 2001).

The luminal absorption of cholesterol requires the partitioning of the sterol into bile salt prior to its transport to the brush border membranes of enterocytes. The uptake of cholesterol is then coupled with that of related plant sterols, but a selective excretion process eliminates the majority of plant sterols. This link has encouraged the proactive use of plant sterols to limit cholesterol absorption. It has been recently shown that ATP-binding cassette transporters G5 and G8, encoded by two highly related genes, are apical pumps that promote partial efflux of cholesterol and lead to nearly complete efflux of plant sterols into the intestinal lumen after their absorption. Mutations in these genes cause sitosterolaemia (Lu *et al.*, 2001). Recent studies have also pointed out an association of p.Tyr54Cys and p.Thr400Lys polymorphisms as well as the p.Met429Val variation at the ABCG8 locus, with higher cholesterol absorption in hypercholesterolaemic Japanese subjects (Miwa *et al.*, 2005). A possible association of the ABCG5 p.Gln640Glu polymorphism with a higher total plasma cholesterol in response to dietary cholesterol supply in subjects homozygous for the E allele has also been reported (Weggemans *et al.*, 2002). Similarly, it has been shown that sequence variants in the ATP binding cassette type A1 also contributed to variations in plasma HDL cholesterol levels in the general population, which underlines the role played by ABC transporters in mediating cholesterol efflux from monocytes (Pajukanta, 2004; Frikke-Schmidt *et al.*, 2004).

The availability of inhibitors able to selectively block cholesterol absorption (ezitimibe for example) have allowed the identification of some other proteins as putative transporters in the intestine. Polymorphisms in the class B type I scavenger receptor (SR-B1) gene have been shown to be associated with lower LDL cholesterol and higher HDL cholesterol in plasma (Acton *et al.*, 1999), but no clear association with intestinal absorption has been demonstrated. More recently, a bioinformatics-genomics approach, screening an expression sequence tags library, proposed the Niemann-Pick C-1 like-1 gene as containing predictive features of a cholesterol transporter (Altmann *et al.*, 2004). The hypothesized demonstration role played by NPC1-L1 in cholesterol absorption has been supported by the demonstration that ezitimibe-resistant patients bear non-synonymous polymorphisms in the *NPC1L1* gene (Wang *et al.*, 2005).

Another hypothesis to explain the broad range of responses to dietary cholesterol is that this variability could result from inter-individual variations in cholesterol neosynthesis. It has been shown, indeed, that an increase in dietary cholesterol can induce a net decrease in cholesterol synthesis (Lin and Connor, 1980; McMurry *et al.*, 1985; Jones *et al.*, 1996). Conversely any decrease in cholesterol synthesis results in change in the absorption/excretion process (Gylling, 2004).

Endogenous synthesis of cholesterol originates from acetyl CoA moieties, products of intracellular degradation of carbohydrates and fatty acids. The enzyme HMG CoA reductase plays a key role in this synthesis and is the target of pharmacological molecules such as statins. It is noteworthy that polymorphisms in genes involved in cholesterol synthesis, absorption and transport may affect statin efficacy, suggesting a high level of integration between these processes. Polymorphisms in the promoter for *ABCG8* or for the *ApoA1* gene have been linked to variations in response to statins (Caslake and Packard, 2004).

In addition, several clues seem to link cholesterol and fatty acid metabolisms more tightly than previously thought, since expression of several genes involved in cholesterol and fatty acids synthesis have been shown to be under the control of a family of transcription factors, the sterol regulatory element binding proteins (SREBP) (Gibbons, 2003). These basic helix–turn–helix–leucine zipper transcription factors are activated by proteolytic cleavages, then targeted to the nucleus where they participate in regulating the expression of several genes involved in cholesterol, fatty acid or glucose synthesis.

One member of this family, SREBP-2, a product of the *SREBF-2* gene, is activated by cholesterol depletion (Brown and Goldstein, 1999), while another member, SREBP-1c, produced from another gene (*SREBF-1*) has been clearly involved in the selective induction of lipogenic enzymes but also in the insulin signal pathway (Shimano *et al.*, 1997; Shimomura *et al.*, 1997; Horton *et al.*, 1998). The third one, SREBP-1a, seems to be more sensitive to nutritional status and involved in both cholesterol and fatty acids synthesis (Shimano *et al.*, 1996). To date, a mutation in the *SREBF-2* gene, resulting in a decrease of SREBP-2 cleavage, has been shown to be associated with elevated plasma LDL cholesterol concentrations in hypercholesterolaemic, but not in normocholesterolaemic subjects (Miserez *et al.*, 2002). This effect is probably due to a decrease in the density of LDL receptors.

Inasmuch as the bulk of circulating cholesterol is transported by LDL, another possible way to explain the heterogeneity of plasma cholesterol in response to diets would be related to a particular responsiveness of LDL metabolism to dietary factors. Several studies have suggested that intestinal cholesterol absorption may be related to the apolipoprotein E phenotype, but certainly through complex interactions with other genes or other nutrients (Kesaniemi *et al.*, 1987; Miettinen *et al.*, 1992). Similarly, some studies that have investigated the role played by the apolipoprotein *A4* gene, provided evidence for a complex interaction between diet and *ApoA-IV* polymorphisms (Weggemans *et al.*, 2000). As an example, on a diet rich in polyunsaturates, fractional cholesterol absorption was lower in carriers of the His variant at the

ApoA-IV locus (p.Gln360His) but only in subjects homozygous for another variant in the same gene, the p.Ser347Thr (Weinberg *et al.*, 2000). Another example is provided by the observation that a low-fat, low-cholesterol diet strategy may be particularly efficient in lowering the plasma LDL cholesterol of those subjects carrying the E4 allelic variant at the apolipoprotein E locus (Dreon *et al.*, 1995). Similarly, response to statin treatment brings us indirect evidence about the role played by several genes in the control of cholesterol homeostasis. Indeed, subjects who respond more efficiently to treatment are those carrying high-risk allelic variants in genes involved in lipoprotein metabolism, such as ApoE, CETP, LPL or hepatic lipase (Dornbrook-Lavender and Pieper, 2003; Zambon *et al.*, 2003)

3.4 Genetic influences on the metabolic syndrome

Although the metabolic syndrome per se is not central to the focus of this review, we must give brief consideration to this major public health concern. The prevalence of the metabolic syndrome as defined by the NCEP-ATP III report is about 23% in the American population and rises to about 43% of elderly people in the USA, while higher prevalence rates can be observed in various ethnic groups around the world (Ford *et al.*, 2002). This syndrome associates obesity, excessive blood pressure, high plasma glucose with disturbances of lipid homeostasis (high plasma triglycerides and low HDL cholesterol).

Numerous epidemiological studies have pointed out the role played by both environmental factors (e.g. lack of physical exercise, smoking) and nutritional factors (calorically dense, low-fibre and high-fat diets) (Zhu *et al.*, 2004). On the other hand, some recent clues that heredity plays an important role came from the discovery of certain rare but major mutations associated with severe forms of glucose impairment (Yki-Jarvinen, 1997). The role played by genetic factors has also been highlighted by several epidemiological studies. It has been shown, for example, that impairment of insulin action could be inherited in the offspring of diabetic probands (Vauhkonen *et al.*, 1998). Similarly, when the various determinants of glucose homeostasis are analysed in different populations, only the resistance of glucose intake, which is directly linked to impaired function of insulin, correlates with genetic background (Ferrannini *et al.*, 2003).

It has long been thought that obesity precedes the metabolic syndrome, but it is now known that this syndrome can be observed in lean subjects, even if its prevalence increases in a graded fashion as body weight increases (St-Onge *et al.*, 2004). Recent findings about the endocrine (but also paracrine and autocrine) function of adipocytes have renewed interest in the topic. Indeed, it has been demonstrated that fat cells are able to secrete pro-inflammatory and insulin resistance-inducing cytokines (TNF-alpha, resistin), as well as molecules acting in concert to facilitate glucose uptake (adiponectin) or the central control of satiety (leptin) (Lafontan, 2005).

The main feature of the metabolic syndrome is an association between dysfunction of energy storage (adipocyte physiology) and insulin resistance in a dramatic vicious circle (Miranda *et al.*, 2005). Insulin resistance results in a decreased translocation of the GLUT4 glucose transporter to the plasma membrane of adipocytes. This would induce a relative glucose deprivation, thus contributing to an adipocyte stress response and secretion of inflammatory and anti-insulinic compounds such as TNF-alpha. Dysfunction of energy storage (overflow) leads to day-long elevated plasma free fatty acid levels and accumulation of triglycerides in muscle and liver, which in turn hinders glucose utilization, thus contributing to the overall insulin resistance. In plasma, beside disturbances of fasting insulin and glucose levels, the main quantitative abnormalities are decreased HDL cholesterol levels and increased VLDL and IDL triglyceride-rich lipoproteins, an abnormality that is exacerbated in the postprandial period (Chen *et al.*, 1993; Mekki *et al.*, 1999).

Another important feature of the metabolic syndrome is explained through the particular pathways of insulin action. This hormone, which is also a growth factor, displays pleiotrophic and tissue-specific effects, so that, within the same cell, metabolic pathways may differ in their response to insulin (Saltiel and Kahn, 2001). This observation supports the hypothesis that fat cell, muscle or liver dysfunctions, as observed in the metabolic syndrome, may be due to a decrease in insulin action for some of them, but in others to the consequence of hyperinsulinaemia.

The extracellular binding of insulin to the insulin receptor induces a conformational change that results in the activation of tyrosine kinase in the intracellular domain of the receptor, which induces the phosphorylation of specific substrates. These substrates are also able to be phosphorylated on seryl residues, which generally counteracts activating effects of the tyrosine phosphorylation (Bouzakri *et al.*, 2003). Two main signalling cascades are initiated, the first through the activation of an insulin-receptor substrate (IRS) that leads to the activation of phosphatidylinositol 3-kinase PI(3)K kinase, and the synthesis of phosphatidyl-3-phosphate. This compound activates several distinct pathways, one of them resulting in the activation of the protein kinase Akt/PKB, which in turn seems to activate several other regulatory proteins; the activities of some of them have been shown to be associated with obesity (Manning, 2004). Downstream of the IRS-PI(3)K pathway lies the insulin-mediated expression of SREBP-1c isoform, which plays an important role in regulation of lipid synthesis in liver, muscle and adipose tissue (Shimano, 2002).

The second signalling cascade activates the MAP kinase pathway and induces mitogenic and pro-inflammatory effects (Muller-Wieland *et al.*, 2001). The tyrosyl residues of the insulin receptor can also be dephosphorylated by protein tyrosine phosphatases (PTP) and null mice for the PTP 1B isoform has been shown to display improved insulin sensitivity and resistance to diet induced obesity (Elchebly *et al.*, 1999). In the metabolic syndrome, pathways leading to the activation of the PI(3)K are blocked while those inducing the MAP kinases pathways remain open and will be hyper-activated by the raised insulin levels that characterize the metabolic syndrome (Cusi *et al.*, 2000). Therefore, some of the features of the metabolic syndrome are due to a relative hyperinsulinaemia, while others are the consequence of insulin resistance.

Accordingly, candidate genes for predisposition to the metabolic syndrome are those involved in the fat cell metabolism, including secreted adipokines, or the insulin signalling pathway acting in liver, muscle or fat cells. Some of them have already been described above, those associated with dyslipidaemia (Laakso, 2004), such as hepatic lipase (Ordovas *et al.*, 2002), CETP (Weitgasser *et al.*, 2004), LPL (Holzl *et al.*, 2002) and apolipoprotein E (Kesaniemi *et al.*, 1992). PPAR gamma, a nuclear receptor that is involved in adipocyte differentiation and is a fatty acid-sensitive gene, will be described below (Baratta *et al.*, 2003). Some others are more specifically linked to insulin resistance. For example, the transmembrane glycoprotein PC-1 has been shown to inhibit *in vitro* insulin-induced tyrosine kinase activity of the insulin receptor. As a matter of fact, a polymorphism of the PC-1 protein, p.Lys121Gln has been correlated with clinical insulin resistance and a high plasma leptin level independently of obesity (Frittitta *et al.*, 2001; Gonzalez Sanchez *et al.*, 2002). But owing to variability in nutritional intake this correlation has been questioned in other studies. Interestingly, a recent study showed that, among individuals homozygous for the p12P variant in the *PPAR* gamma gene, those bearing the Q allelic variant display significantly higher fasting plasma glucose level and lower insulin sensitivity than p121 K carriers (Baratta *et al.*, 2003). Another example is provided by the p.Gly972Arg polymorphism in the *IRS-1* gene that causes carriers of the R variant to have a significantly reduced insulin sensitivity when compared with carriers of the G allelic variant (McGettrick *et al.*, 2005). This insulin resistance is accompanied with several features of the metabolic syndrome, such as increased total triglyceridaemia, decreased plasma HDL or elevated blood pressure. Finally, recent studies have shown that *SREBF-1* gene polymorphisms could be associated with obesity and insulin resistance (Laudes *et al.*, 2004; Eberle *et al.*, 2004).

However, despite the growing interest in the metabolic syndrome, relatively few studies have been focused on the influence of insulin resistance on lipid and lipoprotein response to dietary intervention. Most studies indicate that in patients with metabolic syndrome, responsiveness to dietary intervention is less marked than in lean and insulin-sensitive subjects (Beynen and Katan, 1985; Knopp *et al.*, 1997, 2000). A recent study has also shown that insulin-resistant subjects present a decreased cholesterol absorption (Knopp *et al.*, 2003). These findings are supportive of studies suggesting a role for insulin in the postprandial accumulation of intestinally derived lipoproteins (Harbis *et al.*, 2001, 2004).

3.5 Dietary fatty acids and the regulation of gene expression

In bacteria or unicellular eukaryotic cells, fatty acids (FAs) display their dual role of structural membrane components and suppliers of energy. Supply of FAs leads to the down-regulation of endogenous FA synthesis and to the up-regulation of genes coding for transport and metabolism of FAs. This is a sparing process that is achieved through the binding of acyl-CoA to a specific DNA binding protein that changes its affinity for DNA response elements. In mammals, the expression of genes involved in transport and metabolism appears to be regulated by FAs in a positive or a negative manner. However, the simple bacterial process could provide the paradigm of the regulation of gene expression by FAs. FAs or derivatives depress genes coding for enzymes involved in lipogenesis and activate those that allow the transport and the oxidation of FAs. FA binding to transcription factors modifies their involvement in the transcription process. As a matter of fact, in mammals several genes coding for proteins involved in lipogenesis or weight control such as leptin, are down-regulated. This mechanism may be related to the decrease in hepatic *de novo* lipogenesis that can be observed in animals and humans submitted to a polyunsaturated fatty acid (PUFA)-rich diet. In contrast, other genes are up-regulated, such as those coding for proteins involved in transport and oxidation of FA (*FAT-CD36*, *LPL*, *FABPs*, *CPT 1*). Some other genes are regulated in a tissue-specific way, for example, *PEP-CK* is up-regulated in adipocytes but not in the liver (Antrasferry *et al.*, 1994).

3.5.1 Down-regulation of gene transcription

Our knowledge on the mechanisms by which linoleic acid can depress hepatic lipogenesis has long provided the paradigm of down-regulation of gene expression by FAs. This down-regulation involves a specific effect of PUFA on the expression of fatty acid synthase (*FAS*) and *Spot 14*, whose product was shown to act as a transcription regulator of metabolic genes (Compe *et al.*, 2001). This effect was shown to be restricted to PUFAs and not to mono-unsaturated or saturated FAs (Blake and Clarke, 1990; Jump *et al.*, 1993). In 1998, it was shown that PUFA are able to depress the hepatic pool of the mature form of SREBP 1 and 2 (Worgall *et al.*, 1998). Among genes involved in lipogenesis, *FAS* and *Spot 14*, display SREBP-specific response elements in their promoter (Ren *et al.*, 1997). Down-regulatory effects of PUFAs on *FAS* and *Spot 14* gene expression are thus indirect. Recently, it has been demonstrated that unsaturated FA inhibit transcription of SREBP 1 by interfering with the activity of a nuclear receptor, the liver X receptor (LXR) (Ou *et al.*, 2001). PUFA seem indeed to be involved in a competitive binding with LXR for specific response elements in the SREBF-1 gene promoter (Yoshikawa *et al.*, 2002). In addition, PPAR alpha and LXR alpha can physically interact and antagonize each other, which opens the possibility of multiple cross-regulations between FA and sterols acting respectively as PPAR and LXR ligands.

3.5.2 Up-regulation of gene expression

Nuclear receptors (NRs) are members of a superfamily of transcription factors that share a common domain organization and sequence similitude. To date, over 300 NRs have been cloned. Most of them do not have an identifiable relevant ligand (orphan receptors). Others are ligand-inducible and respond to endogenous or exogenous lipophilic molecules. These factors are able to bind specific response elements in the vicinity of the genes on which they act. The presence of bound ligands induces a transconformation state that makes them recruit co-activators in place of co-repressors that they bind in the absence of ligand. Cross-regulations between different members of this family are due to their ability to dimerize and the fact that they share similar affinity for a small number of co-activators and co-repressors. Here, two of them will be more particularly quoted, PPARs and HNF4, since they are directly linked to the fatty acid regulation of gene expression. However, other nuclear receptors such as thyroid hormone receptors or chicken ovalbumin upstream promoter transcription factors have been consistently shown to be able to bind FAs (Duplus *et al.*, 2000; Duplus and Forest, 2002).

Peroxisome proliferator-activated receptors are members of the superfamily of nuclear receptors, which are ligand-activated transcription factors. In mammals, three subtypes have been described. Their tissue distribution largely differs: PPAR beta is expressed in most cells, while the expression of other subtypes is more restricted (mainly liver, heart and muscle for PPAR alpha and adipokines for PPAR gamma). Rat PPAR alpha cDNA was first cloned from the liver and is the only true peroxisome proliferator. Human PPAR alpha and all subtypes have been named because of high sequence similitude. All of them are transcriptionaly active only after heterodimerization with another nuclear receptor, the 9-*cis* retinoic acid activated retinoid X receptor (RXR). RXR acts as a heterodimerization partner with other nuclear receptors, some of them able to bind lipid derivatives such as thyroid hormone receptors (TR) or LXR, which hints a possible interplay between nuclear receptors with regard to ligand concentrations. In addition, PPARs generally show low ligand specificity, being activated by several long chain saturated or unsaturated fatty acids and by eicosanoids. This is certainly due to a generous pocket that also allows binding to many other endogenous or pharmacological compounds (fibrate or thiazolidinedione).

The ubiquitous expression of PPAR beta made the identification of its function elusive. However, it has recently been shown that a PPAR beta-specific ligand promotes lipid accumulation in human macrophages, which can be considered potentially pro-atherogenic (Vosper *et al.*, 2001). In contrast, the high and almost selective expression of PPAR gamma in adipocytes shows that it is likely to play a major role in the differentiation of these cells (Tontonoz *et al.*, 1994; Grimaldi, 2001; Kliewer *et al.*, 2001; Ferre, 2004). But there is a concern about its role in energy metabolism in these cells (Walczak and Tontonoz, 2002). Some genes (for example, those coding for the glucose transporter GLUT4, the acyl CoA synthase or the phospho-enol-pyruvate-CK) are involved in the activation and esterification of fatty acids and display specific DNA elements able to bind PPAR. However, simply because FA are potential ligands of PPARs does not necessarily imply that transcriptional effects of FA are mediated through these nuclear receptors. This point has been clearly illustrated in the *PEP-CK* gene. For example, several effects induced by FA are PPAR-independent and are probably modulated by other transcription factors (Duplus and Forest, 2002).

The putative role of PPARs as FA-induced nuclear receptors in several cells is more directly supported by studies on PPAR alpha. Indeed, it has been possible to delete this gene in mice and these animals subsequently lost the ability to increase their fatty acids oxidation when treated with fibrate, a PPAR alpha ligand. In addition, although the phenotype of normally fed null mice was not fundamentally different from wild type, starvation induced major differences. Null mice presented an impaired utilization of fatty acids that led to hepatic and cardiac steatosis. These observations are sustained by mechanistic studies on genes that are obviously involved in FA transport, synthesis of CoA derivatives and the subsequent peroxisomal degradation of very long chain fatty acids (the example of the liver acyl CoA oxidase is particularly clear). The expressions of genes coding for some key enzymes involved in mainstream mitochondrial oxidation and synthesis of ketone bodies are also activated by PPAR alpha ligand. The key regulatory enzyme of mitochondrial oxidation is carnitine palmitoyl transferase type I, which allows the activated FA to enter the mitochondria. In primary hepatocytes, the expression of this gene is clearly induced by fibrates and long chain fatty acids, whether saturated or not. Nevertheless, the careful deciphering of regulatory sequences in the vicinity of the *CPT 1* gene demonstrated that FA and fibrates act through different elements, suggesting that the FA-induced overexpression of CPT 1 is PPAR-independent process. This study provides us with another example of the difficulty of unequivocally ascribing the FA-induced regulation of a given gene to PPARs, even when pharmacological effects of PPAR-specific ligands seem to permit such a deduction.

Hepatic Nuclear Factor 4 (HNF-4) has long been considered an orphan receptor until structural studies reported it was able to constitutively bind FAs. Recent studies reported that the transcriptional activity of this receptor could be modulated by long chain FA when a reporter gene was fused with response elements issued from the human ApoC-III promoter (Pastier *et al.*, 2002). This activation was paralleled by the binding of cognate acyl-CoA thioesters to the ligand domain of HNF-4. This process was saturation dependent since palmitoyl-CoA derivative greatly enhanced the transcriptional activity as well as the binding of HNF4 to its specific DNA site, while PUFA and their respective acyl-CoA derivatives displayed a clear inhibition of transcriptional activity, together with a diminished DNA binding. It has also been recently demonstrated that the Apo A-IV gene transcription in enterocyte cell cultures is dependent on the apical supply of complexes of micelles mimicking the composition of duodenal micelles. This increase was clearly abolished when a negative dominant form of HNF-4 was transfected, which strongly suggests the involvement of the nuclear receptor in this regulation (Carriere *et al.*, 2005).

3.6 Conclusions: lipid–gene interactions and personalized nutrition

The literature reviewed in this chapter has shown that the influence of dietary lipids (fat, cholesterol) on metabolic markers and risk factors is markedly influenced by genetic polymorphisms in humans. Current recommendations (to limit total and saturated fat, to reduce cholesterol and to increase monounsaturated and n-3 polyunsaturated fat intake) must be reinforced in a way that reflects the reality of how consumers prepare and eat meals today. However, dietary recommendations that have been made to date on the basis of a whole population should be updated to take into account individual responsiveness to nutrients or dietary patterns, which is based on various genetic susceptibilities.

It is worth recognizing that, until recently, most research started from pathological conditions and their associated predictive markers. The main way to elucidate nutrient–gene interaction has been to study disturbances of such markers with regard to genetic polymorphisms. It is not unrealistic to imagine that the search for earlier health markers could also represent a step toward predictive nutrigenomics and personalized nutrition. To date, our knowledge in nutrigenomics comes from small-scale intervention studies that have underscored the potential of this approach. Moreover, too many contradictory results have been obtained from these studies. It has become necessary to implement strategies that will provide more robust findings, building on the information obtained during the first decade of the nutrigenomics era.

The following suggestions can be made. First, the size of the population sample needed to test the gene–nutrient interaction is far larger than the one usually used in the nutrition field. Statistical tools must be developed to deal with a huge number of different data, such as phenotypic, dietetic and gene–gene interactions. To collect this information, database capacity must be improved in order to classify the number of various data that will be generated. Secondly, in this field, collaborative research performed simultaneously in several countries becomes a necessity, which implies strictly standardized protocols and the integrating of disparate databases, as exemplified in the Lipgene project (http://www.lipgene.tcd.ie). Thirdly, studies on gene-diet interactions also need the collection of a large number of dietary records and the availability of accurate and fully documented databases of food nutrients composition that take into account new products from food industry. The formation of such a database is taking place within another FP6-funded project, EuroFIR (project number FP6-513944, website http://www.eurofir.net/).

The second point that this chapter highlighted deals with the different regulating effects of various fatty acids on important metabolic pathways, organ functions or whole body homeostasis. The recent knowledge that individual fatty acids (or their derivatives) specifically regulate gene transcription is of huge importance and provides a strong rationale for exploring transcription mechanisms and their regulation. Indeed it is clear that the classical nutritional approach in humans, as described above, must be accompanied by mechanistic and experimental studies, with special emphasis put on the use of sustained animal models in dietary experiments. This approach has also to take into account the network of cross-regulations occurring within responsive cells, which implies the use of bioinformatics.

3.7 References

ACTON, S., OSGOOD, D., DONOGHUE, M., CORELLA, D., POCOVI, M., CENARRO, A., MOZAS, P., KEILTY, J., SQUAZZO, S., WOOLF, E. A. and ORDOVAS, J. M. (1999) *Arterioscler Thromb Vasc Biol*, **19**, 1734–43.

AGREN, J. J., VALVE, R., VIDGREN, H., LAAKSO, M. and UUSITUPA, M. (1998) *Arterioscler Thromb Vasc Biol*, **18**, 1606–10.

ALTMANN, S. W., DAVIS, H. R., JR., ZHU, L. J., YAO, X., HOOS, L. M., TETZLOFF, G., IYER, S. P., MAGUIRE, M., GOLOVKO, A., ZENG, M., WANG, L., MURGOLO, N. and GRAZIANO, M. P. (2004) *Science*, **303**, 1201–4.

ANTRASFERRY J., LEBIGOT G., ROBIN P., ROBIN D. and FOREST C. (1994) *Biochem Biophys Res Commun*, **203**, 385–91.

ASZTALOS, B. F., ROHEIM, P. S., MILANI, R. L., LEFEVRE, M., MCNAMARA, J. R., HORVATH, K. V. and SCHAEFER, E. J. (2000) *Arterioscler Thromb Vasc Biol*, **20**, 2670–76.

ASZTALOS, B. F., HORVATH, K. V., MCNAMARA, J. R., ROHEIM, P. S., RUBINSTEIN, J. J. and SCHAEFER, E. J. (2002) *Atherosclerosis*, **164**, 361–9.

BAIER, L. J., SACCHETTINI, J. C., KNOWLER, W. C., EADS, J., PAOLISSO, G., TATARANNI, P. A., MOCHIZUKI, H., BENNETT, P. H., BOGARDUS, C. and PROCHAZKA, M. (1995) *J Clin Invest*, **95**, 1281–7.

BARATTA, R., DI PAOLA, R., SPAMPINATO, D., FINI, G., MARUCCI, A., COCO, A., VIGNERI, R., FRITTITTA, L. and TRISCHITTA, V. (2003) *J Mol Med*, **81**, 718–23.

BEYNEN, A. C. and KATAN, M. B. (1985) *Atherosclerosis*, **54**, 157–66.

BEYNEN, A. C., KATAN, M. B. and VAN ZUTPHEN, L. F. (1987) *Adv Lipid Res*, **22**, 115–71.

BLAKE, W. L. and CLARKE, S. D. (1990) *J Nutr*, **120**, 1727–9.

BLANKENBERG, S., RUPPRECHT, H. J., BICKEL, C., JIANG, X. C., POIRIER, O., LACKNER, K. J., MEYER, J., CAMBIEN, F. and TIRET, L. (2003) *J Am Coll Cardiol*, **41**, 1983–9.

BOSNER, M. S., LANGE, L. G., STENSON, W. F. AND OSTLUND, R. E., JR (1999) *J Lipid Res*, **40**, 302–8.

BOUZAKRI, K., ROQUES, M., GUAL, P., ESPINOSA, S., GUEBRE-EGZIABHER, F., RIOU, J. P., LAVILLE, M., LE MARCHAND-BRUSTEL, Y., TANTI, J. F. and VIDAL, H. (2003) *Diabetes*, **52**, 1319–25.

BROUSSEAU, M. E., O'CONNOR, J. J., JR, ORDOVAS, J. M., COLLINS, D., OTVOS, J. D., MASSOV, T., MCNAMARA, J. R., RUBINS, H. B., ROBINS, S. J. and SCHAEFER, E. J. (2002) *Arterioscler Thromb Vasc Biol*, **22**, 1148–54.

BROWN, M. S. and GOLDSTEIN, J. L. (1974) *Proc Natl Acad Sci USA*, **71**, 788–92.

BROWN, M. S. and GOLDSTEIN, J. L. (1999) *Proc Natl Acad Sci USA*, **96**, 11041–8.

CARMENA-RAMON, R., ASCASO, J. F., REAL, J. T., ORDOVAS, J. M. and CARMENA, R. (1998) *Arterioscler Thromb Vasc Biol*, **18**, 1266–74.

CARRIERE, V., VIDAL, R., LAZOU, K., LACASA, M., DELERS, F., RIBEIRO, A., ROUSSET, M., CHAMBAZ, J. and LACORTE, J. M. (2005) *J Biol Chem*, **280**, 5406–13.

CASLAKE, M. J. and PACKARD, C. J. (2004) *Curr Opin Lipidol*, **15**, 387–92.

CHEN, Y. D., SWAMI, S., SKOWRONSKI, R., COULSTON, A. and REAVEN, G. M. (1993) *J Clin Endocrinol Metab*, **76**, 172–7.

COMPE, E., DE SOUSA, G., FRANCOIS, K., ROCHE, R., RAHMANI, R., TORRESANI, J., RAYMONDJEAN, M. and PLANELLS, R. (2001) *Biochem J*, **358**, 175–83.

CORDAIN, L., MILLER, J. B., EATON, S. B., MANN, N., HOLT, S. H. and SPETH, J. D. (2000) *Am J Clin Nutr*, **71**, 682–92.

CORELLA, D., TUCKER, K., LAHOZ, C., COLTELL, O., CUPPLES, L. A., WILSON, P. W., SCHAEFER, E. J. and ORDOVAS, J. M. (2001) *Am J Clin Nutr*, **73**, 736–45.

CUSI, K., MAEZONO, K., OSMAN, A., PENDERGRASS, M., PATTI, M. E., PRATIPANAWATR, T., DEFRONZO, R. A., KAHN, C. R. and MANDARINO, L. J. (2000) *J Clin Invest*, **105**, 311–20.

DE GROOTH, G. J., ZERBA, K. E., HUANG, S. P., TSUCHIHASHI, Z., KIRCHGESSNER, T., BELDER, R., VISHNUPAD, P., HU, B., KLERKX, A. H., ZWINDERMAN, A. H., JUKEMA, J. W., SACKS, F. M., KASTELEIN, J. J. and KUIVENHOVEN, J. A. (2004) *J Am Coll Cardiol*, **43**, 854–7.

DORNBROOK-LAVENDER, K. A. and PIEPER, J. A. (2003) *Cardiovasc Drugs Ther*, **17**, 75–82.

DREON, D. M., FERNSTROM, H. A., MILLER, B. and KRAUSS, R. M. (1995) *Arterioscler Thromb Vasc Biol*, **15**, 105–11.

DUPLUS, E. and FOREST, C. (2002) *Biochem Pharmacol*, **64**, 893–901.

DUPLUS, E., GLORIAN, M. and FOREST, C. (2000) *J. Biol. Chem.*, **275**, 30749–52.

EBERLE, D., CLEMENT, K., MEYRE, D., SAHBATOU, M., VAXILLAIRE, M., LE GALL, A., FERRE, P., BASDEVANT, A., FROGUEL, P. and FOUFELLE, F. (2004) *Diabetes*, **53**, 2153–7.

ELCHEBLY, M., PAYETTE, P., MICHALISZYN, E., CROMLISH, W., COLLINS, S., LOY, A. L., NORMANDIN, D., CHENG, A., HIMMS-HAGEN, J., CHAN, C. C., RAMACHANDRAN, C., GRESSER, M. J., TREMBLAY, M. L. and KENNEDY, B. P. (1999) *Science*, **283**, 1544–8.

ERKKILA, A. T., SARKKINEN, E. S., LINDI, V., LEHTO, S., LAAKSO, M. and UUSITUPA, M. I. (2001) *Am J Clin Nutr*, **73**, 746–52.

FERRANNINI, E., GASTALDELLI, A., MATSUDA, M., MIYAZAKI, Y., PETTITI, M., GLASS, L. and DEFRONZO, R. A. (2003) *J Clin Endocrinol Metab*, **88**, 3251–7.

FERRE, P. (2004) *Diabetes*, **53** Suppl 1, S43–50.

FORD, E. S., GILES, W. H. and DIETZ, W. H. (2002) *JAMA*, **287**, 356–9.

FRANK, P. G. and MARCEL, Y. L. (2000) *J Lipid Res*, **41**, 853–72.

FRIKKE-SCHMIDT, R., NORDESTGAARD, B. G., JENSEN, G. B. and TYBJAERG-HANSEN, A. (2004) *J Clin Invest*, **114**, 1343–53.

FRITTITTA, L., BARATTA, R., SPAMPINATO, D., DI PAOLA, R., PIZZUTI, A., VIGNERI, R. and TRISCHITTA, V. (2001) *J Clin Endocrinol Metab*, **86**, 5888–91.

GERDES, C., FISHER, R. M., NICAUD, V., BOER, J., HUMPHRIES, S. E., TALMUD, P. J. and FAERGEMAN, O. (1997) *Circulation*, **96**, 733–40.

GIBBONS, G. F. (2003) *Prog Lipid Res*, **42**, 479–97.

GINSBERG, H. N., KARMALLY, W., SIDDIQUI, M., HOLLERAN, S., TALL, A. R., RUMSEY, S. C., DECKELBAUM, R. J., BLANER, W. S. and RAMAKRISHNAN, R. (1994) *Arterioscler Thromb*, **14**, 576–86.

GINSBERG, H. N., KARMALLY, W., SIDDIQUI, M., HOLLERAN, S., TALL, A. R., BLANER, W. S. and RAMAKRISHNAN, R. (1995) *Arterioscler Thromb Vasc Biol*, **15**, 169–78.

GONZALEZ SANCHEZ, J. L., SERRANO RIOS, M., FERNANDEZ PEREZ, C., LAAKSO, M. and MARTINEZ LARRAD, M. T. (2002) *Eur J Endocrinol*, **147**, 495–501.

GREGG, R. E. and WETTERAU, J. R. (1994) *Curr Opin Lipidol*, **5**, 81–6.

GRIMALDI, P. A. (2001) *Prog Lipid Res*, **40**, 269–81.

GYLLING, H. (2004) *Int J Clin Pract*, **58**, 859–66.

GYLLING, H. and MIETTINEN, T. A. (2002) *J Lipid Res*, **43**, 1472–6.

HARBIS, A., DEFOORT, C., NARBONNE, H., JUHEL, C., SENFT, M., LATGE, C., DELENNE, B.,

PORTUGAL, H., ATLAN-GEPNER, C., VIALETTES, B. and LAIRON, D. (2001) *Diabetes*, **50**, 462–9.

HARBIS, A., PERDREAU, S., VINCENT-BAUDRY, S., CHARBONNIER, M., BERNARD, M. C., RACCAH, D., SENFT, M., LOREC, A. M., DEFOORT, C., PORTUGAL, H., VINOY, S., LANG, V. and LAIRON, D. (2004) *Am J Clin Nutr*, **80**, 896–902.

HEGELE, R. A. (1998) *Clin Biochem*, **31**, 609–12.

HEGELE, R. A., WOLEVER, T. M., STORY, J. A., CONNELLY, P. W. and JENKINS, D. J. (1997) *Eur J Clin Invest*, **27**, 857–62.

HOCKEY, K. J., ANDERSON, R. A., COOK, V. R., HANTGAN, R. R. and WEINBERG, R. B. (2001) *J Lipid Res*, **42**, 211–17.

HOLZL, B., IGLSEDER, B., SANDHOFER, A., MALAIMARE, L., LANG, J., PAULWEBER, B. and SANDHOFER, F. (2002) *Diabetologia*, **45**, 378–84.

HORTON, J. D., SHIMOMURA, I., BROWN, M. S., HAMMER, R. E., GOLDSTEIN, J. L. and SHIMANO, H. (1998) *J Clin Invest*, **101**, 2331–9.

HUMPHRIES, S. E., TALMUD, P. J., COX, C., SUTHERLAND, W. and MANN, J. (1996) *Q J Med*, **89**, 671–80.

JANSEN, S., LOPEZ-MIRANDA, J., ORDOVAS, J. M., ZAMBRANA, J. L., MARIN, C., OSTOS, M. A., CASTRO, P., McPHERSON, R., LOPEZ SEGURA, F., BLANCO, A., JIMENEZ PEREPEREZ, J. A. and PEREZ-JIMENEZ, F. (1997) *J Lipid Res*, **38**, 1995–2002.

JONES, P. J., PAPPU, A. S., HATCHER, L., LI, Z. C., ILLINGWORTH, D. R. and CONNOR, W. E. (1996) *Arterioscler Thromb Vasc Biol*, **16**, 1222–8.

JUMP, D., CLARKE, S., MACDOUGALD, O. and THELEN, A. (1993) *Proc Natl Acad Sci USA*, **90**, 8454–8.

KESANIEMI, Y. A., EHNHOLM, C. and MIETTINEN, T. A. (1987) *J Clin Invest*, **80**, 578–81.

KESANIEMI, Y. A., LILJA, M., KERVINEN, K. and RANTALA, A. (1992) *Ann Med*, **24**, 461–4.

KESTIN, M., CLIFTON, P. M., ROUSE, I. L. and NESTEL, P. J. (1989) *Am J Clin Nutr*, **50**, 528–32.

KLIEWER, S. A., XU, H. E., LAMBERT, M. H. and WILLSON, T. M. (2001) *Recent Prog Horm Res*, **56**, 239–65.

KNOPP, R. H., WALDEN, C. E., RETZLAFF, B. M., McCANN, B. S., DOWDY, A. A., ALBERS, J. J., GEY, G.O. and COOPER, M. N. (1997) *JAMA*, **278**, 1509–15.

KNOPP, R. H., RETZLAFF, B., WALDEN, C., FISH, B., BUCK, B. and McCANN, B. (2000) *Proc Soc Exp Biol Med*, **225**, 191–9.

KNOPP, R. H., RETZLAFF, B., FISH, B., WALDEN, C., WALLICK, S., ANDERSON, M., AIKAWA, K. and KAHN, S. E. (2003) *Arterioscler Thromb Vasc Biol*, **23**, 1437–43.

LAAKSO, M. (2004) *Curr Opin Lipidol*, **15**, 115–20.

LAFONTAN, M. (2005) *Annu Rev Pharmacol Toxicol*, **45**, 119–46.

LAUDES, M., BARROSO, I., LUAN, J., SOOS, M. A., YEO, G., MEIRHAEGHE, A., LOGIE, L., VIDAL-PUIG, A., SCHAFER, A. J., WAREHAM, N. J. and O'RAHILLY, S. (2004) *Diabetes*, **53**, 842–6.

LIN, D. S. AND CONNOR, W. E. (1980) *J Lipid Res*, **21**, 1042–52.

LOPEZ-MIRANDA, J., ORDOVAS, J. M., OSTOS, M. A., MARIN, C., JANSEN, S., SALAS, J., BLANCO-MOLINA, A., JIMENEZ-PEREPEREZ, J. A., LOPEZ-SEGURA, F. and PEREZ-JIMENEZ, F. (1997) *Arterioscler Thromb Vasc Biol*, **17**, 1765–73.

LU, K., LEE, M. H., HAZARD, S., BROOKS-WILSON, A., HIDAKA, H., KOJIMA, H., OSE, L., STALENHOEF, A. F., MIETINNEN, T., BJORKHEM, I., BRUCKERT, E., PANDYA, A., BREWER, H. B., JR., SALEN, G., DEAN, M., SRIVASTAVA, A. and PATEL, S. B. (2001) *Am J Hum Genet*, **69**, 278–90.

MANNING, B. D. (2004) *J Cell Biol*, **167**, 399–403.

MASSON, L. F. and McNEILL, G. (2005) *Curr Opin Lipidol*, **16**, 61–7.

MASSON, L. F., McNEILL, G. and AVENELL, A. (2003) *Am J Clin Nutr*, **77**, 1098–111.

McGETTRICK, A. J., FEENER, E. P. and KAHN, C. R. (2005) *J Biol Chem*, **280**, 6441–6.

McMURRY, M. P., CONNOR, W. E., LIN, D. S., CERQUEIRA, M. T. and CONNOR, S. L. (1985) *Am J Clin Nutr*, **41**, 1289–98.

McNAMARA, D. J. (1987) *Annu Rev Nutr*, **7**, 273–90.

McNAMARA, D. J. (1995) *Can J Cardiol*, **11** Suppl G, 123G–126G.

MEKKI, N., DUBOIS, C., CHARBONNIER, M., CARA, L., SENFT, M., PAULI, A. M., PORTUGAL, H., GASSIN, A. L., LAFONT, H. and LAIRON, D. (1997) *Am J Clin Nutr*, **66**, 1443–51.

MEKKI, N., CHRISTOFILIS, M. A., CHARBONNIER, M., ATLAN-GEPNER, C., DEFOORT, C., JUHEL, C., BOREL, P., PORTUGAL, H., PAULI, A. M., VIALETTES, B. and LAIRON, D. (1999) *J Clin Endocrinol Metab*, **84**, 184–91.

MERO, N., SUURINKEROINEN, L., SYVANNE, M., KNUDSEN, P., YKI-JARVINEN, H. and TASKINEN, M. R. (1999) *J Lipid Res*, **40**, 1663–70.

MIETTINEN, T. A., GYLLING, H., VANHANEN, H. and OLLUS, A. (1992) *Arterioscler Thromb*, **12**, 1044–52.

MIRANDA, P. J., DEFRONZO, R. A., CALIFF, R. M. and GUYTON, J. R. (2005) *Am Heart J*, **149**, 33–45.

MISEREZ, A. R., MULLER, P. Y., BARELLA, L., BARELLA, S., STAEHELIN, H. B., LEITERSDORF, E., KARK, J. D. and FRIEDLANDER, Y. (2002) *Atherosclerosis*, **164**, 15–26.

MIWA, K., INAZU, A., KOBAYASHI, J., HIGASHIKATA, T., NOHARA, A., KAWASHIRI, M., KATSUDA, S., TAKATA, M., KOIZUMI, J. and MABUCHI, H. (2005) *Clin Sci (Lond)*, **109**, 183–8.

MULLER-WIELAND, D., KNEBEL, B., AVCI, H., LEHR, S., LAUDES, M., RISTOW, M., KRONE, W. and KOTZKA, J. (2001) *Int J Obes Relat Metab Disord*, **25** Suppl 1, S35–7.

ORDOVAS, J. M. (2001) *Curr Atheroscler Rep*, **3**, 200–208.

ORDOVAS, J. M., CORELLA, D., DEMISSIE, S., CUPPLES, L. A., COUTURE, P., COLTELL, O., WILSON, P. W., SCHAEFER, E. J. and TUCKER, K. L. (2002) *Circulation*, **106**, 2315–21.

OSTLUND, R. E., JR., BOSNER, M. S. and STENSON, W. F. (1999) *J Lipid Res*, **40**, 1453–8.

OU, J., TU, H., SHAN, B., LUK, A., DEBOSE-BOYD, R. A., BASHRNAKOV, Y., GOLDSTEIN, J. L. and BROWN, M. S. (2001) *Proc Natl Acad Sci USA*, **98**, 6027–32.

PAJUKANTA, P. (2004) *J Clin Invest*, **114**, 1244–7.

PASTIER, D., LACORTE, J. M., CHAMBAZ, J., CARDOT, P. and RIBEIRO, A. (2002) *J Biol Chem*, **277**, 15199–206.

PEELMAN, F., VERSCHELDE, J. L., VANLOO, B., AMPE, C., LABEUR, C., TAVERNIER, J., VANDEKERCKHOVE, J. and ROSSENEU, M. (1999) *J Lipid Res*, **40**, 59–69.

PRATLEY, R. E., BAIER, L., PAN, D. A., SALBE, A. D., STORLIEN, L., RAVUSSIN, E. and BOGARDUS, C. (2000) *J Lipid Res*, **41**, 2002–8.

RANTALA, M., RANTALA, T. T., SAVOLAINEN, M. J., FRIEDLANDER, Y. and KESANIEMI, Y. A. (2000) *Am J Clin Nutr*, **71**, 713–24.

REN, B., THELEN, A. P., PETERS, J. M., GONZALEZ, F. J. and JUMP, D. B. (1997) *J Biol Chem*, **272**, 26827–32.

REZNIK, Y., POUSSE, P., HERROU, M., MORELLO, R., MAHOUDEAU, J., DROSDOWSKY, M. A. and FRADIN, S. (1996) *Metabolism*, **45**, 63–71.

ROOSBEEK, S., VANLOO, B., DUVERGER, N., CASTER, H., BREYNE, J., DE BEUN, I., PATEL, H., VANDEKERCKHOVE, J., SHOULDERS, C., ROSSENEU, M. and PEELMAN, F. (2001) *J Lipid Res*, **42**, 31–40.

SALTIEL, A. R. and KAHN, C. R. (2001) *Nature*, **414**, 799–806.

SCHAEFER, E. J., LAMON-FAVA, S., JOHNSON, S., ORDOVAS, J. M., SCHAEFER, M. M., CASTELLI, W. P. and WILSON, P. W. (1994) *Arterioscler Thromb*, **14**, 1105–13.

SEHAYEK, E., NATH, C., HEINEMANN, T., McGEE, M., SEIDMAN, C. E., SAMUEL, P. and BRESLOW, J. L. (1998) *J Lipid Res*, **39**, 2415–22.

SENTI, M., BOSCH, M., AUBO, C., ELOSUA, R., MASIA, R. and MARRUGAT, J. (2000) *Atherosclerosis*, **150**, 135–41.

SHIMANO, H. (2002) *Vitam Horm*, **65**, 167–94.

SHIMANO, H., HORTON, J. D., HAMMER, R. E., SHIMOMURA, I., BROWN, M. S. and GOLDSTEIN, J. L. (1996) *J Clin Invest*, **98**, 1575–84.

SHIMANO, H., HORTON, J. D., SHIMOMURA, I., HAMMER, R. E., BROWN, M. S. and GOLDSTEIN, J. L. (1997) *J Clin Invest*, **99**, 846–54.

SHIMOMURA, I., SHIMANO, H., HORTON, J. D., GOLDSTEIN, J. L. and BROWN, M. S. (1997) *J Clin Invest*, **99**, 838–45.

SING, C. F. and DAVIGNON, J. (1985) *Am J Hum Genet*, **37**, 268–85.

ST-ONGE, M. P., JANSSEN, I. and HEYMSFIELD, S. B. (2004) *Diabetes Care*, **27**, 2222–8.

THOMPSON, J. F., LIRA, M. E., DURHAM, L. K., CLARK, R. W., BAMBERGER, M. J. and MILOS, P. M. (2003) *Atherosclerosis*, **167**, 195–204.

TONTONOZ, P., HU, E. and SPIEGELMAN, B. M. (1994) *Cell*, **79**, 1147–56.

VAUHKONEN, I., NISKANEN, L., VANNINEN, E., KAINULAINEN, S., UUSITUPA, M. and LAAKSO, M. (1998) *J Clin Invest*, **101**, 86–96.

VIALETTES, B., REYNIER, P., ATLAN-GEPNER, C., MEKKI, N., LESLUYES-MAZZOCHI, L., LUC, G., LAIRON, D. and MALTHIERY, Y. (2000) *Br J Nutr*, **83**, 615–22.

VORSTER, H. H., BENADE, A. J., BARNARD, H. C., LOCKE, M. M., SILVIS, N., VENTER, C. S., SMUTS, C. M., ENGELBRECHT, G. P. and MARAIS, M. P. (1992) *Am J Clin Nutr*, **55**, 400–10.

VOSPER, H., PATEL, L., GRAHAM, T. L., KHOUDOLI, G. A., HILL, A., MACPHEE, C. H., PINTO, I., SMITH, S. A., SUCKLING, K. E., WOLF, C. R. and PALMER, C. N. A. (2001) *J. Biol. Chem.*, **276**, 44258–65.

WALCZAK, R. and TONTONOZ, P. (2002) *J. Lipid Res.*, **43**, 177–86.

WANG, J., WILLIAMS, C. M. and HEGELE, R. A. (2005) *Clin Genet*, **67**, 175–7.

WEGGEMANS, R. M., ZOCK, P. L., MEYBOOM, S., FUNKE, H. and KATAN, M. B. (2000) *J Lipid Res*, **41**, 1623–8.

WEGGEMANS, R. M., ZOCK, P. L. and KATAN, M. B. (2001) *Am J Clin Nutr*, **73**, 885–91.

WEGGEMANS, R. M., ZOCK, P. L., TAI, E. S., ORDOVAS, J. M., MOLHUIZEN, H. O. and KATAN, M. B. (2002) *Clin Genet*, **62**, 226–9.

WEINBERG, R. B., GEISSINGER, B. W., KASALA, K., HOCKEY, K. J., TERRY, J. G., EASTER, L. and CROUSE, J. R. (2000) *J Lipid Res*, **41**, 2035–41.

WEITGASSER, R., GALVAN, G., MALAIMARE, L., DERFLINGER, I., HEDEGGER, M., LANG, J., IGLSEDER, B., LADURNER, G. and PAULWEBER, B. (2004) *Biomed Pharmacother*, **58**, 619–27.

WORGALL, T. S., STURLEY, S. L., SEO, T., OSBORNE, T. F. and DECKELBAUM, R. J. (1998) *J. Biol. Chem.*, **273**, 25537–40.

YE, S. Q. and KWITEROVICH, P. O., JR. (2000) *Am J Clin Nutr*, **72**, 1275S–84S.

YKI-JARVINEN, H. (1997) *Lancet*, **349**, 516–17.

YOSHIKAWA, T., SHIMANO, H., YAHAGI, N., IDE, T., AMEMIYA-KUDO, M., MATSUZAKA, T., NAKAKUKI, M., TOMITA, S., OKAZAKI, H., TAMURA, Y., IIZUKA, Y., OHASHI, K., TAKAHASHI, A., SONE, H., OSUGA JI, J., GOTODA, T., ISHIBASHI, S. and YAMADA, N. (2002) *J Biol Chem*, **277**, 1705–11.

ZAMBON, A., DEEB, S. S., PAULETTO, P., CREPALDI, G. and BRUNZELL, J. D. (2003) *Curr Opin Lipidol*, **14**, 179–89.

ZHANG, K., ZHANG, S., ZHENG, K., HOU, Y., LIAO, L., HE, Y., ZHANG, L., NEBERT, D. W., SHI, J., SU, Z. and XIAO, C. (2004) *Biochem Biophys Res Commun*, **318**, 4–10.

ZHU, S., ST-ONGE, M. P., HESHKA, S. and HEYMSFIELD, S. B. (2004) *Metabolism*, **53**, 1503–11.

4

Health benefits of monounsaturated fatty acids

J. López-Miranda, P. Pérez-Martínez and F. Pérez-Jiménez, Hospital Universitario Reina Sofia, Cordoba, Spain

4.1 Introduction

Currently, much is known about the effect on lipid metabolism of the principal fatty acids in the human diet (Mensink and Katan, 1992). Based on this knowledge, dietary recommendations have been made for the population with the aim of reducing cardiovascular risk. Given that the most noteworthy effect is that saturated fatty acids (SFAs) increase plasma levels of total cholesterol and low-density lipoprotein (LDL) cholesterol, it is widely accepted that a healthy diet should contain a limited amount of this nutrient.

One of the dietary models is the Therapeutic Lifestyle Changes Diet (TLCD), recommended by the National Cholesterol Education Program (NCEP), in the Adult Treatment Panel III, with <7% SFA, up to 10% of polyunsaturated fatty acids (PUFAs) and up to 10% monounsaturated fatty acids (MUFAs) (NCEP, 2001). Moreover, the NCEP now recommends a higher intake of MUFAs, in accordance with the experience of the Mediterranean diet. Historically, this diet has been associated with a lower rate of cardiovascular disease and cancer in those populations that consume it (Willett *et al.*, 1995). This type of diet is similar to the TLCD, since the majority of calories come from foods of vegetable origin and the intake of SFA and cholesterol remains low. Furthermore, in the Mediterranean diet, the total fat intake is not substantial and need not be limited, as long as MUFAs are predominant. Oleic acid (*cis* C18:1) makes up 92% of the MUFAs present in foods, and almost 60–80% of oleic acid intake comes from olive oil. Much has been learned about this topic since 1995, indicating that diet has pleiotropic effects that reach far beyond its action on plasma lipoproteins (Kris-Etherton, 1999).

4.2 Lipoprotein metabolism

In the mid-1980s, investigators began to debate the question of the ideal substitute for SFA calories: carbohydrate or unsaturated fatty acids, specifically MUFAs under stable weight conditions. The results of two similar studies conducted by Grundy (1986) and Mensink and Katan (1987) reported a similar total cholesterol-lowering effect of both a high-fat diet (40% of energy) rich in MUFA and low in SFAs and a low-fat/carbohydrate-rich diet. Although both diets lowered total and LDL cholesterol, the high-MUFA diet did not lower high-density lipoprotein (HDL) cholesterol or increase triglycerides, as did the carbohydrate-rich diet. The carbohydrate-rich diet lowered HDL cholesterol by 14–22% and markedly elevated triglycerides (22–39%).

Since these pioneering studies, a number of subsequent studies have reported similar results (Grundy *et al.*, 1988; Ginsberg *et al.*, 1990). More recently, the DELTA Study reported that a Step 1 diet and a high-MUFA diet low in SFA and cholesterol, both lowered total and LDL cholesterol levels by 5.5% and 7%, respectively, compared with an average American diet (AAD) rich in SFA in subjects with a low HDL cholesterol level, moderately elevated triglycerides, or elevated insulin levels (Ginsberg *et al.*, 1998). Triglycerides increased by 12% and 7% on the Step 1 diet compared with the high-MUFA diet and the AAD, respectively. Interestingly, plasma triglycerides were lower on the high-MUFA diet (by 4%) than on the AAD. Although HDL cholesterol decreased on both cholesterol-lowering diets compared with the AAD, the decrease in HDL cholesterol was less on the high-MUFA diet (4.3%) than on the Step 1 diet (7.2%). When MUFA substitutes SFA, the most important effect is a decrease in LDL cholesterol at a level comparable to low-fat diets, with up to 30% of total calories provided by fat and 55–60% of total calories as CHO. An additional benefit is that the HDL cholesterol is maintained at higher levels when SFA rather than PUFA or CHO is replaced by MUFA in the diet (Mensink *et al.*, 1989; Mata *et al.*, 1992; Gardner and Kraemer, 1995; Perez-Jimenez *et al.*, 1995) (Table 4.1). Thus, the high-MUFA Mediterranean diet may be a better nutritional option than the low-fat, high-CHO diet, for substituting a Westernized diet enriched in SFA, considering that low levels of HDL cholesterol are frequent in populations with low total fat consumption.

A well-designed study performed in healthy subjects by Kris-Etherton *et al.* (1999) is illustrative of both the assortment of MUFA-rich foods that can be incorporated into a healthy diet and the beneficial effect of MUFA diets on serum triglycerides when substituted for CHO. These investigators compared the average American diet with four cholesterol-lowering diets: the NCEP Step II diet and three different MUFA diets. The four diets had a similar cholesterol-lowering effect but, compared with those in the average American diet, triglycerides concentrations were 11% higher with the Step II diet and were 13% lower with the MUFA diets. The HDL cholesterol level was preserved with the high-MUFA, while it was 4% lower with the Step II diet (Kris-Etherton *et al.*, 1999).

Table 4.1 Expected healthy effects with the replacement of dietary monounsaturated fat for saturated fat. CHO: carbohydrates

Level of evidence	Type of effect
Demonstrated by dietary intervention trials in different populations	1. A more favourable lipid profile, with a decrease in LDL cholesterol plasma levels. Moreover, HDL cholesterol is higher than with the replacement by CHO 2. Reduction *in vitro* oxidation of LDL obtained from subjects fed with MUFA-rich diets 3. Improvement of glucose metabolism in normal subjects and type 2 diabetic patients. MUFAs result in a lower insulin requirement and plasma glucose concentration compared with the replacement by CHO
Suggested by few dietary intervention trials or with *in vitro* experiments	1. Reduced activation of monocytes by oxidized LDL obtained from subjects fed with MUFA-rich diets. 2. A 3–10% reduction in systolic and diastolic blood pressure, in normotensive and hypertensive subjects. 3. Changes in arterial wall components (Table 4.2). 4. The promotion of a less prothrombotic environment, influencing different thrombogenic factors (Tables 4.3 and 4.4)

In comparison with low-fat diets, modest triglyceride reductions and/or HDL cholesterol increases have been observed as well after consumption of diets containing MUFA-rich nuts, such as macadamia nuts (Curb *et al.*, 2000) and pecans (Rajaram *et al.*, 2001). Thus, both in diabetic and in healthy subjects, natural food-based MUFA regimes may be preferable to a low-fat diet because of more favourable effects on TAG-rich lipoproteins and HDL cholesterol, with an attendant decrease of the cardiovascular risk profile. However, there exists no evidence that the reduction of HDL cholesterol, related with low-fat diets, favours the onset of coronary heart disease (Knuiman *et al.*, 1982).

Both Keys (1965) and Hegsted *et al.* (1965) analysed data from controlled feeding studies and developed similar blood cholesterol predictive equations. MUFAs did not affect total cholesterol levels, but SFA raised them. PUFAs lowered total cholesterol half as much as SFA raised it. More recent analyses confirmed these findings, although there is some suggestion that MUFAs elicit a cholesterol-lowering effect that is less than that observed for PUFAs (Mensink and Katan, 1992; Yu *et al.*, 1995). In support of these findings, Howard *et al.* (1995) found greater reductions in total cholesterol levels with PUFAs versus MUFAs ($p < 0.05$) in a controlled-feeding study. However, other controlled-feeding studies, as well as a study with free-living subjects, observed comparable total and LDL cholesterol-lowering effects of these fatty acids (Ginsberg *et al.*, 1994; Gardner and Kraemer, 1995) when 4–14% of energy of each fatty acid class was substituted for the other. Likewise, in a meta-analysis of results of 14 studies published between 1983 and 1994, diets high in oils enriched in

MUFAs versus PUFA elicited similar effects on total, LDL and HDL cholesterol, whereas the PUFA-enriched oil had a slight triglyceride-lowering effect (Gardner and Kraemer, 1995). Thus, the cholesterolaemic effects of MUFA versus PUFA substitution for dietary SFA are comparable.

In addition, in patients with diabetes mellitus, Garg's meta-analysis of ten studies (Garg, 1998) showed that the net changes in fasting plasma concentrations of TAG, VLDL cholesterol, HDL cholesterol and LDL cholesterol with consumption of a high-MUFA diet were a 19% reduction, a 22.5% reduction, a 4% increase and a 0% change, respectively.

4.2.1 Postprandial lipaemia

Postprandial lipaemia, defined by the extent and duration of the rise in plasma TAG after a fatty meal, is a state during which the TAG metabolic capacity is under challenge. Many studies have supported the concept that circulating TAG-rich lipoproteins after meals are significant contributors to the development of atherosclerosis. Postprandial lipaemia is influenced by the amount and type of dietary fat present in the test meal, as well as other dietary components including fibre, glucose, starch and alcohol (Williams, 1998).

Most studies with n-3 PUFA-rich fats showed a reduced postprandial lipaemia when ingested in the daily diet or as a single meal (Weintraub *et al.*, 1988; Tinker *et al.*, 1999) compared with other fat sources. Comparisons of the effects of n-6 PUFA-rich oils with olive oil n-9 monounsaturated fatty acids or MUFA showed lower (de Bruin *et al.*, 1993) or comparable (Lichtenstein *et al.*, 1993; Tholstrup *et al.*, 2001) magnitudes of postprandial lipaemia. There is physiological evidence that different MUFA-rich oils can lead to similar plasma lipid and lipoprotein profiles in fasting healthy subjects, but can produce different functional and postprandial responses. Recently Abia *et al.* (2001) showed that virgin olive oil as compared to a high oleic sunflower oil intake reduced the postprandial TAG lipoprotein response. This suggests that factors other than the oleic acid content may be responsible for the different metabolic effects. Chylomicrons formed after olive oil feeding appear to enter the circulation more rapidly, and to be cleared at a faster rate, than those formed after intake of fats rich in SFAs (Roche *et al.*, 1998) or rich in PUFAs, such as safflower oil. Accelerated chylomicron metabolism would actually make olive oil less atherogenic even if the overall magnitude of postprandial lipaemia was similar to that elicited by other fatty meals.

The habitual diet of an individual may also influence the postprandial response. Until recently, few studies had investigated the influence of background diet on the postprandial response. Silva *et al.* (2003) compared a diet high in SFAs (reference diet) with diets containing an increasing proportion of MUFAs in place of SFAs using a parallel design. Compared with the reference diet, the two levels of MUFA intake led to a marked reduction in apoB-48 production following the test meal, which suggested that chylomicron particle size was increased following the moderate- and high-MUFA diets. The authors concluded that a high-MUFA diet results in the production of chylomicrons of a larger size. However, Rivellese *et al.* (2003) could find no difference in post-prandial lipaemia on a diet high in MUFA compared with diets high in SFAa.

4.2.2 LDL particle size

One of the untoward consequences of a prolonged residence time of TAG-rich lipoproteins in the circulation is enhanced lipid exchange between lipoprotein classes, leading to cholesterol depletion of LDL. These lipoprotein particles (small, dense LDL, as opposed to large, buoyant LDL) are prone to oxidation and enter the arterial wall more readily than larger particles, accelerating the development of atherosclerosis. LDL particle size and subclass pattern might be influenced by dietary fat. Until now, research on this topic has focused on the quantity rather than the quality of dietary fat. Several studies have consistently shown that low-fat diets lead to a decrease in mean LDL size compared with high fat diets (Krauss and Dreon, 1995). Dreon and colleagues (1998) investigated the effect of nutrient intakes on LDL size and subclass pattern, and found a positive correlation between dietary SFA content and LDL peak particle diameter. Such an association was not apparent for MUFA or PUFA.

In studies using isoenergetic diets with a varying proportion of CHO and reciprocal changes in the proportion of fat at a fixed MUFA content, a strong linear correlation was observed between decreased fat/increased CHO intakes and prevalence of small, dense LDL in healthy men (Krauss, 2001). This is supported by the results of a study in obese women that compared two hypocaloric diets, a high-CHO diet and a high-MUFA diet based on olive oil, which showed a decrease of the dense LDL fraction in the MUFA group (Zambon *et al.*, 1999). However, in the study of Luscombe *et al.* (1999) with diabetic subjects, no differences in LDL size were observed with diets varying in fat content by up to 14%. In addition, Moreno *et al.* (2004) showed recently that a Mediterranean diet, high in MUFAs, increases LDL particle size compared with a CHO-rich diet, and this effect is dependent on apoE genotypes.

4.3 LDL oxidation

Substantial evidence exists to suggest that LDL may undergo oxidative modification *in vivo* and that this process may be critical in the initiation and evolution of atherosclerosis (Witztum and Steinberg, 1991). Dietary fat is one of the most important factors determining plasma LDL cholesterol concentrations, and diet can modulate susceptibility of LDL to oxidative modification. This effect has been attributed to diet-induced changes in the concentrations of PUFAs and antioxidants in the LDL particle. The particles rich in MUFAs have been shown to be less susceptible to oxidative modification compared with LDL particles enriched with n-6 PUFA (Parthasarathy *et al.*, 1990; Berry *et al.*, 1991; Reaven *et al.*, 1991, 1993; Bonanome *et al.*, 1992; Abbey *et al.*, 1993) (Table 4.1).

Reaven *et al.* (1996) compared the effects of n-6 PUFA with the effects of MUFA on the susceptibility of LDL to oxidative modification. Healthy volunteers received either linoleic or oleic-enriched diets, or continued with their usual American diets for 6 weeks. The authors concluded that oleic-enriched diets decrease the susceptibility of LDL to lipid peroxidation. Baroni *et al.* (1999) studied the effects of feeding MUFA versus PUFA-enriched diets on LDL composition in hypercholesterolaemic patients. Antioxidant values remained constant during the study, while the concentration of MUFA in LDL particles increased 11% and PUFA decreased 10% following an olive oil diet. They conclude that oleic-enriched LDL was more resistant to oxidative modifications as measured by different peroxidation parameters.

Consumption of a range of dietary antioxidants may be beneficial in protecting LDL against oxidative modification. Wiseman *et al.* (1996) studied the effect of polyphenol antioxidants on the susceptibility of LDL to oxidation in New Zealand white rabbits. All diets comprised 17% energy as MUFA, but oils with different polyphenol contents were used to provide the dietary source of oleic acid: refined olive oil, extra virgin olive oil and Trisun high-oleic sunflower oil. The lag phase in isolated LDL was significantly increased in the high polyphenol, extra virgin olive oil group. This could suggest that phenolic compounds, which are present only in extra virgin olive oil, may contribute to the endogenous antioxidant capacity of LDL (Wiseman *et al.*, 2002). In accordance with these data, Caruso *et al.* (1999) demonstrated the efficacy of virgin olive oil phenolic compounds in preventing oxidative modifications of human LDL oxidized by UV light *in vitro*.

Surprisingly, few formal feeding trials have examined the effects of high-CHO versus high-MUFA diets on LDL oxidizability. In a recent study, Rodriguez-Villar *et al.* (2004) found a similar lag time in LDL isolated from well-controlled diabetic subjects after CHO-rich and MUFA-rich diets with a 12% difference in daily energy from fat. On the other hand, Gumbiner *et al.* (1998) found that the LDL particles of obese diabetic subjects were less susceptible to oxidation after a MUFA-rich diet than after a CHO-rich diet. Four studies assessed LDL oxidation in healthy, free-living individuals who were prescribed natural diets high in CHO and high in MUFA, with <12% difference in fat content between diets (Berry *et al.*, 1992; Perez-Jimenez *et al.*, 1999; Castro *et al.*, 2000; Hargrove *et al.*, 2001). Compared with the CHO-rich diets, the MUFA-rich diets either reduced the susceptibility of LDL to oxidation (Perez-Jimenez *et al.*, 1999) or had no effect. However, an antioxidant effect of alpha-tocopherol in MUFA-rich foods, such as almonds (Berry *et al.*, 1992) and high-oleic-acid sunflower oil (Castro *et al.*, 2000), might have contributed to the increased resistance of LDL to oxidation.

4.4 Endothelial function

The endothelium plays an important role in the regulation of vascular tone through the release of vasodilator and vasoconstrictor substances (Vane *et al.*,

1990). Furthermore, endothelial cells secrete multiple metabolites involved in coagulation, fibrinolysis and the adhesion and transendothelial migration of circulating leukocytes into the vascular wall, such as vascular cell adhesion molecule-1 (VCAM-1), intercellular adhesion molecule-1 (ICAM-1) and P-selectin, all of which are involved in the development of atherosclerosis (Ross, 1999).

Some findings suggest that nutrients, including MUFAs, may modulate atherogenesis, by affecting different arterial wall components. Recently, in an *in vitro* model of early atherogenesis based on cultured endothelial cells stimulated by cytokines, Carluccio *et al.* (1999) demonstrated that the incorporation of oleic acid in total cell lipids decreased the expression of several endothelial leukocyte adhesion molecules (Table 4.2). Oleic acid also brings about a parallel reduction in messenger RNA for VCAM-1, by interfering with the activation of the most important transcription factor controlling endothelial activation, nuclear factor-kappa B. In addition, Mata *et al.* (1996) conducted a dietary intervention study in 42 healthy men and women, who were subjected to four consecutive dietary periods, differing in the fat content of SFA, MUFA and PUFA (n-6 and n-3). LDL induction of monocyte adhesion to endothelial cells was lower during the MUFA phase than during the other periods (Mata *et al.*, 1996).

To confirm that dietary fat influences the proinflammatory properties of mildly oxidized LDL, Tsimikas *et al.* (1999) isolated LDL from healthy subjects after consumption of diets enriched in either oleic or linoleic acid. When exposed to oxidative stress, the LDL enriched in oleic acid promoted less monocyte chemotaxis (52% lower) and reduced monocyte adhesion (77%), compared with linoleic-enriched LDL (Table 4.2). Furthermore, in healthy middle-aged men entered a double-blind, randomized, controlled trial in which they consumed either a MUFA diet or a control diet, there was a significant decrease in the expression of ICAM-1 by peripheral blood mononuclear cells from subjects consuming the MUFA diet (Yaqoob *et al.*, 1998). The recent observation that the ingestion of a high-MUFA diet based on olive oil had no

Table 4.2 Changes in arterial wall components, related with MUFA

Variables studied	Described possible effects
1. Endothelial cells exposed to oleic acid-enriched LDL	1. Decreased expression in vascular cell adhesion molecule-1 (VCAM-1)
2. Monocytes exposed to oleic acid-enriched LDL	2. Less endothelial cell adhesion and a lower chemotactic activity
3. Vasomotor response during MUFA intake	3. A reduction in endothelium-dependent vaso-dilatation, in hypercholesterolaemic patients
4. Reduction in plasma levels of endothelial markers	4. P-selectin, von Willebrand factor, PAI-1, and Tissue Factor Pathway Inhibitor (TFPI)
5. Smooth muscle cells exposed to sera from volunteers fed with MUFA-enriched diets	5. Less ^{3}H-thymidine incorporation into DNA of cultured smooth muscle cells

effect or reduced the expression of the nuclear transcription factor kappa-B in mononuclear cells as opposed to the stimulatory effect of PUFA (Toborek *et al.*, 2002) and SAFA (Bellido *et al.*, 2004), provides a new and conceptually attractive aspect of the putative antiatherogenic effects of MUFA at the molecular level.

The regulatory function of endothelium is altered in hypercholesterolaemia, and endothelial dysfunction plays a central role in the development of atherosclerosis (Celermajer, 1997). Diet is the cornerstone of the treatment of hypercholesterolaemia and studies in animals have shown that dietary therapies restore endothelium-dependent vasodilatation to normal (Harrison *et al.*, 1987). However, the information available in humans is scarce and mainly obtained with n-3 PUFA rich diets (Goode *et al.*, 1997; Mori *et al.*, 2000). We carried out a dietary intervention study in 22 white hypercholesterolaemic males consisting of a baseline SFA phase and two randomized-crossover dietary periods: a low-fat diet and a high MUFA Mediterranean diet, from olive oil (Fuentes *et al.*, 2001). Using the SFA-rich period as a reference, we observed significantly increased flow-mediated (endothelium-dependent) dilatation during the Mediterranean diet. Plasma P-selectin levels were lower during both the Mediterranean diet and the low-fat diet, but not during the SFA-diet (Table 4.1). In addition, Esposito *et al.* (2004) found that a Mediterranean-style diet improved the endothelial function and vascular inflammatory markers in patients with the metabolic syndrome. Ryan *et al.* (2000) showed that a diet rich in olive oil attenuated the endothelial dysfunction present during consumption of a baseline diet high in PUFA. Finally, Vogel *et al.* (2000) showed that a meal with vegetables and olive oil, but not olive oil alone, attenuated the postprandial endothelial dysfunction that follows a fatty meal, implying that improved vascular reactivity was due to antioxidants in vegetables. On the other hand, single fatty meals rich both in MUFAs from high oleic acid sunflower oil (Ong *et al.*, 1999) and in SFAs impaired postprandial endothelial function in comparison with single high-CHO meals.

Proliferation of smooth muscle cells (SMCs) plays an important role in the progression of atherosclerotic lesions. To investigate the effect of dietary fat on the proliferation of these cells, Mata *et al.* (1997) studied 24 healthy men and women who were placed on four consecutive diets: SFA-rich diet, MUFA-rich diet, n-6 PUFA rich diet, and n-3 PUFA rich diet. Human coronary SMCs were cultured and induced by sera derived from the different groups. ^{3}H-Thymidine incorporation into DNA was significantly reduced during the MUFA and n-6 PUFA periods, but not during the n-3 PUFA diet versus the SFA diet (Table 4.2).

4.5 Dietary monounsaturated fat and haemostasis

Atherosclerosis is a complex pathogenic process. In recent years we have seen important developments in the study of the role of thrombotic phenomena in the biology of atheroma plaque. One of the most interesting new lines of study proposes the formation of the occlusive thrombus on a biologically disposed plaque, the vulnerable or high-risk plaque, which brings about a sudden interruption of arterial flow, triggering the primary signs of vascular disease: acute myocardial infarction, unstable angina and sudden cardiac death. Sudden occlusion occurs when a thrombus forms on a ruptured or fissured plaque, and this is a key factor in setting off the clotting cascade (Fuster *et al.*, 1992).

4.5.1 Platelet function

The ingestion of n-3 fatty acids could influence haemostasis, especially by prolonging template bleeding time, but also by exerting some beneficial effects on erythrocyte flexibility and reducing platelet aggregation. However, it appears unlikely that n-3 fatty acids lower fibrinogen or interact with the fibrinolytic system directly (Schmidt *et al.*, 1990; Knapp, 1997). Furthermore, the influence of other dietary unsaturated fatty acids such as n-6 PUFA and MUFA on thrombosis is less well understood. Sirtori and co-workers (1986) described a change in platelet function characterized by reduced sensitivity to collagen during the consumption of an olive oil-enriched diet, while sensitivity to arachidonic acid decreased during a corn oil-enriched diet. The experiment was conducted in a free-living population, which was fed diets enriched with both vegetable oils over two consecutive periods (Sirtori *et al.*, 1986). These findings were confirmed recently by Smith *et al.* (2003) who compared two MUFA-rich diets, a moderate-MUFA and a high-MUFA diet in which 16 g and 32 g of dietary SFA/100 g total fatty acids were substituted with MUFA respectively. Platelet responses to ADP and arachidonic acid differed with time on the two diets; at 16 weeks, platelet aggregatory response to ADP was significantly lower on the high-MUFA than on the moderate-MUFA diet; ADP responses were also significantly lower within this group at 8 and 16 weeks compared with the high-SFA diet (Table 4.3).

Table 4.3 Effects of high monounsaturated fat intake in humans on platelet function and eicosanoid pathway

Haemostatic parameters	Expected changes
Platelet aggregation	Reduction of collagen-induced aggregability Reduction of ADP-induced aggregability Decrease of thromboxane B2 production
Von Willebrand factor	Decrease in plasma levels
Thromboxane B2	Decrease of *in vitro* thromboxane B_2 production in platelet samples Decrease in the urinary excretion of 11-dehydro-thromboxane B_2 Decrease of plasma thromboxane B_2 levels in subjects consuming a virgin olive oil-enriched diet as compared to a high oleic acid sunflower oil diet

In another study, total lipids of Greek olive oils and seed oils of four kinds, namely, soybean, corn, sunflower and sesame oil, were separated into total polar lipids and total neutral lipids via a novel extraction procedure. Each lipid fraction from oils was tested *in vitro* for the capacity to induce or to inhibit washed rabbit platelet aggregation. Comparison between olive and seed oils supports the superiority of olive oil, as high levels of platelet activating factor antagonists were detected, mainly in total polar lipid (Karantonis *et al.*, 2002). In an experimental study on rats, animals fed an olive oil-enriched diet showed a significant delay in the thrombotic occlusion of the 'aortic loop', a lower incidence of venous thrombosis and a prolonged bleeding time in comparison with the control group fed the usual diet (Brzosko *et al.*, 2002). Furthermore, a recent study evaluated the effect of dietary supplementation with virgin olive oil in an experimental model with rabbits fed an atherogenic diet. Animals fed the virgin olive oil diet, compared with the SFA diet group, showed decreased platelet hyperactivity and subendothelial thrombogenicity (De La Cruz *et al.*, 2000).

Eicosatrienoic acid is potentially synthesized from oleic acid and it has been suggested that this fatty acid acts as a precursor for eicosanoids of a less inflammatory mixture, although this is speculative. Although the effect of eicosatrienoic acid on cyclooxygenase is poorly understood, as is the effect on lipoxygenase, this fatty acid has been suggested to inhibit thromboxane B_2 (TXB_2) and PGE_2 synthesis, resulting in a situation similar to that produced by an increased intake of long chain n-3 fatty acids from fish oil (Sirtori *et al.*, 1986; Lerner *et al.*, 1995). This could explain Sirtori's findings in the study mentioned above, where they observed a decrease of *in vitro* TXB_2 production in platelet samples obtained during the ingestion of olive oil, but not during the corn oil-enriched diet (Sirtori *et al.*, 1986). Likewise, in a study conducted on rats, the administration of olive oil was seen to induce a decrease in TXB2 plasma levels (Navarro *et al.*, 1992). Furthermore, in the comparative dietary trial with different fatty acid compositions mentioned above, the authors observed a decrease in the urinary excretion of 11-dehydro-thromboxane B_2, a TXB_2 metabolite, during the MUFA phase compared with the n-6 fatty acid dietary period, suggesting that dietary MUFA has an effect on this eicosanoid pathway (Lahoz *et al.*, 1997).

Olive oil is composed not only of fatty acids but numerous minor components of which the polyphenols are a significant category. A recent study compared the effects of two monounsaturated oils, virgin olive oil and high-oleic-acid sunflower oil, on eicosanoid production and TXB_2 in 14 non-obese post-menopausal women. Serum peroxides and TXB_2 levels in stimulated platelet-rich plasma were significantly higher after the high-oleic-acid sunflower oil diet than after the extra virgin olive oil diet (Oubina *et al.*, 2001). These findings suggest that differences in the type of minor compounds, as well as in the concentration of linoleic acid, in both these monounsaturated oils may play an important role in modulating eicosanoid production. Other new studies have shown that the polyphenols present in olive oil induce inhibition of platelet aggregation to a degree comparable to that observed with resveratrol and quercetin (Togna *et al.*, 2003).

The combined intake of foods rich in MUFA and n-3 PUFA from fish and vegetable sources is characteristic of the Mediterranean diet, and this combination may have beneficial effects that go beyond the consumption of each in isolation, as recently noted by Vognild *et al.* (1998). In this study the influence of various dietary marine oils and olive oil on platelets was investigated in 266 healthy volunteers who consumed 15 ml/day of cod liver oil, whale blubber oil, mixtures of seal blubber oil and cod liver oil, or olive oil and cod liver oil for 12 weeks. Lipopolysaccharide-stimulated blood tended to generate less TXB_2 in the cod liver oil and olive oil groups. The combination of cod liver oil and olive oil may produce better effects than these oils given separately. In addition, a combined high-MUFA and marine n-3 PUFA diet induced a significant lowering of FIIc, FIXc, FXc, FVIIc, FVIIa, FXIIa, PAI-1, plasma viscosity and platelet activity, but led to an increase in fibrinogen, as compared with a low-fat complex carbohydrate- and dietary fibre-rich diet (Junker *et al.*, 2001).

A coagulation component associated with the formation of platelet thrombus is vWF (von Willebrand factor). vWF could participate in arterial thrombosis, binding to platelet membrane glycoproteins in both adhesion and aggregation, leading to thrombus formation in high shear stress rates. In a study conducted on subjects with type 2 diabetes mellitus, vWF was seen to decrease during the consumption of a very high-fat diet, and with a high content of MUFA (30% of total calories) (Rasmussen *et al.*, 1994). Furthermore, a similar decrease was observed by us in healthy normolipaemic young males, during the consumption of a high-MUFA Mediterranean diet while no changes in vWF were observed during a low-fat, high-CHO enriched diet (Perez-Jimenez *et al.*, 1999).

4.5.2 Coagulation factors

With regard to the effect of dietary fatty acids on other thrombogenic factors, several dietary intervention studies have shown that Factor VII (FVII), a key protein in thrombosis and a risk factor for CHD, is indeed influenced by diet. An increase in FVII was observed during the chronic intake of a high-SFA diet, as was the postprandial activation of coagulant Factor VII (FVIIc) during acute intake (Mennen *et al.*, 1996; Marckmann *et al.*, 1998). These changes suggest that SFA may shift the haemostatic steady state toward hypercoagulability, with adverse consequences in individuals at risk of acute coronary events. However, the effects of different kinds of fatty acids may be different (Sanders, 1996). In a 4-week intervention trial on 38 healthy volunteers, a decrease in FVIIc was observed during the consumption of a high-MUFA diet compared with an SFA diet and n-6 PUFA diet (Turpeinen and Mutanen, 1999). The same effect was evidenced in the comparison of specific dietary fatty acids (lauric acid, palmitic acid and oleic acid) in women and men fed with three different diets for 6 weeks (Temme *et al.*, 1999).

Table 4.4 Effects of high monounsaturated fat intake in humans on coagulation factors

Haemostatic parameters	Expected changes
Tissue factor	Reduced expression in mononuclear cells Reduction of Tissue Factor Plasma Inhibitor
Factor VII	Chronic effect: reduction in Factor VII plasma levels Acute effect: less activation after MUFA intake
Factors XII and X	Reduction of Factor XIIc, XIIa and Xc
Fibrinolysis	Reduction in PAI-1 plasma levels

The reducing effect of the MUFA-enriched diet on FVII was also explored by Larsen *et al.* (1999) in a comparative crossover intervention trial. The trial was divided into three different dietary periods: a virgin olive oil-enriched diet, a sunflower oil-enriched diet and a rapeseed oil-enriched diet. There were significant differences between the diets regarding fasting plasma values of FVII protein, FVIIc and activated FVII (FVIIa), compared with baseline diet. These data suggest that MUFA diets favour a less thrombogenic environment. In a recent study 58 healthy students received either a 4-week rapeseed oil, an olive oil or a sunflower oil diet (Table 4.4). With the olive oil diet, a reduction of coagulation factors VIIc, XIIc, XIIa and Xc was found, whereas sunflower oil led to lower values of coagulation factors XIIc, XIIa and Ixc (Junker *et al.*, 2001).

4.5.3 Postprandial coagulation factors

The selective effect of MUFA on postprandial activation of FVII appears to be less evident. A postprandial increase of FVIIa and FVIIc has been observed during the intake of fat with different high-fat meals in normolipaemic and in hypertrygliceridaemic subjects (Oakley *et al.*, 1998; Sanders *et al.*, 1996, 1999; Sanders, 1996). Meals rich in MUFA were shown not to differ from meals rich in PUFA or SFA with regard to acute effects on postprandial plasma FVII (Larsen *et al.*, 1997; Roche and Gibney, 1997). Yet other work describes more pronounced responses of FVIIc to test meals rich in MUFA compared with meals rich in SFA (Oakley *et al.*, 1998; Sanders *et al.*, 1999). However, certain data suggest that the background diet could influence this FVII postprandial activation (Roche *et al.*, 1998).

The potential influence of diets habitually rich in MUFA on postprandial FVII was illustrated by the observation of different postprandial patterns of FVIIc in a cross-cultural study involving northern and southern European males. Again no significant effect of test meal composition was found (SFA *vs* MUFA), but FVIIc was significantly greater 8 h postprandially in northern Europeans than in southern Europeans (Zampelas *et al.*, 1998). In turn, the study by Roche *et al.* (1998), cited earlier, demonstrated significantly lower postprandial FVIIa and FVIIag concentrations after approximately 40% of the dietary SFA was replaced with MUFA in an 8-week crossover dietary intervention study. In a fat test meal conducted on the final day of the three-diet period of the trial, the mean postprandial peak concentrations of FVIIa showed an 18% reduction after a 3-week olive oil dietary period versus a sunflower oil diet and a 15% reduction versus a rapeseed oil diet, with no change in FVIIc (Larsen *et al.*, 1999). However, in a recent study previously described (Smith *et al.*, 2003), the postprandial factor VIIc response was lower than on the high-MUFA diet compared with an SFA-rich diet.

These findings were confirmed recently by Silva *et al.* (2003) who compared two MUFA-rich diets, a moderate-MUFA and a high-MUFA diet. The postprandial increases in FVIIc and FVIIa were 18% and 17% lower respectively on the moderate MUFA diet. Postprandial increases in FVIIc and FVIIa were 50% and 29% lower on the high-MUFA diet, and the area under the postprandial FVIIc response curve was also lower on the high-MUFA diet.

4.5.4 Tissue factor

Tissue factor (TF) is a transmembrane glycoprotein linked to factor VII. The activation and expression of TF in the macrophages have been related to the coagulant activity of the lesion, which favours the development of acute coronary syndrome. *In vitro* studies have revealed that fatty acids can influence lipopolysaccharide (LPS)-induced TF expression in monocytes while PUFA inhibits LPS-induced TF expression in monocytes and macrophages (Tremoli *et al.*, 1994a). This has been confirmed in monocytes of hypertriglyceridaemic patients during the ingestion of n-3 fatty acids (Tremoli *et al.*, 1994b). Moreover, the isocaloric replacement of a SFA diet by a MUFA or a low-fat, high-CHO diet in healthy subjects reduced TF expression in monocytes obtained during the different dietary phases (Bravo-Herrera *et al.*, 2004). Tissue Factor Pathway Inhibitor (TFPI) is an activated factor X-dependent inhibitor of TF-induced coagulation. The main role of TFPI seems to be to inhibit small amounts of TF, which are probably essential for maintaining a normal haemostatic balance. A previous study has shown that TFPI in the plasma of crab-eating monkeys increases notably in response to a high-cholesterol diet (Abumiya *et al.*, 1994).

The effect of diets enriched with fat from different sources was explored by Larsen *et al.* (1999) in a randomized crossover study with three dietary periods: an olive oil-enriched diet, a sunflower oil diet and a rapeseed oil diet. The influence of dietary intervention on TFPI plasma levels was null. In contrast, we have shown more recently that the isocaloric replacement of a palm oil-enriched diet or a low-fat diet by a Mediterranean diet had a reducing effect on plasma TFPI (Perez-Jimenez *et al.*, 1999). Circulating plasma TFPI levels have been found to modulate the activity of the TF-dependent coagulation cascade. Free TFPI presents high anticoagulant activity and its plasma level correlates with unfavourable outcomes in unstable angina. Total TFPI represents mainly the lipid-bound form, which seems to have a poor anticoagulant activity. Total TFPI correlated strongly with LDL-C (Kato, 2002). The decrease in total TFPI plasma levels observed in the study of Perez-Jimenez *et al.* is difficult to interpret. It could reflect a reduction of anticoagulant activity. On the other hand, it has previously been suggested that it may reflect an increase in the protease on the endothelial surface, and TFPI may be a marker of endothelial cell dysfunction. Furthermore, since total TFPI strongly correlated with LDL-C, the decrease of total TFPI levels observed during the high-MUFA diet as compared with the high-SFA diet could be associated with the decrease of LDL-C levels (Morange *et al.*, 2001).

4.5.5 Fibrinolysis

In the stabilization and progress of thrombus, fibrinolysis plays an important role and is regulated by the equilibrium between the tissue plasminogen activator (t-PA) and its strongest natural inhibitor, PAI-1. Few studies have been conducted to determine the influence of dietary factors on fibrinolysis, although certain data suggest its importance in the development of atherothrombosis. Administration of a diet rich in n-3 fatty acids caused an increase in plasma PAI-1 both in healthy individuals and in those with diabetes, suggesting an impairment of fibrinolytic activity (Marckmann *et al.*, 1991; Fumeron *et al.*, 1991).

Studies to investigate the effect of MUFA on fibrinolysis are scarce. We carried out a study on 21 young, healthy male volunteers, who followed two low-fat diets and two high-MUFA diets from incorporating virgin olive oil. The study demonstrated a decrease in plasma PAI-1 levels with both oleic acid-enriched diets. Plasma levels of fibrinogen, thrombin–antithrombin complexes, plasminogen, α_2 antiplasmin and t-PA did not differ significantly among the experimental diets used in this study (Lopez-Segura *et al.*, 1996). The effect of a high-MUFA olive oil-rich diet on PAI-1 has been explored more recently by us with a different experimental design. In an intervention study trial comparing the isocaloric substitution of a SFA-rich diet for a low-fat diet or a high-MUFA Mediterranean diet enriched with olive oil, both cardioprotective diets decreased PAI-1 plasma levels. The reducing effect was higher during the Mediterranean diet (Perez-Jimenez *et al.*, 1999) (Table 4.4).

The positive findings of the Mediterranean diet were confirmed in another intervention trial with a free-living population in Italy, which compared the effects of substituting an urban diet (rich in SFA) for a rural Mediterranean diet. Consumption of the Mediterranean diet induced a decrease in both PAI-1 and F-VII plasma levels in both men and women. Both groups returned to previous plasma levels when changing back to their original diets, suggesting the positive effects of the Mediterranean diet on thrombogenic risk (Avellone *et al.*, 1998). In contrast to the beneficial effects of replacing an SFA diet with a MUFA diet, the comparative effects of two unsaturated fats (one enriched with linoleic acid and the other with oleic acid) demonstrated a similar effect on PAI-1 plasma levels in a two-phase intervention trial with 38 healthy humans (Turpeinen and Mutanen, 1999). Furthermore, Niskanen *et al.* (1997) also failed to demonstrate a decrease in PAI-1 plasma levels with either a MUFA-rich diet or a low-fat diet, in impaired glucose tolerance subjects. On the other hand, contrary to the data indicated on the effects of chronic consumption of different diets on fasting PAI-1 plasma levels, neither the amount nor type of fat during the postprandial state influenced PAI-1, t-PA or D-dimer concentration (Oakley *et al.*, 1998).

In summary, MUFA diets might decrease a prothrombotic environment, modifying different haemostatic components. The high-MUFA diets reduce platelet aggregation by reduction of collagen and ADP-induced aggregability, and by decrease of TXB_2 production. Furthermore, a high-MUFA diet decreases VWF plasma levels, reduces tissue factor expression in mononuclear cells, reduces total Factor VII and PAI-1 plasma levels and induces a lower postprandial activation of Factor VII.

4.6 Blood pressure

Multiple dietary factors influence blood pressure. A positive relationship has been found between blood pressure and salt consumption (Sacks *et al.*, 2001), high intake of SFA (Stamler *et al.*, 1996) and alcohol (Puddey *et al.*, 1987), whereas vegetables and dairy products have a negative influence (Appel *et al.*, 1997). The qualitative effect of different types of fat is less well known. Evidence from observational epidemiological studies and several small trials suggest that supplementation of the diet with n-3 polyunsaturated fatty acid can reduce blood pressure (Appel *et al.*, 1993).

The effects of MUFAs on blood pressure have received scant attention. There are two aspects to consider in regards to the possible relationship between blood pressure and MUFAs. On the one hand, we must consider the specific effects that the consumption of this type of fat can have on blood pressure rates in the population and on the other hand, the possible influence of high MUFA intake on the risks associated with hypertension. Firstly, hypotensive effects of MUFA have been suggested in different epidemiological studies among populations with a high intake of this kind of fat (Keys, 1970; Williams *et al.*, 1987; Rubba *et al.*, 1987; Stamler *et al.*, 1997; Psaltopoulou *et al.*, 2004; Panagiotakos *et al.*, 2003).

Although limited in number, intervention studies that suggest a hypotensive effect when SFA is substituted by MUFA are of special interest. In one of the first studies carried out, it was demonstrated that the isocaloric substitution of a diet rich in SFA by a low-fat, high-CHO diet, or a high MUFA-enriched diet, similarly reduced blood pressure in both men and women (Mensink *et al.*, 1988), and it was confirmed in other studies in healthy subjects (Table 4.1). Moreover, a significant decrease in blood pressure was also observed, when comparing the consumption of a Mediterranean diet with a low-fat diet (Salas *et al.*, 1999). In addition, the multicentre KANWU study, has shown that a moderate shift from SFA to MUFA significantly reduces diastolic blood pressure. On the other hand, a moderate supplementation of long-chain n-3 PUFA for 3 months had no effect on blood pressure (Vessby *et al.*, 2001). A similar hypotensive effect was observed by Rasmussen and coworkers (1993) in type 2 diabetic patients.

The beneficial effects, due to the dietary enrichment with MUFA, contrast with the results of an intervention trial in a small hypertensive population. In this study, a decrease in blood pressure was observed only with a MUFA-rich diet where olive oil was the principal source of MUFA, versus another diet with the same concentration of MUFA but where high-oleic sunflower oil was the source of fatty acids (Ruiz-Gutierrez *et al.*, 1996). The difference in the hypotensive effect was attributed to the non-fat components present in virgin olive oil. However, the small size of the sample population, 16 participants, could limit the interpretation of the results. In one interesting trial, a diet rich in MUFAs lowered systolic and diastolic blood pressure by 8 and 6 mmHg, respectively (Ferrara *et al.*, 2000). This double-blind, randomized crossover study evaluated a possible difference between antihypertensive effects of MUFA (extra-virgin olive oil) and PUFA (sunflower oil). All patients receiving the PUFA diet required antihypertensive treatment, whereas eight of those receiving the MUFA diet needed no drug therapy. In conclusion, a slight reduction in saturated fat intake, along with the use of extra-virgin olive oil, markedly lowers daily antihypertensive dosage requirement, possibly through enhanced nitric oxide levels stimulated by polyphenols (Ferrara *et al.*, 2000).

There are a growing number of studies indicating that antioxidants may be responsible for some of the protective effects of virgin olive oil (Moline *et al.*, 2000; Giugliano, 2000). In concordance with this hypothesis, Perona *et al.* (2004) have suggested that dietary virgin olive oil compared with sunflower oil proved to be helpful in reducing the systolic pressure of treated hypertensive elderly subjects. Recently, Esposito *et al.* (2004) have demonstrated, in a randomized, single blind trial, conducted among 180 patients with the metabolic syndrome, that the consumption of a Mediterranean-style diet was associated with a significant reduction of blood pressure. With this information we are led to believe that diets rich in MUFA may induce a hypotensive effect that is more potent than that observed for in other unsaturated enriched diets. Nevertheless, more intervention trials are needed before we can ascertain to what extent they are beneficial and in which subgroups they would be most effective. The possible mechanisms of the high-MUFA diet on blood pressure are unknown. One possible reason is that the consumption of a high-MUFA diet is associated with improvement of endothelial function and a significant reduction of markers of systemic vascular inflammation, resulting in a vasodilator effect.

4.7 Energy balance

Body fatness is probably the principal modifiable risk factor for the development of diabetes and metabolic syndrome. Traditionally, hypocaloric diets intended for weight loss are high in CHO and low in fat. A common perception is that dietary fat of any kind is fattening, while low-fat diets have slimming properties.

Thus, in spite of the accumulating evidence of the cardiovascular health benefits of diets high in MUFAs, nutrition experts are still reluctant to recommend them as an alternative to low-fat diets. However, as reviewed (Shah and Garg, 1996, Seidell, 1998), there is no evidence of weight gain with high-fat compared with high-CHO diets under isoenergetic conditions. This concept is supported by the results of parallel-design studies that compared high-CHO and high-MUFA energy-restricted diets in obese subjects with (Heilbronn *et al.*, 1999) or without diabetes (Golay *et al.*, 1996; McManus *et al.*, 2001) for outcomes of weight loss and metabolic control. These studies included various sources of MUFA (oleic acid-rich oils and fats, peanuts and tree nuts) in the high-fat diet groups, with between-diet differences in fat content ranging from 15% to 27% of energy. All three studies showed that it was energy restriction, not diet composition, that determined weight loss, which was similar with the two dietary approaches. The study of McManus *et al.* (2001) showed superior long-term participation and adherence, with consequent improvements in weight loss, in the high-fat (35% of energy) group than in the low-fat (20% of energy) one. This was due to the higher palatability of a diet containing daily portions of products that are not traditional 'diet foods', such as olive oil, peanuts, peanut butter and mixed nuts. Two meta-analyses (Yu-Poth *et al.*, 1999; Astrup *et al.*, 2000) compiled data on body weight from randomized, controlled studies that compared *ad libitum* energy diets high in either total fat or CHO on a number of health outcomes in non-obese, non-diabetic subjects. The results favour low-fat diets for weight maintenance in normal-weight individuals or weight loss in the overweight, but a reduction of SFA, not MUFA intake, was the major component of the CHO-for-fat exchange in the studies reviewed.

The long-term outcome, however, of *ad libitum* reduced-fat diets for weight control is dismal (Swinburn *et al.*, 2001), supporting the notion that attaining a permanent change in eating habits related to obesity is a most difficult task. In addition, moderate-fat weight loss (from MUFA) and weight-maintenance diets improve the cardiovascular disease risk profile on the basis of favourable changes in lipids and lipoproteins (Pelkman *et al.*, 2004). At the molecular level, Rodríguez *et al.* (2002) recently demonstrated upregulation of uncoupling protein genes (that is, enhanced mitochondrial fatty acid oxidation and thermogenesis) by olive oil feeding in rat adipose tissue and skeletal muscle. This is important, as increased heat production by specific fatty acids provides a mechanism to improve energy balance by decreasing the efficiency of fat deposition, thus targeting the core of the problem in obesity and diabetes. Studies comparing high-MUFA diets and high-CHO diets with *ad libitum* energy intake are needed to evaluate their efficacy in weight reduction and maintenance of weight loss.

4.8 Carbohydrate metabolism

The primary question under consideration in the current review is whether diets high in carbohydrate (CHO) or unsaturated fatty acids have a more beneficial influence on the metabolism of glucose. Studies examining the effects of modulating total dietary fat and CHO can be difficult to compare because investigators have employed variable end-points, diet composition, duration, methodologies and different design.

For years, the development of type 2 diabetes mellitus, metabolic syndrome and insulin resistance have been found to be related to high caloric intake, especially saturated fatty acids (SFAs), and it is usually associated with excess weight and obesity (Reaven, 2003). For this reason, research in the 1960s, pointed out that a diet higher in CHO (up to 60–70% of total energy), complemented by a reduction in the daily intake of cholesterol and an increase in the consumption of fibre, could be used by people with diabetes. The studies have usually shown that substituting total fat (with high content of SFA) with CHO results in an improvement in mediated-glucose disposal and insulin secretion (Brunzell *et al.*, 1971; O'Dea *et al.*, 1989; Borkman *et al.*, 1991).

The possibility that a diet with a high complex CHO intake might improve glucose metabolic control and lipid profile was of great interest. However, it soon became a concern that these diets could have negative effects on diabetic patients since they could raise the plasma levels of triglycerides and lower HDL cholesterol plasma levels (NIH, 1987). Although the findings were initially thought to be transitory, they were confirmed by several subsequent studies (Garg *et al.*, 1992; Parillo *et al.*, 1992; Blades and Garg, 1995). This led to the belief that CHO intake could favour the appearance of features of insulin resistance syndrome, owing to an increase in CHO intake, which would necessitate higher levels of hormone to maintain glucose homeostasis. Furthermore, recently studies have produced variable results with no consistent detrimental effects of high-CHO diets on insulin sensitivity. Thus, Gerhard *et al.* (2004) have shown, an *ad libitum*, low-fat, high-fibre, high-complex CHO diet resulted in greater weight loss than did a high-MUFA diet, and the former did not increase plasma triglyceride concentrations from baseline or worsen glycaemic control in patients with type 2 diabetes mellitus. However, this result is in contrast to previous reports that low-fat, high-CHO diets may cause deterioration in glycaemic control in type 2 diabetes (Parillo *et al.*, 1992).

Experience with healthy Mediterranean populations, having a low rate of ischaemic coronary heart disease, explains the great interest placed on the study of the effects of MUFA on CHO metabolism. One of the first studies, carried out by Garg *et al.* (1988), showed that feeding type 2 diabetic patients with a high-fat diet enriched in MUFA (50% fat and 33% of calories as MUFA) resulted in a lower insulin requirement, lower plasma glucose concentration and lower triglyceride plasma concentration versus a low-fat, high-CHO diet (60% CHO, 25% fat and 9% as MUFA). Using a similar design, Bonanome *et al.* (1991) failed to demonstrate this improvement. However, different studies since 1995 have confirmed the initial data, showing that MUFA-enriched diets reduce the requirement for insulin and decrease plasma concentration of glucose and insulin. By replacing complex CHO with MUFA in the diet, Parillo *et al.* (1992) found a decrease in plasma triglyceride, postprandial plasma glucose and insulin concentrations, with higher insulin mediated glucose-disposal using the euglycemic hyperinsulinaemic clamp method. Additional studies in people with diabetes have shown lower fasting blood glucose, lower average blood glucose and lower peak blood glucose levels, during a normal meal cycle and 24-h urinary excretion (Rasmussen *et al.*, 1993).

At the end of the 1990s, a meta-analysis of various studies comparing these two approaches to diet therapy, low-fat, high-CHO diet or high-MUFA diet, in patients with type 2 diabetes, revealed that high-MUFA diets improve lipoprotein profiles as well as glycaemic control, while having no effect on fasting insulin and glycated haemoglobin concentration (Garg, 1998) (Table 4.1). Since Garg's meta-analysis, the results of various randomized crossover studies comparing the effect of the two dietary approaches on glycaemic control in diabetic patients have been reported. These studies, carried out by Rodriguez-Villar *et al.* (2000) and Luscombe *et al.* (1999), showed no differences in glycaemic control after a high-CHO diet with fat limited to 23–30% of energy compared with a high-MUFA diet with a total fat content up of 40%. Furthermore, Thomsen *et al.* (1999) have demonstrated that isocaloric diets rich in MUFAs or CHO, respectively, seem to have similar effects on cardiovascular risk factors in persons at high risk of developing type 2 diabetes mellitus. No differences in insulin sensitivity were found in healthy young subjects (Perez-Jimenez *et al.*, 2001) after a high-CHO diet and a high-MUFA diet.

Many aspects of the diet composition have been considered to be important in the modulation of insulin resistance, but in the past years, more attention has been given to the ability of the quality of dietary fat, independent of the total amount, to influence insulin sensitivity and, throughout this, the risk of type 2 diabetes. The fact that a diet rich in CHO is accompanied by an increase in glycaemia and insulin, when compared with the MUFA-enriched diet, may be due to the fact that CHO increases peripheral insulin resistance. However, studies performed on insulin sensitivity, using the euglycaemic, hyperinsulinaemic glucose clamp method, have demonstrated that CHO-enriched diets, compared with MUFA-diets, caused either no change or a decrease in insulin sensitivity in type 2 diabetic patients and in healthy subjects (Garg *et al.*, 1992; Garg, 1994; Berry, 1997; Lichtenstein and Schwab, 2000; Perez-Jimenez *et al.*, 2001). Thus, an alternative explanation for the decrease in insulin requirements, with MUFA diets, is the reduction in glucose availability and, consequently, the needs for insulin. Moreover, in the KANWU study, Vessby *et al.* (2001) showed that a change in the proportions of dietary fatty acid, decreasing SFA and increasing MUFA, improves insulin sensitivity but has no effect on insulin secretion in healthy subjects. In conclusion, with respect to dietary fat composition, diets enriched in SFA may increase insulin resistance, whereas a MUFA-enriched diet appears to improve insulin sensitivity. On the other hand, a high-CHO diet is an adequate alternative for improving glucose metabolism in healthy young men and women.

In summary, there is substantial evidence that in patients with type 2 diabetes mellitus, metabolic syndrome and insulin resistance, diets with a relatively high fat content based on MUFA provide a degree of metabolic control that is similar or even better than that obtained with high-CHO diets.

4.9 MUFA and cardiovascular risk

Diet, and especially its fat content, can have a varying influence upon cardiovascular risk factors and on mechanisms related to the onset and progression of atheroma plaques. The final aim of preventing and treating coronary arteriosclerosis is to reduce the risk of new heart attacks and mortality from them. In spite of this, research studies into the effects of dietary intervention on the clinical course of the disease are few in number and have only provided significant results in secondary prevention of the disease (Brousseau and Schaefer, 2000). Intervention studies researching the preventive effects of the traditional Mediterranean dietary model, i.e. a high concentration of total fat from MUFA, do not exist .

In a trial conducted on patients with coronary heart disease, the effect of a diet rich in *n*-3 alpha-linolenic acid, referred to as the Mediterranean diet, was studied (de Lorgeril *et al.*, 1994). This diet was accompanied by a 70% reduction in cardiovascular risk, much higher than the reduction observed in previous studies with hypolipaemic drugs or other dietary models. However, the above-mentioned study does not establish the beneficial effects of the traditional Mediterranean diet, which is high in fat and MUFA, since the principal modification in the experimental group was not an increase in the concentration of MUFA but rather alpha-linolenic acid.

The most consistent epidemiological evidence in support of the benefits of consuming these fatty acids lies in observational studies, especially the Seven Countries Study (Keys *et al.*, 1986) and the data from the Nurseś Health Study (Hu *et al.*, 1997). In the 15-year death rate in the Seven Countries Study comprising 11 579 men, all coronary heart disease death rates were low in cohorts consuming olive oil as the main fat. In the 14-year follow-up of the population included in the Nurseś Health Study, a 5% increase in energy intake from MUFA, as compared with an equivalent energy intake from SFA, was associated with a relative risk of coronary disease of 0.81 (95% confidence interval, 0.65 to 1.00; $p = 0.05$). The greater protective effect of PUFA was also reported with a relative risk of 0.62 for every 5% increase in energy from PUFA (Hu *et al.*, 1997). There are other controlled epidemiological studies with confounding factors that have confirmed the protective effect of MUFA in different populations (Artaud-Wild *et al.*, 1993; Pietinen *et al.*, 1997). However, this protective effect has not been confirmed by the data from the Framingham Heart Study or other studies (McGee *et al.*, 1984; Posner *et al.*, 1991). This may be due to the lack of control over confounding factors or because there exist other factors, associated with lifestyle or a higher consumption of other nutrients, in subjects and populations with a higher consumption of MUFA-enriched diets.

4.10 Dietary monounsaturated fat and cancer

The great interest during the past several decades on the relationship between diet and cancer derives from the large variations on rates of specific cancer among countries, coupled with the dramatic changes in the incidence of these conditions among populations emigrating to regions with different rates. Mediterranean populations are known to be partially protected against coronary heart disease and certain types of cancers (Trichopoulou and Critselis, 2004; La Vecchia, 2004). Their dietary habits with low intake of saturated and polyunsaturated fats together with the high intake of oleic acid, n-3 fatty acids, fibre and natural antioxidants have been proposed to explain this protection (Bingham and Riboli, 2004).

Previous studies have shown that the switch from a diet high in MUFA to a diet containing a high proportion of SFA may have contributed to the rise in cancer incidences observed in different populations. There is evidence that MUFA have cancer chemoprotective effects. Recently, Bartsch *et al.* (2002) have suggested that molecular pathways to cancer involve multiple genetic changes, whereby extensive oxyradical damage causes mutations in cancer-related genes and leads to a cycle of cell death and regeneration. Besides direct oxidative DNA-damage, nitrogen species and reactive oxygen can induce etheno-DNA adducts mainly via *trans*-4-hydroxy-2-nonenal, generated as the major aldehyde by lipid peroxidation of PUFA. In contrast, previous studies with oleic acid show that the biomarkers for oxidative stress and lipid peroxidation are decreased compared with n-6 PUFA, suggesting a favourable effect in prevention and development of certain cancer types affected by diet. In concordance with this study, Hughes-Fulford *et al.* (2001) have found that the essential fatty acid, linoleic acid, and arachidonic acid stimulate tumour growth while eicosapentaenoic acid and oleic acid inhibit growth of PC-3 human prostate tumour cells *in vitro*.

Analytic epidemiological studies generally fail to detect a positive association of total fat intake with risk of colorectal cancer (Howe *et al.*, 1997). On the other hand, recently, Llor *et al.* (2003) have observed that supplementation with olive oil results in an early down regulation of *cox-2* followed by a decrease in *Bcl-2* expression, important mediators of colorectal cancer development (Willett, 1997; Llor *et al.*, 2003). Thus, olive oil is capable of influencing crucial processes responsible for colorectal cancer development. In concordance with this, Braga *et al.* (1998) have observed that there was some evidence that olive oil decreased the risk of colorectal carcinoma compared with other fat types. It has been suggested in at least three case-control studies conducted in Spain, Italy and Greece, that olive oil, which has a high MUFA content, may be associated with decreased risk of breast cancer (Willett, 1997). An analysis of data from a cohort in Sweden also suggested that MUFA may be associated with decreased risk of breast cancer, although interpretation of the results of this study is complicated by the fact that the major sources of MUFAs in the Swedish diet are also the main sources of SFAs (Wolk *et al.*, 1998). Overall, these observations suggest that a high-MUFA diet may decrease the risk of breast cancer, although more work is necessary before such inferences can be made with confidence.

Emerging data suggest that the strong protective associations reported for olive oil intake in dietary studies may be due to some other protective components. A multinational study carried out by Simonsen *et al.* (1998) in five European centres shows that the protective effect reported for olive oil intake may be due to components contained in the unsaponificable fraction of the oil. Compelling data from *in vitro* and *in vivo* laboratory studies, epidemiological investigations and human clinical trials indicate that antioxidants present in the unsaponificable fraction of olive oil have important effects on cancer chemoprevention and therapy (Stark and Madar, 2002). These compounds may interfere in several of the steps that lead to the development of malignant tumours, including protecting DNA from oxidative damage, inhibiting carcinogen activation and activating carcinogen detoxifying systems. In addition, some studies have reported that antioxidants enhance the apoptosis induced by standard chemotherapeutic agents employed for the management of some cancers (Chinery *et al.*, 1997; Pathak *et al.*, 2002). In summary, this evidence shows that the amount and quality of dietary fat exert a clear influence on the aetiology of cancer.

4.11 Future trends

In recent years the interest in MUFA as the principal source of dietary fat, has focused on the elucidation of its healthy cardiovascular effects, when substituting for the saturated fatty acid, especially effects on the lipid profile but also other biological effects. Furthermore, research is now actively in progress to clarify the comparative effect of this kind of fat, when substituting for complex carbohydrates, on insulin resistance syndrome, obesity and metabolic syndrome. However, in future a number of important questions must be clarified, including the following:

- Human intervention trials to test the effects of MUFA-enriched diets, compared with high-carbohydrate diets, on coronary heart disease, evaluated with clinical end-points. It could also be interesting to test the different effects of diets that provide a low fat content or a high fat content, both with MUFA as the principal source of energy.
- To clarify the comparative healthy effect of MUFA provided by different sources, looking for a potential interaction between different nutrients present in different MUFA-rich foods. An example could be the contrast between MUFA from animal or vegetal sources, or the comparison of oils from different origins, such as olive oil or plant-refined oils, with different micro-nutrient compositions.
- Future studies must focus on uncovering the mechanisms by which a high-MUFA diet exerts its beneficial effects. The application of available func-

tional genomic, proteomic, metabonomic, metabolomic, lipomic platforms and systems biology approaches will facilitate a comprehensive understanding of MUFA health effects. Furthermore, this information, in the context of general population, could provide information to identify those subgroups who might benefit from specific dietary patterns.

- Special effort must be provided by food technology to reduce the proportion of SFA in foods and increase that of MUFA, while avoiding the presence of *trans* fatty acids. This is especially important in the case of the principal fat provider foods, including milk and dairy, meat and tropical fats.

4.12 Sources of further information

- *Prevention of Coronary Heart Disease: Diet, Lifestyle and Risk Factors in the Seven Countries Study*, edited by Daan Kromhout, Alessandro Menotti and Henry Blackburn, 2002, 267 pages. Kluwer Academic Publishers, Norwell, MA.
- *Nutrient-Gene Interactions in Health and Disease*, edited by Naïma Moustaïd-Moussa and Carolyn D. Berdanier, 2001, 472 pages. CRC Press, Boca Raton, FL.
- *Nutritional Health – Strategies for Dietary Prevention*, edited by T Wilson and NJ Temple, 2001, 352 pages. Humana Press Inc, Totowa, NJ.
- *The Mediterranean Diet: Constituents and Health Promotion*, edited by Antonia-Leda Matalas, Antonis Zampelas, Vassilis Stavrinos and Ira Wolinsky, 2001, 389 pages. CRC Press, Boca Raton, FL.
- *Fatty Acids: Physiologic and Behavioral Functions*, edited by David I. Mostofsky, Shlomo Yehuda and Norman Salem, Jr, 2001, 435 pages. Humana Press, Totowa, NJ.
- 'UK Food Standards Agency *cis*-monounsaturated fatty acid workshop report', Sanderson P, Gill JM, Packard CJ, Sanders TA, Vessby B, Williams CM, *Br J Nutr.* 2002; **88**(1): 99–104.
- 'Atherosclerosis – epidemiological studies on the health effects of a Mediterranean diet', Kok FJ, Kromhout D, *Eur J Nutr.* 2004; **43** Suppl 1:I/2–5.
- 'Dietary *cis*-monounsaturated fatty acids and metabolic control in type 2 diabetes', Ros E, *Am J Clin Nutr.* 2003; **78** (3 Suppl): 617S–625S.
- 'The degree of unsaturation of dietary fatty acids and the development of atherosclerosis (review)', Moreno JJ, Mitjavila MT, *J Nutr Biochem.* 2003; **14**(4): 182–95.
- 'Dietary monounsaturated versus polyunsaturated fatty acids: which is really better for protection from coronary heart disease?', Lada AT, Rudel LL, *Curr Opin Lipidol* 2003; **14**(1): 41–6.
- 'Relationship of dietary fat to glucose metabolism', Lichtenstein AH, Schwab US', *Atherosclerosis* 2000; **150**(2): 227–43.
- 'Fatty acid modulation of endothelial activation', De Caterina R, Liao JK, Libby P, *Am J Clin Nutr.* 2000; **71** (1 Suppl): 213S–23S.

4.13 Conclusions

From the previous information we can conclude that the effect of a high intake of MUFAs results in a wide range of health benefits beyond cholesterol, raising great interest in the possible preventive effects of this type of diet on cardiovascular risk. MUFA-enriched diets reduce the requirement for insulin and decrease plasma concentration of glucose and insulin, in type 2 diabetic patients, compared with the effect of high-SFA and low-fat, high-CHO diets. Moreover, certain data show that this dietary model could have a hypotensive effect, similar to that observed with the intake of other unsaturated fat enriched diets. Furthermore, substantial evidence suggests that oleic-enriched LDL are more resistant to oxidative modifications and dietary MUFA could influence different components and functions related with the endothelium. This includes endothelium-dependent vasodilatation and a reduced capacity of oleic-enriched LDL to promote the adhesion and chemotaxis of monocytes. On the other hand, MUFA-enriched diet decreases the prothrombotic environment, modifying platelet adhesion, coagulation and fibrinolysis. Specially relevant is its reducing effect on PAI-1 plasma levels, resulting in an increase in fibrinolytic ratio, t-PA:PAI-1. Finally, certain observational epidemiological studies suggest that a high intake of MUFA is associated with reduced coronary risk and reduced prevalence of cancer, although other dietary and environmental factors could interact, confusing the interpretation of the results.

4.14 Acknowledgements

This work was supported by research grants from the CICYT, the Spanish Ministry of Health (FIS), Fundación Cultural 'Hospital Reina Sofía-Cajasur', Consejerías de Educación, Salud y Agricultura y Pesca, de la Junta de Andalucía, Servicio Andaluz de Salud and Diputación de Córdoba.

4.15 References

ABBEY, M., BELLING, G. B., NOAKES, M., HIRATA, F. and NESTEL, P. J. (1993) Oxidation of low-density lipoproteins: intraindividual variability and the effect of dietary linoleate supplementation *Am J Clin Nutr*, **57** (3), 391–8.

ABIA, R., PACHECO, Y. M., PERONA, J. S., MONTERO, E., MURIANA, F. J. and RUIZ-GUTIERREZ, V. (2001) The metabolic availability of dietary triacylglycerols from two high oleic oils during the postprandial period does not depend on the amount of oleic acid ingested by healthy men *J Nutr*, **131** (1), 59–65.

ABUMIYA, T., NAKAMURA, S., TAKENAKA, A., TAKENAKA, O., YOSHIKUNI, Y., MIYAMOTO, S., KIMURA, T., ENJYOJI, K. and KATO, H. (1994) Response of plasma tissue factor pathway inhibitor to diet-induced hypercholesterolemia in crab-eating monkeys *Arterioscler Thromb*, **14** (3), 483–8.

APPEL, L. J., MILLER, E. R., 3RD, SEIDLER, A. J. and WHELTON, P. K. (1993) Does supplementation of diet with 'fish oil' reduce blood pressure? A meta-analysis of controlled clinical trials *Arch Intern Med*, **153** (12), 1429–38.

APPEL, L. J., MOORE, T. J., OBARZANEK, E., VOLLMER, W. M., SVETKEY, L. P., SACKS, F. M., BRAY, G. A., VOGT, T. M., CUTLER, J. A., WINDHAUSER, M. M., LIN, P. H. and KARANJA, N. (1997) A clinical trial of the effects of dietary patterns on blood pressure. DASH Collaborative Research Group *N Engl J Med*, **336** (16), 1117–24.

ARTAUD-WILD, S. M., CONNOR, S. L., SEXTON, G. and CONNOR, W. E. (1993) Differences in coronary mortality can be explained by differences in cholesterol and saturated fat intakes in 40 countries but not in France and Finland. A paradox *Circulation*, **88** (6), 2771–9.

ASTRUP, A., RYAN, L., GRUNWALD, G. K., STORGAARD, M., SARIS, W., MELANSON, E. and HILL, J.O. (2000) The role of dietary fat in body fatness: evidence from a preliminary meta-analysis of ad libitum low-fat dietary intervention studies *Br J Nutr*, **83** Suppl 1 S25–32.

AVELLONE, G., DI GARBO, V., CORDOVA, R., SCALFFIDI, L. and BOMPIANI, G.D. (1998) Effects of Mediterranean diet on lipid, coagulative and fibrinolytic parameters in two randomly selected population samples in Western Sicily *Nutr Metab Cardiovasc Dis*, **8**, 287–96.

BARONI, S. S., AMELIO, M., SANGIORGI, Z., GADDI, A. and BATTINO, M. (1999) Solid monounsaturated diet lowers LDL unsaturation trait and oxidisability in hypercholesterolemic (type IIb) patients *Free Radic Res*, **30** (4), 275–85.

BARTSCH, H., NAIR, J. and OWEN, R. W. (2002) Exocyclic DNA adducts as oxidative stress markers in colon carcinogenesis: potential role of lipid peroxidation, dietary fat and antioxidants *Biol Chem*, **383** (6), 915–21.

BELLIDO, C., LOPEZ-MIRANDA, J., BLANCO-COLIO, L. M., PEREZ-MARTINEZ, P., MURIANA, F. J., MATIN-VENTURA, J. L., MARIN, C., GOMEZ, P., FUENTES, F., EGIDO, J. and PEREZ JIMENEZ, F. (2004) Butter and walnut, but not olive oil, intake elicits postprandial activation of nuclear transcription factor kB in peripheral blood mononuclear cells from healthy men. *Am J Clin Nutr*, **80** (6), 1487–91.

BERRY, E. M. (1997) Dietary fatty acids in the management of diabetes mellitus *Am J Clin Nutr*, **66** (4 Suppl), 991S–997S.

BERRY, E. M., EISENBERG, S., HARATZ, D., FRIEDLANDER, Y., NORMAN, Y., KAUFMANN, N. A. and STEIN, Y. (1991) Effects of diets rich in monounsaturated fatty acids on plasma lipoproteins – the Jerusalem Nutrition Study: high MUFAs vs high PUFAs *Am J Clin Nutr*, **53** (4), 899–907.

BERRY, E. M., EISENBERG, S., FRIEDLANDER, Y., HARATS, D., KAUFMANN, N. A., NORMAN, Y. and STEIN, Y. (1992) Effects of diets rich in monounsaturated fatty acids on plasma lipoproteins – the Jerusalem Nutrition Study. II. Monounsaturated fatty acids vs carbohydrates *Am J Clin Nutr*, **56** (2), 394–403.

BINGHAM, S. and RIBOLI, E. (2004) Diet and cancer – the European Prospective Investigation into Cancer and Nutrition *Nat Rev Cancer*, **4** (3), 206–15.

BLADES, B. and GARG, A. (1995) Mechanisms of increase in plasma triacylglycerol concentrations as a result of high carbohydrate intakes in patients with non-insulin-dependent diabetes mellitus *Am J Clin Nutr*, **62** (5), 996–1002.

BONANOME, A., VISONA, A., LUSIANI, L., BELTRAMELLO, G., CONFORTIN, L., BIFFANTI, S., SORGATO, F., COSTA, F. and PAGNAN, A. (1991) Carbohydrate and lipid metabolism in patients with non-insulin-dependent diabetes mellitus: effects of a low-fat, high-carbohydrate diet vs a diet high in monounsaturated fatty acids *Am J Clin Nutr*, **54** (3), 586–90.

BONANOME, A., PAGNAN, A., BIFFANTI, S., OPPORTUNO, A., SORGATO, F., DORELLA, M., MAIORINO, M. and URSINI, F. (1992) Effect of dietary monounsaturated and polyunsaturated fatty acids on the susceptibility of plasma low density lipoproteins to oxidative modification *Arterioscler Thromb*, **12** (4), 529–33.

BORKMAN, M., CAMPBELL, L. V., CHISHOLM, D. J. and STORLIEN, L. H. (1991) Comparison of the effects on insulin sensitivity of high carbohydrate and high fat diets in normal subjects *J Clin Endocrinol Metab*, **72** (2), 432–7.

BRAGA, C., LA VECCHIA, C., FRANCESCHI, S., NEGRI, E., PARPINEL, M., DECARLI, A., GIACOSA, A. and TRICHOPOULOS, D. (1998) Olive oil, other seasoning fats, and the risk of colorectal carcinoma *Cancer*, **82** (3), 448–53.

BRAVO-HERRERA, M. D., LOPEZ-MIRANDA, J., MARIN, C., GOMEZ, P., GOMEZ, M. J., MORENO, J. A., PEREZ-MARTINEZ, P., BLANCO, A., JIMENEZ-GOMEZ, Y. and PEREZ-JIMENEZ, F. (2004) Tissue factor expression is decreased in monocytes obtained from blood during Mediterranean or high carbohydrate diets *Nutr Metab Cardiovasc Dis*, **14** (3), 128–32.

BROUSSEAU, M. E. and SCHAEFER, E. J. (2000) Diet and coronary heart disease: clinical trials *Curr Atheroscler Rep*, **2** (6), 487–93.

BRUNZELL, J. D., LERNER, R. L., HAZZARD, W. R., PORTE, D., JR. and BIERMAN, E. L. (1971) Improved glucose tolerance with high carbohydrate feeding in mild diabetes *N Engl J Med*, **284** (10), 521–4.

BRZOSKO, S., DE CURTIS, A., MURZILLI, S., DE GAETANO, G., DONATI, M. B. and IACOVIELLO, L. (2002) Effect of extra virgin olive oil on experimental thrombosis and primary hemostasis in rats *Nutr Metab Cardiovasc Dis*, **12** (6), 337–42.

CARLUCCIO, M. A., MASSARO, M., BONFRATE, C., SICULELLA, L., MAFFIA, M., NICOLARDI, G., DISTANTE, A., STORELLI, C. and DE CATERINA, R. (1999) Oleic acid inhibits endothelial activation: a direct vascular antiatherogenic mechanism of a nutritional component in the Mediterranean diet *Arterioscler Thromb Vasc Biol*, **19** (2), 220–28.

CARUSO, D., BERRA, B., GIAVARINI, F., CORTESI, N., FEDELI, E. and GALLI, G. (1999) Effect of virgin olive oil phenolic compounds on *in vitro* oxidation of human low density lipoproteins *Nutr Metab Cardiovasc Dis*, **9** (3), 102–7.

CASTRO, P., MIRANDA, J. L., GOMEZ, P., ESCALANTE, D. M., SEGURA, F. L., MARTIN, A., FUENTES, F., BLANCO, A., ORDOVAS, J. M. and JIMENEZ, F. P. (2000) Comparison of an oleic acid enriched-diet vs NCEP-I diet on LDL susceptibility to oxidative modifications *Eur J Clin Nutr*, **54** (1), 61–7.

CELERMAJER, D. S. (1997) Endothelial dysfunction: does it matter? Is it reversible? *J Am Coll Cardiol*, **30** (2), 325–33.

CHINERY, R., BROCKMAN, J. A., PEELER, M. O., SHYR, Y., BEAUCHAMP, R. D. and COFFEY, R. J. (1997) Antioxidants enhance the cytotoxicity of chemotherapeutic agents in colorectal cancer: a p53-independent induction of p21WAF1/CIP1 via C/EBPbeta *Nat Med*, **3** (11), 1233–41.

CURB, J. D., WERGOWSKE, G., DOBBS, J. C., ABBOTT, R. D. and HUANG, B. (2000) Serum lipid effects of a high-monounsaturated fat diet based on macadamia nuts *Arch Intern Med*, **160** (8), 1154–8.

DE BRUIN, T. W., BROUWER, C. B., VAN LINDE-SIBENIUS TRIP, M., JANSEN, H. and ERKELENS, D.W. (1993) Different postprandial metabolism of olive oil and soybean oil: a possible mechanism of the high-density lipoprotein conserving effect of olive oil *Am J Clin Nutr*, **58** (4), 477–83.

DE LA CRUZ, J. P., VILLALOBOS, M. A., CARMONA, J. A., MARTIN-ROMERO, M., SMITH-AGREDA, J.

M. and DE LA CUESTA, F. S. (2000) Antithrombotic potential of olive oil administration in rabbits with elevated cholesterol *Thromb Res*, **100** (4), 305–15.

DE LORGERIL, M., RENAUD, S., MAMELLE, N., SALEN, P., MARTIN, J. L., MONJAUD, I., GUIDOLLET, J., TOUBOUL, P. and DELAYE, J. (1994) Mediterranean alpha-linolenic acid-rich diet in secondary prevention of coronary heart disease *Lancet*, **343** (8911), 1454–9.

DREON, D. M., FERNSTROM, H. A., CAMPOS, H., BLANCHE, P., WILLIAMS, P. T. and KRAUSS, R. M. (1998) Change in dietary saturated fat intake is correlated with change in mass of large low-density-lipoprotein particles in men *Am J Clin Nutr*, **67** (5), 828–36.

ESPOSITO, K., MARFELLA, R., CIOTOLA, M., DI PALO, C., GIUGLIANO, F., GIUGLIANO, G., D'ARMIENTO, M., D'ANDREA, F. and GIUGLIANO, D. (2004) Effect of a Mediterranean-style diet on endothelial dysfunction and markers of vascular inflammation in the metabolic syndrome: a randomized trial *JAMA*, **292** (12), 1440—46.

FERRARA, L. A., RAIMONDI, A. S., D'EPISCOPO, L., GUIDA, L., DELLO RUSSO, A. and MAROTTA, T. (2000) Olive oil and reduced need for antihypertensive medications *Arch Intern Med*, **160** (6), 837–42.

FUENTES, F., LOPEZ-MIRANDA, J., SANCHEZ, E., SANCHEZ, F., PAEZ, J., PAZ-ROJAS, E., MARIN, C., GOMEZ, P., JIMENEZ-PEREPEREZ, J., ORDOVAS, J. M. and PEREZ-JIMENEZ, F. (2001) Mediterranean and low-fat diets improve endothelial function in hypercholesterolemic men *Ann Intern Med*, **134** (12), 1115–19.

FUMERON, F., BRIGANT, L., OLLIVIER, V., DE PROST, D., DRISS, F., DARCET, P., BARD, J. M., PARRA, H. J., FRUCHART, J. C. and APFELBAUM, M. (1991) n-3 polyunsaturated fatty acids raise low-density lipoproteins, high-density lipoprotein 2, and plasminogen-activator inhibitor in healthy young men *Am J Clin Nutr*, **54** (1), 118–22.

FUSTER, V., BADIMON, L., BADIMON, J. J. and CHESEBRO, J. H. (1992) The pathogenesis of coronary artery disease and the acute coronary syndromes (1) *N Engl J Med*, **326** (4), 242–50.

GARDNER, C. D. and KRAEMER, H. C. (1995) Monounsaturated versus polyunsaturated dietary fat and serum lipids. A meta-analysis *Arterioscler Thromb Vasc Biol*, **15** (11), 1917–27.

GARG, A. (1994) High-monounsaturated fat diet for diabetic patients. Is it time to change the current dietary recommendations? *Diabetes Care*, **17** (3), 242–6.

GARG, A. (1998) High-monounsaturated-fat diets for patients with diabetes mellitus: a meta-analysis *Am J Clin Nutr*, **67** (3 Suppl), 577S–582S.

GARG, A., BONANOME, A., GRUNDY, S. M., ZHANG, Z. J. and UNGER, R. H. (1988) Comparison of a high-carbohydrate diet with a high-monounsaturated-fat diet in patients with non-insulin-dependent diabetes mellitus *N Engl J Med*, **319** (13), 829–34.

GARG, A., GRUNDY, S. M. and UNGER, R. H. (1992) Comparison of effects of high and low carbohydrate diets on plasma lipoproteins and insulin sensitivity in patients with mild NIDDM *Diabetes*, **41** (10), 1278–85.

GERHARD, G. T., AHMANN, A., MEEUWS, K., MCMURRY, M. P., DUELL, P. B. and CONNOR, W. E. (2004) Effects of a low-fat diet compared with those of a high-monounsaturated fat diet on body weight, plasma lipids and lipoproteins, and glycemic control in type 2 diabetes *Am J Clin Nutr*, **80** (3), 668–73.

GINSBERG, H. N., BARR, S. L., GILBERT, A., KARMALLY, W., DECKELBAUM, R., KAPLAN, K., RAMAKRISHNAN, R., HOLLERAN, S. and DELL, R. B. (1990) Reduction of plasma cholesterol levels in normal men on an American Heart Association Step 1 diet or a Step 1 diet with added monounsaturated fat *N Engl J Med*, **322** (9), 574–9.

GINSBERG, H. N., KARMALLY, W., BARR, S. L., JOHNSON, C., HOLLERAN, S. and RAMAKRISHNAN,

R. (1994) Effects of increasing dietary polyunsaturated fatty acids within the guidelines of the AHA step 1 diet on plasma lipid and lipoprotein levels in normal males *Arterioscler Thromb*, **14** (6), 892–901.

GINSBERG, H. N., KRIS-ETHERTON, P., DENNIS, B., ELMER, P. J., ERSHOW, A., LEFEVRE, M., PEARSON, T., ROHEIM, P., RAMAKRISHNAN, R., REED, R., STEWART, K., STEWART, P., PHILLIPS, K. and ANDERSON, N. (1998) Effects of reducing dietary saturated fatty acids on plasma lipids and lipoproteins in healthy subjects: the DELTA Study, protocol 1 *Arterioscler Thromb Vasc Biol*, **18** (3), 441–9.

GIUGLIANO, D. (2000) Dietary antioxidants for cardiovascular prevention *Nutr Metab Cardiovasc Dis*, **10** (1), 38–44.

GOLAY, A., ALLAZ, A. F., MOREL, Y., DE TONNAC, N., TANKOVA, S. and REAVEN, G. (1996) Similar weight loss with low- or high-carbohydrate diets *Am J Clin Nutr*, **63** (2), 174–8.

GOODE, G. K., GARCIA, S. and HEAGERTY, A. M. (1997) Dietary supplementation with marine fish oil improves *in vitro* small artery endothelial function in hypercholesterolemic patients: a double-blind placebo-controlled study *Circulation*, **96** (9), 2802–7.

GRUNDY, S. M. (1986) Comparison of monounsaturated fatty acids and carbohydrates for lowering plasma cholesterol *N Engl J Med*, **314** (12), 745–8.

GRUNDY, S. M., FLORENTIN, L., NIX, D. and WHELAN, M. F. (1988) Comparison of monounsaturated fatty acids and carbohydrates for reducing raised levels of plasma cholesterol in man *Am J Clin Nutr*, **47** (6), 965–9.

GUMBINER, B., LOW, C. C. and REAVEN, P. D. (1998) Effects of a monounsaturated fatty acid-enriched hypocaloric diet on cardiovascular risk factors in obese patients with type 2 diabetes *Diabetes Care*, **21** (1), 9–15.

HARGROVE, R. L., ETHERTON, T. D., PEARSON, T. A., HARRISON, E. H. and KRIS-ETHERTON, P. M. (2001) Low fat and high monounsaturated fat diets decrease human low density lipoprotein oxidative susceptibility *in vitro J Nutr*, **131** (6), 1758–63.

HARRISON, D. G., ARMSTRONG, M. L., FREIMAN, P. C. and HEISTAD, D. D. (1987) Restoration of endothelium-dependent relaxation by dietary treatment of atherosclerosis *J Clin Invest*, **80** (6), 1808–11.

HEGSTED, D. M., McGANDY, R. B., MYERS, M. L. and STARE, F. J. (1965) Quantitative effects of dietary fat on serum cholesterol in man *Am J Clin Nutr*, **17** (5), 281–95.

HEILBRONN, L. K., NOAKES, M. and CLIFTON, P. M. (1999) Effect of energy restriction, weight loss, and diet composition on plasma lipids and glucose in patients with type 2 diabetes *Diabetes Care*, **22** (6), 889–95.

HOWARD, B. V., HANNAH, J. S., HEISER, C. C., JABLONSKI, K. A., PAIDI, M. C., ALARIF, L., ROBBINS, D. C. and HOWARD, W. J. (1995) Polyunsaturated fatty acids result in greater cholesterol lowering and less triacylglycerol elevation than do monounsaturated fatty acids in a dose–response comparison in a multiracial study group *Am J Clin Nutr*, **62** (2), 392–402.

HOWE, G. R., ARONSON, K. J., BENITO, E., CASTELLETO, R., CORNEE, J., DUFFY, S., GALLAGHER, R. P., ISCOVICH, J. M., DENG-AO, J., KAAKS, R., KUNE, G. A., KUNE, S., LEE, H. P., LEE, M., MILLER, A. B., PETERS, R. K., POTTER, J. D., RIBOLI, E., SLATTERY, M. L., TRICHOPOULOS, D., TUYNS, A., TZONOU, A., WATSON, L. F., WHITTEMORE, A. S., SHU, Z. *et al.* (1997) The relationship between dietary fat intake and risk of colorectal cancer: evidence from the combined analysis of 13 case-control studies *Cancer Causes Control*, **8** (2), 215–28.

HU, F. B., STAMPFER, M. J., MANSON, J. E., RIMM, E., COLDITZ, G. A., ROSNER, B. A., HENNEKENS, C.H. and WILLETT, W. C. (1997) Dietary fat intake and the risk of coronary heart disease in women *N Engl J Med*, **337** (21), 1491–9.

HUGHES-FULFORD, M., CHEN, Y. and TJANDRAWINATA, R. R. (2001) Fatty acid regulates gene expression and growth of human prostate cancer PC-3 cells *Carcinogenesis*, **22** (5), 701–7.

JUNKER, R., KRATZ, M., NEUFELD, M., ERREN, M., NOFER, J. R., SCHULTE, H., NOWAK-GOTTL, U., ASSMANN, G. and WAHRBURG, U. (2001) Effects of diets containing olive oil, sunflower oil, or rapeseed oil on the hemostatic system *Thromb Haemost*, **85** (2), 280–86.

KARANTONIS, H. C., ANTONOPOULOU, S. and DEMOPOULOS, C. A. (2002) Antithrombotic lipid minor constituents from vegetable oils. Comparison between olive oils and others *J Agric Food Chem*, **50** (5), 1150–60.

KATO, H. (2002) Regulation of functions of vascular wall cells by tissue factor pathway inhibitor: basic and clinical aspects *Arterioscler Thromb Vasc Biol*, **22** (4), 539–48.

KEYS, A. (1965) Effects of different dietary fats on plasma-lipid levels *Lancet*, **17** 318–19.

KEYS, A. (1970) Coronary heart disease in seven countries *Circulation*, **41** 1–211.

KEYS, A., MENOTTI, A., KARVONEN, M. J., ARAVANIS, C., BLACKBURN, H., BUZINA, R., DJORDJEVIC, B. S., DONTAS, A. S., FIDANZA, F. and KEYS, M. H. (1986) The diet and 15-year death rate in the seven countries study *Am J Epidemiol*, **124** (6), 903–15.

KNAPP, H. R. (1997) Dietary fatty acids in human thrombosis and hemostasis *Am J Clin Nutr*, **65** (5 Suppl), 1687S–1698S.

KNUIMAN, J. T., WEST, C. E. and HAUTVAST, J. G. (1982) Role of diet to HDL-cholesterol and coronary disease: serum total and HDL-cholesterol in boys and men from developing and developed countries *Am Heart J*, **103** (3), 447–8.

KRAUSS, R. M. (2001) Atherogenic lipoprotein phenotype and diet-gene interactions *J Nutr*, **131** (2), 340S–43S.

KRAUSS, R. M. and DREON, D. M. (1995) Low-density-lipoprotein subclasses and response to a low-fat diet in healthy men *Am J Clin Nutr*, **62** (2), 478S–87S.

KRIS-ETHERTON, P. M. (1999) AHA science advisory: monounsaturated fatty acids and risk of cardiovascular disease *J Nutr*, **129** (12), 2280–84.

KRIS-ETHERTON, P. M., PEARSON, T. A., WAN, Y., HARGROVE, R. L., MORIARTY, K., FISHELL, V. and ETHERTON, T. D. (1999) High-monounsaturated fatty acid diets lower both plasma cholesterol and triacylglycerol concentrations *Am J Clin Nutr*, **70** (6), 1009–15.

LAHOZ, C., ALONSO, R., ORDOVAS, J. M., LOPEZ-FARRE, A., DE OYA, M. and MATA, P. (1997) Effects of dietary fat saturation on eicosanoid production, platelet aggregation and blood pressure *Eur J Clin Invest*, **27** (9), 780–87.

LARSEN, L. F., BLADBJERG, E. M., JESPERSEN, J. and MARCKMANN, P. (1997) Effects of dietary fat quality and quantity on postprandial activation of blood coagulation factor VII *Arterioscler Thromb Vasc Biol*, **17** (11), 2904–9.

LARSEN, L. F., JESPERSEN, J. and MARCKMANN, P. (1999) Are olive oil diets antithrombotic? Diets enriched with olive, rapeseed, or sunflower oil affect postprandial factor VII differently *Am J Clin Nutr*, **70** (6), 976–82.

LA VECCHIA, C. (2004) Mediterranean diet and cancer *Public Health Nutr*, **7** (7), 965–8.

LERNER, R., LINDSTROM, P., BERG, A., JOHANSSON, E., ROSENDAHL, K. and PALMBLAD, J. (1995) Development and characterization of essential fatty acid deficiency in human endothelial cells in culture *Proc Natl Acad Sci USA*, **92** (4), 1147–51.

LICHTENSTEIN, A. H. and SCHWAB, U. S. (2000) Relationship of dietary fat to glucose metabolism *Atherosclerosis*, **150** (2), 227–43.

LICHTENSTEIN, A. H., AUSMAN, L. M., CARRASCO, W., JENNER, J. L., GUALTIERI, L. J., GOLDIN,

B. R., ORDOVAS, J. M. and SCHAEFER, E. J. (1993) Effects of canola, corn, and olive oils on fasting and postprandial plasma lipoproteins in humans as part of a National Cholesterol Education Program Step 2 diet *Arterioscler Thromb*, **13** (10), 1533–42.

LLOR, X., PONS, E., ROCA, A., ALVAREZ, M., MANE, J., FERNANDEZ-BANARES, F. and GASSULL, M. A. (2003) The effects of fish oil, olive oil, oleic acid and linoleic acid on colorectal neoplastic processes *Clin Nutr*, **22** (1), 71–9.

LOPEZ-SEGURA, F., VELASCO, F., LOPEZ-MIRANDA, J., CASTRO, P., LOPEZ-PEDRERA, R., BLANCO, A., JIMENEZ-PEREPEREZ, J., TORRES, A., TRUJILLO, J., ORDOVAS, J. M. and PEREZ-JIMENEZ, F. (1996) Monounsaturated fatty acid-enriched diet decreases plasma plasminogen activator inhibitor type 1 *Arterioscler Thromb Vasc Biol*, **16** (1), 82–8.

LUSCOMBE, N. D., NOAKES, M. and CLIFTON, P. M. (1999) Diets high and low in glycemic index versus high monounsaturated fat diets: effects on glucose and lipid metabolism in NIDDM *Eur J Clin Nutr*, **53** (6), 473–8.

MARCKMANN, P., JESPERSEN, J., LETH, T. and SANDSTROM, B. (1991) Effect of fish diet versus meat diet on blood lipids, coagulation and fibrinolysis in healthy young men *J Intern Med*, **229** (4), 317–23.

MARCKMANN, P., BLADBJERG, E. M. and JESPERSEN, J. (1998) Diet and blood coagulation factor VII – a key protein in arterial thrombosis *Eur J Clin Nutr*, **52** (2), 75–84.

MATA, P., ALVAREZ-SALA, L. A., RUBIO, M. J., NUNO, J. and DE OYA, M. (1992) Effects of long-term monounsaturated- vs polyunsaturated-enriched diets on lipoproteins in healthy men and women *Am J Clin Nutr*, **55** (4), 846–50.

MATA, P., ALONSO, R., LOPEZ-FARRE, A., ORDOVAS, J. M., LAHOZ, C., GARCES, C., CARAMELO, C., CODOCEO, R., BLAZQUEZ, E. and DE OYA, M. (1996) Effect of dietary fat saturation on LDL oxidation and monocyte adhesion to human endothelial cells in vitro *Arterioscler Thromb Vasc Biol*, **16** (11), 1347–55.

MATA, P., VARELA, O., ALONSO, R., LAHOZ, C., DE OYA, M. and BADIMON, L. (1997) Monounsaturated and polyunsaturated n-6 fatty acid-enriched diets modify LDL oxidation and decrease human coronary smooth muscle cell DNA synthesis *Arterioscler Thromb Vasc Biol*, **17** (10), 2088–95.

McGEE, D. L., REED, D. M., YANO, K., KAGAN, A. and TILLOTSON, J. (1984) Ten-year incidence of coronary heart disease in the Honolulu Heart Program. Relationship to nutrient intake *Am J Epidemiol*, **119** (5), 667–76.

McMANUS, K., ANTINORO, L. and SACKS, F. (2001) A randomized controlled trial of a moderate-fat, low-energy diet compared with a low fat, low-energy diet for weight loss in overweight adults *Int J Obes Relat Metab Disord*, **25** (10), 1503–11.

MENNEN, L. I., SCHOUTEN, E. G., GROBBEE, D. E. and KLUFT, C. (1996) Coagulation factor VII, dietary fat and blood lipids: a review *Thromb Haemost*, **76** (4), 492–9.

MENSINK, R. P. and KATAN, M. B. (1987) Effect of monounsaturated fatty acids versus complex carbohydrates on high-density lipoproteins in healthy men and women *Lancet*, **1** (8525), 122–5.

MENSINK, R. P. and KATAN, M. B. (1992) Effect of dietary fatty acids on serum lipids and lipoproteins. A meta-analysis of 27 trials *Arterioscler Thromb*, **12** (8), 911–19.

MENSINK, R. P., JANSSEN, M. C. and KATAN, M. B. (1988) Effect on blood pressure of two diets differing in total fat but not in saturated and polyunsaturated fatty acids in healthy volunteers *Am J Clin Nutr*, **47** (6), 976–80.

MENSINK, R. P., DE GROOT, M. J., VAN DEN BROEKE, L. T., SEVERIJNEN-NOBELS, A. P., DEMACKER, P. N. and KATAN, M. B. (1989) Effects of monounsaturated fatty acids v complex carbohydrates on serum lipoproteins and apoproteins in healthy men and women *Metabolism*, **38** (2), 172–8.

MOLINE, J., BUKHAROVICH, I. F., WOLFF, M. S. and PHILLIPS, R. (2000) Dietary flavonoids and hypertension: is there a link? *Med Hypotheses*, **55** (4), 306–9.

MORANGE, P. E., RENUCCI, J. F., CHARLES, M. A., AILLAUD, M. F., GIRAUD, F., GRIMAUX, M. and JUHAN-VAGUE, I. (2001) Plasma levels of free and total TFPI, relationship with cardiovascular risk factors and endothelial cell markers *Thromb Haemost*, **85** (6), 999–1003.

MORENO, J. A., PEREZ-JIMENEZ, F., MARIN, C., GOMEZ, P., PEREZ-MARTINEZ, P., MORENO, R., BELLIDO, C., FUENTES, F. and LOPEZ-MIRANDA, J. (2004) The effect of dietary fat on LDL size is influenced by apolipoprotein E genotype in healthy subjects *J Nutr*, **134** (10), 2517–22.

MORI, T. A., WATTS, G. F., BURKE, V., HILME, E., PUDDEY, I. B. and BEILIN, L. J. (2000) Differential effects of eicosapentaenoic acid and docosahexaenoic acid on vascular reactivity of the forearm microcirculation in hyperlipidemic, overweight men *Circulation*, **102** (11), 1264–9.

NAVARRO, M. D., HORTELANO, P., PERIAGO, J. L. and PITA, M. L. (1992) Effect of dietary olive and sunflower oils on the lipid composition of the aorta and platelets and on blood eicosanoids in rats *Arterioscler Thromb*, **12** (7), 830–35.

NCEP (2001) Executive Summary of The Third Report of The National Cholesterol Education Program (NCEP) Expert Panel on Detection, Evaluation, And Treatment of High Blood Cholesterol In Adults (Adult Treatment Panel III) *JAMA*, **285** (19), 2486–97.

NIH (1987) Consensus Development Conference on Diet and Exercise in Non-Insulin-Dependent Diabetes Mellitus. National Institutes of Health *Diabetes Care*, **10** (5), 639–44.

NISKANEN, L., SCHWAB, U. S., SARKKINEN, E. S., KRUSIUS, T., VAHTERA, E. and UUSITUPA, M. I. (1997) Effects of dietary fat modification on fibrinogen, factor VII, and plasminogen activator inhibitor-1 activity in subjects with impaired glucose tolerance *Metabolism*, **46** (6), 666–72.

OAKLEY, F. R., SANDERS, T. A. and MILLER, G. J. (1998) Postprandial effects of an oleic acid-rich oil compared with butter on clotting factor VII and fibrinolysis in healthy men *Am J Clin Nutr*, **68** (6), 1202–7.

O'DEA, K., TRAIANEDES, K., IRELAND, P., NIALL, M., SADLER, J., HOPPER, J. and DE LUISE, M. (1989) The effects of diet differing in fat, carbohydrate, and fiber on carbohydrate and lipid metabolism in type II diabetes *J Am Diet Assoc*, **89** (8), 1076–86.

ONG, P. J., DEAN, T. S., HAYWARD, C. S., DELLA MONICA, P. L., SANDERS, T. A. and COLLINS, P. (1999) Effect of fat and carbohydrate consumption on endothelial function *Lancet*, **354** (9196), 2134.

OUBINA, P., SANCHEZ-MUNIZ, F. J., RODENAS, S. and CUESTA, C. (2001) Eicosanoid production, thrombogenic ratio, and serum and LDL peroxides in normo- and hypercholesterolaemic post-menopausal women consuming two oleic acid-rich diets with different content of minor components *Br J Nutr*, **85** (1), 41–7.

PANAGIOTAKOS, D. B., PITSAVOS, C. H., CHRYSOHOOU, C., SKOUMAS, J., PAPADIMITRIOU, L., STEFANADIS, C. and TOUTOUZAS, P. K. (2003) Status and management of hypertension in Greece: role of the adoption of a Mediterranean diet: the Attica study *J Hypertens*, **21** (8), 1483–9.

PARILLO, M., RIVELLESE, A. A., CIARDULLO, A. V., CAPALDO, B., GIACCO, A., GENOVESE, S. and RICCARDI, G. (1992) A high-monounsaturated-fat/low-carbohydrate diet improves peripheral insulin sensitivity in non-insulin-dependent diabetic patients *Metabolism*, **41** (12), 1373–8.

PARTHASARATHY, S., KHOO, J. C., MILLER, E., BARNETT, J., WITZTUM, J. L. and STEINBERG, D. (1990) Low density lipoprotein rich in oleic acid is protected against oxidative modification: implications for dietary prevention of atherosclerosis *Proc Natl Acad Sci USA*, **87** (10), 3894–8.

PATHAK, A. K., SINGH, N., KHANNA, N., REDDY, V. G., PRASAD, K. N. and KOCHUPILLAI, V. (2002) Potentiation of the effect of paclitaxel and carboplatin by antioxidant mixture on human lung cancer h520 cells *J Am Coll Nutr*, **21** (5), 416–21.

PELKMAN, C. L., FISHELL, V. K., MADDOX, D. H., PEARSON, T. A., MAUGER, D. T. and KRIS-ETHERTON, P. M. (2004) Effects of moderate-fat (from monounsaturated fat) and low-fat weight-loss diets on the serum lipid profile in overweight and obese men and women *Am J Clin Nutr*, **79** (2), 204–12.

PEREZ-JIMENEZ, F., ESPINO, A., LOPEZ-SEGURA, F., BLANCO, J., RUIZ-GUTIERREZ, V., PRADA, J. L., LOPEZ-MIRANDA, J., JIMENEZ-PEREPEREZ, J. and ORDOVAS, J. M. (1995) Lipoprotein concentrations in normolipidemic males consuming oleic acid-rich diets from two different sources: olive oil and oleic acid-rich sunflower oil *Am J Clin Nutr*, **62** (4), 769–75.

PEREZ-JIMENEZ, F., CASTRO, P., LOPEZ-MIRANDA, J., PAZ-ROJAS, E., BLANCO, A., LOPEZ-SEGURA, F., VELASCO, F., MARIN, C., FUENTES, F. and ORDOVAS, J. M. (1999) Circulating levels of endothelial function are modulated by dietary monounsaturated fat *Atherosclerosis*, **145** (2), 351–8.

PEREZ-JIMENEZ, F., LOPEZ-MIRANDA, J., PINILLOS, M. D., GOMEZ, P., PAZ-ROJAS, E., MONTILLA, P., MARIN, C., VELASCO, M. J., BLANCO-MOLINA, A., JIMENEZ PEREPEREZ, J. A. and ORDOVAS, J. M. (2001) A Mediterranean and a high-carbohydrate diet improve glucose metabolism in healthy young persons *Diabetologia*, **44** (11), 2038–43.

PERONA, J. S., CANIZARES, J., MONTERO, E., SANCHEZ-DOMINGUEZ, J. M., CATALA, A. and RUIZ-GUTIERREZ, V. (2004) Virgin olive oil reduces blood pressure in hypertensive elderly subjects *Clin Nutr*, **23** (5), 1113–21.

PIETINEN, P., ASCHERIO, A., KORHONEN, P., HARTMAN, A. M., WILLETT, W. C., ALBANES, D. and VIRTAMO, J. (1997) Intake of fatty acids and risk of coronary heart disease in a cohort of Finnish men. The Alpha-Tocopherol, Beta-Carotene Cancer Prevention Study *Am J Epidemiol*, **145** (10), 876–87.

POSNER, B. M., COBB, J. L., BELANGER, A. J., CUPPLES, L. A., D'AGOSTINO, R. B. and STOKES, J., 3RD (1991) Dietary lipid predictors of coronary heart disease in men. The Framingham Study *Arch Intern Med*, **151** (6), 1181–7.

PSALTOPOULOU, T., NASKA, A., ORFANOS, P., TRICHOPOULOS, D., MOUNTOKALAKIS, T. and TRICHOPOULOU, A. (2004) Olive oil, the Mediterranean diet, and arterial blood pressure: the Greek European Prospective Investigation into Cancer and Nutrition (EPIC) study *Am J Clin Nutr*, **80** (4), 1012–18.

PUDDEY, I. B., BEILIN, L. J. and VANDONGEN, R. (1987) Regular alcohol use raises blood pressure in treated hypertensive subjects. A randomised controlled trial *Lancet*, **1** (8534), 647–51.

RAJARAM, S., BURKE, K., CONNELL, B., MYINT, T. and SABATE, J. (2001) A monounsaturated fatty acid-rich pecan-enriched diet favorably alters the serum lipid profile of healthy men and women *J Nutr*, **131** (9), 2275–9.

RASMUSSEN, O. W., THOMSEN, C., HANSEN, K. W., VESTERLUND, M., WINTHER, E. and HERMANSEN, K. (1993) Effects on blood pressure, glucose, and lipid levels of a high-monounsaturated fat diet compared with a high-carbohydrate diet in NIDDM subjects *Diabetes Care*, **16** (12), 1565–71.

RASMUSSEN, O., THOMSEN, C., INGERSLEV, J. and HERMANSEN, K. (1994) Decrease in von

Willebrand factor levels after a high-monounsaturated-fat diet in non-insulin-dependent diabetic subjects *Metabolism*, **43** (11), 1406–9.

REAVEN, G. M. (2003) The insulin resistance syndrome *Curr Atheroscler Rep*, **5** (5), 364–71.

REAVEN, P., PARTHASARATHY, S., GRASSE, B. J., MILLER, E., ALMAZAN, F., MATTSON, F. H., KHOO, J. C., STEINBERG, D. and WITZTUM, J. L. (1991) Feasibility of using an oleate-rich diet to reduce the susceptibility of low-density lipoprotein to oxidative modification in humans *Am J Clin Nutr*, **54** (4), 701–6.

REAVEN, P., PARTHASARATHY, S., GRASSE, B. J., MILLER, E., STEINBERG, D. and WITZTUM, J. L. (1993) Effects of oleate-rich and linoleate-rich diets on the susceptibility of low density lipoprotein to oxidative modification in mildly hypercholesterolemic subjects *J Clin Invest*, **91** (2), 668–76.

REAVEN, P., GRASSE, B. and BARNETT, J. (1996) Effect of antioxidants alone and in combination with monounsaturated fatty acid-enriched diets on lipoprotein oxidation *Arterioscler Thromb Vasc Biol*, **16** (12), 1465–72.

RIVELLESE, A. A., MAFFETTONE, A., VESSBY, B., UUSITUPA, M., HERMANSEN, K., BERGLUND, L., LOUHERANTA, A., MEYER, B. J. and RICCARDI, G. (2003) Effects of dietary saturated, monounsaturated and n-3 fatty acids on fasting lipoproteins, LDL size and post-prandial lipid metabolism in healthy subjects *Atherosclerosis*, **167** (1), 149–58.

ROCHE, H. M. and GIBNEY, M. J. (1997) Postprandial coagulation factor VII activity: the effect of monounsaturated fatty acids *Br J Nutr*, **77** (4), 537–49.

ROCHE, H. M., ZAMPELAS, A., KNAPPER, J. M., WEBB, D., BROOKS, C., JACKSON, K. G., WRIGHT, J. W., GOULD, B. J., KAFATOS, A., GIBNEY, M. J. and WILLIAMS, C. M. (1998) Effect of long-term olive oil dietary intervention on postprandial triacylglycerol and factor VII metabolism *Am J Clin Nutr*, **68** (3), 552–60.

RODRIGUEZ, V. M., PORTILLO, M. P., PICO, C., MACARULLA, M. T. and PALOU, A. (2002) Olive oil feeding up-regulates uncoupling protein genes in rat brown adipose tissue and skeletal muscle *Am J Clin Nutr*, **75** (2), 213–20.

RODRIGUEZ-VILLAR, C., MANZANARES, J. M., CASALS, E., PEREZ-HERAS, A., ZAMBON, D., GOMIS, R. and ROS, E. (2000) High-monounsaturated fat, olive oil-rich diet has effects similar to a high-carbohydrate diet on fasting and postprandial state and metabolic profiles of patients with type 2 diabetes *Metabolism*, **49** (12), 1511–17.

RODRIGUEZ-VILLAR, C., PEREZ-HERAS, A., MERCADE, I., CASALS, E. and ROS, E. (2004) Comparison of a high-carbohydrate and a high-monounsaturated fat, olive oil-rich diet on the susceptibility of LDL to oxidative modification in subjects with Type 2 diabetes mellitus *Diabet Med*, **21** (2), 142–9.

ROSS, R. (1999) Atherosclerosis – an inflammatory disease *N Engl J Med*, **340** (2), 115–26.

RUBBA, P., MANCINI, M., FIDANZA, F., GAUTIERO, G., SALO, M., NIKKARI, T., ELTON, R. and OLIVER, M. F. (1987) Adipose tissue fatty acids and blood pressure in middle-aged men from southern Italy *Int J Epidemiol*, **16** (4), 528–31.

RUIZ-GUTIERREZ, V., MURIANA, F. J., GUERRERO, A., CERT, A. M. and VILLAR, J. (1996) Plasma lipids, erythrocyte membrane lipids and blood pressure of hypertensive women after ingestion of dietary oleic acid from two different sources *J Hypertens*, **14** (12), 1483–90.

RYAN, M., McINERNEY, D., OWENS, D., COLLINS, P., JOHNSON, A. and TOMKIN, G. H. (2000) Diabetes and the Mediterranean diet: a beneficial effect of oleic acid on insulin sensitivity, adipocyte glucose transport and endothelium-dependent vasoreactivity *Qjm*, **93** (2), 85–91.

SACKS, F. M., SVETKEY, L. P., VOLLMER, W. M., APPEL, L. J., BRAY, G. A., HARSHA, D.,

OBARZANEK, E., CONLIN, P. R., MILLER, E. R., 3RD, SIMONS-MORTON, D. G., KARANJA, N. and LIN, P. H. (2001) Effects on blood pressure of reduced dietary sodium and the Dietary Approaches to Stop Hypertension (DASH) diet. DASH – Sodium Collaborative Research Group *N Engl J Med*, **344** (1), 3–10.

SALAS, J., LOPEZ MIRANDA, J., JANSEN, S., ZAMBRANA, J. L., CASTRO, P., PANIAGUA, J. A., BLANCO, A., LOPEZ SEGURA, F., JIMENEZ PEREPEREZ, J. A., PEREZ JIMENEZ, F. and PEREPEREZ, J. A. (1999) The diet rich in monounsaturated fat modifies in a beneficial way carbohydrate metabolism and arterial pressure *Med Clin (Barc)*, **113** (20), 765–9.

SANDERS, T. A. (1996) Effects of unsaturated fatty acids on blood clotting and fibrinolysis *Curr Opin Lipidol*, **7** (1), 20–23.

SANDERS, T. A., MILLER, G. J., DE GRASS, T. and YAHIA, N. (1996) Postprandial activation of coagulant factor VII by long-chain dietary fatty acids *Thromb Haemost*, **76** (3), 369–71.

SANDERS, T. A., DE GRASSI, T., MILLER, G. J. and HUMPHRIES, S. E. (1999) Dietary oleic and palmitic acids and postprandial factor VII in middle-aged men heterozygous and homozygous for factor VII R353Q polymorphism *Am J Clin Nutr*, **69** (2), 220–25.

SCHMIDT, E. B., VARMING, K., ERNST, E., MADSEN, P. and DYERBERG, J. (1990) Dose–response studies on the effect of n-3 polyunsaturated fatty acids on lipids and haemostasis *Thromb Haemost*, **63** (1), 1–5.

SEIDELL, J. C. (1998) Dietary fat and obesity: an epidemiologic perspective *Am J Clin Nutr*, **67** (3 Suppl), 546S–550S.

SHAH, M. and GARG, A. (1996) High-fat and high-carbohydrate diets and energy balance *Diabetes Care*, **19** (10), 1142–52.

SILVA, K. D., KELLY, C. N., JONES, A. E., SMITH, R. D., WOOTTON, S. A., MILLER, G. J. and WILLIAMS, C. M. (2003) Chylomicron particle size and number, factor VII activation and dietary monounsaturated fatty acids *Atherosclerosis*, **166** (1), 73–84.

SIMONSEN, N. R., FERNANDEZ-CREHUET NAVAJAS, J., MARTIN-MORENO, J. M., STRAIN, J. J., HUTTUNEN, J. K., MARTIN, B. C., THAMM, M., KARDINAAL, A. F., VAN'T VEER, P., KOK, F. J. and KOHLMEIER, L. (1998) Tissue stores of individual monounsaturated fatty acids and breast cancer: the EURAMIC study. European Community Multicenter Study on Antioxidants, Myocardial Infarction, and Breast Cancer *Am J Clin Nutr*, **68** (1), 134–41.

SIRTORI, C. R., TREMOLI, E., GATTI, E., MONTANARI, G., SIRTORI, M., COLLI, S., GIANFRANCESCHI, G., MADERNA, P., DENTONE, C. Z. and TESTOLIN, G. (1986) Controlled evaluation of fat intake in the Mediterranean diet: comparative activities of olive oil and corn oil on plasma lipids and platelets in high-risk patients *Am J Clin Nutr*, **44** (5), 635–42.

SMITH, R. D., KELLY, C. N., FIELDING, B. A., HAUTON, D., SILVA, K. D., NYDAHL, M. C., MILLER, G. J. and WILLIAMS, C. M. (2003) Long-term monounsaturated fatty acid diets reduce platelet aggregation in healthy young subjects *Br J Nutr*, **90** (3), 597–606.

STAMLER, J., CAGGIULA, A., GRANDITS, G. A., KJELSBERG, M. and CUTLER, J. A. (1996) Relationship to blood pressure of combinations of dietary macronutrients. Findings of the Multiple Risk Factor Intervention Trial (MRFIT) *Circulation*, **94** (10), 2417–23.

STAMLER, J., CAGGIULA, A. W. and GRANDITS, G. A. (1997) Relation of body mass and alcohol, nutrient, fiber, and caffeine intakes to blood pressure in the special intervention and usual care groups in the Multiple Risk Factor Intervention Trial *Am J Clin Nutr*, **65** (1 Suppl), 338S–365S.

STARK, A. H. and MADAR, Z. (2002) Olive oil as a functional food: epidemiology and nutritional approaches *Nutr Rev*, **60** (6), 170–76.

SWINBURN, B. A., METCALF, P. A. and LEY, S. J. (2001) Long-term (5-year) effects of a reduced-fat diet intervention in individuals with glucose intolerance *Diabetes Care*, **24** (4), 619–24.

TEMME, E. H., MENSINK, R. P. and HORNSTRA, G. (1999) Effects of diets enriched in lauric, palmitic or oleic acids on blood coagulation and fibrinolysis *Thromb Haemost*, **81** (2), 259–63.

THOLSTRUP, T., SANDSTROM, B., BYSTED, A. and HOLMER, G. (2001) Effect of 6 dietary fatty acids on the postprandial lipid profile, plasma fatty acids, lipoprotein lipase, and cholesterol ester transfer activities in healthy young men *Am J Clin Nutr*, **73** (2), 198–208.

THOMSEN, C., RASMUSSEN, O., CHRISTIANSEN, C., PEDERSEN, E., VESTERLUND, M., STORM, H., INGERSLEV, J. and HERMANSEN, K. (1999) Comparison of the effects of a monounsaturated fat diet and a high carbohydrate diet on cardiovascular risk factors in first degree relatives to type-2 diabetic subjects *Eur J Clin Nutr*, **53** (10), 818–23.

TINKER, L. F., PARKS, E. J., BEHR, S. R., SCHNEEMAN, B. O. and DAVIS, P. A. (1999) (n-3) fatty acid supplementation in moderately hypertriglyceridemic adults changes postprandial lipid and apolipoprotein B responses to a standardized test meal *J Nutr*, **129** (6), 1126–34.

TOBOREK, M., LEE, Y. W., GARRIDO, R., KAISER, S. and HENNIG, B. (2002) Unsaturated fatty acids selectively induce an inflammatory environment in human endothelial cells *Am J Clin Nutr*, **75** (1), 119–25.

TOGNA, G. I., TOGNA, A. R., FRANCONI, M., MARRA, C. and GUISO, M. (2003) Olive oil isochromans inhibit human platelet reactivity *J Nutr*, **133** (8), 2532–6.

TREMOLI, E., ELIGINI, S., COLLI, S., MADERNA, P., MARANGONI, F., ANGELI, M. T., SIRTORI, C. R. and GALLI, C. (1994a) Effects of omega 3 fatty acid ethyl esters on monocyte tissue factor expression *World Rev Nutr Diet*, **76**, 55–9.

TREMOLI, E., ELIGINI, S., COLLI, S., MADERNA, P., RISE, P., PAZZUCCONI, F., MARANGONI, F., SIRTORI, C. R. and GALLI, C. (1994b) n-3 fatty acid ethyl ester administration to healthy subjects and to hypertriglyceridemic patients reduces tissue factor activity in adherent monocytes *Arterioscler Thromb*, **14** (10), 1600–608.

TRICHOPOULOU, A. and CRITSELIS, E. (2004) Mediterranean diet and longevity *Eur J Cancer Prev*, **13** (5), 453–6.

TSIMIKAS, S., PHILIS-TSIMIKAS, A., ALEXOPOULOS, S., SIGARI, F., LEE, C. and REAVEN, P. D. (1999) LDL isolated from Greek subjects on a typical diet or from American subjects on an oleate-supplemented diet induces less monocyte chemotaxis and adhesion when exposed to oxidative stress *Arterioscler Thromb Vasc Biol*, **19** (1), 122–30.

TURPEINEN, A. M. and MUTANEN, M. (1999) Similar effects of diets high in oleic or linoleic acids on coagulation and fibrinolytic factors in healthy humans *Nutr Metab Cardiovasc Dis*, **9** (2), 65–72.

VANE, J. R., ANGGARD, E. E. and BOTTING, R. M. (1990) Regulatory functions of the vascular endothelium *N Engl J Med*, **323** (1), 27–36.

VESSBY, B., UNSITUPA, M., HERMANSEN, K., RICCARDI, G., RIVELLESE, A. A., TAPSELL, L. C., NALSEN, C., BERGLUND, L., LOUHERANTA, A., RASMUSSEN, B. M., CALVERT, G. D., MAFFETONE, A., PEDERSEN, E., GUSTAFSSON, I. B. and STORLIEN, L. H. (2001) Substituting dietary saturated for monounsaturated fat impairs insulin sensitivity in healthy men and women: The KANWU Study *Diabetologia*, **44** (3), 312–19.

VOGEL, R. A., CORRETTI, M. C. and PLOTNICK, G. D. (2000) The postprandial effect of components of the Mediterranean diet on endothelial function *J Am Coll Cardiol*,

36 (5), 1455–60.

VOGNILD, E., ELVEVOLL, E. O., BROX, J., OLSEN, R. L., BARSTAD, H., AURSAND, M. and OSTERUD, B. (1998) Effects of dietary marine oils and olive oil on fatty acid composition, platelet membrane fluidity, platelet responses, and serum lipids in healthy humans *Lipids*, **33** (4), 427–36.

WEINTRAUB, M. S., ZECHNER, R., BROWN, A., EISENBERG, S. and BRESLOW, J. L. (1988) Dietary polyunsaturated fats of the W-6 and W-3 series reduce postprandial lipoprotein levels. Chronic and acute effects of fat saturation on postprandial lipoprotein metabolism *J Clin Invest*, **82** (6), 1884–93.

WILLETT, W. C. (1997) Specific fatty acids and risks of breast and prostate cancer: dietary intake *Am J Clin Nutr*, **66** (6 Suppl), 1557S–1563S.

WILLETT, W. C., SACKS, F., TRICHOPOULOU, A., DRESCHER, G., FERRO-LUZZI, A., HELSING, E. and TRICHOPOULOS, D. (1995) Mediterranean diet pyramid: a cultural model for healthy eating *Am J Clin Nutr*, **61** (6 Suppl), 1402S–1406S.

WILLIAMS, C. M. (1998) Dietary interventions affecting chylomicron and chylomicron remnant clearance *Atherosclerosis*, **141** Suppl 1, S87–92.

WILLIAMS, P. T., FORTMANN, S. P., TERRY, R. B., GARAY, S. C., VRANIZAN, K. M., ELLSWORTH, N. and WOOD, P. D. (1987) Associations of dietary fat, regional adiposity, and blood pressure in men *JAMA*, **257** (23), 3251–6.

WISEMAN, S. A., MATHOT, J. N., DE FOUW, N. J. and TIJBURG, L. B. (1996) Dietary non-tocopherol antioxidants present in extra virgin olive oil increase the resistance of low density lipoproteins to oxidation in rabbits *Atherosclerosis*, **120** (1–2), 15–23.

WISEMAN, S. A., TIJBURG, L. B. and VAN DE PUT, F. H. (2002) Olive oil phenolics protect LDL and spare vitamin E in the hamster *Lipids*, **37** (11), 1053–7.

WITZTUM, J. L. and STEINBERG, D. (1991) Role of oxidized low density lipoprotein in atherogenesis *J Clin Invest*, **88** (6), 1785–92.

WOLK, A., BERGSTROM, R., HUNTER, D., WILLETT, W., LJUNG, H., HOLMBERG, L., BERGKVIST, L., BRUCE, A. and ADAMI, H. O. (1998) A prospective study of association of mono-unsaturated fat and other types of fat with risk of breast cancer *Arch Intern Med*, **158** (1), 41–5.

YAQOOB, P., KNAPPER, J. A., WEBB, D. H., WILLIAMS, C. M., NEWSHOLME, E. A. and CALDER, P. C. (1998) Effect of olive oil on immune function in middle-aged men *Am J Clin Nutr*, **67** (1), 129–35.

YU, S., DERR, J., ETHERTON, T. D. and KRIS-ETHERTON, P. M. (1995) Plasma cholesterol-predictive equations demonstrate that stearic acid is neutral and monounsaturated fatty acids are hypocholesterolemic *Am J Clin Nutr*, **61** (5), 1129–39.

YU-POTH, S., ZHAO, G., ETHERTON, T., NAGLAK, M., JONNALAGADDA, S. and KRIS-ETHERTON, P.M. (1999) Effects of the National Cholesterol Education Program's Step I and Step II dietary intervention programs on cardiovascular disease risk factors: a meta-analysis *Am J Clin Nutr*, **69** (4), 632–46.

ZAMBON, A., SARTORE, G., PASSERA, D., FRANCINI-PESENTI, F., BASSI, A., BASSO, C., ZAMBON, S., MANZATO, E. and CREPALDI, G. (1999) Effects of hypocaloric dietary treatment enriched in oleic acid on LDL and HDL subclass distribution in mildly obese women *J Intern Med*, **246** (2), 191–201.

ZAMPELAS, A., ROCHE, H., KNAPPER, J. M., JACKSON, K. G., TORNARITIS, M., HATZIS, C., GIBNEY, M. J., KAFATOS, A., GOULD, B. J., WRIGHT, J. and WILLIAMS, C. M. (1998) Differences in postprandial lipaemic response between Northern and Southern Europeans *Atherosclerosis*, **139** (1), 83–93.

5

Health benefits of polyunsaturated fatty acids (PUFAs)

A. M. Minihane and J. A. Lovegrove, University of Reading, UK

5.1 Introduction

Recent FAO (2004) data, based on food production, import and export figures indicates that total fat contributes an average of 35.3% of total energy intake across the 25 EU member states, with a range of 26.5–41.7%. Owing to a general unavailability of reliable food survey data, the contribution of polyunsaturated fatty acids (PUFAs) to total fat intake in Europe is difficult to assess. In the UK, data derived from the recent National Diet and Nutrition Survey of UK adults (2003) indicate that PUFA constitutes 18% of total fat intake and contributes 6.4% (n-6 PUFA 5.4%, n-3 PUFA 1.0%) of total dietary energy, with long chain n-3 PUFA intakes of 0.1 g/day representing only 0.1%. PUFAs play diverse roles in human nutrition. Two PUFAs, namely linoleic acid and α-linolenic acid, cannot be synthesised in mammalian tissues and are therefore essential macronutrients. Lack of these essential fatty acids in animals leads to typical scaling of the skin, growth retardation and impaired reproduction (Burr and Mildred, 1929). Similar skin symptoms have been described in human infants fed artificial milk formula and in patients on long-term intravenous nutrition, but essential fatty acid deficiency is rarely observed in humans consuming mixed diets.

Essential and non-essential PUFAs are integral components of cell membrane phospholipids, and serve as precursors to a group of hormone-like inflammatory mediators, called the eicosanoids. Furthermore recent research has demonstrated the ability of the long chain PUFA to regulate cell metabolism at the nuclear level by acting as modulators of a range of transcription factors. This impact on gene regulation is thought to provide in part the metabolic link between dietary PUFA intake, health and the progression of chronic diseases.

5.2 Polyunsaturated fatty acid structure, dietary sources and biosynthesis

5.2.1 PUFA structure

Polyunsaturated fatty acids are hydrocarbon chains containing two or more double bonds. The characterisation of PUFAs as either an n-3 PUFA or n-6 PUFA refers to the position of the first double bond relative to the methyl end of the fatty acid. In nature, double bonds are usually in the *cis* (bent) format. However, approximately 2–5% of the fatty acids present in ruminant milk and meat and 5–20% in hydrogenated oils are in the *trans* (straight) orientation. Figure 5.1 depicts a typical PUFA structure, with Table 5.1 listing the main PUFAs in the diet and biological tissues.

A further subclass of PUFAs is the conjugated linoleic acids (CLA). CLAs are a group of 18-carbon PUFA isomers, which lack a methyl group between adjacent double bonds, with 80–90% of dietary CLA present as the *cis*-9 *trans*-11 isomer (c9, t11 CLA). Dairy products are the principal source of these PUFAs, with intakes of only 0.1–0.2 g per day. The issue of the role of CLA in human health and in the development of chronic disease is the subject of Chapter 8 and will therefore not form part of the current chapter.

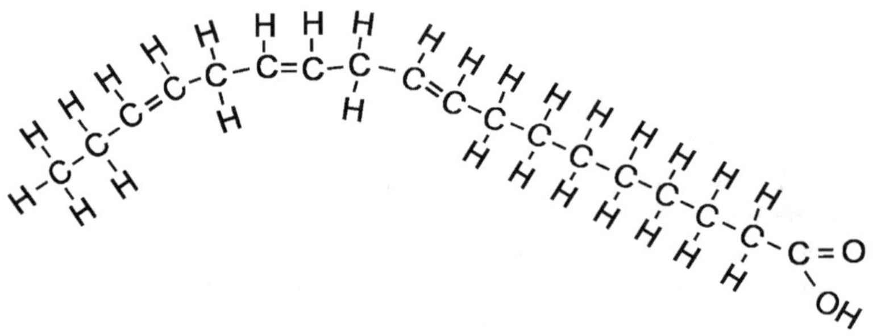

Linoleic acid C18:3 (n-3) – 2 *cis* double bonds

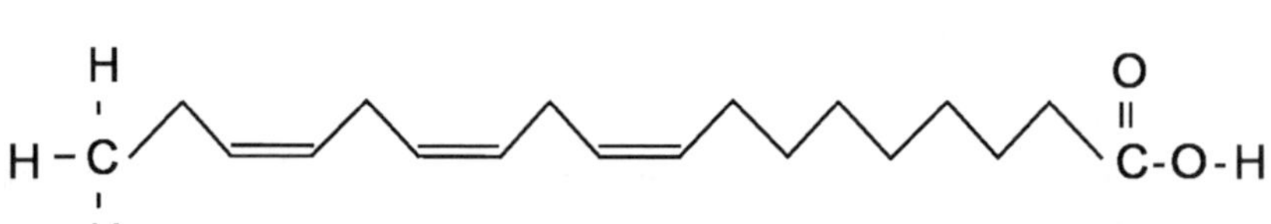

Simple linear representation of linoleic acid

Fig. 5.1 Diagram of the structure of a polyunsaturated fatty acid (PUFA).

Table 5.1 Principal polyunsaturated acids (PUFAs) in foods and biological tissues

Fatty acid	Structural title	Commonly used abbreviation
Linoleic acid	C18:2-*cis* (n-6)	LA
α-linolenic acid	C18:3-*cis* (n-3)	ALNA
γ-linolenic acid	C18:3-*cis* (n-6)	GLA
Arachidonic	C20:4-*cis* (n-6)	AA
Eicosapentaenoic acid	C20:5-*cis* (n-3)	EPA
Docosapentaenoic acid	C22:5-*cis* (n-3)	DPA
Docosahexaenoic acid	C22:6-cis (n-3)	DHA

5.2.2 Polyunsaturated fatty acid content of oil sources

Table 5.2 gives the fatty acid composition of common oil sources. As can be seen the seed oils are rich in PUFAs, with commonly consumed sunflower oil and soybean oil containing approximately 60% of total fatty acids as PUFA. The ratio of n-6:n-3 PUFA varies considerably depending on the oil source with rapeseed oil and soybean oil being relatively rich in n-3 PUFA, and oils such as sunflower oil containing predominantly n-6 PUFA. Oily fish represent the richest dietary source of the long chain (LC) n-3 PUFA, eicosapentaenoic acid (EPA) and docosahexaenoic acid (DHA), with a small contribution from meats. However, it is likely that genetic engineering will provide a vegetable oil source within the next 10 years (Chapter 20). Fatty acid composition, in addition to being an important determinant of the 'health' properties of any individual fat source, has major impacts on the physical properties of fat in foodstuffs. Over the last 30–40 years the hydrogenation of oils such as soybean oil, has been a widely used process by the food industry, to produce a more solid fat source, with lower susceptibility to oxidation and therefore an extended shelf-life. However, as indicated in Table 5.2, industrial hydrogenation can increase the *trans* fatty acid content of the product by 10–20 fold. With the realisation of the deleterious impact of *trans* fatty acids (TFAs) on disease pathology, there has been a major focus on reducing the TFA in processed foods (see Chapter 21).

5.2.3 Long chain (LC) PUFA biosynthesis

Linoleic (LA, C18:2, n-6) and α-linolenic (ALNA, C18:3, n-3) acids are the precursors for the n-6 and n-3 fatty acid families respectively, and are considered essential fatty acids as the mammalian body does not contain the desaturase enzymes (Δ12 and Δ15 desaturases respectively) to insert double bonds beyond the C9 position. Therefore a dietary supply is necessary. It is estimated that human requirements for these fatty acids are 1% and 0.2% of daily energy intake (Department of Health, 1994). As can be seen from Fig. 5.2, both the n-6 and n-3 fatty acid precursors use the same enzymes to coordinate the elongation and desaturation into their longer chain products arachidonic acid (AA) and EPA respectively, a process which occurs predominantly in the liver.

Table 5.2 The fatty acid profile of selected commercially available vegetable oils[1]

Food	SFA	C12:0–C16:0	MUFA	PUFA	n-6 PUFA	n-3 PUFA	TFA
Coconut	86.5	70.4	6.0	1.5	1.5	0	tr
Cottonseed	26.1	23.2	18.3	50.2	50.1	0.1	< 1.0
Groundnut (peanut)	20.0	10.9	44.4	31.0	31.0	0	< 1.0
Olive	14.3	10.1	73.0	8.2	7.5	0.7	< 1.0
Palm	47.8	42.8	37.1	10.4	10.1	0.3	tr
Rapeseed	6.6	4.2	59.2	29.3	19.7	9.6	< 1.0
Sesame	14.6	8.6	37.5	43.4	43.1	0.3	< 1.0
Soybean	15.6	10.8	21.2	58.8	51.5	7.3	< 1.0
Sunflower	12.0	6.3	20.5	63.3	63.2	0.1	< 1.0
Commercial fish oils	24.6	19.8	28.6	41.7	0.6	41.6	1.0
Lard	40.6	25.8	43.0	9.8	9.2	0.5	tr
Palm olein	45.1	41.4	42.3	9.6	9.5	0.1	< 1
Partially hydrogenated rapeseed	11.5	5.0	79	8.3	8.0	0.3	19
Partially hydrogenated soybean	16	8.7	50	32	30.1	1.9	20
High oleic (HO) sunflower[2]	10	3.4	81	9	9	0.1	< 1
High oleic (HO) rapeseed[3]	7.0	3.7	77.3	15.3	8	0.3	tr

1. The values given in the table are average values, with the fatty acid profile of the native oils varying depending on a number of factors, including climate, geography, state of ripeness, etc. and species of fish and season for fish oils. For the hydrogenated oils, the fatty acid composition of the end product can vary greatly depending on the hydrogenation conditions
2. Trisun
3. Natreon
SFA, saturated fatty acids; MUFA, monounsaturated fatty acids; PUFA, polyunsaturated fatty acids; TFA, *trans* fatty acids

In the majority of European countries the dietary intake of LA is several fold higher than the intake of ALNA. There has been speculation that this may favour the n-6 biosynthetic pathway and arachidonic acid (AA) production, which has been suggested to adversely impact on whole body inflammation and coagulation. However, there is still considerable uncertainty regarding the impact of the dietary n-6:n-3 PUFA ratio on the biosynthetic pathways of the longer chain PUFAs.

5.3 Metabolism of fatty acids

5.3.1 Cellular metabolism of fatty acids

On reaching their target tissue, fatty acids transported in the bloodstream within lipoproteins or bound to albumin gain access to cells by a receptor-driven saturable process. Although specific receptors and transporters have not as yet

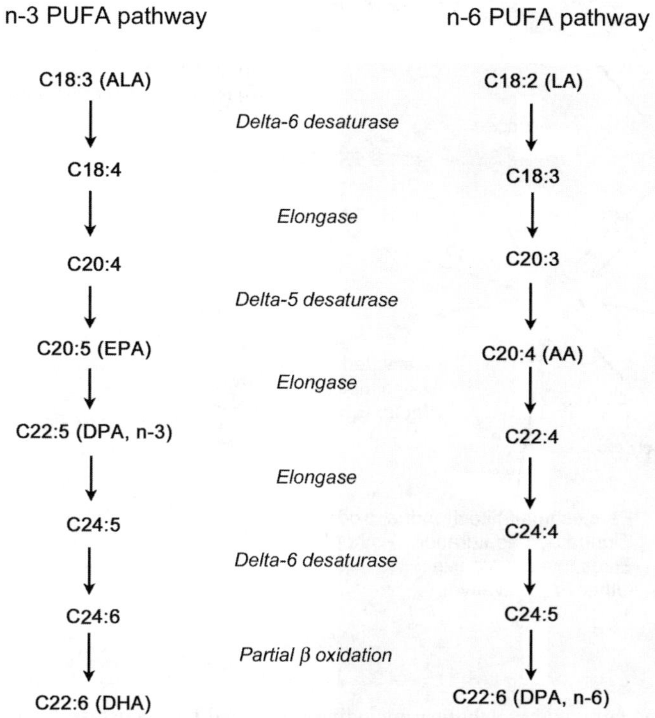

Fig. 5.2 Long chain polyunsaturated fatty acid (LC-PUFA) biosynthetic pathways (*ALA, alpha-linolenic acid: EPA, eicosapentaenoic acid: DPA, docosapentaenoic acid: DHA, docosahexaenoic acid: LA, linoleic acid: AA, arachidonic acid*).

been fully characterised, it is thought that an albumin receptor and one or more fatty acid transporters (FAT) may be involved (Berk and Stump, 1999; Motojima *et al.*, 1998). The fatty acids are metabolised into fatty acyl-CoA-thioesters (FA-CoA) and transported intracellularly bound to fatty acid binding proteins (FABPs) where the FA have a number of potential metabolic fates (Fig. 5.3) including:

- cellular energy production via peroxisomal or mitochondrial β-oxidation;
- incorporated into membrane lipids such as phospholipids or sphingolipids. The chain length and degree of unsaturation of the fatty acids within the bilayer has a large impact on the physical properties of the membrane, altering membrane fluidity and therefore function;
- re-esterified into triglycerides – in adipose tissue, TG stored in fat droplets serves as a fatty acid reserve;
- elongated and/or desaturated to form other fatty acids as per Fig. 5.2 above;
- metabolised into cell signalling lipid derivatives such as eicosanoids (section 5.3.2);

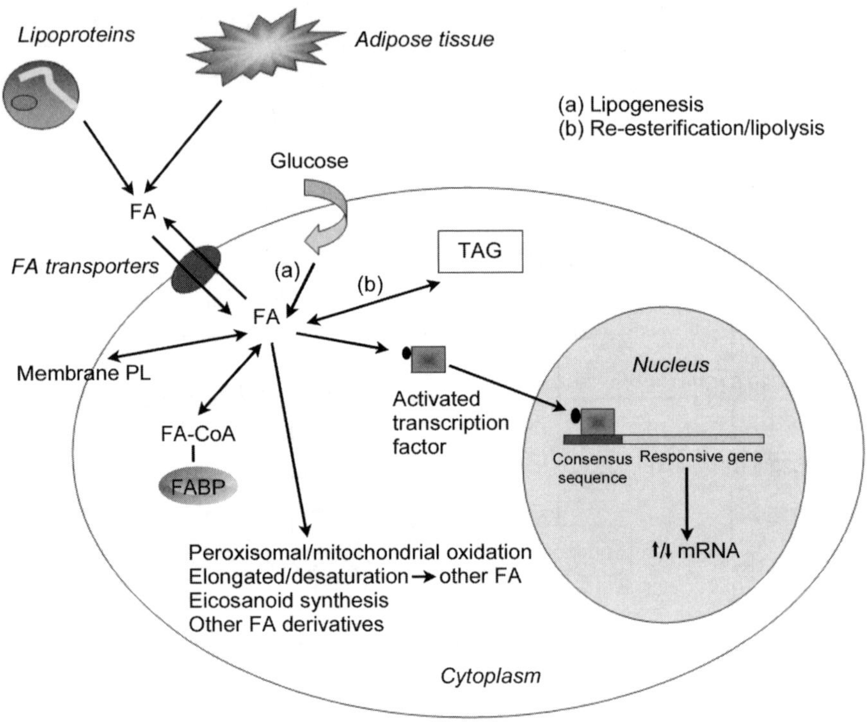

Fig. 5.3 Cellular fatty acid metabolism including postulated mechanisms of action on gene expression (*FA, fatty acid: PL, phospholipids: TAG, triglycerides: FABP, fatty acid binding protein: FA-CoA, fatty acyl-CoA*).

- serve as a ligand for transcription factors which subsequently translocate to the nucleus and impact on the expression of target genes (Section 5.3.3).

5.3.2 Fatty acids in cell signalling

A variety of fatty acid derivatives such as inositol phospholipids and the sphingolipid second messenger serve to convert extracellular signals into intracellular responses. Furthermore membrane PUFA, in particular the C20 and C22 PUFAs, are the precursors of a variety of hormone-like compounds known collectively as eicosanoids (Fig. 5.3). These locally acting, rapidly metabolised compounds mediate a variety of cellular functions including smooth muscle contraction/vascular reactivity, platelet aggregation and coagulation, inflammation, leukocyte adhesion and chemotaxis (Fig. 5.4). A full understanding of the range of eicosanoids produced and their cellular mechanism of action is currently lacking.

The main precursor for the synthesis of eicosanoids is arachidonic acid (c20:4,n-6), which is released from membrane phospholipids by phospholipase A, following an appropriate stimulus and metabolised by lipoxygenases or by cyclooxygenase, as illustrated in Fig. 5.4. Metabolism by lipoxygenases gives

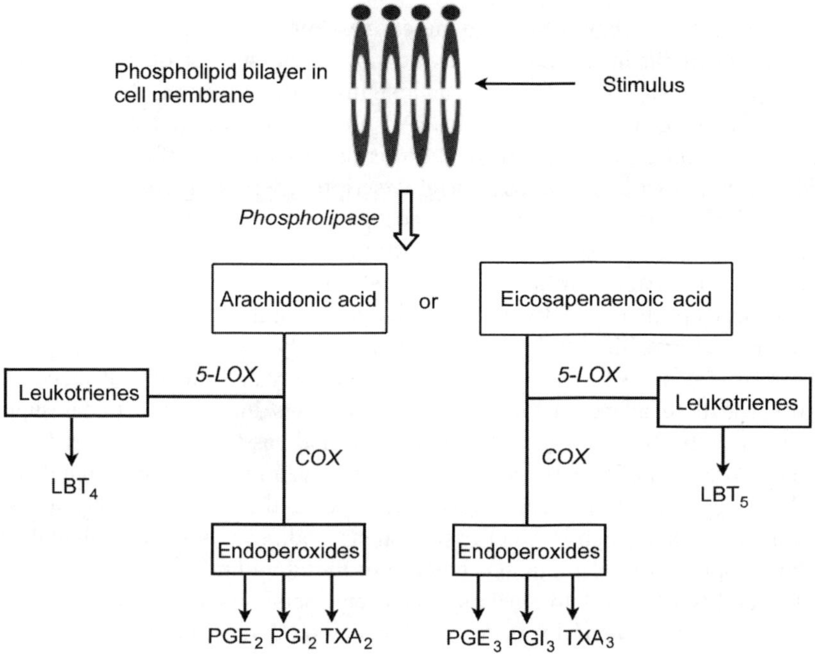

Fig. 5.4 Oxidative metabolism of arachidonic acid and eicosapentaenoic acid producing the eicosanoids which include the prostaglandins, prostacyclins, thromboxanes and leukotrienes (*PGE, prostaglandins: PGI, prostacyclins: TXA, thromboxanes: LBT, leukotrienes: COX, cyclooxygenase: LOX, lipoxygenase*).

rise to leukotrienes, lipoxins and hydroxy fatty acids, while metabolism by cyclooxygenase gives rise to prostaglandins, thromboxanes and prostacyclins.

Although arachidonic acid is regarded as the main precursor of eicosanoids, a separate family of eicosanoids is derived from the 20-carbon n-3 polyunsaturated fatty acid, EPA (Fig. 5.4). EPA incorporated into biological membranes can replace arachidonic acid to some degree. This has two consequences. First, the replacement of arachidonic acid in the membranes of eicosanoid-synthesising cells by EPA results in a decrease in the production of arachidonic acid-derived eicosanoids. Second, there appears to be production of selected EPA-derived eicosanoids.

The physiological significance of the n-3 polyunsaturated fatty acid-derived eicosanoids is of considerable interest, but is relatively poorly understood. Some studies have demonstrated that the EPA-derived eicosanoids are less potent than those derived from arachidonic acid. For example, leukotriene C_4, derived from arachidonic acid, is a chemotactic factor with approximately 10-fold higher activity than leukotriene C_5, which is derived from EPA (Lewis *et al.*, 1986). This impact on eicosanoid metabolism has formed the basis of suggestions that the LC n-3 polyunsaturated fatty acids possess anti-inflammatory and immunomodulatory properties (Section 5.7).

5.3.3 Fatty acid regulation of gene expression

The impact of fat intake on gene expression is the subject of more extensive discussion in Chapter 3. However, as a significant proportion of the impact of PUFAs, and in particular n-3 PUFA, on lipoprotein and adipose tissue metabolism and on endothelial function, is due to a direct effect of these fatty acids on gene expression rates, a brief description will be given here.

In order to maintain cellular homeostasis and in order to be adaptive to extracellular events, expression of the 30 000 genes that encode for all cellular proteins needs to be carefully orchestrated. Over the past 30–40 years it has become evident that the fatty acid composition within the cell, and in particular the PUFA composition, either directly or indirectly regulates the expression of numerous genes. As this is reflective of whole body and dietary fat intake, this allows a cell to adapt its transcriptional processes in response to fat supply. Research in this area is in its relative infancy, and has for the most part focused on the expression of hepatic genes directly involved in fatty acid metabolism or lipid transport as lipoproteins. However, data on the ability of fatty acids to module gene expression in other tissues such as adipose tissue, endothelial cells and macrophages is beginning to emerge in the literature.

The ability of PUFA to alter macronutrient metabolism was first recognised over 35 years ago, when it was observed that a diet deficient in LA enhanced the concentration of a number of lipogenic enzymes (Allman and Gibson, 1969). A large number of subsequent studies have verified these earlier findings with a range of dietary PUFAs and in particular the LC n-3 PUFAs, EPA and DHA, shown to suppress lipogenesis by increasing peroxisomal β-oxidation gene expression and inhibiting the concentration of enzymes involved in glucose metabolism and fatty acid biosynthesis such as fatty acid synthetase (FAS), glucose 6 phosphate dehydrogenase (G6PDH), L-pyruvate kinase (L-PK), glucose transporter-4 and more recently Δ-5 and Δ-6 desaturase (Cho *et al.*, 1999; Clarke, 2001; Duplus *et al.*, 2000; Forest *et al.*, 1997, Power *et al.*, 1997; Wahle *et al.*, 2003). In adipose tissue, PUFA content has been shown to alter adipocyte maturation (adipogenesis), lipid uptake (lipogenesis) and adipokines, with knock-on effects on adipose tissue mass and topography, fuel partitioning, insulin sensitivity and appetite control (Chambrier *et al.*, 2002; Sampath and Ntambi, 2004).

Peroxisome proliferator-activated receptors (PPARs)

Early work failed to identify the molecular targets responsible for the effect of PUFAs on modulation of gene transcription and translation. The cloning of the peroxisome proliferator activating receptors (PPARs) in 1990 (Issemann and Green, 1990), led to the discovery in 1992 (Auwerx, 1992), that this group of nuclear receptors provided one of the mechanisms whereby PUFA co-ordinately suppressed genes involved in lipid biosynthesis.

Similar to other nuclear receptors PPARs possess both a ligand and DNA binding domain (Hihi *et al.*, 2002; Jump and Clark, 1999; Wahle *et al.*, 2003). Upon activation by ligands, PPARs translocate to the nucleus and bind to a specific DNA sequence, referred to as a PPAR-response element (PPRE) in the promoter region of target genes, resulting in an up- or down- regulation of gene expression.

The PPAR family consists of three specific receptors, PPARα, PPARδ and PPARγ which differ in their tissue distribution and ligand specificity. PPARα is known to exert its effect mainly in liver and muscle cells where it is centrally involved in glucose and fat homeostasis. PPARγ modulates gene expression in tumour and adipose tissue. In adipose tissue PPARγ activation is associated with adipocyte maturation and lipid storage as triglycerides. Both PPARα and PPARγ are expressed in the arterial wall by both endothelial cells and macrophages, and their activation in these tissues inhibits the expression of inflammatory genes and induces the expression of genes involved in cholesterol efflux from macrophages such as apoE and the *ABCA1* genes (Beisiegel *et al.*, 2003). PPARδ appears to be expressed in a variety of tissues. However its specific role is not currently understood.

The n-3 PUFAs, in particular EPA and DHA, are thought to be more potent than the n-6 PUFA as activators of PPARα (Clarke, 2001; Power and Newsholme, 1997). Although not as yet fully understood, it is thought that an array of PUFA derivatives, including specific eicosanoids and oxidised lipids such as 8S-hydroxyeicosatetraenoic acid, bind PPARα with one or two orders of magnitude higher affinity than the native fatty acids and are therefore far more potent activators of PPARα-dependent genes (Krey *et al.*, 1997).

Alternative transcription factors

Although PPARs were originally thought of as the mediator of all the PUFA effects on gene expression, evidence quickly emerged to suggest that other transcription factors may be involved. PUFAs are known to suppress hepatic lipogenesis and the expression of the lipogenic S14 and FAS genes *in vivo* or in hepatocytes derived from PPAR$\alpha^{-/-}$ mice (Sessler and Ntambi, 1998). Furthermore the expression of PPAR-α in the human liver is relatively low (Palmer *et al.*, 1998). Although research in this area is at present incomplete, it is likely that a large proportion of the impact of PUFA on gene expression is due to more recently identified and studied transcription factors including, sterol regulatory element-binding protein (SREBP), hepatocyte nuclear factor 4 (HNF-4), nuclear factor-Y (NF-Y) and nuclear factor κB (NF-κB).

5.4 Cardiovascular disease

On average cardiovascular disease, which includes cardiovascular disease and stroke, accounts for about half of total mortality in Europe, 55% of deaths in women and 43% in men, with the ratios of cardiovascular to total mortality varying from 35% to 60% between western and eastern Europe (British Heart Foundation, 2000).

5.4.1 Overview of dietary fat and cardiovascular risk

Dietary fat composition is a major modifiable factor contributing to a range of physiological processes involved in disease pathology such as lipoprotein metabolism, endothelial dysfunction, plaque structure, vascular reactivity and blood pressure, insulin sensitivity and adipose tissue metabolism and topography.

In the 1960s epidemiological evidence linking a high saturated fat (SFA) and low PUFA content of the diet with elevated circulating total cholesterol (TC) and low-density lipoprotein cholesterol (LDL-C) led to recommendations for the replacing of SFA with PUFA as a public health strategy to reduce the population burden of CVD (Hegsted *et al.*, 1965; Keys *et al.*, 1965). Over the past 50 years there have been enormous advances in our understanding of the pathophysiology of disease and its association to dietary fat composition.

A relatively recently recognised risk factor for CHD is an elevated level of circulating triglycerides (TG) in both the fasted and fed (postprandial) state (Alberti and Zimmet, 1998; Patsch *et al.*, 1992; Steinberg *et al.*, 1996b). In addition to TG-rich lipoprotein directly sequestering lipid into the developing atherosclerotic plaque (Rapp *et al.*, 1994), and impacting on endothelial and platelet function, high levels of TG affect the atherogenicity of other lipoproteins, resulting in a reduction in HDL cholesterol levels and an increase in the proportion of LDL as the atherogenic LDL-3 particle. This combined dyslipidaemia of elevated TG, low HDL-C and a high proportion of LDL-3 is referred to as an 'atherogenic lipoprotein phenotype' and it is the dyslipidaemia commonly observed in diabetics and those with the metabolic syndrome (Austin *et al.*, 1990). With the worldwide incidence of diabetes expected to increase from 150 million to 300 million between 2000 and 2025, the prevalence of ALP, which is associated with a two- or threefold increased CHD risk (Griffin *et al.*, 1994), is rapidly increasing. As will be discussed in Section 5.4.3 high-dose long chain n-3 PUFA provides an effective hypotriglyceridaemic agent with potencies comparable to pharmacological treatments, such as fibrates.

5.4.2 Long chain n-3 PUFA and CHD mortality

Evidence for the ability of the LC n-3 PUFAs to reduce risk of CHD initially emerged from the Greenland Inuits where death from acute myocardial infarction was several fold lower than age- and sex-matched Danes (Dyerberg, 1982), despite a high total fat intake. These findings were attributed to a high intake of LC n-3 PUFA of 5–15 g/day, consumed as seal and whale meat rich in EPA and DHA (Kromhout *et al.*, 1985). Since these early findings there has been extensive cohort and prospective epidemiological evidence from studies such as the *Zupthen Study* (Kromhout *et al.*, 1985), *Multiple Risk Factor Intervention Trial* (Dolecek, 1992), *US Physicians' Health Study* (Albert *et al.*, 1998) and the *Nurses' Health Study* (Hu *et al.*, 2002) linking high fish and LC n-3 PUFA intake with reduced risk of CHD and fatal and non-fatal MI. For example, in the case-control analysis among apparently healthy men who were followed for up to 17 years in the *Physicians' Health Study,* the adjusted relative risk (RR) of sudden death was 0.19 in the lowest versus the highest quartile of blood LC n-3 PUFA (Albert *et al.*, 2002). However, some inconsistencies in the literature do exist, with Ascherio and coworkers in a 6-year follow-up of 45 000 healthy males, noting no difference in risk of CHD between those who consumed one or two portions of fish per week versus those who consumed five or six (Ascherio *et al.*, 1995).

Three secondary prevention trials have generally confirmed an association between increased LC n-3 PUFA intake and reduced acute coronary mortality (Burr *et al.*, 1989; GISSI, 1999; R. B. Singh *et al.*, 1997). The largest of these trials conducted among 11 324 Italian post-MI males reported a 45% decrease from sudden cardiac death and a 20% reduction in all cause mortality in the LC n-3 PUFA intervention group (850 mg of LC n-3 PUFA per day), with no significant impact on MI incidence observed (GISSI, 1999). However, this study also reported the little publicised increase in the mortality from strokes in the n-3 PUFA group, possibly due to an increase in haemorrhagic strokes. In the diet and reinfarction trial (DART) LC n-3 PUFA intakes of 0.8 g/day resulted in 29% fewer total deaths in the 2-year follow-up period (Burr *et al.*, 1989), with no impact on reinfarction rates. In both of these studies where participant intakes of EPA + DHA were < 1 g/day, no impact on MI was evident. Increased post-MI survival was attributed to the anti-arrhythmic action of EPA and DHA in heart muscle tissue, resulting in a reduction in ischaemia-induced fibrillation (irregular and rapid heart beat). This anti-arrhythmic action has subsequently been repeatedly observed in animal models and cultured cardiomyocytes (Leaf and Xiao, 2001; Nair *et al.*, 1997). However, the most recently published prospective study, does not agree with the findings of the earlier studies (Burr *et al.*, 2003). In this study, 3114 men with angina were studied prospectively for up to ten years. The consumption of two portions of oily fish per week, or an equivalent amount consumed as fish oil capsules resulted in hazard ratios of 1.26 and 1.54 for cardiac death and sudden cardiac death.

In addition to an impact on post-MI survival, LC n-3 PUFAs may have a positive effect on the pathological process which leads to CVD, i.e. atherosclerosis, as summarised in Table 5.3. A large number of intervention studies examining the benefit of fish oil fatty acids on CHD risk markers have focused on lipoprotein metabolism and thrombosis as the primary outcomes. Generally these studies have fed large doses of EPA + DHA (3–4 g/day, equivalent to one or two portions of oily fish/day) for relatively short intervention periods. Intervention trials using more modest realistic EPA + DHA intakes are needed.

5.4.3 Long chain n-3 PUFA intake and CHD risk markers

LC n-3 PUFA and triglyceride metabolism

One of the principal benefits of dietary LC n-3 PUFA is its ability to reduce fasting and postprandial (non-fasting) plasma TG concentrations, in both healthy (Schmidt *et al.*, 1990) and hyperlipidaemic patients (Harris *et al.*, 1991;

Table 5.3 Potential mechanisms whereby long chain n-3 PUFAs may protect against cardiovascular risk

- Anti-arrhythmic
- ↓ Thrombosis
- ↓ Platelet aggregation
- Anti-inflammatory by ↓ production of inflammatory eicosanoids and cytokines
- ↓ Production of adhesion molecules and chemoattractants
- ↓ Smooth muscle proliferation
- Modest ↓ blood pressure
- ↑ NO production
- ↑ Endothelial induced vasodilatation
- ↓ Fasting and postprandial triglyceride levels
- ↑ Plaque stability

Minihane *et al.*, 2000; Roche and Gibney, 2000) at intakes of > 3 g LC n-3 PUFA per day. For example, in the study by Minihane *et al.* (2000), the consumption of fish oils providing 3 g EPA + DHA/day reduced fasting and postprandial TG levels by 35% and 23% with an associated 26% reduction in the % LDL as LDL-3. However, studies testing doses of LC n-3 PUFA of less than 2.5 g/day have reported less consistent findings. Lovegrove and colleagues (Brady *et al.*, 2004; Lovegrove *et al.*, 2004) reported a significant reduction in fasting plasma TG after supplementation with 2.5 g/day LC n-3 PUFA in Caucasian and British Asian groups, which supported data by Indu and Ghafoorunissa (1992). In contrast other studies have failed to demonstrate a hypotrigylceridaemic effect at this level of intake (Conquer and Holub, 1998; Higgins *et al.*, 2001; Lovegrove *et al.*, 1997; Sorensen *et al.*, 1998).

Although most studies have fed fish oils containing EPA + DHA simultaneously, a limited number examining the differential effect of EPA and DHA has observed that both fatty acids have hypotrigylceridaemic properties with DHA being more potent than EPA (Buckley *et al.*, 2004; Hansen *et al.*, 1998; Mori *et al.*, 2000a).

A number of mechanisms are thought to be responsible for the TG lowering, including an increased rate of β-oxidation and reduced lipogenesis in the liver, increased lipoprotein lipase (Khan *et al.*, 2002) and apoE (Buckley *et al.*, 2004) and reduced apoC3 expressions, effects in large part mediated through the impact of the LC n-3 PUFA on transcription factor activity.

LC n-3 PUFA and other physiological risk factors of coronary heart disease

Within the micro-environment of the artery wall, fish oil fatty acids are thought to have numerous anti-atherogenic effects. Although some inconsistencies exist in the literature, these fatty acids have been shown to reduce chemoattractant and adhesion molecule expression on endothelial cells, thereby reducing leukocyte and smooth muscle migration into the arterial intima (Calder, 2004; Miles *et al.*, 2001; Wallace *et al.*, 1995). Increased tissue levels are also associated with a localised anti-inflammatory effects mediated by a decreased cytokine synthesis, a shift in eicosanoid synthesis towards the less potent EPA derivatives (Fig. 5.4) and an increased endothelial NO production (Okuda *et al.*, 1997). This impact on NO synthesis is thought to be in part responsible for the positive impact of LC n-3 PUFA supplementation on vascular reactivity reported in human volunteers (Khan *et al.*, 2003; Mori *et al.*, 2000a). For example, in a study conducted by Khan *et al.*, (2003), tuna oil supplementation for 8 months (1.7 g EPA + DHA/day) resulted in a significant 12% reduction in vascular reactivity in adults. Increased NO levels are also thought in part to explain the positive impact of fish oils on platelet aggregation and thrombosis which have been frequently observed at intake of EPA/DHA of > 2 g/day (Connor and Connor, 1997; Kristensen *et al.*, 2001). However, the shift in eicosanoid from the potent promoter of aggregation thromboxane A2 (TXA_2) towards the weaker EPA derived pro-aggregator TXA_3 may make a significant contribution (Calder and Grimble, 2002; Mantzioris *et al.*, 2000; von Schacky and Weber, 1985).

Although the protective effect of EPA + DHA against acute cardiovascular events has been attributed to its anti-arrhythmic action, the ability of these fatty acids to improve plaque stability and therefore reduce the likelihood of plaque rupture has also been suggested (Calder, 2004; Thies *et al.*, 2003). In a recent intervention study the provision of 1.4 g EPA + DHA per day for a supplementation period of 7–189 days (median 42) resulted in reduced inflammation and thin fibrous cap incidence and decreased macrophage infiltration in the carotid artery, events which would contribute to plaque stability (Thies *et al.*, 2003).

5.4.5 α-linolenic acid and CHD risk

With a general lack of acceptability of oily fish, ever-reducing worldwide fish oils stocks, and the technological challenges of fortifying commonly consumed food with unsaturated EPA/DHA, there has been recent research interest in the CVD benefits of α-linolenic acid as a source of endogenously synthesised EPA and DHA (as previous discussed in Section 5.2.3). In the Lyon secondary prevention trial the substantial reduction in coronary events and death in subjects following a Mediterranean-style diet was attributed to the inclusion of an α-linolenic acid-rich margarine, although it is likely that the increased fish, reduced meat, increased fibre and fruit and vegetable intake advice contributed to the observed benefits (de Lorgeril *et al.*, 1994). Two prospective observational studies reported a protective effect of increased dietary ALNA intake on the relative risk from fatal CHD (Ascherio *et al.*, 1996; Hu *et al.*, 1999). However, intervention studies investigating the individual impact of α-linolenic acid on CHD risk factors have in general failed to observe a benefit (Bemelmans *et al.*, 2002; Finnegan *et al.*, 2003a,b). For example, the consumption of 4.5 or 9.5 g α-linolenic acid/day for 6 months showed little benefit on lipoprotein metabolism, markers of thrombosis, inflammation or immune cell function in UK adults (Finnegan *et al.*, 2003a,b). An explanation for this lack of effect is that the endogenous biological conversion of dietary ALNA to LC n-3 PUFAs is relatively inefficient, with conversion ratios of α-linolenic acid into

EPA of approximately 7:1 on a molar basis (Burdge *et al.*, 2003; Emken *et al.*, 1994; Finnegan *et al.*, 2003a), and subsequent conversion to DHA almost negligible (Emken *et al.*, 1994; Finnegan *et al.*, 2003b; Vermunt *et al.*, 2000).

5.4.5 n-6 PUFA and CHD risk

Most research on n-6 PUFA and CHD risk has highlighted the benefit of n-6 PUFA on the blood cholesterol profiles when it replaces saturated fat in the diet (Gardner and Kraemer, 1995; Keys, 1970; Mensink and Katan, 1992) (see Chapter 1). Furthermore a high meal n-6 PUFA versus saturated fat content is associated with enhanced postprandial triglyceride clearance (Jackson *et al.*, 2002; Juhel *et al.*, 1999; Weintraub *et al.*, 1988; Zampelas *et al.*, 1994a). Intakes of n-6 PUFA intakes > 10% dietary energy are not recommended as it is associated with a decrease in HDL-cholesterol levels

Although there have been numerous studies investigating the significance of the n-6:n-3 PUFA ratio of the diet on blood lipid profiles, few effects of realistic alterations in this ratio have been reported (Brady *et al.*, 2004; Gronn *et al.*, 1991). Although data are currently lacking, it is likely that the ratio of these two PUFA families may well be important in relation to other risk factors, such as inflammation and coagulation, where the predominance of the linoleic to arachidonic acid biosynthetic pathway may result in a more pro-aggregatory, pro-inflammatory eicosanoid profile (Section 5.7).

5.4.6 PUFA intake and oxidative stress

A potential deleterious effect of increased intake of dietary unsaturated PUFAs, in particular EPA and DHA which contain five and six double bonds respectively, is an increase in whole body oxidative stress. PUFA oxidation leads to increased lipid peroxides and aldehyde breakdown products, which can lead to localised damage to cell membranes, protein or nucleic acids (DNA) (Alexander-North *et al.*, 1994). Data from human intervention studies investigating the effect of EPA + DHA supplementation (1–5 g/day) have reported increased thiobarbituric acid-reactive substances (TBARs), conjugated dienes and LDL oxidation and a decrease of antioxidant vitamins (Brown and Wahle, 1990; D'Aquino *et al.*, 1991; Kubo *et al.*, 1997; Leigh-Firbank *et al.*, 2002; Palozza *et al.*, 1996) although a limited number of studies have reported no effect (Frankel *et al.*, 1994; Nenseter *et al.*, 1992).

The consequential effect on CHD risk of an increased oxidative stress afforded by increased LC n-3 PUFA intake is, however, unclear. It is known that oxidative stress-associated free radicals and reactive oxygen and nitrogen species are integrally involved in almost all stages of atherogenesis included endothelial damage, inflammatory responses LDL oxidation and smooth muscle proliferation and migration (Glass and Witztum, 2001). In contrast, lipid peroxidation of other metabolic derivatives of EPA + DHA have been shown to be more potent ligands for the PPAR family of transcription factors than their parent fatty acids (Section 5.3.3) (Krey *et al.*, 1997). Furthermore the potential of increased LC n-3 PUFA to increase whole body lipid peroxidation may be counterbalanced by the reported positive impact of these fatty acids on glutathione peroxidase (GPx) activity and/or gene expression (Crosby *et al.*, 1996; Lemaitre *et al.*, 1997; Venkatraman *et al.*, 1994). Further clarification is needed.

5.5 Insulin resistance

Hepatic and systemic insulin resistance is considered to be the central biochemical defect of diabetes and the metabolic syndrome. Studies in cell culture, animal models and humans have consistently demonstrated that high dietary and membrane saturated fat is associated with a loss of insulin sensitivity and reduced tissue glucose disposal (Feskens *et al.*, 1995; Rivellese, 2000; Vessby, 2003).

Animal studies have consistently demonstrated improvements in insulin action following LC n-3 PUFA (Behme, 1996; D'Alessandro *et al.*, 2002) with EPA + DHA being shown in part to reverse the adverse effects of saturated fats (Alsaif and Duwaihy, 2004; Storlien *et al.*, 1996). However, many of the studies have used extreme EPA + DHA intakes which would not be achievable by dietary means in humans. Postulated mechanisms for these putative beneficial effects on insulin action include alterations in cell membrane composition and fluidity impacting on insulin receptor affinity and improved glucose transport into cells via glucose transporters (Lovejoy, 2002; Vessby *et al.*, 2000). In addition LC n-3 PUFA may elicit their insulin-sensitising effects via activation of transcription factors, such as PPARγ in adipose tissue (section 5.3.3).

Prospective studies in humans have also suggested a protective effect of fish intake on insulin resistance (Feskens *et al.*, 1991). However, results from relatively short-term intervention studies in diabetic, obese, hypertensive, hyperlipidaemeic and 'healthy' volunteers have proved disappointing (Brady *et al.*, 2004; Eritsland *et al.*, 1994; Fasching *et al.*, 1991; Toft *et al.*, 1995; Vessby *et al.*, 2001). In contrast, in the KANWU study Vessby and colleagues (2001) noted that the substitution of saturated fat with MUFA for three months had a significant impact on insulin action in healthy volunteers, with no added benefit associated with the supplementation of 2.6 g EPA + DHA/day for three months. Similarly Lovegrove and colleagues observed no change in insulin sensitivity in healthy Caucasian and Indian Asian volunteers following exposure to a fish oil supplement providing 2.5 g of EPA + DHA per day (Brady *et al.*, 2004; Lovegrove *et al.*, 2004). Furthermore the investigators observed no impact of the n-6:n-3 PUFA ratio of the diet (9 or 16) on membrane EPA/DHA incorporation or insulin action in the study groups (Minihane *et al.*, 2005).

The impact of n-6 PUFA and α-linolenic acid on insulin action have been less well studied relative to EPA + DHA. High saturated fat and low linoleic acid concentrations have been consistently observed in the serum cholesterol esters of newly diagnosed type 2 diabetics (Vessby, 2000). Intervention studies feeding linseed oil, rapeseed and corn oil have to date failed to demonstrate a benefit of n-6 PUFAs or the short chain n-3 PUFA on insulin sensitivity and/or glucose disposal (Fasching *et al.*, 1996; McManus *et al.*, 1996; Toft *et al.*, 1995; Vessby *et al.*, 2000).

5.6 Colorectal cancer

The majority of evidence to date indicates dietary fat intake may be an important modulator of colorectal cancer development and progression. Evidence for a link with cancer at other sites is weaker and will not be considered here.

Colorectal cancer is the second most common cancer in Western societies and its incidence shows regular increases of between 3% and 7% annually. According to the latest estimates, worldwide an estimated one million cases of colorectal cancer are diagnosed annually (Globocan, 2001) mostly in industrialised countries (IARC, 2000) and it is estimated that over a third of cases are associated with factors relating to the Western diet. Both the type and amount of fat consumed have been linked to colorectal cancer aetiology.

5.6.1 Long chain n-3 PUFA and cancer

Epidemiological studies reveal a significantly lower incidence of colorectal cancer in Greenland Eskimo and Japanese populations following their traditional diet characteristically high in n-3 PUFA (Anti *et al.*, 1992; Bingham, 1998). Most population-based human studies show little or no association between more modest n-3 PUFA intakes and colorectal cancer, although limited data on short-term biomarker studies in humans suggest high fish oil intake could offer some protection (Dommels *et al.*, 2002). In a recent meta-analysis, increased levels of tissue EPA were reported to protect against colorectal cancer, whereas the evidence for DHA, ALNA and n-6:n-3 PUFA ratio were unconvincing (Nkondjock *et al.*, 2003). Limited intervention data are available on n-3 PUFA and human cancer development. However a high dose of n-3 PUFA (4.1 g of EPA and 3.6 g DHA per day) given to patients with sporadic adenomatous colorectal polyps reported a significant reduction in the percentage of cells in the S-phase in the upper crypt of the rectal mucosa (Anti *et al.*, 1992). Results from animal studies indicate that the incidence of chemically induced colon tumours or growth of transplanted mice and human tumours in mice is significantly lower in those animals fed fish oil enriched diets compared to saturated and vegetable oil-enriched diets (Rao *et al.*, 2001; Singh *et al.*, 1988). However, the high doses of EPA + DHA and the model used make extrapolation to humans difficult. Although the data are encouraging, more research is required to determine the effects of LC n-3 PUFA intake on colorectal cancer prevention and progression before recommendations can be made for n-3 PUFA use in the treatment of cancer.

5.6.2 Possible mechanisms of LC n-3 PUFA and colorectal cancer

The available evidence of the mechanisms of action of LC n-3 PUFA and reduction on colorectal cancer indicate that they act at the initiation and the post-initiation phase (Roynette *et al.*, 2004). These include intralumenal effects such as reducing the production of reactive and genotoxic secondary bile acids (Rao *et al.*, 1996) and indirectly modulating the enzyme orthnithine decarboxylase, which is responsible for the production of colonic carcinogenic polyamines, by reducing bile salt levels intraluminally (Rao and Reddy, 1993). Intracellular factors are also believed to have a significant impact on the reduction afforded by LC n-3 PUFA ingestion. Arachidonic acid-derived prostaglandins (2-series, PGE_2) are considered as colon tumour promoters and n-3 PUFA modulation of their synthesis has been reported (Calder *et al.*, 1998; Rao *et al.*, 1996). In addition, DHA has been shown to inhibit the inducible isoform of nitric oxide synthetase (iNOS), believed to be a tumour promoter, in Caco-3 cells (Narayanan *et al.*, 2003). Furthermore, LC n-3 PUFA modulate Ras protein expression and activity by reducing the intracellular Ras levels which interfere with the post-translational modification necessary for membrane binding and activity, effecting malignant transformation (Collett *et al.*, 2001; Davidson *et al.*, 2000). LC n-3 PUFA can also promote apoptosis by a number of different mechanisms, including modulation of proteins involved with apoptosis (Davidson *et al.*, 2000) and by reducing the activity of COX-2, which inhibits apoptosis (Singh *et al.*, 1997). In addition the modulatory effects of n-3 PUFA on the immune system could also have a beneficial impact on carcinogenesis.

5.6.3 n-6 PUFA and cancer

There is evidence that the effect of the n-6 PUFA class in relation to cancer development have an opposing effect to n-3 PUFA in animal and cell studies. Nkondjonk reported that tissue and dietary AA might be associated with an increased risk, whereas evidence for other n-6 PUFA, such as LA, was not convincing (Nkondjock *et al.*, 2003). In addition, data from the 24 European countries study reported a high dietary n-6:n-3 PUFA ratio was a risk factor for colon cancer (Caygill & Hill, 1995). There is also supportive evidence in short-term biomarker studies in humans reporting n-6 PUFA supplementation may increase risk of colorectal carcinogenesis (Dommels *et al.*, 2002). Results from animal models indicate that n-6 PUFA have a tumour-enhancing effect (Singh *et al.*, 1997; Rao *et al.*, 2001). However, the *in vitro* data are inconclusive.

Possible mechanisms of n-6 PUFA action have been hypothesised to be predominantly during the post-initiation phase. Prostaglandins, specifically the 2-series (PGE_2), are considered as colon tumour promoters derived from the n-6 PUFA, AA (Sheng *et al.*, 1998).

5.6.4 Cachexia

Cachexia, the catabolic state that develops in the late stages of most cancers, is associated with depletion of adipose tissue, skeletal muscle and finally functional proteins in the myocardium and pulmonary parenchyma. This tissue loss appears to arise not only from decreased food intake, but also from the production of catabolic factors, including cytokines and a peptide termed proteolysis inducing factor (PIF), by certain tumours (Todorov *et al.*, 1996). Fatty acids have been found to have anti-cachectic effects in animal models and in human intervention studies. The effect seems to be structurally specific, with EPA reported to be actively anti-cachectic, whereas other n-3 PUFA such as DHA or alpha-linolenic acid (ALNA) were without effect (Tisdale, 1996). The anti-lipolytic effect of EPA arose from the inhibition of the elevation of cyclic AMP in adipocytes in response to the lipid mobilising factors (Tisdale, 1996). EPA also inhibited skeletal muscle degradation by modulating the PGE2 response and inhibiting ATP/ubiquitin-dependent muscle proteolysis in a murine model (Calder *et al.*, 1998; Tisdale and Dhesi, 1990; Whitehouse *et al.*, 2001). This association between EPA supplementation and a reduction in cachexia has also been demonstrated in human studies and was related to acute phase and metabolic response (Barber *et al.*, 1999). Therefore the evidence seems to support a beneficial effect of EPA in cancer initiation and progression and in the debilitating symptoms of cancer cachexia.

5.7 Inflammation and autoimmune diseases

An inappropriate or dysfunctional inflammatory response or activation of immune T cells underlies acute and chronic inflammatory conditions such as rheumatoid arthritis, inflammatory bowel disease (IBD), asthma and psoriasis. As mentioned previously, eicosanoids are important mediators of inflammation (Section 5.3.2). Arachidonic acid-derived thromboxane A_2 (TXA_2) and leukotriene B_4 (LTB_4) are pro-inflammatory agents, being potent vasoconstrictors and inducers of leukocyte chemotaxis and adherence respectively, relative to their EPA-derived TAX_3 and LTB_5. Inflammatory cytokines predominantly produced by monocytes/macrophages and adipose tissue, including tumour necrosis factor-alpha (TNF-α), interleukin 1 (IL-1) and IL-6, are also integrally involved in inflammation, mediating acute phase protein synthesis and activating T and B lymphocyte activity.

The benefit of EPA + DHA to protect against chronic inflammatory disorders was initially recognised in Greenland Inuits who experienced a low incidence of conditions such as psiorasis and arthritis compared with age and gender-matched Danish adults (Kromann and Green, 1980). Experimental evidence accumulating in the last two decades has indicated that decreased dietary n-6:n-3 PUFA ratio and increased LC n-3 PUFA may help ameliorate the symptoms and allow a reduction in the use of anti-inflammatory medications in individuals with chronic inflammatory conditions (Prescott and Calder, 2004; Simopoulos, 2002a).

The anti-inflammatory effects of EPA + DHA have been attributed to a shift in eicosanoid metabolism and a decreased expression of cyclooxygenase 2

(COX-2), TNF-α, IL-1 and IL-6 (Caughey *et al.*, 1996; Endres *et al.*, 1989; Simopoulos, 2002). Caughey *et al.* (1996) demonstrated that diets enriched with flaxseed (a rich dietary sources of ALNA) decreased cytokine production (TNF-α, IL-1β) by about 30% in 4 weeks with a >70% reduction evident following fish oil supplementation.

In patients with rheumatoid arthritis there is a consistent body of evidence indicating that EPA + DHA supplementation is associated with a reduction in clinical symptoms including number of tender joints and use of analgesic anti-inflammatory drugs and decreased circulating cytokines and pro-inflammatory eicosanoids such as LTB_4 (Fortin *et al.*, 1995; James and Cleland, 1997; Simopoulos, 2002a). James and Cleland (1997) have suggested that those with arthritis should have an n-3 nutritional status index of EPA > 1.5% of total cell phospholipid fatty acid and > 3% plasma phospholipid fatty acids. At these EPA levels the authors noted significant reductions in TNF-α and IL-1β and a higher discontinuation of the use of non-steroidal anti-inflammatory medications by patients attending clinic. The evidence for other autoimmune conditions is conflicting and less convincing, often because of the relatively small subject number in intervention trials and the complication of the concurrent use of a wide range of medications. However, a number of studies do indicate that increased EPA + DHA may result in modest improvements in asthmatic sufferers, and in those with IBD and psoriasis (Allen, 1991; Belluzzi *et al.*, 1996; Broughton *et al.*, 1997).

5.8 Cognitive function

The lipid content of the retina and brain are highly enriched in both DHA and AA (Horrocks and Yeo, 1999). Owing to the rapid accretion of these fatty acids in the brain during the third trimester of pregnancy and early postnatal period, when brain growth is maximal, the infant is particularly vulnerable to the effects of fatty acid deficiencies. There is controversy at present as to whether infant formulas that do not contain DHA or AA are sufficient for adequate brain growth. Several published studies in which infants have been randomly assigned to milk formulas that contain DHA, both DHA and AA, or low levels of these LC PUFA, have suggested improved cognition in the DHA/AA-supplemented groups. Although there was no effect on visual recognition, pre-term infants fed DHA-supplemented diets showed shorter look durations, indicating improved visual attention (Carlson and Werkman, 1996; Werkman and Carlson, 1996). In addition a subsequent study has shown improved problem solving in 10-month-old term infants fed on diets supplemented with DHA and AA compared with those on a very low n-3 PUFA content (Willatts *et al.*, 1998). However lower language scores have been reported in 14-month-old term infants fed formulas supplemented with DHA (Scott *et al.*, 1998), although these effects seemed to be transient and the predictive validity of early language with respect to later cognitive function is controversial (Wainwright, 2000). Studies in cognitive function are very problematic, as performance on cognitive measures (learning and memory) may be confounded by alterations in non-cognitive functions (emotionality and arousal) or an inadequate sensory and motor skill (Wainwright, 2000). However, there is evidence that DHA plays a unique role in the function of excitable membranes (Carlson and Neuringer, 1999) and is intricately involved with many aspects of brain function (Horrocks and Yeo, 1999).

In addition to brain development, the LC n-3 PUFA content of the brain may be important in the pathology of neuropsychiatric disorders such as depression, bi-polar disorder and excessive aggressive behaviour (Hibbeln, 1998; Stoll *et al.*, 1999). Furthermore low LC n-3 PUFA status has been observed in age-related dementia, notably Alzheimer's disease (Tully *et al.*, 2003), with Morris and co-workers (2003) observing that total intake of n-3 PUFA and DHA but not EPA was predictive of AD development in a 7-year prospective trial. Further research is needed to determine the ability of increased LC n-3 PUFA intake to delay or prevent the onset of dementia.

5.9 Recommendations for population fat intake

At present, population guidelines for fat intake are largely based on the known association between dietary fat composition and CVD, in particular fasting lipid levels. Table 5.4 lists the current WHO/FAO (2003) and UK guidelines (Department of Health, 1994; Food Standards Agency and Department of Health, 2004).

Table 5.4 Current recommendations for dietary fat intake

Fat component	FAO/WHO (2003)	COMA (1994)/ SACN (2004) – UK
Total fat	Up to 35% energy in highly active groups, with a diet rich in fruit, vegetables legumes and wholegrain cereals, otherwise lower	< 35% food energy (<33% including alcohol)
Saturated fat	< 10% total energy, < 7% in high risk individuals	< 11% total energy (<10% including alcohol)
Trans fatty acid	< 1% total energy	< 2% total energy
Total MUFA	No recommendation	No recommendation
Total PUFA	6–10% total energy	No further increase
n-6:n-3 PUFA ratio	2.5:1-8:1	–
LC n-3 PUFA	No specific recommendation: 'Eat fish once or twice a week'	0.45 g/day

PUFA, polyunsaturated fatty acids; MUFA, monounsaturated fatty acids; LC n-3 PUFA-long chain n-3 polyunsaturated fatty acids; COMA, Committee of Medical Aspects of Food Policy; SACN, Scientific Advisory Committee on Nutrition.

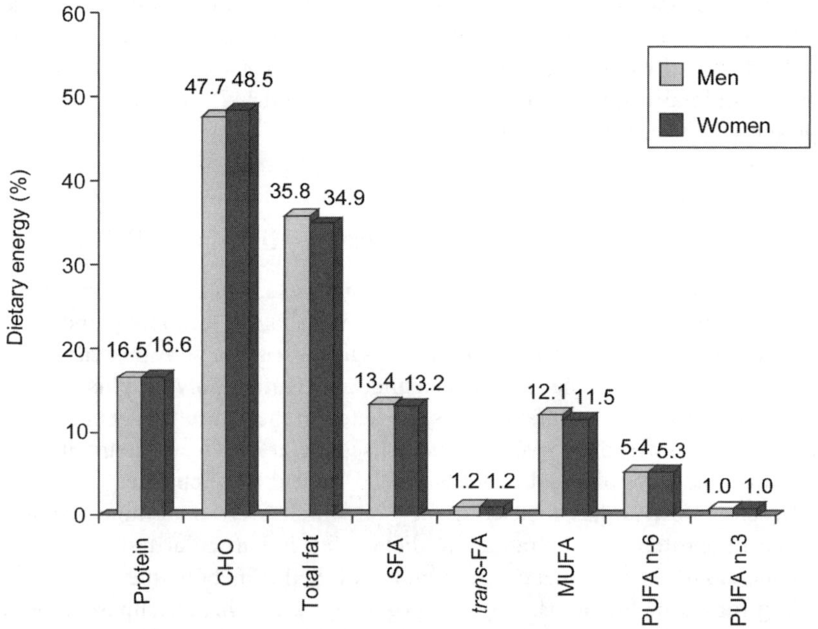

Fig. 5.5 Mean population macronutrient intake in the UK (National Diet and Nutrition Survey, 2003) (*CHO, carbohydrate: SFA, saturated fatty acids: PUFA, polyunsaturated fatty acid, MUFA, monounsaturated fatty acids*).

In general it is recommended that energy derived from fat should not exceed 35% of total food energy, with the WHO/FAO recommending lower intakes for the majority of the population. Currently in the UK average fat intakes of 35.8% and 34.9% of food energy are evident in men and women respectively (Fig. 5.5), with only 43% of men and 50% of women with intakes lower than the recommendations (Food Standards Agency, 2003). For saturated fats (SFA) only 12% of men and 17% of women meet the < 10% of energy from saturated fat target, with > 40% of UK adults with intakes of SFA > 14% of energy (Food Standards Agency, 2003). Although the average intakes of *trans* fatty acids of 1.2% are evident in the UK, 60% of individuals have intakes over the FAO/WHO recommendation of < 1% dietary energy. Intakes of LC n-3 PUFA are low in the UK, with average population intakes estimated to be less than 0.1 g/day.

Current recommendations in the UK to increase LC n-3 PUFA intakes to 0.45 g/day is based on the consumption of two portions of fish per week, one oily, with the recommendation based on a recent review of the nutritional and toxicological data (Food Standards Agency and Department of Health, 2004). The report states that this recommendation is also suitable for pregnant and lactating women, with a note suggesting the avoidance of certain species of fish such as marlin, swordfish and shark, owing to concerns regarding heavy metal contamination.

Regarding specific recommendations on the n-6:n-3 PUFA ratio of the diet, it is likely that the available scientific literature is currently not sufficiently established to draw up a specific recommendation. The current WHO guidelines suggest an intake of n-6 and n-3 PUFA of 5–8% and 1–2% of daily energy to be optimal (WHO Europe, 2003) (Table 5.4).

5.10 Genotype and responsiveness to dietary PUFA changes

Dietary recommendations as given above are based on the assessment of the 'average' group responses to dietary fat change. It is becoming increasingly recognised that responsiveness to diet is highly variable, with this variability in part due to common genetic variants, single nucleotide polymorphisms (SNPs). Although in its relevant infancy, it is predicted in the future that genetic profiles may be used as part of an overall personalised dietary advice strategy, in order to maximise the physiological benefits gained from dietary change.

Research to date has focused mainly on which SNPs determine response of fasting lipoprotein concentrations to dietary fat, in particular reduced saturated and increased PUFA intakes. A number of SNPs in both the promoter and coding region of the apoB, apoC3, apoA1, apoE and hepatic lipase gene have emerged as being potentially important (Humphries *et al.*, 1996; Ordovas and Schaefer, 2000; Ordovas *et al.*, 2002; Rantala *et al.*, 2000). The genetic determinants of responsiveness to altered dietary LC n-3 PUFA are largely unknown. However, in a study conducted by Minihane *et al.* (2000), where the impact of 3 g EPA + DHA on fasting and postprandial lipid metabolism was determined in adult males, significant 35%, 23% and 26% decreases in fasting TG, postprandial TG and % LDL as LDL-3 were evident, with a borderline significant increase in LDL-C ($P = 0.054$). Retrospective data analysis according to *apoE* genotype indicated a significant 16% in LDL-C in *apoE4* carriers (25–27% UK population) whereas significantly greater post-supplementation postprandial TG clearance was evident in the *apoE2* subgroup (12–15% UK population). It is likely that the large variability in responsiveness of other physiological determinants of chronic disease to dietary PUFA is also in large part determined by genetics and there is currently much research focused on gaining an understanding of diet–genotype–disease relationships.

5.11 Conclusion and future trends

Conclusive evidence exists that reduction of saturated fats in the diet and *trans* fatty acids are associated with a significant improvement in the blood lipid profile. Although less conclusive, there is substantial evidence from animal trials and accumulating evidence from observational and intervention studies in humans to suggest that such a strategy would also be associated with improved insulin sensitivity and glucose disposal. With the recent worldwide 'epidemic' of diabetes, a continued public health focus to minimise population saturated : unsaturated (MUFA + PUFA) dietary ratio is essential.

The long chain n-3 PUFAs at intakes of 0.5–1.0 g per day undoubtedly offer protection against fatal acute cardiac events. At intakes greater than 3 g per day positive impacts on physiological processes that contribute to CHD risk have been observed, although the clinical impact of changes evident at lower, more realistic levels of intake, remains uncertain. Although work in animals showed immense promise, repeated intervention trials of up to 3 months' duration have failed to demonstrate any impact of EPA + DHA supplementation on insulin action in humans. With respect to colorectal cancer and chronic inflammatory conditions, emerging evidence is demonstrating that a high dietary n-6:n-3 PUFA ratio and low intakes of LC n-3 PUFA may make a modest contribution to disease pathology, with the association in part mediated through altered eicosanoid production.

Despite the recognised association between dietary saturated : unsaturated fatty acid ratio, n-6 : n-3 PUFA ratio and LC n-3 PUFA and the development of chronic diseases, large proportions of European populations are not meeting the national dietary targets for fat intake. The efficacy of dietary strategies to reduce the population burden of major chronic diseases such as CVD, cancers and diabetes requires:

- ongoing scientific research into diet–disease relationships;
- effective strategies to disseminate research findings to the general population;
- a well-informed and motivated consumer;
- the provision of accessible, acceptable food products with an 'enhanced' fatty acid profile.

In the future, the provision of personalised advice, potentially including genetic information, would undoubtedly improve consumer motivation and strive to maximise the benefit of dietary change through choice of strategy to suit the individual.

5.12 References

ALBERT CM, HENNEKENS CH, O'DONNELL CJ, AJANI UA, CAREY VJ, WILLETT WC, RUSKIN JN & MANSON JE (1998) Fish consumption and risk of sudden cardiac death. *Journal of the American Medical Association* **279**, 23–28.

ALBERT CM, CAMPOS H, STAMPFER MJ, RIDKER PM, MANSON JE, WILLETT WC & MA J (2002) Blood levels of long-chain n-3 fatty acids and the risk of sudden death. *New England Journal of Medicine* **346**, 1113–1118.

ALBERTI KG & ZIMMET PZ (1998) Definition, diagnosis and classification of diabetes mellitus and its complications. Part 1: diagnosis and classification of diabetes mellitus provisional report of a WHO consultation. *Diabetes Medicine* **15**, 539–553.

ALEXANDER-NORTH LS, NORTH JA, KIMINYO KP, BUETTNER GR & SPECTOR AA (1994) Polyunsaturated fatty-acids increase lipid radical formation induced by oxidant stress in endothelial-cells. *Journal of Lipid Research* **35**, 1773–1785.

ALLEN BR (1991) Fish oil in combination with other therapies in the treatment of psoriasis. In *Health effects of omega-3 polyunsaturated fatty acids in seafoods*, pp. 436–445 [Simopoulos AP, Martin RE, Barlow SM, eds]. Basel: Karger.

ALLMANN DW & GIBSON DW (1969) Fatty acid synthesis during early linoleic deficiency in the mouse. *Journal of Lipid Research* **6**, 51–62.

ALSAIF MA & DUWAIHY MMS (2004) Influence of dietary fat quantity and composition on glucose tolerance and insulin sensitivity in rats. *Nutrition Research* **24**, 417–425.

ANTI M, MARRA G, ARMELAO F, BARTOLI GM, FICARELLI R, PERCESEPE A, DEVITIS I, MARIA G, SOFO L, RAPACCINI GL, GENTILONI N, PICCIONI E & MIGGIANO G (1992) Effect of omega-3-fatty-acids on rectal mucosal cell-proliferation in subjects at risk for colon cancer. *Gastroenterology* **103**, 883–891.

ASCHERIO A, RIMM EB, STAMPFER MJ, GIOVANNUCCI MD & WILLETT WC (1995) Dietary intake of marine n-3 fatty acids, fish intake and the risk of coronary disease among men. *New England Journal of Medicine* **332**, 977–983.

ASCHERIO A, RIMM EB, GIOVANNUCCI EL, SPIEGELMAN D, STAMPFER M & WILLETT WC (1996) Dietary fat and risk of coronary heart disease in men: cohort follow up study in the United States. *British Medical Journal* **313**, 84–90.

AUSTIN MA, KING MC, VRANIGAN KM & KRAUSS RM (1990) Atherogenic lipoprotein phenotype: a proposed genetic marker for coronary heart disease risk. *Circulation* **82**, 495–506.

AUWERX J (1992) Regulation of gene expression by fatty acids and fibric acid derivatives: an integrative role for peroxisome proliferators activated receptor. The Belgian Endocrine Society Lecture. *Hormone Research* **38**, 269–277.

BARBER MD, ROSS JA, VOSS AC, TISDALE MJ & FEARON KCH (1999) The effect of an oral nutritional supplement enriched with fish oil on weight loss in patients with pancreatic cancer. *British Journal of Cancer* **81**, 80–86.

BEHME MT (1996) Dietary fish oil induces insulin sensitivity in miniature pigs. *Journal of Nutrition* **126**, 1549–1553.

BEISIEGEL U, HEEREN J & SCHNIEDERS F (2003) Fatty acids and gene expression. In *Molecular Nutrition* [Zempleni J, ed.]. Wallingford, UK: CABI.

BELLUZZI A, BRIGNOLA C, CAMPIERI M, PERA A, BOSCHI S & MIGLIOLI M (1996) Effect of an enteric-coated fish-oil preparation on relapses in Crohn's disease. *New England Journal of Medicine* **334**, 1557–1560.

BEMELMANS WJ, BROER J, FESKENS EJ, SMIT AJ, MUSKIET FA, LEFRANDT JD, BOM VJ, MAY JF & MEYBOOM-DE JONG B (2002) Effect of an increased intake of alpha-linolenic acid and group nutritional education on cardiovascular risk factors: the Mediterranean alpha-linolenic enriched Groningen dietary intervention (MARGARIN) study. *American Journal of Clinical Nutrition* **75**, 221–227.

BERK PD & STUMP DD (1999) Mechanism of cellular uptake of long chain free fatty acids. *Molecular and Cellular Biochemistry* **192**, 17–31.

BINGHAM SA (1998) Epidemiology of colorectal cancer. In *Encyclopedia of human nutrition*, pp. 230–235 [Strain J, Sadler M, Caballero B, eds]. New York: Academic Press.

BRADY LM, LOVEGROVE SS, LESAUVAGE SV, GOWER BA, MINIHANE AM, WILLIAMS CM & LOVEGROVE JA (2004) Increased n-6 polyunsaturated fatty acids do not attenuate the effects of long-chain n-3 polyunsaturated fatty acids on insulin sensitivity or triacylglycerol reduction in Indian Asians. *Am J Clin Nutr* **79**, 983–991.

BRITISH HEART FOUNDATION (BHF) (2000) *European Cardiovascular Statistics*. London: BHF.

BROUGHTON KS, JOHNSON CS, PACE BK, LIEBMAN M & KLEPPINGER KM (1997) Reduced asthma symptoms with n-3 fatty acid ingestion are related to 5-series leukotriene production. *American Journal of Clinical Nutrition* **65**, 1011–1017.

BROWN JE & WAHLE KWJ (1990) Effect of fish-oil and vitamin-E supplementation on lipid-peroxidation and whole-blood aggregation in man. *Clinica Chimica Acta* **193**, 147–156.

BUCKLEY R, SHEWRING B, TURNER R, YAQOOB P & MINIHANE AM (2004) Circulating triacylglycerol and apoE levels in response to EPA and docosahexaenoic acid supplementation in adult human subjects. *British Journal of Nutrition* **92**, 477–483.

BURDGE GC, FINNEGAN YE, MINIHANE AM, WILLIAMS CM & WOOTTON SA (2003) Effect of altered dietary n-3 fatty acid intake upon plasma lipid fatty acid composition, conversion of [13C]alpha-linolenic acid to longer-chain fatty acids and partitioning towards beta-oxidation in older men. *British Journal of Nutrition* **90**, 311–321.

BURR GO & MILDRED MM (1929) A new deficiency disease produced by the rapid exclusion of fat from the diet. *Journal of Biological Chemistry* **82**, 345–367.

BURR ML, FEHILY AM, GILBERT JF, ROGERS S, HOLLIDAY RM, SWEETNAM PM, ELWOOD PC & DEADMAN NM (1989) Effects of changes in fat, fish, and fibre intakes on death and myocardial reinfarction: diet and reinfarction trial (DART). *Lancet* **2**, 757–761.

BURR ML, ASHFIELD-WATT PAL, DUNSTAN FDJ, FEHILY AM, ASHTON T & ZOTOS PC (2003) Lack of benefit of dietary advice to men with angina: results of a controlled trial. *European Journal of Clinical Nutrition* **57**, 193–200.

CALDER PC (2004) n-3 fatty acids and cardiovascular disease: evidence explained and mechanisms explored. *Clinical Science* **107**, 1–11.

CALDER PC & GRIMBLE RF (2002) Polyunsaturated fatty acids, inflammation and immunity. *European Journal of Clinical Nutrition* **56**, S14–S19.

CALDER PC, DAVIS J, YAQOOB P, PALA H, THIES F & NEWSHOLME EA (1998) Dietary fish oil suppresses human colon tumour growth in athymic mice. *Clinical Science* **94**, 303–311.

CARLSON SE & NEURINGER M (1999) Polyunsaturated fatty acid status and neurodevelopment: a summary and critical analysis of the literature. *Lipids* **34**, 171–178.

CARLSON SE & WERKMAN SH (1996) A randomized trial of visual attention of preterm infants fed docosahexaenoic acid until two months. *Lipids* **31**, 85–90.

CAUGHEY GE, MANTZIORIS E, GIBSON RA, CLELAND LG & JAMES MJ (1996) The effect on human tumor necrosis factor alpha and interleukin 1 beta production of diets enriched in n-3 fatty acids from vegetable oil or fish oil. *American Journal of Clinical Nutrition* **63**, 116–122.

CAYGILL CPJ & HILL MJ (1995) Fish, n-3 fatty-acids and human colorectal and breast-cancer mortality. *European Journal of Cancer Prevention* **4**, 329–332.

CHAMBRIER C, BASTARD JP, RIEUSSET J, CHEVILLOTTE E, BONNEFONT-ROUSSELOT D, THEROND P, HAINQUE B, RIOU JP, LAVILLE M & VIDAL H (2002) Eicosapentaenoic acid induces mRNA expression of peroxisome proliferator-activated receptor gamma. *Obesity Research* **10**, 518–525.

CHO HP, NAKAMURA MT & CLARKE SD (1999) Cloning, expression and fatty acid regulation of the human delta-5 desaturase. *Journal of Biological Chemistry* **274**, 37335–37339.

CLARKE SD (2001) Polyunsaturated fatty acid regulation and gene transcription: a molecular mechanism to improve the metabolic syndrome. *Journal of Nutrition* **131**, 1129–1132.

COLLETT ED, DAVIDSON LA, FAN YY, LUPTON JR & CHAPKIN RS (2001) n-6 and n-3 polyunsaturated fatty acids differentially modulate oncogenic *Ras* activation in colonocytes. *American Journal of Physiology – Cell Physiology* **280**, C1066–C1075.

CONNOR SL & CONNOR WE (1997) Are fish oils beneficial in the prevention and treatment of coronary artery disease? *American Journal of Clinical Nutrition* **66**, S1020–S1031.

CONQUER JA & HOLUB BJ (1998) Effect of supplementation with different doses of DHA on the levels of circulating DHA as non-esterified fatty acid in subjects of Asian Indian background. *Journal of Lipid Research* **39**, 286–292.

CROSBY AJ, WAHLE KWJ & DUTHIE GG (1996) Modulation of glutathione peroxidase activity in human vascular endothelial cells by fatty acids and the cytokine interleukin-1 beta. *Biochimica et Biophysica Acta – Lipids and Lipid Metabolism* **1303**, 187–192.

D'ALESSANDRO ME, L LOMBARDO YB & CHICCO A (2002) Effect of fish oil on insulin sensitivity and metabolic fate of glucose in the skeletal muscle of normal rats. *Annals of Nutrition Metabolism* **46**, 114–120.

D'AQUINO M, BENEDETTI PC, DIFELICE M, GENTILI V, TOMASSI G, MAIORINO M & URSINI F (1991) Effect of fish oil and coconut oil on antioxidant defense system and lipid-peroxidation in rat-liver. *Free Radical Research Communications* **12-3**, 147–152.

DAVIDSON LA, BROWN RE, CHANG WCL, MORRIS JS, WANG NY, CARROLL RJ, TURNER ND, LUPTON JR & CHAPKIN RS (2000) Morphodensitometric analysis of protein kinase C beta(II) expression in rat colon: modulation by diet and relation to in situ cell proliferation and apoptosis. *Carcinogenesis* **21**, 1513–1519.

DE LORGERIL M, RENAUD S, MAMELLE N, SALEN P, MARTIN JL, MONJAUD I, GUIDOLLET J, TOUBOUL P & DELAYE J (1994) Mediterranean alpha-linolenic acid-rich diet in secondary prevention of coronary heart disease. *Lancet* **343**, 1445–1454.

DEPARTMENT OF HEALTH (1994) *Committee of Medical Aspects of Food Policy (COMA): Nutritional aspects of cardiovascular disease*. London: HMSO.

DOLECEK TA (1992) Epidemiological evidence of relationships between dietary polyunsaturated fatty acids and mortality in the Multiple Risk Factor Intervention Trial. *Proceedings of the Society of Experimental Biology and Medicine* **200**, 177–182.

DOMMELS YEM, ALINK GM, VAN BLADEREN PJ & VAN OMMEN B (2002) Dietary n-6 and n-3 polyunsaturated fatty acids and colorectal carcinogenesis: results from cultured colon cells, animal models and human studies. *Environmental Toxicology and Pharmacology* **11**, 297–308.

DUPLUS E, GLORIAN M, FOREST C (2000) Fatty acid regulation of gene transcription. *Journal of Biological Chemistry* **275** (40), 30749–30752.

DYERBERG JAB, H. O (1982) A hypothesis on the development of acute myocardial infarction in Greenlanders. *Scandinavian Journal of Laboratory Investigation* **161**, 7–13.

EMKEN EA, ADLOF RO & GULLEY RM (1994) Dietary linoleic-acid influences desaturation and acylation of deuterium-labeled linoleic and linolenic acids in young-adult males. *Biochimica Et Biophysica Acta – Lipids and Lipid Metabolism* **1213**, 277–288.

ENDRES S, GHORBANI R, KELLEY VE, GEORGILIS K, LONNEMANN G, VAN DER MEER JW, CANNON JG, ROGERS TS, KLEMPNER MS, WEBER PC *et al.* (1989) The effect of dietary supplementation with n-3 polyunsaturated fatty acids on the synthesis of interleukin-1 and tumor necrosis factor by mononuclear cells. *New England Journal of Medicine* **320**, 265–271.

ERITSLAND J, SELJEFLOT I, ABDELNOOR M, ARNESEN H & TORJESEN PA (1994) Long-term effects of n-3 fatty-acids on serum-lipids and glycemic control. *Scandinavian Journal of Clinical & Laboratory Investigation* **54**, 273–280.

FAO (2004) *Percentage of total energy from fat by country, 1971–2001, Europe*. Rome: FAO.

FASCHING P, RATHEISER K, WALDHAUSL W, ROHAC M, OSTERRODE W, NOWOTNY P & VIERHAPPER H (1991) Metabolic effects of fish-oil supplementation in patients with impaired glucose-tolerance. *Diabetes* **40**, 583–589.

FASCHING P, RATHEISER K, SCHEEWEISS B, ROHAC M, NOWOTNY P & WALDHAUSL W (1996) No effect of short-term dietary supplementation of saturated and poly- and mono-unsaturated fatty acids on insulin secretion and sensitivity in healthy men. *Annals of Nutrition and Metabolism* **40**, 116–122.

FESKENS EJM, BOWLES CH & KROMHOUT D (1991) Inverse association between fish intake and risk of glucose-intolerance in normoglycemic elderly men and women. *Diabetes Care* **14**, 935–941.

FESKENS EJM, VIRTANEN SM, RASANEN L, TUOMILEHTO J, STENGARD J, PEKKANEN J, NISSINEN A & KROMHOUT D (1995) Dietary factors determining diabetes and impaired glucose-tolerance – a 20-year follow-up of the Finnish and Dutch cohorts of the 7-Countries Study. *Diabetes Care* **18**, 1104–1112.

FINNEGAN YE, HOWARTH D, MINIHANE AM, KEW S, MILLER GJ, CALDER PC & WILLIAMS CM (2003a) Plant and marine derived (n-3) polyunsaturated fatty acids do not affect blood coagulation and fibrinolytic factors in moderately hyperlipidemic humans. *Journal of Nutrition* **133**, 2210–2213.

FINNEGAN YE, MINIHANE AM, LEIGH-FIRBANK EC, KEW S, MEIJER GW, MUGGLI R, CALDER PC & WILLIAMS CM (2003b) Plant- and marine-derived n-3 polyunsaturated fatty acids have differential effects on fasting and postprandial blood lipid concentrations and on the susceptibility of LDL to oxidative modification in moderately hyperlipidemic subjects. *American Journal of Clinical Nutrition* **77**, 783–795.

FOOD STANDARDS AGENCY (2003) *National Diet and Nutrition Survey: adults aged 19 to 64 years* [G Swan, ed.]. London: TSO.

FOOD STANDARDS AGENCY AND DEPARTMENT OF HEALTH: SCIENTIFIC ADVISORY COMMITTEE ON NUTRITION (SACN) AND COMMITTEE ON TOXICITY (2004) *Advice on fish consumption: benefits and risks*. London: TSO.

FOREST C, FRANCKHAUSER S, GLORIAN M, ANTRAS-FERRY J, ROBIN D & ROBIN P (1997) Regulation of gene transcription by fatty acids, fibrates and prostaglandins: the phosphoenolpyruvate carboxykinase gene as a model. *Prostaglandins Leukotrienes and Essential Fatty Acids* **57**, 47–56.

FORTIN PR, LEW RA, LIANG MH, WRIGHT EA, BECKETT LA, CHALMERS TC & SPERLING RI (1995) Validation of a meta-analysis: the effects of fish oil in rheumatoid arthritis. *Journal of Clinical Epidemiology* **48**, 1379–1390.

FRANKEL EN, PARKS EJ, XU R, SCHNEEMAN BO, DAVIS PA & GERMAN JB (1994) Effect of n-3 fatty acid-rich fish-oil supplementation on the oxidation of low-density lipoproteins. *Lipids* **29**, 233–236.

GISSI (1999) Dietary supplementation with n-3 polyunsaturated fatty acids and vitamin E after myocardial infarction: results of the GISSI-Prevenzione trial. Gruppo Italiano per lo Studio della Sopravvivenza nell'Infarto miocardico. *Lancet* **354**, 447–455.

GLASS CK & WITZTUM JL (2001) Atherosclerosis: the road ahead. *Cell* **104**, 503–516.

GLOBOCAN (2001) Cancer Incidence, Mortality and Prevalence Worldwide (2000 estimates). Lyon, France: International Agency for Research on Cancer (www.dep.iarc.fr).

GRIFFIN BA, FREEMAN DJ, TAIT GW, THOMSON J, CASLAKE MJ, PACKARD CJ & SHEPHERD J (1994) Role of plasma triglyceride in the regulation of plasma low density lipoprotein (LDL) subfractions: relative contribution of small, dense LDL to coronary heart disease risk. *Atherosclerosis* **106**, 241–253.

GRONN M, GORBITZ C, CHRISTENSEN E, LEVORSEN A, OSE L, HAGVE TA & CHRISTOPHERSEN BO (1991) Dietary n-6 fatty-acids inhibit the incorporation of dietary n-3 fatty-acids in thrombocyte and serum phospholipids in humans – a controlled dietetic study. *Scandinavian Journal of Clinical & Laboratory Investigation* **51**, 255–263.

HANSEN JB, GRIMSGAARD S, NILSEN H, NORDOY A & BONAA KH (1998) Effects of highly purified eicosapentaenoic acid and docosahexaenoic acid on fatty acid absorption, incorporation into serum phospholipids and postprandial triglyceridemia. *Lipids* **33**, 131–138.

HARRIS WS, WINDSOR SL & DUJOVNE CA (1991) Effects of four doses of n-3 fatty acids given to hyperlipidemic patients for six months. *J Am Coll Nutr* **10**, 220–227.

HEGSTED DM, MCGANDY RM, MYERS ML & STARE FJ (1965) Quantitative effects of dietary fat on serum cholesterol in man. *American Journal of Clinical Nutrition* **17**, 281–295.

HIBBELN JR (1998) Fish oil consumption and major depression. *Lancet* **351**, 1213.

HIGGINS S, CARROLL YL, MCCARTHY SN, CORRIDAN BM, ROCHE HM, WALLACE JM, O'BRIEN NM & MORRISSEY PA (2001) Susceptibility of LDL to oxidative modification in healthy volunteers supplemented with low doses of n-3 polyunsaturated fatty acids. *British Journal of Nutrition* **85**, 23–31.

HIHI AK, MICHALIK L & WAHLI W (2002) PPARs: transcriptional effectors of fatty acids and their derivatives. *Cell and Molecular Life Sciences* **59**, 790–798.

HORROCKS LA & YEO YK (1999) Health benefits of docosahexaenoic acid (DHA). *Pharmacological Research* **40**, 211–225.

HU FB, STAMPFER MJ, MANSON JE, RIMM EB, WOLK A, COLDITZ GA, HENNEKENS CH & WILLETT WC (1999) Dietary intake of alpha-linolenic acid and risk of fatal ischemic heart disease among women. *American Journal of Clinical Nutrition* **69**, 890–897.

HU FB, BRONNER L, WILLETT WC, STAMPFER MJ, REXRODE KM, ALBERT CM, HUNTER D & MANSON JE (2002) Fish and omega-3 fatty acid intake and risk of coronary heart disease in women. *Journal of the American Medical Association* **287**, 1815–1821.

HUMPHRIES SE, TALMUD P, COX C, SUTHERLAND W & MANN J (1996) Genetic factors affecting the consistency and magnitude of changes in plasma cholesterol in response to dietary challenge. *Quarterly Journal of Medicine* **86**, 671–680.

IARC (2000) *Cancer incidence, mortality and prevalence worldwide – 2000 estimates.* Lyon: IARC Press.

INDU M & GHAFOORUNISSA (1992) n-3 fatty acids in Indian diets – comparison of the effects of precursor (alpha-linoleic acid) vs product (long chain n-3 polyunsaturated acids). *Nutrition Research* **12**, 569–582.

ISSEMANN I & GREEN S (1990) Activation of a member of the steroid hormone receptor superfamily by peroxisome proliferators. *Nature* **347**, 645–650.

JACKSON KG, ROBERTSON MD, FIELDING BA, FRAYN KN & WILLIAMS CM (2002) Olive oil increases the number of triacylglycerol-rich chylomicron particles compared with other oils: an effect retained when a second standard meal is fed. *American Journal of Clinical Nutrition* **76**, 942–949.

JAMES MJ & CLELAND L (1997) Dietary n-3 fatty acids and therapy for rheumatoid arthritis. *Seminars in Arthritis and Rheumatism* **27**, 85–97.

JUHEL C, SENFT M, PAFUMI Y, GIRARD-GLOBA A, LEVY E, LAFONT H & LAIRON D (1999) Acute ingestion of different dietary fatty acid species modulates postprandial lipid responses in New Zealand white rabbits. *Journal of Nutritional Biochemistry* **10**, 458–466.

JUMP DB & CLARK SD (1999) Regulation of gene expression by dietary fat. *Annual Reviews in Nutrition* **19**, 63–90.

KEYS A (1970) Coronary heart disease in seven countries. *Circulation* **164**, 1912–1919.

KEYS A, ANDERSON J & GRANDE F (1965) Serum cholesterol responses to changes in diet: particular saturated fatty acids in the diet. *Metabolism* **14**, 776–787.

KHAN F, ELHERIK K, BOLTON-SMITH C, BARR R, HILL A, MURRIE I & BELCH JJF (2003) The effects of dietary fatty acid supplementation on endothelial function and vascular tone in healthy subjects. *Cardiovascular Research* **59**, 955–962.

KHAN S, MINIHANE A, TALMUD PJ, WRIGHT JW, MURPHY MC, WILLIAMS CM & GRIFFIN BA (2002) Dietary long-chain n-3 PUFAs increase LPL gene expression in adipose tissue of subjects with an atherogenic lipoprotein phenotype. *Journal of Lipid Research* **43**, 979–985.

KREY G, BRAISSANT O, L'HORSET F, KALKHOVEN E, PERROUD M, PARKER MG & WAHLI W (1997) Fatty acids, eicosanoids, and hypolipidemic agents identified as ligands of peroxisome proliferator-activated receptors by coactivator-dependent receptor ligand assay. *Molecular Endocrinology* **11**, 779–791.

KRISTENSEN SD, IVERSEN A & SCHMIDT EB (2001) n-3 polyunsaturated fatty acids and coronary thrombosis. *Lipids* **36**, S79–S82.

KROMANN N & GREEN A (1980) Epidemiological studies in the Upernavik district, Greenland. Incidence of some chronic diseases 1950–1974. *Acta Medica Scandinavica* **208**, 401–408.

KROMHOUT D, BOSSCHIETER EB & DE LEZENNE COULANDER C (1985) The inverse relation between fish consumption and 20-year mortality from coronary heart disease. *New England Journal of Medicine* **312**, 1205–1209.

KUBO K, SAITO M, TADOKORO T & MAEKAWA A (1997) Changes in susceptibility of tissues to lipid peroxidation after ingestion of various levels of docosahexaenoic acid and vitamin E. *British Journal of Nutrition* **78**, 655–669.

LEAF A & XIAO F (2001) The modulation of ionic currents in excitable tissues by n-3 polyunsaturated fatty acids. *Journal of Membrane Biology* **184**, 263–271.

LEIGH-FIRBANK EC, MINIHANE AM, LEAKE DS, WRIGHT JW, MURPHY MC, GRIFFIN BA & WILLIAMS CM (2002) Eicosapentaenoic acid and docosahexaenoic acid from fish oils: differential associations with lipid responses. *British Journal of Nutrition* **87**, 435–445.

LEMAITRE D, VERICEL E, POLETTE A & LAGARDE M (1997) Effects of fatty acids on human platelet glutathione peroxidase: possible role of oxidative stress. *Biochemical Pharmacology* **53**, 479–486.

LEWIS RA, LEE TH & AUSTEN KF (1986) Effects of omega-3 fatty acids on the generation of products of 5-lipooxygenase pathway. In: *Health effects of polyunsaturated fatty acids in seafoods*. Orlando: Academic Press.

LOVEGROVE JA, BROOKS CN, MURPHY MC, GOULD BJ & WILLIAMS CM (1997) Use of manufactured foods enriched with fish oils as a means of increasing long-chain n-3 polyunsaturated fatty acid intake. *British Journal of Nutrition* **78**, 223–236.

LOVEGROVE JA, LOVEGROVE SS, LESAUVAGE SV, BRADY LM, SAINI N, MINIHANE AM, WILLIAMS CM, BURDGE GC, FINNEGAN YE & WOOTTON SA (2004) Moderate fish-oil supplementation reverses low-platelet, long-chain n-3 polyunsaturated fatty acid status and reduces plasma triacylglycerol concentrations in British Indo-Asians. *American Journal of Clinical Nutrition* **79**, 974–982.

LOVEJOY JC (2002) The influence of dietary fat on insulin resistance. *Current Diabetic Reports* **2**, 435–440.

MANTZIORIS E, CLELAND LG, GIBSON RA, NEUMANN MA, DEMASI M & JAMES MJ (2000) Biochemical effects of a diet containing foods enriched with n-3 fatty acids. *American Journal of Clinical Nutrition* **72**, 42–48.

McMANUS RM, JUMPSON J, FINEGOOD DT, CLANDININ MT & RYAN EA (1996) A comparison of the effects of n-3 fatty acids from linseed oil and fish oil in well-controlled type II diabetes. *Diabetes Care* **19**, 463–467.

MENSINK RP & KATAN M (1992) Effect of dietary fatty acids on serum lipids and lipoproteins. A meta-analysis of 27 trials. *Arteriosclerosis and Thrombosis* **12**, 911–919.

MILES EA, THIES F, WALLACE FA, POWELL JR, HURST TL, NEWSHOLME EA & CALDER PC (2001) Influence of age and dietary fish oil on plasma soluble adhesion molecule concentrations. *Clinical Science* **100**, 91–100.

MINIHANE AM, KHAN S, LEIGH-FIRBANK EC, TALMUD P, WRIGHT JW, MURPHY MC, GRIFFIN BA & WILLIAMS CM (2000) ApoE polymorphism and fish oil supplementation in subjects with an atherogenic lipoprotein phenotype. *Arteriosclerosis Thrombosis and Vascular Biology* **20**, 1990–1997.

MINIHANE AM, BRADY L, LOVEGROVE SS, LESAUVAGE SV, WILLIAMS CM & LOVEGROVE JA (2005) Lack of effect of dietary n-6:n-3 PUFA ratio on plasma lipids and markers of insulin responses in Indian Asians living in the UK. *European Journal of Nutrition* **44**, 26–32.

MORI TA, BURKE V, PUDDEY IB, WATTS GF, O'NEAL DN, BEST JD & BEILIN LJ (2000a) Purified eicosapentaenoic and docosahexaenoic acids have differential effects on serum lipids and lipoproteins, LDL particle size, glucose, and insulin in mildly hyperlipidemic men. *American Journal of Clinical Nutrition* **71**, 1085–1094.

MORI TA, WATTS GF, BURKE V, HILME E, PUDDEY IB, BEILIN LJ (2000b) Differential effects of eicosapentaenoic acid and docosahexaenoic acid on vascular reactivity of the forearm microcirculation in hyperlipidemic, overweight men. *Circulation* **102**, 1264–1269.

MORRIS MC, EVANS DA, BIENIAS JL, TANGNEY CC, BENNETT DA, WILSON RS, AGGARWAL N & SCHNEIDER J (2003) Consumption of fish and n-3 fatty acids and risk of incident Alzheimer disease. *Archives of Neurology* **60**, 940–946.

MOTOJIMA K, PASSILLY P, PETERS JM, GONZALEZ FJ & LATRUFFE N (1998) Expression of putative fatty acid transporter genes are regulated by peroxisome proliferator-activated receptor alpha and gamma activators in a tissue- and inducer-specific manner. *Journal of Biological Chemistry* **273**, 16710–16714

NAIR SSD, LEITCH JW, FALCONER J & GARG ML (1997) Prevention of cardiac arrhythmia by dietary (n-3) polyunsaturated fatty acids and their mechanism of action. *Journal of Nutrition* **127**, 383–393.

NARAYANAN BA, NARAYANAN NK, SIMI B & REDDY BS (2003) Modulation of inducible nitric oxide synthase and related proinflammatory genes by the omega-3 fatty acid docosahexaenoic acid in human colon cancer cells. *Cancer Research* **63**, 972–979.

NATIONAL DIET AND NUTRITION SURVEY (2003) *The National Diet and Nutrition Survey: Adults 19–64 years*, HMSO, London.

NENSETER MS, RUSTAN AC, LUNDKATZ S, SOYLAND E, MAELANDSMO G, PHILLIPS MC & DREVON CA (1992) Effect of dietary supplementation with n-3 polyunsaturated fatty-acids on physical-properties and metabolism of low-density-lipoprotein in humans. *Arteriosclerosis and Thrombosis* **12**, 369–379.

NKONDJOCK A, SHATENSTEIN B, MAISONNEUVE P & GHADIRIAN P (2003) Specific fatty acids and human colorectal cancer: an overview. *Cancer Detection and Prevention* **27**, 55–66.

OKUDA Y, KAWASHIMA K, SAWADA T, TSURUMARU K, ASANO M, SUZUKI S, SOMA M, NAKAJIMA T & YAMASHITA K (1997) Eicosapentaenoic acid enhances nitric oxide production by cultured human endothelial cells. *Biochemical and Biophysical Research Communications* **232**, 487–491.

ORDOVAS JM & SCHAEFER EJ (2000) Genetic determinants of plasma lipid response to dietary intervention: the role of the ApoA1/C3/A4 gene cluster and the ApoE gene. *British Journal of Nutrition* **83**, S127–S136.

ORDOVAS JM, CORELLA D, CUPPLES LA, DEMISSIE S, KELLEHER A, COLTELL O, WILSON PW, SCHAEFER EJ & TUCKER K (2002) Polyunsaturated fatty acids modulate the effects of the APOA1 G-A polymorphism on HDL-cholesterol concentrations in a sex-specific manner: the Framingham Study. *American Journal of Clinical Nutrition* **75**, 38–46.

PALMER CN, HU MF, GRIFFIN KJ, RAUCY JL & JOHNSON EF (1998) Peroxisome proliferator activated receptor-alpha expression in human liver. *Molecular Pharmacology* **53**, 14–22.

PALOZZA P, SGARLATA E, LUBERTO C, PICCIONI E, ANTI M, MARRA G, ARMELAO F, FRANCESCHELLI P & BARTOLI GM (1996) n-3 fatty acids induce oxidative modifications in human erythrocytes depending on dose and duration of dietary supplementation. *American Journal of Clinical Nutrition* **64**, 297–304.

PATSCH JR, MIESENBOCK G, HOPFERWIESER T, MUHLBERGER V, KNAPP E, DUNN JK, GOTTO AM, JR. & PATSCH W (1992) Relation of triglyceride metabolism and coronary artery disease. Studies in the postprandial state. *Arteriosclerosis and Thrombosis* **12**, 1336–1345.

POWER GW & NEWSHOLME EA (1997) Dietary fatty acids influence the activity and metabolic control of mitochondrial carnitine palmitoyltransferase I in rat heart and skeletal muscle. *Journal of Nutrition* **127**, 2142–2150.

PRESCOTT SL & CALDER PC (2004) N-3 polyunsaturated fatty acids and allergic disease. *Current Opinions in Nutrition and Metabolic Care* **7**, 123–129.

RANTALA M, RANTALA TT, SAVOLAINEN MJ, FRIEDLANDER Y & KESANIEMI YA (2000) *American Journal of Clinical Nutrition* **71**, 713–724.

RAO CV & REDDY BS (1993) Modulating effect of amount and types of dietary-fat on ornithine decarboxylase, tyrosine protein-kinase and prostaglandins production during colon carcinogenesis in male F344 rats. *Carcinogenesis* **14**, 1327–1333.

RAO CV, SIMI B, WYNN TT, GARR K & REDDY BS (1996) Modulating effect of amount and types of dietary fat on colonic mucosal phospholipase A(2), phosphatidylinositol-specific phospholipase C activities, and cyclooxygenase metabolite formation during different stages of colon tumor promotion in male F344 rats. *Cancer Research* **56**, 532–537.

RAO CV, HIROSE Y, INDRANIE C & REDDY BS (2001) Modulation of experimental colon tumorigenesis by types and amounts of dietary fatty acids. *Cancer Research* **61**, 1927–1933.

RAPP JH, LESPINE A, HAMILTON RL, COLYVAS N, CHAUMETON AH, TWEEDIE-HARDMAN J, KOTITE L, KUNITAKE ST, HAVEL RJ & KANE JP (1994) Triglyceride-rich lipoproteins isolated by selected-affinity anti-apolipoprotein B immunosorption from human atherosclerotic plaque. *Arteriosclerosis and Thrombosis* **14**, 1767–1774.

RIVELLESE AA (2000) Effects of omega-3 fatty acids on carbohydrate and lipid metabolism in healthy people: the KANWU study. *Diabetologia* **43**, 11.

ROCHE HM & GIBNEY MJ (2000) Effect of long-chain n-3 polyunsaturated fatty acids on fasting and postprandial triacylglycerol metabolism. *American Journal of Clinical Nutrition* **71**, 232S–237S.

ROYNETTE CE, CALDER PC, DUPERTUIS YM & PICHARD C (2004) n-3 Polyunsaturated fatty acids and colon cancer prevention. *Clinical Nutrition* **23**, 139–151.

SAMPATH H & NTAMBI JM (2004) Polyunsaturated fatty acid regulation of gene expression. *Nutrition Reviews* **62**, 333–339.

SCHMIDT EB, NIELSEN LK, PEDERSEN JO, KORNERUP HJ & DYERBERG J (1990) The effect of n-3 polyunsaturated fatty acids on lipids, platelet function, coagulation, fibrinolysis and monocyte chemotaxis in patients with hypertension. *Clinical Chimica Acta* **189**, 25–32.

SCOTT DT, JANOWSKY JS, CARROLL RE, TAYLOR JA, AUESTAD N & MONTALTO MB (1998) Formula supplementation with long-chain polyunsaturated fatty acids: Are there developmental benefits? *Pediatrics* **102**, e59.

SESSLER AM & NTAMBI JM (1998) Polyunsaturated fatty acid regulation of gene expression. *Journal of Nutrition* **128**, 923–926.

SHENG HM, SHAO JY, MORROW JD, BEAUCHAMP RD & DUBOIS RN (1998) Modulation of apoptosis and Bcl-2 expression by prostaglandin E-2 in human colon cancer cells. *Cancer Research* **58**, 362–366.

SIMOPOULOS AP (2002a) Omega-3 fatty acids in inflammation and autoimmune diseases. *Journal of the American College of Nutrition* **21**, 495–505

SIMOPOULOS AP (2002b) The importance of the ratio of omega-6/omega-3 essential fatty acids. *Biomedicine & Pharmacotherapy* **56**, 365–379.

SINGH J, HAMID R & REDDY BS (1997) Dietary fat and colon cancer: modulation of cyclooxygenase-2 by types and amount of dietary fat during the postinitiation stage of colon carcinogenesis. *Cancer Research* **57**, 3465–3470.

SINGH NP, MCCOY MT, TICE RR & SCHNEIDER EL (1988) A simple technique for quantitation of low-levels of DNA damage in individual cells. *Experimental Cell Research* **175**, 184–191.

SINGH RB, NIAZ MA, SHARMA JP, KUMAR R, RASTOGI V & MOSHIRI M (1997) Randomized, double-blind, placebo-controlled trial of fish oil and mustard oil in patients with suspected acute myocardial infarction: the Indian experiment of infarct survival – 4. *Cardiovascular Drugs Therapy* **11**, 485–491.

SORENSEN NS, MARCKMANN P, HOY CE, VAN DUYVENVOORDE W & PRINCEN HM (1998) Effect of fish-oil-enriched margarine on plasma lipids, low-density-lipoprotein particle composition, size, and susceptibility to oxidation. *American Journal of Clinical Nutrition* **68**, 235–241.

STEINBERG HO, CHAKER H, LEAMING R, JOHNSON A, BRECHTEL G & BARON AD (1996) Obesity/insulin resistance is associated with endothelial dysfunction. Implications for the syndrome of insulin resistance. *Journal of Clinical Investigation* **97**, 2601–2610.

STOLL AL, SEVERUS WE, FREEMAN MP, RUETER S, ZBOYAN HA, DIAMOND E, CRESS KK & MARANGELL LB (1999) Omega 3 fatty acids in bipolar disorder: a preliminary double-blind, placebo-controlled trial. *Archives of General Psychiatry* **56**, 413–416.

STORLIEN LH, PAN DA, KRIKETOS AD, OCONNOR J, CATERSON ID, COONEY GJ, JENKINS AB & BAUR LA (1996) Skeletal muscle membrane lipids and insulin resistance. *Lipids* **31**, S261–S265.

THIES F, GARRY JMC, YAQOOB P, RERKASEM K, WILLIAMS J, SHEARMAN CP, GALLAGHER PJ, CALDER PC & GRIMBLE RF (2003) Association of n-3 polyunsaturated fatty acids with stability of atherosclerotic plaques: a randomised controlled trial. *Lancet* **361**, 477–485.

TISDALE MJ (1996) Inhibition of lipolysis and muscle protein degradation by EPA in cancer cachexia. *Nutrition* **12**, S31–S33.

TISDALE MJ & DHESI JK (1990) Inhibition of weight-loss by omega-3-fatty-acids in an experimental cachexia model. *Cancer Research* **50**, 5022–5026.

TODOROV P, CARIUK P, McDEVITT T, COLES B, FEARON K & TISDALE M (1996) Characterization of a cancer cachectic factor. *Nature* **379**, 739–742.

TOFT I, BONAA KH, INGEBRETSEN OC, NORDOY A & JENSSEN T (1995) Effects of N-3 polyunsaturated fatty-acids on glucose-homeostasis and blood-pressure in essential-hypertension – a randomized, controlled trial. *Annals of Internal Medicine* **123**, 911–918.

TULLY AM, ROCHE H, DOYLE R, FALLON C, BRUCE I, LAWLOR B, COAKLEY D & GIBNEY MJ (2003) Low serum cholesteryl ester-docosahexaenoic acid levels in Alzheimer's disease: a case-control study. *British Journal of Nutrition* **89**, 483–489.

VENKATRAMAN JT, CHANDRASEKAR B, KIM JD & FERNANDES G (1994) Effects of n-3 and n-6 fatty-acids on the activities and expression of hepatic antioxidant enzymes in autoimmune-prone Nzbxnzw F1-mice. *Lipids* **29**, 561–568.

VERMUNT SHF, MENSINK RP, SIMONIS MMG & HORNSTRA G (2000) Effects of dietary alpha-linolenic acid on the conversion and oxidation of C-13-alpha-linolenic acid. *Lipids* **35**, 137–142.

VESSBY B (2000). Dietary fat and insulin action in humans. *British Journal of Nutrition* **83**, S91–S96.

VESSBY B (2003) Dietary fat, fatty acid composition in plasma and the metabolic syndrome. *Current Opinion in Lipidology* **14**, 15–19.

VESSBY B, KARLSTROM B, OHRVALL M, JARVI A, ANDERSSON A & BASU S (2000) Diet, nutrition and diabetes mellitus. *Upsala Journal of Medical Sciences* **105**, 151–160.

VESSBY B, UNSITUPA M, HERMANSEN K, RICCARDI G, RIVELLESE AA, TAPSELL LC, NALSEN C, BERGLUND L, LOUHERANTA A, RASMUSSEN BM, CALVERT GD, MAFFETONE A, PEDERSEN E, GUSTAFSSON IB, STORLIEN LH; KANWU STUDY (2001) Substituting dietary saturated for monounsaturated fat impairs insulin sensitivity in healthy men and women: the KANWU Study. *Diabetologia* **44**, 312–319.

WAHLE KWJ, ROTONDO D & HEYS SD (2003) Polyunsaturated fatty acids and gene expression in mammalian systems. *Proceedings of the Nutrition Society* **62**, 349–360.

WAINWRIGHT P (2000) Nutrition and behaviour: the role of n-3 fatty acids in cognitive function. *British Journal of Nutrition* **83**, 337–339.

WALLACE JMW, TURLEY E, GILMORE WS, STRAIN JJ (1995) Dietary fish oil supplementation alters leukocyte function and cytokine production in healthy women. *Arteriosclerosis Thrombosis and Vascular Biology* **15**, 185–189.

WEINTRAUB MS, ZECHNER R, BROWN A, EISENBERG S & BRESLOW JL (1988) Dietary polyunsaturated fats of the w-6 and w-3 series reduce postprandial lipoprotein levels – chronic and acute effects of fat saturation on postprandial lipoprotein metabolism. *Journal of Clinical Investigation* **82**, 1884–1893.

WERKMAN SH & CARLSON SE (1996) A randomized trial of visual attention of preterm infants fed docosahexaenoic acid until nine months. *Lipids* **31**, 91–97.

WHITEHOUSE AS, SMITH HJ, DRAKE JL & TISDALE MJ (2001) Mechanism of attenuation of skeletal muscle protein catabolism in cancer cachexia by eicosapentaenoic acid. *Cancer Research* **61**, 3604–3609.

WHO EUROPE (2003) *Food based dietary guidelines in the WHO European region*, Eur/03/

5045414. Copenhagen: WHO.

WHO/FAO EXPERT CONSULTATION (2003) *Diet nutrition and the prevention of chronic diseases*: WHO technical report series 916. Geneva: WHO.

WILLATTS P, FORSYTH JS, DIMODUGNO MK, VARMA S & COLVIN M (1998) Influence of long-chain polyunsaturated fatty acids on infant cognitive function. *Lipids* **33**, 973–980.

ZAMPELAS A, PEEL AS, GOULD BJ, WRIGHT J & WILLIAMS CM (1994a) Polyunsaturated fatty-acids of the n-6 and n-3 series – effects on postprandial lipid and apolipoprotein levels in healthy men. *European Journal of Clinical Nutrition* **48**, 842–848.

6

Dietary fat and obesity

P. Schrauwen and W. H. M. Saris, Maastricht University, The Netherlands

6.1 Introduction

Obesity is an increasing problem in affluent societies. By definition, the development of obesity is characterized by a mismatch between energy intake and energy expenditure. Apart from genetic factors that have been suggested to lead to obesity, the rapid development of obesity in Western societies has mostly been attributed to a reduction in levels of physical activity and an increase in the consumption of high-fat, energy-dense (fast) foods. Although many studies have tried to explain what the role of dietary fat is in the obesity epidemic, there is still no consensus on this topic.

In this chapter we will review the evidence for a causal role for dietary fat in the development of obesity. In Section 6.1.1 we will describe the current prevalence of obesity and its associated problems and in Section 6.1.2 we will explain why obesity, by definition, is linked to a positive fat balance. In Section 6.2 epidemiological data on fat intake, fat quality and obesity prevalence will be reviewed to examine if evidence exists that these two parameters are interrelated. Although epidemiological data can be useful to identify a potential relationship between fat intake and the development of obesity, many confounding factors should be taken into account in interpreting these types of data. Therefore, intervention studies manipulating dietary fat intake are better suited to test the role of dietary fat in the development of obesity.

In Section 6.3 we will review the evidence derived from intervention studies that have manipulated dietary fat intake (Section 6.3.1), dietary fatty acid composition in the form of CLA supplementation (Section 6.3.2) or dietary fatty acid chain length (Section 6.3.2) and have used body weight as the primary outcome variable. Alongside long-term intervention studies of body weight and composition, many studies have also been performed that examine the effect of short-term manipulation of dietary fat quantity and quality on obesity-related parameters.

In Section 6.4, we will review data on the effect of dietary fat quantity on energy intake (Section 6.4.1) and energy expenditure/fat oxidation (Sections 6.4.2 and 6.4.3), whereas in Section 6.4.4 the role of dietary fat quality on energy metabolism will be discussed. The chapter will end with a brief discussion on the implications of the findings for food processors (Section 6.5) and on potential future trends (Section 6.6).

6.1.1 Obesity: definition and problems

The prevalence of obesity is still increasing in affluent societies. For example, in the United States the number of people older than 20 years with obesity, defined as a body mass index (BMI) of > 30 kg/m^2, increased from 13% in 1960 to 30% in the year 2000, according to the latest NHANES survey (Flegal *et al.*, 2002). Moreover, the overall prevalence in people over 20 years with a BMI > 25 kg/m^2, which is considered to represent overweight, equalled 64% according to this survey. These increases in prevalence of obesity in adults are not only seen in affluent societies but recently also in developing countries. Even more dramatically, the prevalence of obesity in children between 6 and 19 years increased from 4% in the 1960s to 15% in 2000 in the United States (Ogden *et al.*, 2002). Obesity increases the risk for a number of health-threatening diseases and it is expected that obesity will become the number one cause of mortality in the future and be an enormous burden on the health care system in affluent societies. Obesity is accompanied by an increased risk for type 2 diabetes mellitus, high blood pressure, high cholesterol, asthma, arthritis and cardiovascular complications. For example, the number of subjects suffering from type 2 diabetes mellitus doubled between 1980 and 2002 in the United States, reaching a prevalence of 5.9% in 2002. The major question thus remains how we can explain this dramatic increase in the prevalence of obesity.

By definition, the development of obesity and overweight is characterized by a positive energy balance. Therefore, to explain the increase in the prevalence of obesity, either average energy intake or energy expenditure, or both must have been changed in the overall population over the last 20–30 years. Indeed, the rapid increase in the prevalence of obesity is often ascribed to the changing lifestyle characteristics in Westernized societies, among which are the consumption of high-fat, energy-dense diets and a reduction in physical activity. Nevertheless, it should be kept in mind that the regulation of body weight in humans is very strict and well controlled, especially when considering that food is available at any place and any time in our Western society. For example, an average person with a body weight of 75 kg will expend ~10 MJ/day. For such a person, a weight gain of 5 kg in one year requires a positive energy balance of 150 MJ/year or 400 kJ/day, meaning a difference between energy intake and energy expenditure of only 4%. This theoretical calculation indicates that the current increase in the prevalence of obesity must be attributed to very small changes in energy intake and/or expenditure, indicating that despite this increase in obesity prevalence, in general humans are still relatively good in regulating their energy balance. Nevertheless, there are large differences between individuals, probably because of genetic variability in predisposition to obesity. Based on overfeeding studies in identical twins, it was calculated that the efficiency to convert surplus energy towards fat storage varies by a factor of 3 among subjects (Saris, 2004). This result indicates that some individuals within the population are much more susceptible than others to gain weight in our current hostile environment, in which there is abundant food availability and no need to be active.

6.1.2 Energy balance versus fat balance

Although obesity is, by using BMI, defined as an excess body weight, the real problem is an excess in body fat mass. In this respect, the development of obesity concerns a positive fat rather than a positive energy balance per se. However, numerous investigations have shown that in the long term, an imbalance between energy intake and energy expenditure is reflected in a positive fat balance. In the past 20–30 years many food products have become available that are cheap, palatable and high in fat content. Since dietary fat is the most energy-dense macronutrient, with about 38 kJ/g (in comparison: carbohydrate and protein only provide about 17 kJ/g), an increase in dietary fat intake can easily promote an increase in energy intake and thus result in overconsumption. In addition, in humans, there is evidence for a clear substrate hierarchy for utilization of macronutrients, in which fat balance is least regulated. For example, the human body responds only very slowly by increasing fat oxidation when fat intake is increased (Schrauwen *et al.*, 1997a; Thomas *et al.*, 1992), leading to a deposition of dietary fat into the fat stores. On the other hand, the storage capacity for carbohydrate and protein in the human body is limited and therefore carbohydrate and protein oxidation are very well and rapidly adjusted to their respective intake (Abbott *et al.*, 1988). As a consequence, a positive energy balance will be reflected in a positive fat balance.

6.2 Epidemiological associations

6.2.1 Trends in fat intake and body weight

As outlined above, the increasing prevalence of obesity worldwide has been attributed to an increase in high-energy dense and fatty food together with a reduction in energy expenditure during physical activity. Many cross-sectional studies have been performed, which attempt to link (self-reported) fat intake with body fatness or body weight. However, data from these studies are not consistent, with some studies showing the expected positive association (Dreon *et al.*, 1988; Lissner *et al.*, 1987; Romieu *et al.*, 1988; Tremblay *et al.*, 1989) whereas other studies find no association between fat intake and body fatness (Lissner and Heitmann, 1995; Slattery *et al.*, 1992). Also, results from prospective studies are not consistent. For example, Colditz *et al.* (1990) found that the percentage of dietary fat was not related to weight gain, but previous weight was positively related to a high fat intake. In a study of Heitmann *et al.* (1995) dietary fat intake was positively associated with weight gain, but only in women with a predisposition to obesity. Another approach used to study the relationship between dietary fat intake and body weight is by comparing average fat intake and body mass (or BMI) between different populations. In an analysis of data obtained from 20 countries, Bray and Popkin (1998) reported a large, significant positive association between dietary fat consumption and the percentage of people in the population being overweight. A major comment on that study, however, was that there was a large range in socio-economic status across the 20 different countries which introduces many confounding factors such as food availability and physical activity. Comparison of dietary fat intake (as energy%) and BMI between European countries, in which smaller variations in socio-economic status were evident, revealed no association between the two variables in men, and even a negative association in women (Lissner and Heitmann, 1995).

As a consequence of the recommendations to reduce fat intake, the market for low-fat food expanded rapidly in the 1990s (Leveille and Finley, 1997). Based on subjects self-recording, the actual intake of fat expressed as a percentage of energy has decreased significantly over the past decade (Kennedy *et al.*, 1999), whereas the prevalence of obesity has continued to rise. Similarly, with the increasing popularity of lower-fat products, food intake statistics have shown a decrease in dietary fat intake although the prevalence of obesity is rising (NHANESIII, 1994; Willett, 1998), and this is referred to as the so-called fat paradox (Willett, 1998). Therefore, the scientific evidence for the relationship between dietary fat intake and the prevalence of obesity has been seriously challenged in recent years. For example, Katan *et al.* (1997a) questioned the importance of low-fat, high-carbohydrate diets in the prevention and treatment of obesity and provided evidence that reduction of fat intake resulted in only a very limited weight reduction of a few kilograms body weight. However, we should consider figures for self-reported intake with great caution owing to the evidence for systematic under-reporting of energy and fat. This occurs in a significant proportion of whole population but appears to be more marked in the obese resulting in systematic bias in the data (Heitmann and Lissner, 1995; Heitmann *et al.*, 2000). The reported reduction in fat intake in the United States coincides with large campaigns to promote the reduction of fat intake and this is likely to contribute to greater prevalence of under-reporting especially in overweight and obese subjects.. Goris *et al.* (2000) measured total food intake in 30 obese subjects and compared it with total energy expenditure, as measured with the doubly labelled water technique. With this approach, they were able to show a mismatch between energy expenditure and food intake of 37%. In

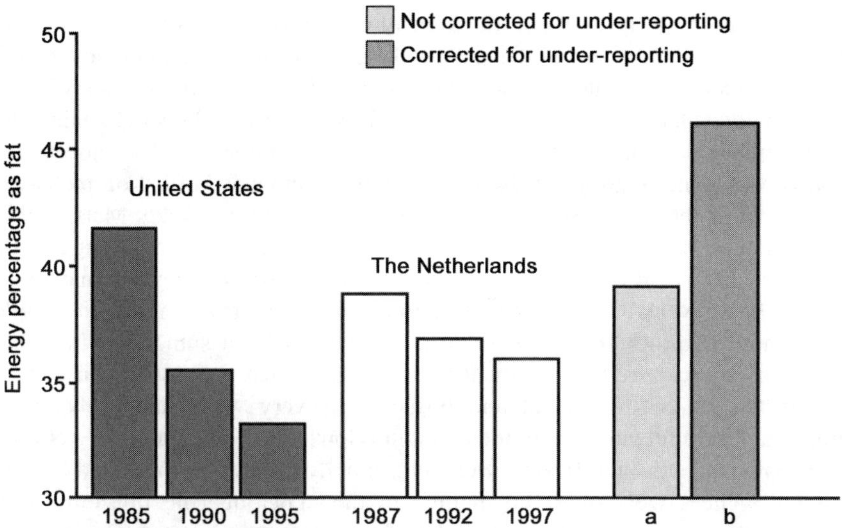

Fig. 6.1 Percentages of energy from fat as measured in the USA (1985—1990–1995) and the Netherlands (1987–1992–1997). A and B are percentages of energy from fat reported by 30 Dutch obese men (Goris *et al.*, 2000), with (b) and without (a) correction for underreporting. Adapted from Westerterp and Goris (2002).

addition, subjects lost body weight during the study period, indicating that subjects under-ate during the study (26%). Water intake was also lower than water loss, indicating that part of the under-reporting was due to under-recording (12%). Interestingly, the reported percentage of energy from fat was related to the level of under-reporting. This study shows that obese subjects indeed under-report their fat intake, and this may have important consequences for the interpretation of epidemiological observations in a period when health campaigns promote a low fat intake. This is illustrated in Fig. 6.1, which shows the reported proportion of energy from fat in national food consumption studies in The Netherlands and in the United States, and the percentage of energy from fat in 30 Dutch obese men (Goris *et al.*, 2000), with and without correction for under-reporting.

This massive systematic under-reporting can also be concluded from the food production figures as recently presented in the report on Diet, Nutrition and the Prevention of Chronic Diseases from the WHO FAO, where edible fat production and available food energy steadily rose over the last decades (Nishida *et al.*, 2004). For instance, the available fat per capita per day rose in the USA from 117 to 143 g between 1967 and 1997. Although the waste of food has increased substantially, it probably did not do so at the same rate as the increase in production. In summary, based on the published results so far it can be concluded that a high fat intake can be considered as a risk factor for overconsumption and thus weight gain.

6.2.2 Dietary fatty acid composition and obesity

In addition to the amount of dietary fat, the composition of the fatty acids in the diet has also been related to the development of obesity. In particular, PUFA-enriched diets have been suggested to be able to prevent body weight gain, when they replace saturated fatty acids in the diet. In animals, it has indeed been shown that a diet high in saturates has a more pronounced effect on increase in body fatness than a highly PUFA-enriched diet (Hill *et al.*, 1992; Matsuo *et al.*, 1995; Pan *et al.*, 1994). Also in humans some evidence exists to suggest that saturated fatty acids in particular induce obesity. Thus, in a large human cohort in the USA a weak but positive correlation between saturated fat intake and BMI was found (Colditz *et al.*, 1990). In a study in Spanish subjects, with a high intake of unsaturated fatty acids, it was concluded that the association between specific types of dietary fat and obesity was very weak and probably not important in the regulation of body weight (Gonzalez *et al.*, 2000). In a study of 128 male subjects, significant differences in body fatness (as measured by waist circumference) were observed in men in the upper quartile of saturated fat intake, whereas high intakes of PUFA had no effect on adiposity (Doucet *et al.*, 1998). Also in some older studies, positive correlations between saturated fat intake (assessed by 7-day diet records) and percentage body fat were reported in 155 sedentary obese subjects, but no such correlation with PUFA was observed (Dreon *et al.*, 1988). Taken together, these studies do indicate that saturated fat may be more fattening in humans compared with polyunsaturates, although the number of studies is still very limited and in general the associations found between saturated fat intake and obesity are rather weak.

6.3 Intervention studies: managing fat intake to control obesity

6.3.1 Long-term manipulation of the fat/carbohydrate ratio to control body weight

From epidemiological data it is difficult to determine whether fat intake is related to the development of obesity, mainly because of the problem of under-reporting of food intake, and in particular, fat intake. Therefore, intervention studies with high *vs* low fat diets are more informative in examining the question whether the proportion of energy from fat in the diet influences body weight. Several studies have been published on the effects of *ad libitum* reduction of fat intake on body weight. We performed a large-scale, long-term, randomized controlled trial (the CARMEN multi-centre trial) on the role of the carbohydrate/fat ratio as well as the simple versus complex carbohydrate content of the diet, on body weight regulation. This study involved 398 moderately overweight subjects in five different countries (Saris *et al.*, 2000) and investigated the effect on energy intake, body weight and blood lipids, of 6 months *ad libitum* intake of low-fat diets (reduction of $\approx$10 energy%) rich in either simple or complex carbohydrates. The results showed that both the low-fat, high-

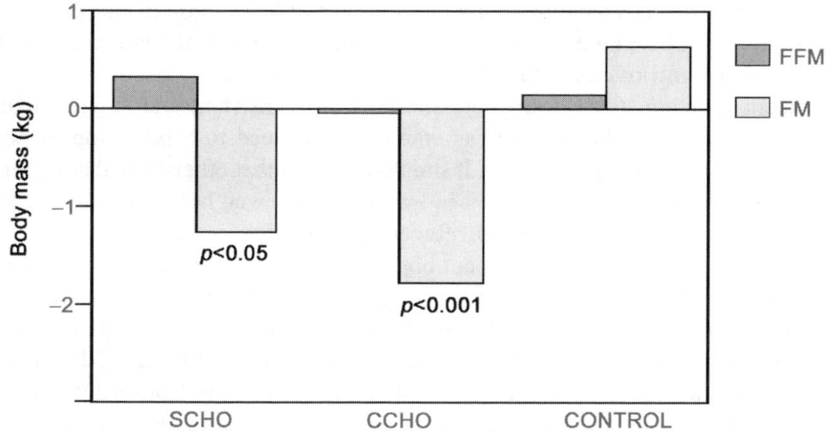

Fig. 6.2 Changes (kg) in fat-free mass (FFM) and fat mass (FM) during a 6 months intervention trial with 398 moderately obese adults on a low-fat, high simple carbohydrate diet (SCHO), low-fat, high complex carbohydrate (CCHO) or normal fat, carbohydrate diet (CONTROL). Adapted from Saris *et al.* (2000).

carbohydrate diets reduced body weight significantly by 1.6 kg (for high simple carbohydrates) and 2.4 kg (for high complex) compared with a control normal-fat, normal-carbohydrate diet (Fig. 6.2).

The findings from the CARMEN study underline the importance of the public health measures aimed to reduce fat intake. A decrease in body weight of 2–3 kg by means of a general reduction in fat intake of approximately 10 energy% in the general population could reduce the prevalence of obesity from 25% to 15% (Astrup *et al.*, 2000a). Further evidence for this comes from four meta-analyses on this topic. Astrup *et al.* (2000b) selected controlled intervention studies lasting more than 2 months that compared *ad libitum* low-fat diets with either medium-fat diets or subjects' habitual diets. All studies were published between 1966 and 1998 and involved 1728 individuals. The low-fat diet resulted in a 2.55 kg greater weight loss compared to the control diet. Simple correlation analysis revealed that baseline body weight and the reduction in the percentage dietary fat (in energy%) were the major determinants for the weight loss (Astrup *et al.*, 2000b). The same authors later updated their initial meta-analysis by excluding those studies where physical activity was promoted, and including some more recent studies (Astrup *et al.*, 2000a). In total 1910 individuals were included and on average the dietary fat reduction was 10 energy% in the low-fat interventions. Again, the low-fat intervention groups showed a greater weight loss than the control groups (3.2 kg). Bray and Popkin (1998) conducted a meta-analysis on 28 intervention trials and found that a reduction of dietary fat intake of 10 energy% resulted in a weight loss of 2.9 kg over 6 months. Finally, Yu-Poth *et al.* (1999) performed a meta-analysis on 37 diet intervention studies published between 1981 and 1997 with the objective of evaluating the effect of the National Cholesterol Education Program diet on cardiovascular disease risk factors. In their analysis, they found that for every 1% decrease in energy as total fat, there was a 0.28 kg decrease in body weight. The effect of change in total fat intake on weight loss explained 57% of the total variance.

Taken together, these four meta-analyses are consistent and suggest that a reduction in dietary fat content (as energy%) can lead to a reduction in body weight of about 2–4 kg. However, it should be noted that other diets that result in lower energy intake are as efficient in lowering body weight (Foreyt and Poston, 2002; Jequier and Bray, 2002). Recently, the first results from the EU-NUGENOB were presented concerning the effect of a 600 kcal/day energy restriction, either by a fat-rich (40 energy% fat) or carbohydrate-rich (60 energy% carbohydrate) diet. It was shown that weight loss was identical in both energy-restricted groups, showing again that energy restriction determines weight loss, irrespective of the type of diet used (Nugenob Consortium, 2004). Nevertheless, owing to the higher energy density of fat-rich foods, a reduction in fat intake might be a more convenient and effective practical way to reduce energy intake.

6.3.2 CLA intervention studies

Conjugated linoleic acid is a group of isomers of conjugated dienoic derivates of linoleic acid. The dietary source of CLA for humans is mainly in ruminant meats such as beef and lamb and in dairy products such as milk and cheese. In animals, many studies have shown that CLA can reduce adiposity and lipid content of the body (DeLany *et al.*, 1999; Ostrowska *et al.*, 1999; Park *et al.*, 1997; Sisk *et al.*, 2001; Terpstra *et al.*, 2002; Tsuboyama-Kasaoka *et al.*, 2000; West *et al.*, 1998). However, in humans data are less consistent. When body weight is taken as the outcome measure, the effects of CLA supplementation are rather disappointing. In type 2 diabetic patients who received 6 g/day of CLA, a correlation was observed between body weight change and plasma concentrations of the t10,*c*12-isomer of CLA (Belury *et al.*, 2003), but most other studies did not find an effect of CLA supplementation on body weight (Mougios *et al.*, 2001; Smedman and Vessby, 2001; Zambell *et al.*, 2000). However, several studies do indicate that CLA supplementation affects body fatness. In overweight humans, CLA supplementation for 12 weeks reduced body fat mass when CLA was administered at doses of 3.4 or 6.8 g/day. Similarly, in healthy non-obese men and women, CLA reduced body fat after 12 weeks at doses of 1.8 g/day (Thom *et al.*, 2001), 4.2 g/day (Smedman and Vessby, 2001) or 1.4 g/day for 4 weeks (Mougios *et al.*, 2001). However, other studies do not find an effect of CLA on body fatness (reviewed in Larsen *et al.*, 2003). It should be noted that all these studies had a relatively short duration and no long-term studies on the effect of CLA are yet available. In addition, recent data suggest that CLA supplementation may have adverse side effects, such as producing lipid peroxidation and insulin resistance (Moloney *et al.*, 2004; Riserus *et al.*, 2004a,b). Therefore, clearly more and longer-term studies are needed before conclusions can be drawn on the effectiveness of CLA in body fat regulation. For a more extensive review on the effect of CLA on body weight and composition, please refer to Chapter 8.

6.3.3 Manipulating the fatty acid chain length

In contrast to long chain fatty acids, medium chain fatty acids, with a chain length of 8–12 carbon atoms, can enter the mitochondria for oxidation without the mitochondrial fatty acid transporter CPT1 (Williamson *et al.*, 1968). This enzyme has been regarded as the rate-limiting step in fatty acid oxidation, and consequently the oxidation of medium chain length fatty acids is more rapid compared with long chain fatty acids. In animals, it has been clearly shown that feeding medium chain triglyceride (MCT) rich diets leads to less body weight gain when compared with long chain triglyceride (LCT)-rich diets (Chanez *et al.*, 1991; Hashim and Tantibhedyangkul, 1987; Kaunitz *et al.*, 1958). However, long-term intervention trials on the efficacy of MCT in the prevention of obesity are limited. Tsuji *et al.* (2001) assessed the potential health benefits of MCT compared with LCT in 78 healthy men and women using a double-blind, controlled protocol. They found that in subjects with a BMI > 23 kg/m^2, body weight and body fat were significantly lower on the MCT diet compared with the LCT diet. However, it should be noted that subjects lost weight on both diets and the difference in weight loss between the diets was relatively small (~2 kg/12 weeks). Nosaka *et al.* (2003) provided 73 subjects with margarines containing 5 g/day of either MCT or LCT for 12 weeks. Again, subjects lost weight on both diets, but the loss in body weight was significantly higher in the MCT compared with the LCT group, with a difference of about 1.5 kg over the 12 weeks. A comparable study by the same group of researchers found similar results in 82 subjects who consumed bread enriched with 1.7 g of medium chain fatty acids per day for 12 weeks (Kasai *et al.*, 2003). Krotkiewski (2001) examined the effect of MCT *vs* LCT supplementation during a very low-calorie diet in obese women for 4 weeks. Again, body weight decreased more in the MCT group, but the results were only significant in the first 2 weeks.

St-Onge and coworkers studied the effect of diets rich in either MCT or LCT for 4 weeks in healthy overweight men (St-Onge and Jones, 2003) and obese women (St-Onge *et al.*, 2003). In obese women, MCT did not significantly affect body weight, although changes in energy expenditure were observed (St-Onge *et al.*, 2003). In overweight men, however, MCT decreased body weight to a significantly greater extent compared with LCT, again due to increased energy expenditure and fat oxidation (St-Onge and Jones, 2003). Taken together, results on MCT supplementation are promising and suggest that MCT may be beneficial in the prevention and treatment of obesity. However, there are no long-term (> 12 weeks) intervention studies examining the effect of MCT. In addition, it should be noted that large (> 20–30 g/day) amounts of MCT in the diet can lead to gastrointestinal discomfort and therefore the use of MCT in the diet will be limited to small (<20 g/day) amounts with, if anything, only small effects on body weight.

6.4 Laboratory studies in humans

6.4.1 Manipulation of fat intake: effects on voluntary energy intake

As mentioned before, fat has the highest energy density and is characterized by its high palatability, and therefore dietary fat is often considered to increase energy intake (Klesges *et al.*, 1992; Miller *et al.*, 1990; Prewitt *et al.*, 1991; Verboeket-van de Venne *et al.*, 1996). In the Leeds high-fat study there were 19 times more obese subjects among those habitually consuming a diet high in fat (>45 energy%) than among the consumers with a low fat content of their habitual diet (<35 energy%) (Blundell and Macdiarmid, 1997). Furthermore, numerous studies show that voluntary energy intake is higher on a high-fat diet (Blundell *et al.*, 1993; Lissner and Heitmann, 1995, Lissner *et al.*, 1987; Westerterp *et al.*, 1996). As mentioned above, the most likely reason why high-fat diets lead to over-consumption is because of their high energy density.

It has also been suggested, however, that iso-energetic high-fat diets are more fattening than high-carbohydrate diets, i.e. independent of an effect on energy intake (Horton *et al.*, 1995; Miller *et al.*, 1990; Romieu *et al.*, 1988). For example, Horton *et al.* (1995) showed that carbohydrate overfeeding produced a progressive increase in total energy expenditure, resulting in 75–85% of excess energy being stored, whereas fat overfeeding had minimal effects on total energy expenditure, leading to storage of 90–95% of excess energy. However, apart from a few of these studies, there is limited evidence for such an effect and it has been clearly shown that the fat content of the diet influences body fat only when energy intake is also increased (Westerterp *et al.*, 1996).

The question then remains how the fat content of the diet influences energy intake. One explanation could be that fat has less effect on satiety than carbohydrate and protein, and therefore leads to passive over-consumption (Rolls and Hammer, 1995). However, Saltzman *et al.* (1997) found no difference in voluntary energy intake over a 9-day period between low-fat (20 energy% fat) and high-fat (40 energy% fat) diets, when matched for energy density and palatability. Also Stubbs *et al.* (1996) found that subjects ate a constant amount (weight) of food derived from diets with low (20 energy%), medium (40 energy%) or high (60 energy%) fat content, but with similar energy density. Rolls and Bell (1999) performed a systematic review of studies that compared the effects of fat and carbohydrate on food intake. They indeed concluded that, when the palatability and energy density were kept the same, the fat and carbohydrate content of a preload had similar effects on subsequent food intake. This finding could be interpreted as evidence for the suggestion that dietary fat intake per se does not lead to overeating and obesity (Willett, 1998), as it is not the dietary fat content but the energy density of the food that determines energy intake.

It has been suggested that, because in so-called 'light-products', dietary fat is often replaced by refined sugars, the energy density of these products remains high and therefore the reduction in fat intake is not reflected in a reduction in body weight in individuals nor in the prevalence of obesity in the population

(Katan *et al.*, 1997b). However, this is a misinterpretation of the energy composition and density of the low-fat foods. Replacing 1 g of fat by 1 g of sugar will reduce energy density by more than 50%. This was recently shown in a randomized clinical trial, in which both experimental groups undertook a reduction in fat intake (10 energy%), either by complex carbohydrate or sugar. As expected, both groups showed a similar reduction in dietary energy density (Saris *et al.*, 2000). Therefore, in normal situations, the fat content of the diet remains the major determinant of the energy density of the diet, as was shown by Prentice and Jebb (2003). They found a high correlation between fat content and energy density in a range of fast foods, Gambian foods, supermarket ready meals and supermarket healthy options. Therefore, reducing the fat content of the diet and adding water are the most efficient ways to affect the energy density of the diet, and thereby reduce voluntary energy intake.

6.4.2 The effect of fat supplements on fat oxidation

Apart from the effect of dietary fat content on energy intake, the effect on fat oxidation has also been frequently studied. A low-fat oxidative capacity has been shown to predispose to the development of obesity (Zurlo *et al.*, 1990), and as mentioned before, in the substrate hierarchy fat oxidation has lowest priority (Abbott *et al.*, 1988). Several studies have investigated the effect on substrate oxidation of adding fat to the diet. One of the first of these studies was performed by Flatt *et al.* (1985), who investigated the effect of a low-fat breakfast (11 energy% fat) or a low-fat breakfast with a 50 g fat supplement on postprandial substrate utilization and nutrient balance in seven young men. It was found that substrate oxidation was not influenced by the surplus fat, with a positive fat balance after the fat supplement as a consequence. Similar results were obtained by Bennett *et al.* (1992), who found no effect of adding 50 g of fat to a standard breakfast on fat oxidation during a 18 h period following breakfast. These short-term studies clearly show that excess fat is not oxidized but rather leads to a positive fat balance. Similar effects are observed in medium-term experiments, where the effect of fat surplus on substrate oxidation is studied in respiratory chambers. Schutz *et al.* (1989) studied subjects for two consecutive 24-h periods and in the second 24-h period 106 g of fat was added to the diet. This had no effect on energy expenditure or substrate oxidation, leading to the conclusion that the total fat surplus was stored and fat balance and energy balance were closely correlated.

In an *ad libitum* experiment, Thomas *et al.* (1992) compared the effect of *ad libitum* low- and high-fat diets for 7 days in obese and lean subjects. As expected, voluntary energy intake was higher on the high-fat diets (energy density was not controlled for). Again, fat oxidation was balanced with fat intake after 7 days of a high-fat diet, although fat oxidation was weakly related to fat intake in the lean subjects but not the obese subjects. This again illustrates that a high-fat diet leads to a positive fat balance, an effect that seems to be more pronounced in obese subjects. This is not surprising, as we have discussed before that energy balance is closely related to fat balance and therefore adding fat to a diet (in excess of the energy requirements) will thus lead to energy (fat) storage.

In that respect, the study of Horton *et al.* (1995) is of particular interest. They compared the effect of an excess of energy of 50% during 14 days either in the form of carbohydrate or in the form of fat. It was found that carbohydrate overfeeding produced rapid increases in carbohydrate oxidation, but importantly also in energy expenditure, resulting in an energy storage efficiency of 80%, whereas excess fat did neither increase fat oxidation nor energy expenditure (energy storage efficiency of 96%). As a result, fat balance was more positive after fat overfeeding compared with carbohydrate overfeeding. A similar effect was more recently reported by Dirlewanger *et al.* (2000), who showed an increase in 24-h energy expenditure after carbohydrate overfeeding but not after fat overfeeding. However, another study did not find a difference in energy expenditure after carbohydrate *vs* fat overfeeding for 96 hours (McDevitt *et al.*, 2000). Clearly, more research is needed on this topic to make a valid conclusion.

6.4.3 Iso-energetic low- *vs* high-fat diets and fat balance

Although fat in excess of energy requirements does not stimulate its own oxidation, the question remains whether high-fat diets given in energy balance are able to stimulate fat oxidation. If fat oxidation is not stimulated on an iso-energetic high-fat diet the body relies on its (limited) carbohydrate stores and a reduction in plasma glucose and/or glycogen will lead to feelings of hunger. One of the first studies to examine the effect of iso-energetic low- and high-fat diets was performed by Abbott *et al.* (1990). They studied the acute effect of iso-energetic high- (65 energy% fat) and low-fat diets (20 energy% fat) on 24-h substrate oxidation in Pima Indians. On the high-fat diet, 24-h fat oxidation was similar to fat intake, whereas on the low-fat diet fat oxidation exceeded fat intake. Hill *et al.* (1991) studied lean subjects after 3 and 7 days on high-fat (60 energy% fat) and low-fat (20 energy% fat) diets. On day 3, fat oxidation shifted in the direction of fat intake on both diets, and no further changes in fat oxidation between day 3 and day 7 were observed.

These results indicate that an iso-energetic shift from a low- to a high-fat diet does affect fat oxidation, although the acute adaptation of fat oxidation to fat intake is not complete. Moreover, the increase in fat oxidation on a high-fat diet seems to be blunted in the pre- (or post-) obese state (Astrup *et al.*, 1994; Lean and James, 1988). Verboeket-van de Venne *et al.* (1994) studied the effect of 3 days low-fat (10 energy% fat), medium-fat (30 energy% fat) or high-fat (50 energy% fat) diets on 24-h substrate oxidation in restrained and unrestrained eaters. On the low-fat and medium-fat diets fat oxidation was higher than fat intake, whereas on the high-fat diet fat oxidation matched fat intake. However, the restrained eaters, who are considered to have higher susceptibility to become obese, responded with a smaller increase in fat oxidation on the high-fat diet than the unrestrained eaters.

Most of the above-mentioned studies measured 24-h substrate oxidation after several days of a low- *vs* high-fat diet and in several of these studies energy balance was not reached. We conducted a study to examine the day-to-day adaptation when subjects shifted from a low-fat diet to a high-fat diet for 1 week (Schrauwen *et al.*, 1997a). First subjects consumed a low-fat diet for 3 days at home, after which subjects stayed in the respiration chamber for 5 consecutive days and were fed in energy balance. On the first and second day in the respiration chamber subjects continued to receive the low-fat diet (30 energy% fat) they had eaten at home. At the third day in the respiration chamber subjects transferred to a high-fat diet (60 energy% fat) for 7 days, and were studied in the chamber for the following three days (days 1–3 high fat diet) and on the final day on the high-fat diet (day 7, high-fat diet). On the low-fat diet, subjects were in both energy and substrate balance (i.e. fat oxidation was equal to fat intake). On the high-fat diet we found that fat oxidation continued to increase and only matched fat intake after seven days of the high-fat diet (Fig. 6.3; Schrauwen *et al.*, 1997a). As a result, subjects were in negative carbohydrate balance during the first days on the high-fat diet, and this accumulated up to 150–200 g of carbohydrate over the 7-day period. In a subsequent study, we showed that the adaptation of fat oxidation to a high-fat diet can be accelerated when glycogen levels are acutely lowered via exercise before consuming the high-fat diet

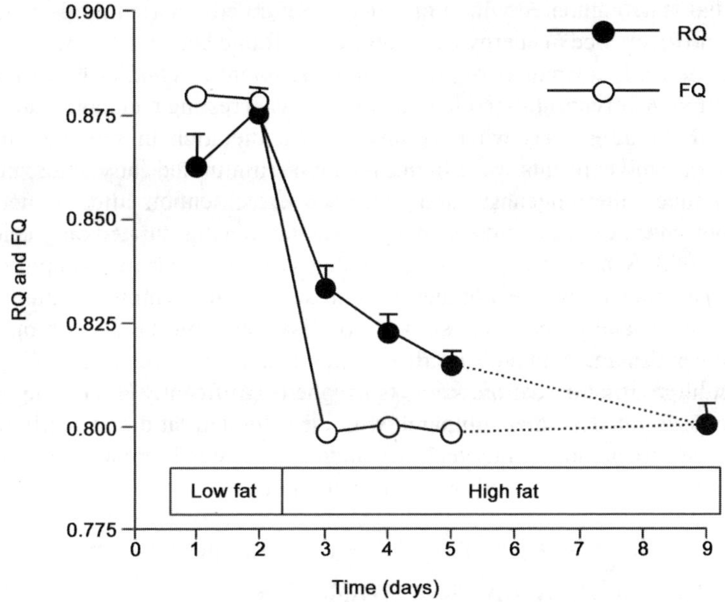

Fig. 6.3 24-h respiratory quotients (RQ) and 24-h food quotients (FQ) as measured in the respiration chamber. Subjects were fed a low-fat diet for 3 days at home and for 2 days while in the respiration chamber (days 1 and 2). Subsequently subjects consumed a high-fat diet for 7 days. Adapted from Schrauwen *et al.* (1997a).

(Schrauwen *et al.*, 1997b, 1998). This illustrates the impact of the carbohydrate balance in the regulation of fat oxidation. Furthermore, it also illustrates that a complete matching of fat oxidation to fat intake on a high-fat diet takes several days, leading to a positive fat balance and reduction in carbohydrate stores, and the latter will most likely lead to overeating under *ad libitum* conditions. In this way, day-to-day variability in dietary fat intake may contribute to the development of overweight over time.

6.4.4 Influence of the degree of saturation of fatty acids on energy metabolism

As mentioned before, there is clear evidence from animal studies that the effect of a diet high in saturated fatty acids in increasing body fatness is more pronounced than with a highly PUFA-enriched diet (Hill *et al.*, 1992; Matsuo *et al.*, 1995; Pan *et al.*, 1994). In humans, data on the effect of diets rich in polyunsaturated fat on energy metabolism is rather limited. Jones and Schoeller (1988) examined the effect of diets with a low *vs* high polyunsaturated : saturated fat ratio for seven days on energy metabolism in humans. It was found that in the postprandial state, polyunsaturated fatty acids had a larger effect on energy expenditure and fat oxidation. In a subsequent study in obese subjects, it was again found that a diet rich in polyunsaturated fatty acids stimulates fat oxidation more in the post-prandial state compared with a diet rich in saturated fatty acids, although in this study no difference in energy expenditure was found between the two diets (Jones *et al.*, 1992). In a small study, van Marken Lichtenbelt *et al.* (1997) showed that diets high in polyunsaturated fatty acids increased resting metabolic rate and diet-induced thermogenesis when compared to a diet rich in saturated fat. More recently, similar results were found for monounsaturated fatty acids, i.e. higher diet-induced thermogenesis and increased fat oxidation after a diet rich in monounsaturated fatty acids compared to a diet rich in saturated fatty acids (Piers *et al.*, 2002; Soares *et al.*, 2004). In another study by the same group, Piers *et al.* (2003) examined the effect of diets rich in saturated fat *vs* monounsaturated fat on body weight and body composition in overweight subjects, using a randomized crossover design. Although no differences could be detected in energy intake, expenditure or fat oxidation, subjects weighed significantly less (−2 kg) after the monounsaturated fat diet compared with the saturated fat diet. Clearly more and longer-term (including intervention) studies are needed to clarify the impact of fatty acid saturation on body weight regulation.

6.5 Implications for food processors

For the food industry, the obesity problem will be an important theme in the future and processors are urged to formulate new food products and consider reformulation of their existing portfolio of products. In contrast to challenges in the past, where for example an outcome parameter such as cardiovascular disease was influenced by exchange of type of dietary fatty acids in the food products, a much more fundamental approach is now needed. Not only will food quality and food safety be issues for food companies but a third factor needs to be included in their strategy: the nutritional factor. The consumer nowadays demands products that can help to keep body weight under control.

A number of criteria are of importance in the process of creating new – or improving existing – products. First, the energy density of food products will be one of the most important factors that needs to be controlled when developing products for the prevention of obesity. Because fats are energy dense the use of dietary fat in food products needs to be reduced, and fat replacers or fat mimics can be of help. Also the use of types of fats with lower energy content or lower metabolic efficacy can positively add nutritional quality of food products. Also increasing the water content is an effective way to lower the energy density of products. In addition to reducing fat content, the type of fat included in food products needs attention, with a preference for polyunsaturated and monounsaturated fatty acids over saturated fatty acids. Although the latter most likely will be of minor importance in relation to body weight regulation, it will certainly be of great benefit in relation to cardiovascular health.

Somewhat beyond the scope of the theme of this book is the importance of portion size. Big portions with high energy content are also an important factor in the regulation of body weight and the food industry should aim to reduce portion size.

6.6 Conclusions and future trends

From the data available in the literature, it seems reasonable to conclude that a high dietary fat intake contributes to the current obesity epidemic. Long-term intervention trials using a reduced fat diet consistently show a small but significant reduction in body weight. However, dietary fat is not the sole food component that can explain the huge increase in obesity prevalence. The most important mechanism through which dietary fat may exert its effect on energy balance is via its effect on energy density. Future research should be focused on studying the effect of low-energy-dense diets in the development of obesity, and campaigns promoting healthy diets should take the energy density into account in their diet recommendations. The food industry could play an important role in the battle against obesity by producing and promoting healthy low-fat, low-energy-dense food products.

Less data are available on the role of fat quality in the development of obesity. Both animal and short-term human studies show that polyunsaturated fatty acids and medium-chain triglycerides are very effective in reducing body fat accumulation and increasing energy expenditure and fat oxidation. However, well-controlled long-term intervention studies on the effect of polyunsaturated and/or medium-chain fatty acids on the regulation of body weight are limited, but such studies are eagerly awaited. Importantly, such long-term intervention studies should also address potential side-effects of these nutrients, as for example CLA supplementation has been suggested to have detrimental effects on insulin sensitivity and medium-chain triglycerides may negatively affect gastrointestinal function. Therefore, long-term intervention studies on these fatty acids should be accompanied by (short-term) experiments examining the underlying mechanisms through which the dietary fat quality may exert positive effects on energy and substrate metabolism, as well as unravelling the pathways that are involved in potential detrimental effects of the nutrient under study. Data from these studies could help the food industry to evaluate their portfolio of products and to develop new functional foods that are able to increase energy metabolism and or fat oxidation and thereby be helpful in the prevention and/or treatment of obesity.

6.7 References

ABBOTT, W. G. H., HOWARD, B. V., CHRISTIN, L., FREYMOND, D., LILLIOJA, S., BOYCE, V. L., ANDERSON, T. E., BOGARDUS, C. & RAVUSSIN, E. (1988) Short-term energy balance: relationship with protein, carbohydrate, and fat balances. *Am J Physiol Endocrinol Metab*, **255**, E332–337.

ABBOTT, W. G., HOWARD, B. V., RUOTOLO, G. & RAVUSSIN, E. (1990) Energy expenditure in humans: effects of dietary fat and carbohydrate. *Am J Physiol Endocrinol Metab*, **258**, E347–351.

ASTRUP, A., BUEMANN, B., CHRISTENSEN, N. J. & TOUBRO, S. (1994) Failure to increase lipid oxidation in response to increasing dietary fat content in formerly obese women. *Am J Physiol*, **266**, E592–599.

ASTRUP, A., GRUNWALD, G. K., MELANSON, E. L., SARIS, W. H. & HILL, J. O. (2000a) The role of low-fat diets in body weight control: a meta-analysis of *ad libitum* dietary intervention studies. *Int J Obes Relat Metab Disord*, **24**, 1545–52.

ASTRUP, A., RYAN, L., GRUNWALD, G. K., STORGAARD, M., SARIS, W., MELANSON, E. & HILL, J. O. (2000b) The role of dietary fat in body fatness: evidence from a preliminary meta-analysis of ad libitum low-fat dietary intervention studies. *Br J Nutr*, **83** Suppl 1, S25–32.

BELURY, M. A., MAHON, A. & BANNI, S. (2003) The conjugated linoleic acid (CLA) isomer, t10*c*12-CLA, is inversely associated with changes in body weight and serum leptin in subjects with type 2 diabetes mellitus. *J Nutr*, **133**, 257S–260S.

BENNETT, C., REED, G. W., PETERS, J. C., ABUMRAD, N. N., SUN, M. & HILL, J. O. (1992) Short-term effects of dietary-fat ingestion on energy expenditure and nutrient balance. *Am J Clin Nutr*, **55**, 1071–1077.

BLUNDELL, J. E. & MACDIARMID, J. I. (1997) Fat as a risk factor for overconsumption: satiation, satiety, and patterns of eating. *J Am Diet Assoc*, **97**, S63–S69.

BLUNDELL, J. E., BURLEY, V. J., COTTON, J. R. & LAWTON, C. L. (1993) Dietary fat and the control of energy intake: evaluating the effects of fat on meal size and postmeal satiety. *Am J Clin Nutr*, **57**, 772S–777S.

BRAY, G. A. & POPKIN, B. M. (1998) Dietary fat intake does affect obesity! *Am J Clin Nutr*, **68**, 1157–73.

CHANEZ, M., BOIS-JOYEUX, B., ARNAUD, M. J. & PERET, J. (1991) Metabolic effects in rats of a diet with a moderate level of medium-chain triglycerides. *J Nutr*, **121**, 585–94.

COLDITZ, G. A., WILLETT, W. C., STAMPFER, M. J., LONDON, S. J., SEGAL, M. R. & SPEIZER, F. E. (1990) Patterns of weight change and their relation to diet in a cohort of healthy women. *Am J Clin Nutr*, **51**, 1100–105.

DELANY, J. P., BLOHM, F., TRUETT, A. A., SCIMECA, J. A. & WEST, D. B. (1999) Conjugated linoleic acid rapidly reduces body fat content in mice without affecting energy intake. *Am J Physiol*, **276**, R1172–9.

DIRLEWANGER, M., DI VETTA, V., GUENAT, E., BATTILANA, P., SEEMATTER, G., SCHNEITER, P., JEQUIER, E. & TAPPY, L. (2000) Effects of short-term carbohydrate or fat overfeeding on energy expenditure and plasma leptin concentrations in healthy female subjects. *Int J Obes Relat Metab Disord*, **24**, 1413–18.

DOUCET, E., ALMERAS, N., WHITE, M. D., DESPRES, J. P., BOUCHARD, C. & TREMBLAY, A. (1998) Dietary fat composition and human adiposity. *Eur J Clin Nutr*, **52**, 2–6.

DREON, D. M., FREY-HEWITT, B., ELLSWORTH, N., WILLIAMS, P. T., TERRY, R. B. & WOOD, P. D. (1988) Dietary fat:carbohydrate ratio and obesity in middle-aged men. *Am J Clin Nutr*, **47**, 995–1000.

FLATT, J. P., RAVUSSIN, E., ACHESON, K. J. & JEQUIER, E. (1985) Effects of dietary fat on postprandial substrate oxidation and on carbohydrate and fat balances. *J Clin Invest*, **76**, 1019–24.

FLEGAL, K. M., CARROLL, M. D., OGDEN, C. L. & JOHNSON, C. L. (2002) Prevalence and trends in obesity among US adults, 1999–2000. *JAMA*, **288**, 1723–7.

FOREYT, J. P. & POSTON, W. S. (2002) Consensus view on the role of dietary fat and obesity. *Am J Med*, **113** Suppl 9B, 60S–62S.

GONZALEZ, C. A., PERA, G., QUIROS, J. R., LASHERAS, C., TORMO, M. J., RODRIGUEZ, M., NAVARRO, C., MARTINEZ, C., DORRONSORO, M., CHIRLAQUE, M. D., BEGUIRISTAIN, J. M., BARRICARTE, A., AMIANO, P. & AGUDO, A. (2000) Types of fat intake and body mass index in a Mediterranean country. *Public Health Nutr*, **3**, 329–36.

GORIS, A. H., WESTERTERP-PLANTENGA, M. S. & WESTERTERP, K. R. (2000) Undereating and underrecording of habitual food intake in obese men: selective underreporting of fat intake. *Am J Clin Nutr*, **71**, 130–34.

HASHIM, S. A. & TANTIBHEDYANGKUL, P. (1987) Medium chain triglyceride in early life: effects on growth of adipose tissue. *Lipids*, **22**, 429–34.

HEITMANN, B. L. & LISSNER, L. (1995) Dietary underreporting by obese individuals – is it specific or non-specific? *BMJ*, **311**, 986–9.

HEITMANN, B. L., LISSNER, L., SORENSEN, T. I. & BENGTSSON, C. (1995) Dietary fat intake and weight gain in women genetically predisposed for obesity. *Am J Clin Nutr*, **61**, 1213–17.

HEITMANN, B. L., LISSNER, L. & OSLER, M. (2000) Do we eat less fat, or just report so? *Int J Obes Relat Metab Disord*, **24**, 435–42.

HILL, J. O., PETERS, J. C., REED, G. W., SCHLUNDT, D. G., SHARP, T. & GREENE, H. L. (1991) Nutrient balance in humans: effects of diet composition. *Am J Clin Nutr*, **54**, 10–17.

HILL, J. O., LIN, D., YAKUBU, F. & PETERS, J. C. (1992) Development of dietary obesity in rats: influence of amount and composition of dietary fat. *Int J Obes Relat Metab Disord*, **16**, 321–33.

HORTON, T. J., DROUGAS, H., BRACHEY, A., REED, G. W., PETERS, J. C. & HILL, J. O. (1995) Fat and carbohydrate overfeeding in humans: Different effects on energy storage. *Am J Clin Nutr*, **62**, 19–29.

JEQUIER, E. & BRAY, G. A. (2002) Low-fat diets are preferred. *Am J Med*, **113** Suppl 9B, 41S–46S.

JONES, P. J. H. & SCHOELLER, D. A. (1988) Polyunsaturated:saturated ratio of diet fat influences energy substrate utilization in the human. *Metabolism*, **37**, 145–51.

JONES, P. J. H., RIDGEN, J. E., TERRY PHANG, P. & LAIRD BIRMINGHAM, C. (1992) Influence of dietary fat polyunsaturated to saturated ratio on energy substrate utilization in obesity. *Metabolism*, **41**, 396–401.

KASAI, M., NOSAKA, N., MAKI, H., NEGISHI, S., AOYAMA, T., NAKAMURA, M., SUZUKI, Y., TSUJI, H., UTO, H., OKAZAKI, M. & KONDO, K. (2003) Effect of dietary medium- and long-chain triacylglycerols (MLCT) on accumulation of body fat in healthy humans. *Asia Pac J Clin Nutr*, **12**, 151–60.

KATAN, M. B., GRUNDY, S. M. & WILLETT, W. C. (1997a) Beyond low-fat diets. *N Eng J Med*, **337**, 563–6.

KATAN, M. B., GRUNDY, S. M. & WILLETT, W. C. (1997b) Should a low-fat, high-carbohydrate diet be recommended for everyone? Beyond low-fat diets. *N Engl J Med*, **337**, 563–6; discussion 566–7.

KAUNITZ, H., SLANETZ, C. A., JOHNSON, R. E., BABAYAN, V. K. & BARSKY, G. (1958) Relation of saturated, medium- and long-chain triglycerides to growth, appetite, thirst and weight maintenance requirements. *J Nutr*, **64**, 513–24.

KENNEDY, E. T., BOWMAN, S. A. & POWELL, R. (1999) Dietary-fat intake in the US population. *J Am Coll Nutr*, **18**, 207–12.

KLESGES, R. C., KLESGES, L. M., HADDOCK, C. K. & ECK, L. H. (1992) A longitudinal analysis of the impact of dietary intake and physical activity on weight change in adults. *Am J Clin Nutr*, **55**, 818–22.

KROTKIEWSKI, M. (2001) Value of VLCD supplementation with medium chain triglycerides. *Int J Obes Relat Metab Disord*, **25**, 1393–400.

LARSEN, T. M., TOUBRO, S. & ASTRUP, A. (2003) Efficacy and safety of dietary supplements containing CLA for the treatment of obesity: evidence from animal and human studies. *J Lipid Res*, **44**, 2234–41.

LEAN, M. E. & JAMES, W. P. (1988) Metabolic effects of isoenergetic nutrient exchange over 24 hours in relation to obesity in women. *Int J Obes*, **12**, 15–27.

LEVEILLE, G. A. & FINLEY, J. W. (1997) Macronutrient substitutes. Description and uses. *Ann N Y Acad Sci*, **819**, 11–21.

LISSNER, L. & HEITMANN, B. L. (1995) Dietary fat and obesity: evidence from epidemiology. *Eur J Clin Nutr*, **49**, 79–90.

LISSNER, L., LEVITSKY, D. A., STRUPP, B. J., KALKWARF, H. J. & ROE, D. A. (1987) Dietary fat and the regulation of energy intake in human subjects. *Am J Clin Nutr*, **46**, 886–892.

MATSUO, T., SHIMOMURA, Y., SAITOH, S., TOKUYAMA, K., TAKEUCHI, H. & SUZUKI, M. (1995) Sympathetic activity is lower in rats fed a beef tallow diet than in rats fed a safflower oil diet. *Metabolism*, **44**, 934–9.

McDEVITT, R. M., POPPITT, S. D., MURGATROYD, P. R. & PRENTICE, A. M. (2000) Macronutrient disposal during controlled overfeeding with glucose, fructose, sucrose, or fat in lean and obese women. *Am J Clin Nutr*, **72**, 369–77.

MILLER, W. C., LINDEMAN, A. K., WALLACE, J. & NIEDERPRUEM, M. (1990) Diet composition, energy intake, and exercise in relation to body fat in men and women. *Am J Clin Nutr*, **52**, 426–30.

MOLONEY, F., YEOW, T. P., MULLEN, A., NOLAN, J. J. & ROCHE, H. M. (2004) Conjugated linoleic acid supplementation, insulin sensitivity, and lipoprotein metabolism in patients with type 2 diabetes mellitus. *Am J Clin Nutr*, **80**, 887–95.

MOUGIOS, V., MATSAKAS, A., PETRIDOU, A., RING, S., SAGREDOS, A., MELISSOPOULOU, A., TSIGILIS, N. & NIKOLAIDIS, M. (2001) Effect of supplementation with conjugated linoleic acid on human serum lipids and body fat. *J Nutr Biochem*, **12**, 585–94.

NHANESIII (1994) From the Centers for Disease Control and Prevention. Prevalence of overweight among adolescents – United States, 1988–1991. *JAMA*, **272**, 1737.

NISHIDA, C., UAUY, R., KUMANYIKA, S. & SHETTY, P. (2004) The joint WHO/FAO expert consultation on diet, nutrition and the prevention of chronic diseases: process, product and policy implications. *Public Health Nutr*, **7**, 245–50.

NOSAKA, N., MAKI, H., SUZUKI, Y., HARUNA, H., OHARA, A., KASAI, M., TSUJI, H., AOYAMA, T., OKAZAKI, M., IGARASHI, O. & KONDO, K. (2003) Effects of margarine containing medium-chain triacylglycerols on body fat reduction in humans. *J Atheroscler Thromb*, **10**, 290–98.

NUGENOB CONSORTIUM, T. (2004) The effect of hypoenergetic diets with a fat energy percent of 20–25 or 40–45 on body weight, blood lipids, insulin and glucose in compliant obese subjects. *Int J Obesity*, **28**, S149.

OGDEN, C. L., FLEGAL, K. M., CARROLL, M. D. & JOHNSON, C. L. (2002) Prevalence and trends in overweight among US children and adolescents, 1999–2000. *JAMA*, **288**, 1728–32.

OSTROWSKA, E., MURALITHARAN, M., CROSS, R. F., BAUMAN, D. E. & DUNSHEA, F. R. (1999) Dietary conjugated linoleic acids increase lean tissue and decrease fat deposition in growing pigs. *J Nutr*, **129**, 2037–42.

PAN, D. A., HULBERT, A. J. & STORLIEN, L. H. (1994) Dietary fats, membrane phospholipids and obesity. *J Nutr*, **124**, 1555–65.

PARK, Y., ALBRIGHT, K. J., LIU, W., STORKSON, J. M., COOK, M. E. & PARIZA, M. W. (1997) Effect of conjugated linoleic acid on body composition in mice. *Lipids*, **32**, 853–8.

PIERS, L. S., WALKER, K. Z., STONEY, R. M., SOARES, M. J. & O'DEA, K. (2002) The influence of the type of dietary fat on postprandial fat oxidation rates: monounsaturated (olive oil) *vs* saturated fat (cream). *Int J Obes Relat Metab Disord*, **26**, 814–21.

PIERS, L. S., WALKER, K. Z., STONEY, R. M., SOARES, M. J. & O'DEA, K. (2003) Substitution of saturated with monounsaturated fat in a 4-week diet affects body weight and composition of overweight and obese men. *Br J Nutr*, **90**, 717–27.

PRENTICE, A. M. & JEBB, S. A. (2003) Fast foods, energy density and obesity: a possible mechanistic link. *Obes Rev*, **4**, 187–94.

PREWITT, T. E., SCHMEISSER, D., BOWEN, P. E., AYE, P., DOLECEK, T. A., LANGENBERG, P., COLE, T. & BRACE, L. (1991) Changes in body weight, body composition, and energy intake in women fed high- and low-fat diets. *Am J Clin Nutr*, **54**, 304–10.

RISERUS, U., SMEDMAN, A., BASU, S. & VESSBY, B. (2004a) Metabolic effects of conjugated linoleic acid in humans: the Swedish experience. *Am J Clin Nutr*, **79**, 1146S–1148S.

RISERUS, U., VESSBY, B., ARNLOV, J. & BASU, S. (2004b) Effects of *cis*-9,*trans*-11 conjugated linoleic acid supplementation on insulin sensitivity, lipid peroxidation, and proinflammatory markers in obese men. *Am J Clin Nutr*, **80**, 279–83.

ROLLS, B. J. & BELL, E. A. (1999) Intake of fat and carbohydrate: role of energy density. *Eur J Clin Nutr*, **53** Suppl 1, S166–73.

ROLLS, B. J. & HAMMER, V. A. (1995) Fat, carbohydrate, and the regulation of energy intake. *Am J Clin Nutr*, **62**, 1086S–1095S.

ROMIEU, I., WILLETT, W. C., STAMPFER, M. J., COLDITZ, G. A., SAMPSON, L., ROSNER, B., HENNEKENS, C. H. & SPEIZER, F. E. (1988) Energy intake and other determinants of relative weight. *Am J Clin Nutr*, **47**, 406-12.

SALTZMAN, E., DALLAL, G. E. & ROBERTS, S. B. (1997) Effect of high-fat and low-fat diets on voluntary energy intake and substrate oxidation: studies in identical twins consuming diets matched for energy density, fiber, and palatability. *Am J Clin Nutr*, **66**, 1332–9.

SARIS, W. H. M. (2004) Focus on the fire of life. *Curr Opin Clin Nutr Metab Care*, **7** (6), 595–7.

SARIS, W. H., ASTRUP, A., PRENTICE, A. M., ZUNFT, H. J., FORMIGUERA, X., VERBOEKET-VAN DE VENNE, W. P., RABEN, A., POPPITT, S. D., SEPPELT, B., JOHNSTON, S., VASILARAS, T. H. & KEOGH, G. F. (2000) Randomized controlled trial of changes in dietary carbohydrate/fat ratio and simple *vs* complex carbohydrates on body weight and blood lipids: the CARMEN study. The Carbohydrate Ratio Management in European National diets. *Int J Obes Relat Metab Disord*, **24**, 1310–18.

SCHRAUWEN, P., VAN MARKEN LICHTENBELT, W. D., SARIS, W. H. & WESTERTERP, K. R. (1997a) Changes in fat oxidation in response to a high-fat diet. *Am J Clin Nutr*, **66**, 276–82.

SCHRAUWEN, P., VAN MARKEN LICHTENBELT, W. D., SARIS, W. H. & WESTERTERP, K. R. (1997b) Role of glycogen-lowering exercise in the change of fat oxidation in response to a high-fat diet. *Am J Physiol*, **273**, E623–9.

SCHRAUWEN, P., LICHTENBELT, W. D., SARIS, W. H. & WESTERTERP, K. R. (1998) Fat balance in obese subjects: role of glycogen stores. *Am J Physiol*, **274**, E1027–33.

SCHUTZ, Y., FLATT, J. P. & JEQUIER, E. (1989) Failure of dietary fat intake to promote fat oxidation: a factor favoring the development of obesity. *Am J Clin Nutr*, **50**, 307–14.

SISK, M. B., HAUSMAN, D. B., MARTIN, R. J. & AZAIN, M. J. (2001) Dietary conjugated linoleic acid reduces adiposity in lean but not obese Zucker rats. *J Nutr*, **131**, 1668–74.

SLATTERY, M. L., MCDONALD, A., BILD, D. E., CAAN, B. J., HILNER, J. E., JACOBS, D. R., JR. & LIU, K. (1992) Associations of body fat and its distribution with dietary intake, physical activity, alcohol, and smoking in blacks and whites. *Am J Clin Nutr*, **55**, 943–9.

SMEDMAN, A. & VESSBY, B. (2001) Conjugated linoleic acid supplementation in humans – metabolic effects. *Lipids*, **36**, 773–81.

SOARES, M. J., CUMMINGS, S. J., MAMO, J. C., KENRICK, M. & PIERS, L. S. (2004) The acute effects of olive oil v. cream on postprandial thermogenesis and substrate oxidation in postmenopausal women. *Br J Nutr*, **91**, 245–52.

ST-ONGE, M. P. & JONES, P. J. (2003) Greater rise in fat oxidation with medium-chain triglyceride consumption relative to long-chain triglyceride is associated with lower initial body weight and greater loss of subcutaneous adipose tissue. *Int J Obes Relat Metab Disord*, **27**, 1565–71.

ST-ONGE, M. P., BOURQUE, C., JONES, P. J., ROSS, R. & PARSONS, W. E. (2003) Medium- versus long-chain triglycerides for 27 days increases fat oxidation and energy expenditure without resulting in changes in body composition in overweight women. *Int J Obes Relat Metab Disord*, **27**, 95–102.

STUBBS, R. J., HARBRON, C. G. & PRENTICE, A. M. (1996) Covert manipulation of the dietary fat to carbohydrate ratio of isoenergetically dense diets: effect on food intake in feeding men *ad libitum*. *Int J Obes*, **20**, 651–60.

TERPSTRA, A. H., BEYNEN, A. C., EVERTS, H., KOCSIS, S., KATAN, M. B. & ZOCK, P. L. (2002) The decrease in body fat in mice fed conjugated linoleic acid is due to increases in energy expenditure and energy loss in the excreta. *J Nutr*, **132**, 940–45.

THOM, E., WADSTEIN, J. & GUDMUNDSEN, O. (2001) Conjugated linoleic acid reduces body fat in healthy exercising humans. *J Int Med Res*, **29**, 392–6.

THOMAS, C. D., PETERS, J. C., REED, G. W., ABUMRAD, N. N., SUN, M. & HILL, J. O. (1992) Nutrient balance and energy expenditure during *ad libitum* feeding of high-fat and high-carbohydrate diets in humans. *Am J Clin Nutr*, **55**, 934–942.

TREMBLAY, A., PLOURDE, G., DESPRES, J. P. & BOUCHARD, C. (1989) Impact of dietary fat content and fat oxidation on energy intake in humans. *Am J Clin Nutr*, **49**, 799–805.

TSUBOYAMA-KASAOKA, N., TAKAHASHI, M., TANEMURA, K., KIM, H. J., TANGE, T., OKUYAMA, H., KASAI, M., IKEMOTO, S. & EZAKI, O. (2000) Conjugated linoleic acid supplementation reduces adipose tissue by apoptosis and develops lipodystrophy in mice. *Diabetes*, **49**, 1534–42.

TSUJI, H., KASAI, M., TAKEUCHI, H., NAKAMURA, M., OKAZAKI, M. & KONDO, K. (2001) Dietary medium-chain triacylglycerols suppress accumulation of body fat in a double-blind, controlled trial in healthy men and women. *J Nutr*, **131**, 2853–9.

VAN MARKEN LICHTENBELT, W. D., MENSINK, R. P. & WESTERTERP, K. R. (1997) The effect of fat composition of the diet on energy metabolism. *Z Ernahrungswiss*, **36**, 303–5.

VERBOEKET-VAN DE VENNE, W. P. H. G., WESTERTERP, K. R. & TEN HOOR, F. (1994) Substrate utilization in man: effects of dietary fat and carbohydrate. *Metabolism*, **43**, 152–6.

VERBOEKET-VAN DE VENNE, W. P. H. G., WESTERTERP, K. R., HERMANS-LIMPENS, T. J. F. M. B., GRAAF, C. D., HOF, K. V. H. & WESTSTRATE, J. A. (1996) Long-term effects of consumption of full-fat or reduced-fat products in healthy non-obese volunteers: assessment of energy expenditure and substrate oxidation. *Metabolism*, **45**, 1004–10.

WEST, D. B., DELANY, J. P., CAMET, P. M., BLOHM, F., TRUETT, A. A. & SCIMECA, J. (1998) Effects of conjugated linoleic acid on body fat and energy metabolism in the mouse. *Am J Physiol*, **275**, R667–72.

WESTERTERP, K. R. & GORIS, A. H. (2002) Validity of the assessment of dietary intake: problems of misreporting. *Curr Opin Clin Nutr Metab Care*, **5**, 489–93.

WESTERTERP, K. R., VERBOEKET-VAN DE VENNE, W. P. H. G., WESTERTERP-PLANTEGA, M. S., VELTHUIS-TE WIERIK, E. J. M., GRAAF, C. D. & WESTSTRATE, J. A. (1996) Dietary fat and body fat: an intervention study. *Int J Obes Relat Metab Disord*, **20**, 1022–6.

WILLETT, W. C. (1998) Is dietary fat a major determinant of body fat? *Am J Clin Nutr*, **67**, 556S–562S.

WILLIAMSON, J. R., BROWNING, E. T., SCHOLZ, R., KREISBERG, R. A. & FRITZ, I. B. (1968) Inhibition of fatty acid stimulation of gluconeogenesis by (+)-decanoylcarnitine in perfused rat liver. *Diabetes*, **17**, 194–208.

YU-POTH, S., ZHAO, G., ETHERTON, T., NAGLAK, M., JONNALAGADDA, S. & KRIS-ETHERTON, P. M. (1999) Effects of the National Cholesterol Education Program's Step I and Step II dietary intervention programs on cardiovascular disease risk factors: a meta-analysis. *Am J Clin Nutr*, **69**, 632–46.

ZAMBELL, K. L., KEIM, N. L., VAN LOAN, M. D., GALE, B., BENITO, P., KELLEY, D. S. & NELSON, G. J. (2000) Conjugated linoleic acid supplementation in humans: effects on body composition and energy expenditure. *Lipids*, **35**, 777–82.

ZURLO, F., LILLIOJA, S., ESPOSITO, D. P. A., NYOMBA, B. L., RAZ, I., SAAD, M. F., SWINBURN, B. A., KNOWLER, W. C., BOGARDUS, C. & RAVUSSIN, E. (1990) Low ratio of fat to carbohydrate oxidation as predictor of weight gain: study of 24-h RQ. *Am J Physiol Endocrinol Metab*, **259**, E650–E657.

7

Specific fatty acids and structured lipids for weight control

M. S. Westerterp-Plantenga, Maastricht University, The Netherlands

7.1 Introduction

Body-weight control means promoting a stable balance between energy intake and energy expenditure. This implies tuning of energy intake to energy requirement, while avoiding accumulating energy storage as fat. Key targets for metabolic intermediates for body-weight management are satiety, thermogenesis, fat oxidation, fat storage, body composition, and energy efficiency. The outcome of targeted interventions include attempts to: (i) sustain satiety even when energy intake is lower than the energy requirement; (ii) prevent a decrease in thermogenesis during, e.g., weight loss; (iii) increase fat oxidation, thus limiting fat storage; (iv) increase energy expenditure by increasing relative fat-free mass; and (v) promote energy inefficiency during body-weight gain or regain.

The role of specific fatty acids and structured lipids as dietary tools in body-weight control focuses on their roles in enhancing satiety with respect to energy intake, thermogenesis and body composition with respect to energy expenditure, and fat oxidation and energy efficiency in relation to energy storage.

7.2 Functionality of lipids

7.2.1 Energy intake and satiety

A better understanding of the mechanisms of satiety will generate ideas about dietary strategies that can stimulate these mechanisms and thus give the subject feelings of satiety without the primary drive for satiety – which is increased food intake. The following sections deal with the mechanisms of satiety.

7.2.1 Central and peripheral mechanisms

Energy expenditure determines the energy requirement,[1–3] and, in principle, energy intake is regulated physiologically by means of hunger and satiety.[4,5] With respect to food intake control in humans, in terms of meal size and meal frequency, two features are worth considering. First is the distinction between satiation and satiety. Satiation refers to the processes that bring a period of eating to an end; these processes influence the size of meals and snacks. Satiety refers to the inhibition of hunger and further eating that arises as a consequence of food ingestion, and determines inter-meal interval, or meal frequency, by determining the next meal initiation. Secondly, the properties of food (and the act of ingesting it) trigger the initiation of the overlapping physiological responses. The quantity and quality of the food determine the intensity and time course of the biological processes generated. This has led to recognition of the different satiating power of different types of food,[4–9] which can be recognized at the level of:

- psychological events (hunger, perception, cravings and hedonic sensations) and behavioral operations (meals, snacks, energy and macronutrient intakes);
- peripheral physiology and metabolic events;
- neuro-transmitter and metabolic interactions in the brain.

The expression of appetite reflects the synchronous operation of events and processes at these three levels. Neural events trigger and guide behavior, but each act of behavior involves a response in the peripheral physiological system; in turn, these physiological events are translated into brain neuro-chemical activity. This brain activity represents the strength of motivation and the willingness to refrain from feeding. Viewed in this way, the psycho-biological system permits an understanding of the interrelationships among behavioral events that comprise eating, peripheral physiology and metabolism and central neuro-chemical processes.[5]

In this respect, the autonomic nervous system and the release of a variety of hormones, such as leptin[10] from the pituitary are currently considered as the main effector systems.[11] In humans, pathological effects such as those observed in craniopharyngioma patients, who show hyperphagia, have been related to dysfunctioning of leptin receptors in the hypothalamus,[12] also indicating the importance of hypothalamic function.

In humans, central and peripheral processes that affect hunger and satiety are signals during and after ingestion of food; respectively leading to sensory specific satiety, sensory satiety, postprandial and post-absorptive satiety. Moreover, hunger and satiety are affected by external factors that also affect energy expenditure, such as physical activity, hypobaric hypoxia and increased environmental temperature decreasing hunger.

7.2.3 Sensory specific satiety

After feeding to satiety, humans reported that the taste of the food on which they had been satiated was almost as intense as when they were hungry, though much less pleasant.[13,14] Analyzing the neural control of feeding in the macaque monkey (*Macaca fascicularis*) by recording the activity of single neurons during feeding has shown that a population of neurons in the lateral hypothalamus respond to the sight and/or taste of food only when the monkey is hungry.[13,14] The modulation of reward of a motivationally relevant sensory stimulus such as the taste of food by motivational state, for example hunger, appears to be an important way in which motivational behavior is controlled.[13–15] The subjective correlate of this modulation is that food tastes pleasant when the subject is hungry, and tastes hedonically neutral when it has been eaten to satiety.[14] Activity in the primary taste area (frontal opercular and insular taste cortices as well as the nucleus of the solitary tract) does not reflect the pleasantness of the taste of a food, but rather its sensory qualities independently of motivational state.[13–16] On the other hand, activity in the secondary taste area (the caudolateral orbitofrontal cortex) and in the lateral hypothalamus are modulated by satiety, and may be related to whether a food tastes pleasant, and to whether the food should be eaten.[13–16]

It was also found in humans that the pleasantness of the taste of food eaten to satiety decreased more than for foods that had not been eaten. This implies that if a variety of foods is available, the total amount consumed will be more than when only one food is offered repeatedly.[17] This effect has been termed 'sensory-specific satiety'.[17] Sensory-specific satiety occurs for the sight as well as for the taste and odor of food.[13]

The enhanced eating when a variety of foods is available may have been advantageous in evolution in ensuring that different foods with important different nutrients were consumed. However, today in humans, when a wide variety of foods are readily available, this can lead to overeating and obesity.

7.2.4 Sensory satiety: effects of linoleic acid

In addition to sensory specific satiety, a relationship between sensory perception and food preference, with respect to satiety, has been shown in rats.[18] Accumulating evidence suggests that dietary fat can be 'tasted' by rats, and that this fat perception seems to be related to fat intake regulation.[18] Gilbertson and co-workers showed that *in vitro* a small concentration (10 μM) of free linoleic acid dose-dependently inhibits the K^+ current of delayed rectifying potassium channels (DRKC) in taste receptor cells of rat tongue epithelium, which indicates an increase in activity of those cells by linoleic acid. Interestingly, the effects were seen only for *cis*-PUFAs (arachidonic, linoleic and linolenic acid). In contrast, the same concentration of free oleic acid did not have an increased activity compared to saline. Furthermore, in a taste aversion test, the ability to perceive this low concentration of linoleic acid by rats was confirmed.[18] Differences in the ability of linoleic acid to inhibit DRKC in tongue epithelium of taste recptor cells between dietary fat-preferring and dietary fat-avoiding rat strains have been shown, in that an increased linoleic acid sensitivity in fat-avoiding rats compared with fat-preferring rats was observed. In addition, when placed on a high-fat diet, the dietary fat-preferring rat strain became rapidly obese, while the dietary fat-avoiding strain reduced their fat intake and remained lean.[18] The hypothesis stresses that in rats, dietary fat intake is reduced by linoleic acid taste sensitivity for perception through the DRKC which may play a role in prevention, and thus in the etiology of obesity.[18,19]

In humans, fat-specific satiety during dinner comprising a meal containing an oil rich in linoleic acid *vs* oil containing oleic acid was shown after a 2-week treatment with one of the oils, but there was no change in general satiety.[20] Moreover, differences in taste perception was also shown in humans using a low concentration of linoleic acid. Tasters appeared to terminate eating a food containing linoleic acid by satiety, whereas non-tasters terminated eating by a decrease in pleasantness of taste.[21]

7.2.5 Satiety in the postprandial phase

With respect to the postprandial phase of satiety, the integrated role of gastric distension, emptying, and contractions within the complex series of physiological and biochemical events surrounding meal patterning is now recognized.[4,22,23] A role of the stomach in hunger and satiety was shown in that increases in hunger ratings were inversely associated with the time that 90% of the test meal had emptied from the stomach.[4] Foods emptying slowly from the stomach have been suggested to sustain satiety and delay the onset of hunger in humans.[4] Gastric emptying may play a role in this relationship, although it is likely that gastric sensations interact with related factors such as the subsequent delayed (and thus prolonged) elevation in blood glucose.[4,24,25] It has been suggested that gastric stretch receptors and contractions indicate the volume of stomach contents to the organism, whereas various peptides secreted from, or induced by, the alimentary tract indicate energy content.

Such peptides include food intake inhibitors such as cholecystokinin (CCK), serotonin (5HT), corticotrophin-releasing factor (CRF), somatostatin, enterostatin, bombesin, glucagon, and glucagon-like peptide (GLP) I and II. GLP-1 for instance, is related to the control of insulin, and to satiety, but its effect is diminished in subjects with visceral (abdominal) obesity.[4] For some of these peptides, it has been questioned whether the experimentally induced reductions in food intake were actually caused by satiety, or by nausea induced by non-physiological quantities of the peptides.[4]

Other peptides believed to stimulate food intake include neuropeptide Y (NPY), galanin and endogenous opiods. It may be that, in general, peptides that reduce food intake signal via the central nervous system to the ventromedial hypothalamus (VMH), and peptides that stimulate food consumption may signal through the central nervous system to the lateral hypothalamus (LH).[4]

The presence of food, particularly fat, in the upper small intestine stimulates the release of CCK, which has both peripheral and central receptors.[26,27] CCK is known to serve regulatory roles in bile secretion, gastric emptying, and the exocrine pancreas. Additionally, CCK relays signals to the brain through the vagus nerve, inhibiting eating behavior in humans and causing meal termination.[28] Conversely, as nutrient delivery to the intestine decreases, CCK release and vagal activity are reduced, so that eating behavior is no longer inhibited. Antagonists to CCK have been shown to increase food intake in rats, whereas CCK stimulants have been shown to decrease food intake in both rats and humans.[4]

In rats, increased transmission of serotonin (5-hydroxytryptophan, 5HT) has been shown to decrease food intake, acting peripherally, and possibly via the central nervous system (CNS) as well. In humans, the hypophagic actions of serotonin have been studied extensively. Synthesis of 5HT in the brain depends on the availability of tryptophan, its amino acid precursor. Thus, dietary factors influencing blood tryptophan concentration may influence 5HT synthesis. Such dietary factors include other amino acids, which compete with 5HT uptake across the blood–brain barrier, and carbohydrate, which may have a diluting effect on tryptophan concentrations. Some data indicate that the hypophagic actions of serotonin work pre-absorptively, possibly through interactions with CCK and enterostatin.[4] Changes in serotonin metabolism have been reported in many cases of individuals with disordered eating, including anorexia, bulimia, obesity and type 2 diabetes mellitus. Some investigators have proposed that serotonin may play a role in macronutrient preferences, including carbohydrate cravings and fat avoidance, but this has been refuted by others.[4]

CRF (corticotrophin-releasing factor), a 41-residue peptide located in neurons throughout the brain, particularly the paraventricular nucleus, is believed to suppress food intake and also to stimulate thermogenesis.[29-31] These actions may occur via the sympathetic nervous system and/or via mediation of the actions of serotonin. Interestingly, alterations in the responses of adrenocorticotrophin hormone (ACTH) and cortisol to CRF have also been reported in some conditions of disturbed eating behavior such as anorexia nervosa.[32] It has also been suggested that CRF, which is stimulated by exercise, may mediate the effects of post-exercise anorexia and elevated energy expenditure, with the effect being strongest immediately following a bout of exercise.[29–31] CRF is also released during the stress response, therefore CRF may be a factor in the down-regulation of food intake during stress, possibly along with noradrenaline.[29–31]

The most potent endogenous appetite stimulant known in humans thus far is neuropeptide Y (NPY), which acts through the central nervous system, possibly through noradrenergic mechanisms.[4] High levels of NPY have been found in the human hypothalamus.[33] In both rats and humans, starvation is associated with elevated levels of NPY which are reversed by refeeding. Some investigators have suggested that disturbed patterns or activity of NPY may occur in patients with anorexia and bulimia nervosa.[4]

Galanin, another peptide with hyperphagic actions, is secreted from the intestine and islets of Langerhans, relaying signals to receptors in the paraventricular nucleus.[34] In both animals and humans, it is recognized that some kinds of stress can reduce food intake (possibly mediated through CRF) whereas other types of stress can stimulate food intake.[34]

Endogenous opioids (beta-endorphin, dynorphin and encephalines) are believed to induce stress-related hyperphagia, acting on several sites in the hypothalamus. Some data, but not all, suggest that these compounds may influence meal size and macronutrient preference (for fat rather than simple carbohydrate) in humans.[35]

7.2.6 Satiety in the postabsorptive phase

Once nutrients cross from the intestinal tract into the blood and become available for metabolism, they may exert post-absorptive regulatory signals sustaining satiety. Satiety and hunger seem to be related to metabolic events surrounding nutrient processing, utilization and storage.[4] Thus, it logically follows that carbohydrate, with its rapid uptake and metabolism, would play important roles in short-term food intake regulation. For example, carbohydrate stores in humans range from approximately 150 to 500 g, depending on body size, exercise, and state of nutriture.[4] This is rather low in relation to the 200 to 500 g of carbohydrate consumed in a typical daily diet. Conversely, the amount of fat and protein in the body are quite high in relation to daily dietary intake. Given each of these relative turnovers, and the complete dependence of the central nervous system (CNS) on glucose as a metabolic fuel, the role of carbohydrate, particularly blood glucose, in the regulation of food intake and energy balance has long been an intense focus of research.[4]

7.2.7 Role of the liver in metabolic control of food intake

Although hepatic metabolic signals are not necessary to maintain food intake and body weight, a large body of evidence indicates that such signals play a role in the control of eating.[36] Total parenteral nutrition and peripheral administration of various metabolites (e.g. glucose, pyruvate, lactate, hydroxybutyrate) generally inhibit eating. On the other hand, metabolic inhibitors such as the glucose antimetabolite 2-deoxy-D-glucose, fatty acid oxidation inhibitors,[37] the fructose analogue 2,5-anhydro-D-mannitol (2,5AM) and the sodium pump inhibitor ouabain have been shown to stimulate eating under various conditions.[36] Many of these effects are particularly pronounced when the substances are infused into the hepatic portal vein, and are markedly attenuated when the hepatic branch of the vagus is disconnected.[36] This suggests that the observed effects on eating originate in the liver and are mediated by hepatic afferent nerves. In addressing these issues, it must be kept in mind that the hepatic afferent nerves involved are also part of a complex network that plays an important role in blood glucose regulation, electrolyte/fluid balance, and other regulatory systems, which may interact with mechanisms of food intake control.[36]

Taken together, satiety is generated by sensory, post-ingestive and post-absorptive mechanisms, that may be targets for sustaining or enhancing satiety while reducing energy intake.

7.3 Metabolic satiety and fat oxidation: effects of conjugated linoleic acid and diacylglycerol

Post-ingestive and post-absorptive mechanisms support the dynamic state of satiety during the inter-meal interval. These mechanisms imply effects on metabolic targets such as 'satiety hormones', thermogenesis and fat oxidation. Thus often satiety is affected in relation to or coinciding with these metabolic targets. Therefore satiety due to post-ingestive or post-absorptive processes is referred to as metabolic satiety.

In the longer term, energy efficiency and body composition can be affected by certain ingredients. The following sections include the scientific evidence for possible beneficial effects for body-weight control from conjugated linoleic acid, respectively diacylglycerol, and illustrate this with possible applications in body weight management research. In addition before dealing with the relative value of high-fat versus low-fat diets in body-weight regulation, the metabolic role of protein is highlighted, since this may well play a role in the effect of diets varying in fat content.

7.3.1 Metabolic satiety and conjugated linoleic acid

Conjugated linoleic acid (CLA) is naturally found in beef, milk and milk products since it is an intermediate in the biohydrogenation of linoleic acid that occurs in the rumen by bacteria.[38,39] CLA refers to a group of positional and geometrical isomers of linoleic acid containing conjugated double bonds. The natural form is predominantly the *cis*-9, *trans*-11 isomer. Numerous physiological effects in relation to body weight control have been attributed to CLA in animals (see also Chapter 8). In different animal models, CLA has been shown to reduce body fat and to increase lean body mass.[40–50] However, effects on body weight are controversial (Chapter 8). Some investigators found reduced body weight after a CLA diet,[47,48,51] whereas others have found no effect[40,43,46–49] or an increase in body weight.[48] Furthermore CLA intake has been associated with increased energy expenditure.[41,46,49] A few human studies on the effect of CLA on body weight, body mass index (BMI), and/or fat mass, showed that though fat mass[50,51] and sagital abdominal diameter[52] were lowered by CLA, this did not result in body weight loss.[51–56] For instance, in healthy overweight humans it was found that CLA supplementation for 1 year reduced body fat mass.[56]

Effects of CLA while subjects are in a state of weight regain is illustrated by the following. After a very low-calorie diet that significantly lowered body weight, percentage body fat, fat mass, fat-free mass, resting metabolic rate, respiratory quotient and plasma glucose, insulin, triacylglycerol, free fatty acids, glycerol, and β-hydroxy butyrate concentrations, CLA (1.8 or 3.6 g/day) was administrated to subjects *vs* placebo during 13 weeks and, as usual, body weight regain took place. However, the regain of fat-free mass was increased by CLA, independently of percentage body weight regain and physical activity. As a consequence of this increased regain of fat free mass by CLA, resting metabolic rate (which is mainly dependent on fat free mass) was increased. Substrate

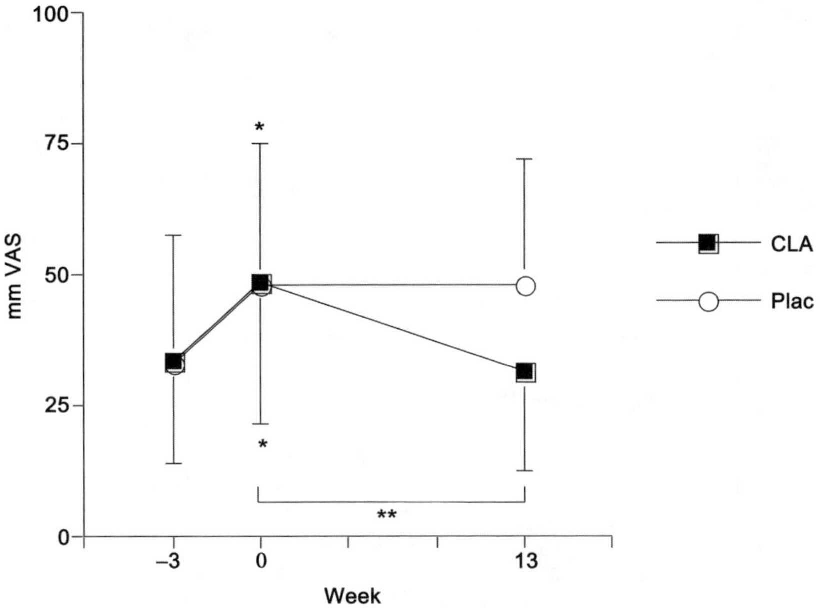

Fig. 7.1 Feelings of hunger measured with an anchored 100 mm visual analogue scale (VAS) before very low calorie diet (VLCD) (–3), after VLCD and before intervention (0) and at 13 weeks of intervention with 1.8 or 3.6 g conjugated linoleic acid/day (CLA, $n = 27$) and 1.8 or 3.6 g placebo/day (oleic acid, $n = 27$). The results are presented as CLA and placebo, with the low and high dosage combined. * Repeated Measures ANOVA for all subjects together showed a significant increase in feelings of hunger from week −3 to week 0 ($p < 0.001$). ** Multiple regression showed that the feeling of hunger during intervention was decreased by CLA compared with placebo (regression coefficient −14.0 (−25.0 − −3), $p < 0.05$). After Kamphuis *et al.*[58]

oxidation and blood plasma parameters were not affected by CLA.[57] Coinciding with the increase in resting metabolic rate, post-absorptive feelings of fullness and satiety were increased and feelings of hunger were decreased after 13 weeks of intervention by CLA compared to placebo, independently of % body weight regain[58] (see Figs 7.1 and 7.2). Thus the increase in satiety coincided with the increased thermogenesis, which was related to increased fat-free mass, the main metabolic target in this respect. However, although the metabolic target was affected by CLA, this did not result in a better weight maintenance compared with the placebo, since dietary restraint tended to increase more and disinhibition tended to decrease more in the placebo group.[57,58]

7.3.2 Metabolic satiety and diacylglycerol

Normal fat intake in the diet is as triacylglycerides (TG), although small amounts of diacylglycerol (DG) are usually present. Studies suggest that modest intakes of DG might have a beneficial effect on lipid metabolism in rats as well

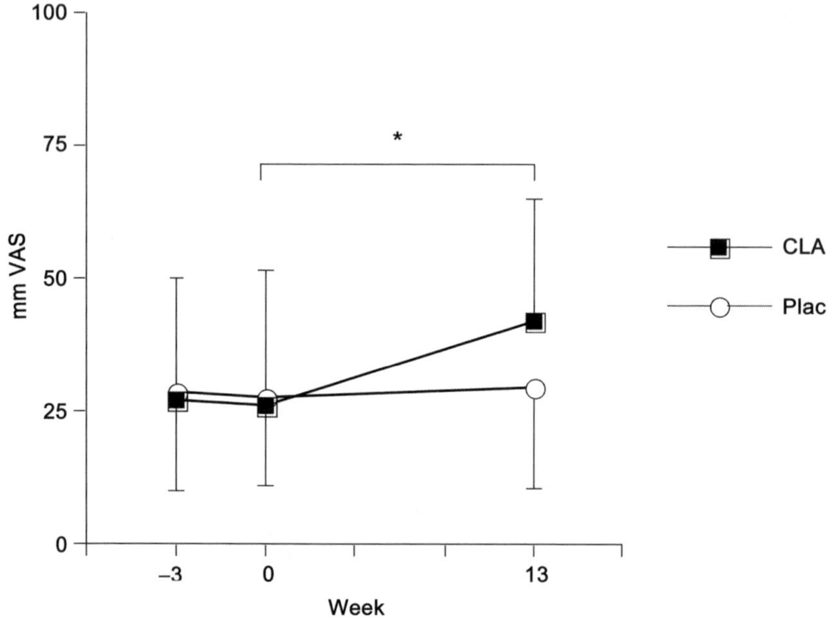

Fig. 7.2 Feelings of satiety measured with an anchored 100 mm visual analogue scale (VAS) before VLCD (−3) after VLCD and before intervention (0) and at 13 weeks of intervention with 1.8 or 3.6 g conjugated linoleic acid/day (CLA, $n = 27$) and 1.8 or 3.6 g placebo/day (oleic acid, $n = 27$). The results are presented as CLA and placebo, with the low and high dosage combined. * Multiple regression showed that the feeling of satiety during intervention was increased by CLA compared with placebo (regression coefficient 12.2 (0.9 − 23.5), $p < 0.05$). After Kamphuis *et al.*[58]

as in humans. Compared with TG, consumption of DG seems to produce lower postprandial elevation of plasma TG concentrations[59,60] in humans and fasting serum TG levels in rats[61,62] and humans.[63] Reduction in total body fat accumulation[64] and visceral fat accumulation[65] in rats and humans[66,67] by DG have also been reported. These effects appear to be most likely attributable to differences in DG utilization, especially promotion of enhanced (postprandial) β-oxidation.[62,67] This is probably due to enhanced post-absorptive availability of free fatty acids in the portal circulation. Notably, DG oil has the same digestion and absorption routes as comparable TG oils, and similar bioavailability and physiological fuel value.[68]

In a respiration-chamber study by Kamphuis *et al.*,[69] effects of partial replacement of TG by DG on substrate oxidation, energy metabolism, respiratory quotient (RQ), relevant blood parameters and measures of appetite were assessed. Fat oxidation appeared to be higher and RQ was lower with DG than with TG. Feelings of hunger, appetite, estimated prospective food intake, and desire to eat were all lower with DG from the second day onwards. Also the mean plasma β-hydroxy-butyrate level was higher with DG. Consumption of

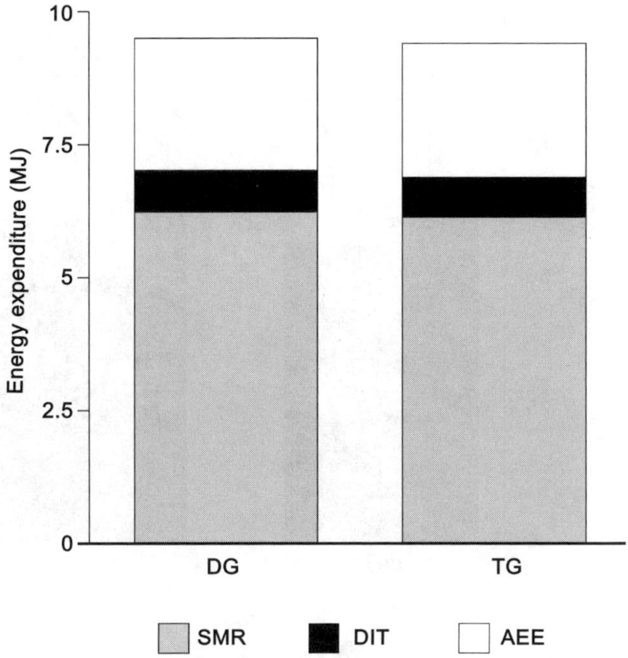

Fig. 7.3 Mean 24 h energy expenditure (EE: 9.5 ± 0.9 and 9.4 ± 0.9 for DG and TG respectively, ns), consisting of sleeping metabolic rate (SMR: 6.3 ± 0.6 and 6.2 ± 0.5 for DG and TG, respectively, ns), diet-induced thermogenesis (DIT: 0.7 ± 0.3 and 0.7 ± 0.2 for DG and TG respectively, ns) and activity-base energy expenditure (AEE: 2.5 ± 0.5 and 2.5 ± 0.4 respectively, ns) of the diacylglyceride-rich oil (DG) intervention and control (triacylglycerides, TG) ($n = 12$). After Kamphuis *et al.*[69]

DG in place of TG did not appear to alter total energy expenditure, but produced metabolic effects, particularly increases in fat oxidation, associated with improved appetite control and energy balance[69] (see Figs 7.3 and 7.4).

Furthermore, recent findings suggest that consumption of diacylglycerol affects lipid metabolism including lowering of plasma triacylglycerol, decreases postprandial lipemia and reduces body fat mass, compared with triacylglycerol. The explanation suggests that as the fatty acids of the two oils are similar, the metabolic differences reside in their structural differences.[70] It is still uncertain whether longer-term consumption of the diacylglycerol oil will lead to persistent and consistent reductions in plasma triacylglycerol and body fat, as has been suggested by a study where diacylglycerol has been exchanged by triacylglycerol as part of a mildly reduced-energy diet.[70,71]

7.3.3 Metabolic satiety and Etomoxir

High-fat diets may stimulate voluntary fat intake. The high palatability of high-fat diets could make overeating more likely, and the high energy density of fat-

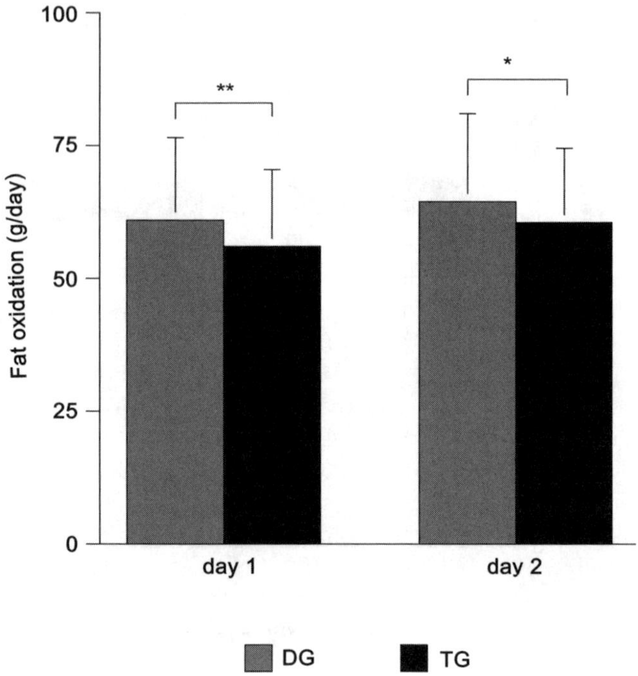

Fig. 7.4 Mean (±SD) fat oxidation (g/day) over day 1 and day 2 of diacylglyceride-rich (DG) and control (triacylglycerol, TG) interventions: * significantly higher than TG ($p < 0.05$, paired t-test, $n = 12$); ** significantly higher than TG ($p = 0.004$, paired t-test, $n = 12$). After Kamphuis *et al.*[69]

rich diets has been shown to increase energy intake,[72] probably by 'passive overeating' (see also Chapter 6). On the other hand, obesity-prone subjects seem to have more difficulties adjusting their fat oxidation when switched to a high-fat intake, favoring storage of fat. Post-obese women failed to increase their fat oxidation appropriately after a 3-day adaptation period to a 50% fat diet, while control subjects could adapt.[73] However, both groups could adapt to a low-fat diet. These results suggest that partitioning of fat between storage and oxidation is important in the development of obesity on a high-fat diet. Interestingly, the oxidation of fuels has been suggested to result in metabolic satiety signals. Evidence for the importance of metabolic satiety signals in food intake regulation comes from studies showing that eating appears to be inversely related to the rate of fuel utilization.[74,75] Fuel oxidation in the liver is thought to provide feedback to the appetite regulating centres of the brain on the energy status of the body (see Section 7.2.7). High metabolism in the liver signals a state where a lot of substrate is available for oxidation and when food intake can thus be decreased. Evidence that, in particular, fat oxidation in the liver can act as a satiety signal comes from studies in which fatty acid oxidation was experimentally manipulated. Ingestion or intragastric administration of medium chain fatty acids (MCTs), which are easily taken up by the liver and are metabolized quickly has been shown to inhibit eating in animals[76,77] and humans.[78,79]

On the other hand, different inhibitors of fatty acid oxidation have been shown to cause an increase in food intake in rats and mice, especially when they are adapted to a high-fat diet.[80,81] An important strategy to inhibit fatty acid oxidation, is to block carnitine *O*-palmitoyltransferase-I, the rate-limiting enzyme in the transport of long chain fatty acids into the mitochondrion, where β-oxidation takes place.

A substance able to do this in humans is Etomoxir. It has been shown clinically that a single dose of Etomoxir increased food intake in a population of young men, habitually eating a high-fat diet,[82] but this occurred in the absence of a detectable decrease in fat oxidation (as measured by indirect calorimetry in a ventilated hood system). In a later study, a respiration chamber was used to measure substrate oxidation after adaptation to a high-fat or a low-fat diet. Changes in substrate oxidation in response to repeated administration of Etomoxir in the high-fat situation were measured. This study showed that in a state of adapted oxidation, administration of Etomoxir resulted in decreased satiety, measured by visual analog scales.[37]

It was shown that fat oxidation was significantly inhibited by Etomoxir and was 13.7% lower than in the placebo situation, while there was a tendency towards an increased carbohydrate oxidation. Moreover, the respiratory quotient (RQ) was significantly different from the food quotient (FQ), when using Etomoxir, revealing that Etomoxir partially reversed the adaptational change in fat oxidation. Carbohydrate balance was negative, and the fat balance was positive. Etomoxir significantly increased 24-h RQ and sleeping RQ compared with the placebo. The repeated administration of Etomoxir resulted in a gradual decrease of fat oxidation.[37]

Although the 24-h hunger and satiety ratings did not differ significantly between the treatments, there was a significant correlation between the differences in satiety ratings and differences of beta-hydroxybutyrate (BHB) concentrations indicating a role of liver fatty acid oxidation in satiety.[36] These correlations show that the subjects who decreased their BHB most in response to Etomoxir also experience a greater decrease in satiety.[37] Taken together, a clear effect of Etomoxir on substrate oxidation was shown, as well as evidence for a role of liver fatty acid oxidation in induction of satiety.[36,37] This may have implications for the lack of satiating power of a low-fat diet, or a diet using fat replacers, such as Olestra.

7.4 The role of high- and low-fat diets

The consequences of high- or low-fat diets may depend to a great extent on the other macronutrients consumed. Until recently, mainly low-fat diets have been promoted to enable weight loss, implying relatively higher carbohydrate and normal protein intakes than on normal mixed diets. These diets seem to have had hardly any long-term success, and, although debated, this may in part be due to the high carbohydrate content. On the other hand, the short-term seemingly positive effects of high-fat, low-carbohydrate diets may well be due to their high protein contents. The following section deals with a long term study using a low-carbohydrate, high-fat, high-protein diet (see also Chapter 6).

7.4.1 High-fat, low-carbohydrate, high-protein diet

The conventional dietary approach to weight management, recommended by the leading research and medical societies, is a high-carbohydrate, low-fat, energy-deficit diet. Yet low-carbohydrate, high-protein, high-fat diets have become increasingly popular, and many best-selling diet books have promoted this approach.[83] A one-year, multicenter, randomized, controlled trial was conducted to evaluate the effect of the low-carbohydrate, high-protein, high-fat Atkins diet on weight loss and risk factors for coronary heart disease in obese persons.[83] The results of this demonstrate that the low-carbohydrate, high-protein, high-fat Atkins diet produces greater weight loss (an absolute difference of approximately 4%) than a conventional high-carbohydrate, low-fat diet for up to 6 months, but that the differences do not persist at one year.[83] The lack of a statistically significant difference between the groups at 1 year is most likely due to greater weight regain in the low-carbohydrate group and the small sample size.

These data suggest that long-term adherence to the low-carbohydrate Atkins diet may be difficult. The difference in weight loss between the two groups in the first 6 months demonstrates an overall greater energy deficit in the low-carbohydrate group, despite unrestricted protein and fat intake in this group and instructions to restrict energy intake in the conventional diet group. When the energy content of an energy-deficit diet is stable, macronutrient composition does not influence weight loss.[83] The mechanism responsible for the decreased energy intake induced by a low-carbohydrate diet with unrestricted protein and fat intake is not known but may be related to the monotony or simplicity of the diet, alterations in plasma or central satiety factors, or other factors that affect appetite and dietary adherence.[83] Ketosis was unlikely to be responsible for the increased weight loss with the low-carbohydrate diet, since no relation between the presence of urinary ketones and weight loss was found.[83] Furthermore, urinary ketones were not present in most subjects on either diet after the first 6 months.[83]

The overall effect of the low-carbohydrate diet in comparison with a conventional diet on the risk of coronary heart disease in our subjects is uncertain. As compared with the conventional diet, the low-carbohydrate diet was associated with a greater improvement in some risk factors for coronary heart disease (serum triglycerides and serum high-density lipoprotein, HDL, cholesterol), but not others (blood pressure, insulin sensitivity, and serum low-density lipoprotein, LDL, cholesterol).[83] Moreover, the clinical significance of the favorable changes in the HDL cholesterol–triglyceride axis in the setting of a high fat intake is not clear. At the present time, there is not enough information to determine whether the beneficial effects of the Atkins diet outweigh its potential adverse effects on the risk of coronary heart disease in obese persons.[83]

Reviewing further studies on 'low-carb diets' it appears that these are usually high in protein (P: 22–49 en%*), low to high in fat (F: 20–68 en%), and low to normal in carbohydrate (CHO: 6–45 en%).[84] Thus high protein is the common denominator. Most subjects appear to lose relatively more weight on a high-protein diet, over 2 weeks to 6 months, irrespective of the CHO proportion; yet there is no difference in weight loss over 1 year.[84] Weight maintenance during 3, 6 and 12 months after weight loss on a high-protein diet appeared to be better, again irrespective of the carbohydrate and fat content.[85,86] In 24-h respiration chamber studies, satiety was higher on a high-protein diet, as was energy expenditure and fat-oxidation; here also the high-protein diet was combined with different levels of carbohydrate.[6] A study comparing effects of a high-protein, high-fat and high-carbohydrate diet showed that all diets were high in protein, and no significant weight loss was observed after 6 months.[87] To our knowledge presently there are no studies known that prove weight loss efficacy of a high-fat, low-carbohydrate diet that is normal in protein. We suggest that the efficacy shown is due to the high protein content of the diets, irrespective of the carbohydrate and fat contents of the diets.

7.5 Weight control, fatty acids and structured lipids: a synthesis

Energy expenditure determines energy requirements, which have to be met by diet or utilization of energy stores. The balance between requirements, intake and expenditure determines whether energy stores are depleted or increased. Since humans are genetically programmed to survive during famine, storing excess energy intake is a strong characteristic, based upon a redundant metabolic system, aiming for a high energy efficiency, i.e. much weight gain with little energy intake. In Westernized societies, famine is absent, thus storing energy is exaggerated. This results in overweight and obesity, together with several co-morbidities. To prevent or treat overweight/obesity, body-weight control needs to be managed in spite of the programmed metabolic system.

In the abundance of a large variety of very attractive foods being available, energy intake needs to be controlled. In addition, the metabolic efficiency of the energy taken in should be low, i.e. that for a given energy intake very little weight gain should occur. Mechanisms to achieve low metabolic efficiency focus on special pathways that finally affect metabolic targets such as thermogenesis and fat oxidation. This often increases satiety as well. The most promising ingredients are those that still affect metabolic targets in the longer term, during weight maintenance, and result in a better body composition together with a higher thermogenesis and fat oxidation. It has been suggested that CLA may improve body composition and reduces appetite, and diacylglycerol seems to be likely to be acting by improving fat oxidation and reducing appetite at the same time.

7.6 Future trends

Unless an unforeseen famine occurs, overweight and obesity will be increasing problems during this century. One future trend will be to characterize subjects with a predisposition to fat storage and lack of dietary-related discipline. This way, possible successes of treatments may be predicted. At the same time refinements in our understanding of the relevant metabolic pathways and the impact of detailed understanding of genetics will take place.

Meanwhile, effects of macronutrient compositions still need to be elucidated in more refined ways: if one aims for a high protein content of the food, how exactly is the fate of carbohydrate and fat affected? One quite blank area of understanding is how taste perception could affect energy intake in a desirable way, i.e. indicating the acceptability of a food, without indicating an increased liking and wanting of the food.

Taken together, with any potential treatment method or ingredient, the subject-specific sensitivity, and the effects on metabolic pathway parameters need to be assessed.

7.7 References

1. WESTERTERP KR, ELBERS JMH (1999). Gender differences, energy balance, and effects of sex steroid hormones on circulating leptin levels. In: Westerterp-Plantenga MS, Steffens AB, Tremblay A (eds). *Regulation of food intake and energy expenditure*. EDRA: Milan; pp 305–324.
2. WESTERTERP KR, GORAN MI (1999). Age and energy balance. In: Westerterp-Plantenga MS, Steffens AB, Tremblay A (eds). *Regulation of food intake and energy expenditure*. EDRA: Milan; pp 325–348.
3. WESTERTERP KR (1999). Exercise and energy balance. (1999). In: Westerterp-Plantenga MS, Steffens AB, Tremblay A (eds). *Regulation of food intake and energy expenditure*. EDRA: Milan, pp 349–361.
4. MELANSON KJ, WESTERTERP-PLANTENGA MS, CAMPFIELD LA, SARIS WHM (1999). Short term regulation of food intake in humans. In: Westerterp-Plantenga MS, Steffens AB, Tremblay A (eds). *Regulation of food intake and energy expenditure*. EDRA: Milan; pp 37–58.
5. HETHERINGTON M, BLUNDELL JE (1999). Eating disorders. In: Westerterp-Plantenga MS, Steffens AB, Tremblay A (eds). *Regulation of food intake and energy expenditure*. EDRA: Milan, pp 98–121.
6. WESTERTERP-PLANTENGA MS, ROLLAND V, WILSON SAJ, WESTERTERP KR (1999). Satiety related to 24h diet-induced thermogenesis during high protein/carbohydrate versus high fat diets, measured in a respiration chamber. *Eur J Clin Nutr*, **53**, 1–8.
7. WESTERTERP-PLANTENGA MS, VERWEGEN CRT (1999). The appetizing effect of an alcohol aperitif in overweight and normal weight humans. *Am J Clin Nutr*, **69**, 205–212.
8. WESTERTERP-PLANTENGA MS, KOVACS EMR, MELANSON KJ (2002). Habitual meal frequency and energy intake regulation in partially temporally isolated men. *Int J Obes Relat Metab Disord*, **26**, 102–110.

9. WESTERTERP-PLANTENGA MS (2001). Analysis of energy density of food in relation to energy intake regulation in humans. *Brit J Nutr*, **85**, 351–361.
10. CAMPFIELD LA, SMITH FJ (1999). OB Protein pathway – a link between adipose tissue mass and central neural networks. In: Westerterp-Plantenga MS, Steffens AB, Tremblay A (eds). *Regulation of food intake and energy expenditure*. EDRA: Milan; pp 85–98.
11. STEFFENS AB, VAN DIJK G (1999). Central nervous control of food intake, metabolism, and body weight. In: Westerterp-Plantenga MS, Steffens AB, Tremblay A (eds). *Regulation of food intake and energy expenditure*. EDRA: Milan; pp 121–134.
12. ROTH C, WILKEN B, HANEFELD F, SCHROTER W, LEONHARDT U (1998). Hyperphagia in children with craniopharyngioma is associated with hyperleptinaemia and a failure in the downregulation of appetite. *Eur J Endocrinol*, **138**, 89–91.
13. ROLLS ET (1999). Taste and olfactory processing in the brain , and its relation to the regulation of food intake. In: Westerterp-Plantenga MS, Steffens AB, Tremblay A (eds). *Regulation of food intake and energy expenditure*. EDRA: Milan; pp 19–36.
14. ROLLS ET, MURZI E, YAXLEY S, THORPE SJ, SIMPSON SJ (1986). Sensory-specific satiety: food-specific reduction in responsiveness of ventral forebrain neurons after feeding in the monkey. *Brain Res*, **368**, 79–86.
15. ROLLS ET, SIENKIEWICZ ZJ, YAXLEY S (1989). Hunger modulates the responses to gustatory stimuli of single neurons in the orbitofrontal cortex. *Europ J Neurosci*, **1**, 53–60.
16. CRITCHLEY HD, ROLLS ET (1996). Hunger and satiety modify the responses of olfactory and visual neurons in the primate orbitofrontal cortex. *J Neurophysiol*, **75**, 1673–1686.
17. ROLLS BJ, ROLLS ET, ROWE EA, SWEENEY K (1981). Sensory specific satiety in man. *Physiol Behav*, **27**, 137–142.
18. GILBERTSON TA, FONTENOT T, LIU L, ZHANG H, MONROE WT (1997). Fatty acid modulation of K+ channels in taste receptor cells: gustatory cues for dietary fat. *Am. J. Physiol.*, **272**, C1203–C1210.
19. GILBERTSON TA, LIU L, YORK DA, BRAY GA (1998). Dietary fat preferences are inversely correlated with peripheral gustatory fatty acid sensitivity. *Ann N Y Acad Sci*, **855**, 165–168.
20. KAMPHUIS MMJW, WESTERTERP-PLANTENGA MS, SARIS WHM (2001). Fat specific satiety in humans for fat high in linoleic acid versus fat high in oleic acid. *Eur J Clin Nutr*, **55**, 499–508.
21. KAMPHUIS MMJW, WESTERTERP-PLANTENGA MS (2001). Taste perception of free fatty acids, i.e. CLA. *Int J Obes and Rel Metab Disord*, **25**, S51.
22. VAN ITALLIE TB (1990). The glucostatic theory 1953–1988: roots and branches. *Int J Obes Rel Metab Disord*, **14**, 1–10.
23. BRAY GA (1996). Static theories in a dynamic world: A glucodynamic theory of food intake. *Obes Res*, **4**, 489–492.
24. LEATHWOOD P, POLLET P (1998). Effects of slow release carbohydrates in the form of bean flakes on the evolution of hunger and satiety in man. *Appetite*, **10**, 1–11.
25. MELANSON KJ, WESTERTERP-PLANTENGA MS, SARIS WHM, CAMPFIELD, LA (1999). Blood glucose patterns and appetite in time-blinded humans: carbohydrate versus fat. *Am J Physiol*, **77** (*Regulatory Integrative Comp Physiol* **46**): R337–R345.
26. FRENCH SJ, MURRAY B, RUMSEY RDE, SEPPLE CP, READ NW (1993). Is cholecystokinin a satiety hormone? Correlations of plasma cholecystokinin with hunger, satiety and gastric emptying in normal volunteers. *Appetite*, **21**, 95–104.

27. SMITH GP, GIBBS J (1985). The satiety effect of cholecystokinin: recent progress and current problems. *Ann N Y Acad Sci*, **448**, 424–430.
28. KISSILEFF HR, PI-SUNYER FX, THORNTON J, SMITH GP (1981). C-terminal octapeptide of cholecystokinin decreases food intake in man. *Am J Clin Nutr*, **34**, 154–160.
29. RICHARD D (1993). Involvement of corticotrophin-releasing factor in the control of food intake and energy expenditure. *Ann N Y Acad Sci*, **456**, 155–172.
30. RICHARD D (1995). Exercise and the neurobiological control of food intake and energy expenditure. *Int J Obes Rel Metab Disord*, **19**, S73–S79.
31. RIVEST S, RICHARD D (1990). Involvement of corticotrophin-releasing factor in the anorexia induced by exercise. *Brain Res Bull*, **25**, 169–172.
32. BERGH C, SODERSTEN P (1996). Anorexia nervosa, self-starvation and the reward of stress. *Nature Med*, **2**, 21–22.
33. ADRIAN TE, ALLEN JM, BLOOM SR, GHATEI MA, ROSSOR MN, ROBERTS GW, CROW TJ, TATEMOTO K, POLAK JM (1983). Neuropeptide Y distribution in the human brain. *Nature*, **306**, 584–586.
34. WOODS SC (1986). Central nervous system control of nutrient homeostasis. In: Bloom F (ed). *Handbook of physiology, Section I: The nervous system Volume 4: Intrinsic regulatory systems of the brain.* American Physiological Society: Bethesda, MD; pp 365–411.
35. STRUBBE JH (1994). Circadian rhythms of food intake. In: Westerterp-Plantenga MS, Fredrix EWHM, Steffens AB (eds*). Food intake and energy expenditure.* CRC Press: London; pp 155–174.
36. LANGHANS W (1999). Metabolic control of food intake. Role of the liver. In: Westerterp-Plantenga MS, Steffens AB, Tremblay A (eds). *Regulation of food intake and energy expenditure*. EDRA: Milan; pp 185–199.
37. HINDERLING VB, SCHRAUWEN P, LANGHANS W, WESTERTERP-PLANTENGA MS (2002). The effect of Etomoxir on 24h substrate oxidation and satiety in humans. *Am J Clin Nutr*, **76**, 141–147.
38. KEPLER CR, TUCKER WP, TOVE SB (1970). Biohydrogenation of unsaturated fatty acids. IV. Substrate specificity and inhibition of linoleate delta-12-*cis*, delta-11-*trans*-isomerase from *Butyrivibrio fibrisolvens*. *J Biol Chem*, **245**(14), 3612–3620.
39. KEPLER CR, TUCKER WP, TOVE SB (1971). Biohydrogenation of unsaturated fatty acids. V. Stereospecificity of proton addition and mechanism of action of linoleic acid delta 12-*cis*, delta 11-*trans*-isomerase from *Butyrivibrio fibrisolvens*. *J Biol Chem*, **246**(9), 2765–2771.
40. PARK Y, ALBRIGHT KJ, LIU W, STORKSON JM, COOK ME, PARIZA MW (1997). Effect of conjugated linoleic acid on body composition in mice. *Lipids*, **32**(8), 853–858.
41. WEST DB, DELANY JP, CAMET PM, BLOHM F, TRUETT AA, SCIMECA J (1998). Effects of conjugated linoleic acid on body fat and energy metabolism in the mouse. *Am J Physiol*, **275**, R667–R672.
42. PARK Y, STORKSON JM, ALBRIGHT KJ, LIU W, PARIZA MW (1999). Evidence that the *trans*-10,*cis*-12 isomer of conjugated linoleic acid induces body composition changes in mice. *Lipids*, **34**(3), 235–241.
43. PARK Y, ALBRIGHT KJ, STORKSON JM, LIU W, COOK ME, PARIZA MW (1999). Changes in body composition in mice during feeding and withdrawal of conjugated linoleic acid. *Lipids*, **34**(3), 243–248.
44. DeLANY JP, BLOHM F, TRUETT AA, SCIMECA JA, WEST DB (1999). Conjugated linoleic acid rapidly reduces body fat content in mice without affecting energy intake. *Am J Physiol*, **276**, R1172–R1179.

45. AZAIN MJ, HAUSMAN DB, SISK MB, FLATT WP, JEWELL DE (2000). Dietary conjugated linoleic acid reduces rat adipose tissue cell size rather than cell number. *J Nutr*, **130**(6), 1548–1554.
46. WEST DB, BLOHM FY, TRUETT AA, DELANY JP (2000). Conjugated linoleic acid persistently increases total energy expenditure in AKR/J mice without increasing uncoupling protein gene expression. *J Nutr*, **130**(10), 2471–2477.
47. SISK MB, HAUSMAN DB, MARTIN RJ, AZAIN MJ (2001). Dietary conjugated linoleic acid reduces adiposity in lean but not obese Zucker rats. *J Nutr*, **131**(6), 1668–1674.
48. MINER JL, CEDERBERG CA, NIELSEN MK, CHEN X, BAILE CA (2001). Conjugated linoleic acid (CLA), body fat, and apoptosis. *Obes Res*, **9**(2), 129–134.
49. OHNUKI K, HARAMIZU S, OKI K, ISHIHARA K, FUSHIKI T (2001). A single oral administration of conjugated linoleic acid enhanced energy metabolism in mice. *Lipids*, **36**(6), 583–587.
50. BLANKSON H, STAKKESTAD JA, FAGERTUN H, THOM E, WADSTEIN J, GUDMUNDSEN O (2000). Conjugated linoleic acid reduces body fat mass in overweight and obese humans. *J Nutr*, **130**(12), 2943–2948.
51. MOUGIOS V, MATSAKAS A, PETRIDOU A, RING S, SAGREDOS A, MELISSOPULOU A, TSIGILIS N, NIKOLAIDIS M (2001). Effect of supplementation with conjugated linoleic acid on human serum lipids and body fat. *J Nutr Biochem*, **12**, 585–594.
52. RISERUS U, BERGLUND L, VESSBY B (2001). Conjugated linoleic acid (CLA) reduced abdominal adipose tissue in obese middle-aged men with signs of the metabolic syndrome: a randomised controlled trial. *Int J Obes Relat Metab Disord*, **25**(8), 1129–1135.
53. BERVEN G, BYE A, HALS O, BLANKSON H, FAGERTUN H, THOM E, WADSTEIN J, GUDMUNDSEN O (2000). Safety of conjugated linoleic acid (CLA) in overweight and obese human volunteers. *Eur J Lipid Sci Technol*, **102**, 455–462.
54. ZAMBELL KL, KEIM NL, VAN LOAN MD, GALE B, BENITO P, KELLEY DS, NELSON GJ (2000). Conjugated linoleic acid supplementation in humans: effects on body composition and energy expenditure. *Lipids*, **35**(7), 777–782.
55. SMEDMAN A, VESSBY B (2001). Conjugated linoleic acid supplementation in humans – metabolic effects. *Lipids*, **36**(8), 773–781.
56. GAULLIER JM, HALSE J, HOYE K, KRISTIANSEN K, FAGERTUN H, VIK H, GUDMUNDSEN O (2004). Conjugated linoleic acid supplementation for 1 y reduces body fat mass in healthy overweight humans. *Am J Clin Nutr*, **79**, 1118–1125.
57. KAMPHUIS MMJW, LEJEUNE MPGM, SARIS WHM, WESTERTERP-PLANTENGA MS (2003). The effect of conjugated linoleic acid supplementation after weight loss on body weight regain, body composition, and resting metabolic rate in overweight subjects. *Int J Obes Relat Metab Disord*, **27**(7), 840–847.
58. KAMPHUIS MMJW, LEJEUNE MPGM, SARIS WHM, WESTERTERP-PLANTENGA MS (2003). Effect of conjugated linoleic acid supplementation after weight loss on appetite and food intake in overweight subjects. *Eur J Clin Nutr*, **57**(10), 1268–1274.
59. TAGUCHI H, WATANABE H, ONIZAWA K, *et al.* (2000). Double-blind controlled study on the effects of dietary diacylglycerol on postprandial serum and chylomicron triacylglycerol responses in healthy humans. *J Am Coll Nutr*, **19**, 789–796.
60. WATANABE H, ONIZAWA K, TAGUCHI H, *et al.* (1997). Effects of diacylglycerols on lipid metabolism in human. *Nippon Yukagaku Kaishi*, **46**, 309–314.
61. HARA K, ONIZAWA K, HONDA H, OTSUJI K, IDE T, MURATA M (1993). Dietary diacylglycerol-dependent reduction in serum triacylglycerol concentration in rats. *Ann Nutr Metab*, **37**, 185–191.

62. MURATA M, IDE T, HARA K (1997). Reciprocal responses to dietary diacylglycerol of hepatic enzymes of fatty acid synthesis and oxidation in the rat. *Br J Nutr*, **77**, 107–121.
63. YAMAMOTO K, ASAKAWA H, TOKUNAGA K, *et al.* (2001). Long-term ingestion of dietary diacylglycerol lowers serum triacylglycerol in type II diabetic patients with hypertriglyceridemia. *J Nutr*, **131**, 3204–3207.
64. WATANABE H, ONIZAWA K, TAGUCHI H, *et al.* (1997). Nutritional characterization of diacylglycerols in rats. *J Japan Oil Chem Soc*, **46**, 301–307.
65. MURASE T, MIZUNO T, OMACHI T, *et al.* (2001). Dietary diacylglycerol suppresses high fat and high sucrose diet- induced body fat accumulation in C57BL/6J mice. *J Lipid Res*, **42**, 372–378.
66. NAGAO T, WATANABE H, GOTO N, *et al.* (2000). Dietary diacylglycerol suppresses accumulation of body fat compared to triacylglycerol in men in a double-blind controlled trial. *J Nutr*, **130**, 792–797.
67. WATANABE H, NAGAO T, GOTO N, *et al.* (1998). Long-term effects of dietary diacylglycerols on body fat metabolism in man. *Nippon Yukagaku Kaishi*, **47**, 369–376.
68. TAGUCHI H, NAGAO T, WATANABE H, *et al.* (2001). Energy value and digestibility of dietary oil containing mainly 1,3-diacylglycerol are similar to those of triacylglycerol. *Lipids*, **36**, 379–382.
69. KAMPHUIS MMJW, MELA DM, WESTERTERP-PLANTENGA MS (2003). Diacylglycerols affect substrate oxidation and appetite in humans. *Am J Clin Nutr*, **77**(5), 1133–1139.
70. TADA N, YOSHIDA H (2003). Diacylglycerol on lipid metabolism. *Curr Opin Lipidol*, **14**, 29–33.
71. MAKI KC, DAVIDSON MH, TSUSHIMA R (2003). Consumption of diacylglycerol oil as part of a mildly reduced-energy diet enhances loss of body weight and fat compared with a triacylglycerol control oil. *Am J Clin Nutr*, **76**, 1230–1236.
72. WESTERTERP KR,VERBOEKET-VAN DE VENNE WPHG,WESTERTERP-PLANTENGA MS, VELTHUIS-TE WIERIK EJM, DE GRAAF C, WESTSTRATE JA (1996). Dietary fat and body fat: an intervention study. *Int J Obes Relat Metab Disord*, **20**, 1022–1026.
73. ASTRUP A, BUEMANN B, CHRISTENSEN NJ, TOUBRO S (1994). Failure to increase lipid oxidation in response to increasing dietary fat content in formerly obese women. *Am J Physiol*, **266**, E592–599.
74. LANGHANS W, EGLI G, SCHARRER E (1985). Regulation of food intake by hepatic oxidative metabolism. *Brain Res Bull*, **15**, 425–428.
75. LANGHANS W, SCHARRER E (1992). *Metabolic control of eating*. Basel: Karger; pp. 1–67.
76. SATABIN P, AUCLAIR E, SERVAN E, LARUE ACHAGIOTIS C, GUEZENNEC CY (1991). Influence of glucose, medium- and long-chain triglyceride gastric loads and forced exercise on food intake and body weight in rats. *Physiol Behav*, **50**, 147–150.
77. FURUSE M, CHOI Y, MABAYO R, OKUMURA J (1992). Feeding behavior in rats fed diets containing medium chain triglyceride. *Physiol Behav*, **52**, 815–817.
78. ROLLS B, GNIZAK N, SUMMERFELD A (1988). Food intake in dieters and nondieters following a liquid meal containing medium-chain triglycerides. *Am J Clin Nutr*, **48**, 66–71.
79. STUBBS RJ, HARBRON CG, PRENTICE AM (1996). Covert manipulation of the dietary fat to carbohydrate ratio of isoenergetically dense diets: effect on food intake in feeding men *ad libitum*. *Int J Obes Relat Metab Disord*, **20**, 651–660.
80. SCHARRER E, LANGHANS W (1986). Control of food intake by fatty acid oxidation. *Am*

J Physiol, **250**, R1003–1006.

81. DEL PRETE E, LUTZ T, ALTHAUS J, SCHARRER E (1998). Inhibitors of fatty acid oxidation (mercaptoacetate, *R*-3-amino-4-trimethylaminobutyric acid) stimulate feeding in mice. *Physiol Behav*, **63**, 751–754.
82. KAHLER A, ZIMMERMANN M, LANGHANS W (1999). Suppression of hepatic fatty acid oxidation and food intake in men. *Nutrition*, **15**, 819–828.
83. FOSTER GD, WYATT HR, HILL JO, MCGUCKIN BG, BRILL C, SELMA MOHAMMED B, SZAPARY PO, M.D., RADER DJ, EDMAN JS, KLEIN S (2003). A randomized trial of a low-carbohydrate diet for obesity. *N Eng J Med*, **348**(21), 2082–2090.
84. HALTON TL, HU FB (2004). The effects of high protein diets on thermogenesis, satiety and weight loss: a critical review. *J Am Coll Nutr*, **23**, 373–385.
85. WESTERTERP-PLANTENGA MS, LEJEUNE MPGM, VAN OOIJEN M, KOVACS EMR (2004). High protein intake sustains weight maintenance after body weight loss in humans. *Int J Obes*, **28**, 57–64.
86. LEJEUNE MPGM, KOVACS EMR, WESTERTERP-PLANTENGA MS (2005). Additional protein intake limits weight regain after weight loss in humans. *Br J Nutr*, **93**, 281–289.
87. McAULEY KA, HOPKINS CM, SMITH KJ, McLAY RT, WILLIAMS SM, TAYLOR RW, MANN JI (2005). Comparison of high-fat and high-protein diets with a high-carbohydrate diet in insulin-resistant obese women. *Diabetologia*, 48, 8–16.

8

Conjugated linoleic acids (CLAs) and health

P. Yaqoob and S. Tricon, University of Reading, UK and G. C. Burdge and P. C. Calder, University of Southampton, UK

8.1 Introduction

Conjugated linoleic acid (CLA) is a collective term for a mixture of positional and geometric isomers of linoleic acid (18:2) in which the two double bonds are conjugated, i.e. contiguous, unlike the double bonds in linoleic acid, which are separated by a methylene group. CLA isomers are mainly present in ruminant animal fat, dairy products and partly hydrogenated vegetable oils. *Cis*-9,*trans*-11 CLA is the main isomer in the human diet, accounting for > 90% of the total CLA intake (Lawson *et al.*, 2001), and is formed in the rumen as an intermediate in the microbial biohydrogenation of linoleic acid to stearic acid, as well as endogenously in mammary tissue from *trans* vaccenic acid (*trans*-11 octadecenoic acid), a precursor of rumen origin (Lock & Bauman, 2004; Fig. 8.1). As much as 70% of the *cis*-9,*trans*-11 CLA in milk is derived from the desaturation of *trans* vaccenic acid by delta-9 desaturase activity in the mammary gland (Lock & Bauman, 2004). The type of feed provided to cows very much influences the CLA content of the milk; the highest levels are obtained from cows grazing fresh pasture rather than feed concentrates, but some supplemental oils can be used to increase the CLA content of milk (Lock & Bauman, 2004). However, supplemental oils do not always result in sustainable elevation of CLA, which could limit their commercial application (see later).

Although diet is the major source of CLA in humans, there is no systematic database for the CLA content of foods and limited data are available on the isomeric distribution of CLA isomers in food, owing to the difficulties in the chromatographic separation of the individual isomers (Sebedio *et al.*, 1999). Total CLA intake has been estimated to be between 52 and 137 mg/day for men and

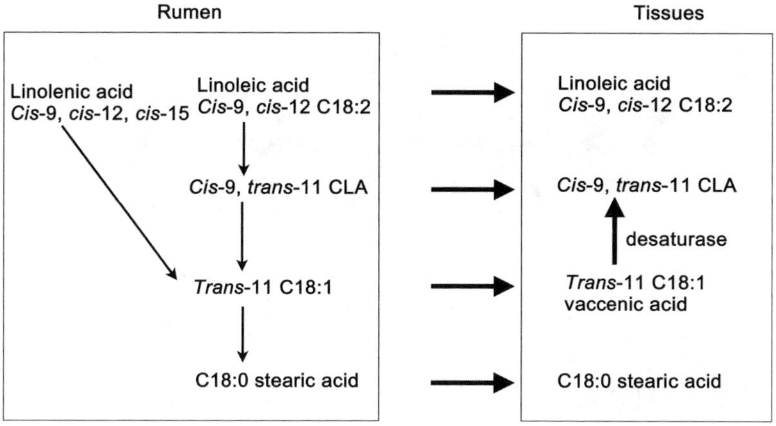

Fig. 8.1 Synthesis of CLA by biohydrogenation in the rumen and desaturation in the mammary gland.

women in the United States, and to average 430 and 350 mg/day for German men and women, respectively (McGuire *et al.*, 1999). Since 1990 there has been increasing interest in CLA, since feeding a mixture of CLA isomers to laboratory animals has been reported to alter tumour growth induced by chemicals (Ip *et al.*, 1991, 1995, 1999; Corl *et al.*, 2003; Chew *et al.*, 1997; Thompson *et al.*, 1997; Belury, 2002), atherogenesis (Lee *et al.*, 1994; Nicolosi *et al.*, 1997), diabetes (Houseknecht *et al.*, 1998), body composition (Park *et al.*, 1997, 1999; West *et al.*, 1998; de Deckere *et al.*, 1999; DeLany *et al.*, 1999; Azain *et al.*, 2000; DeLany & West, 2000; Gavino *et al.*, 2000; Stangl, 2000; Tsuboyama-Kasaoka *et al.*, 2000) and immune cell functions (Cook *et al.*, 1993; Miller *et al.*, 1994; Turek *et al.*, 1997, 1998; Sugano *et al.*, 1998; Hayek *et al.*, 1999; Bassaganya-Riera *et al.*, 2001, 2002; Kelley *et al.*, 2002; Yamasaki *et al.*, 2003). Most of the published studies have used a mixture of CLA isomers that contained the two major forms, *cis*-9,*trans*-11 CLA and *trans*-10,*cis*-12 CLA (Fig. 8.2) in approximately equal amounts, and a number of minor isomers at considerably lower levels. However, emerging evidence indicates that the numerous biological effects are due to the separate actions of the *cis*-9,*trans*-11 and *trans*-10,*cis*-12 isomers (Pariza *et al.*, 2000). This chapter will focus exclusively on human studies and will attempt to define the extent to which the health effects of CLA relating to body composition, blood lipids, insulin sensitivity, immune function and breast cancer reported in animal studies also occur in human subjects.

8.2 CLA and body composition

The body-fat lowering effect of CLA observed in experimental animals has led to the idea that CLA could be used as a tool in body weight management in humans. Eighteen studies in humans have been published so far, but the results

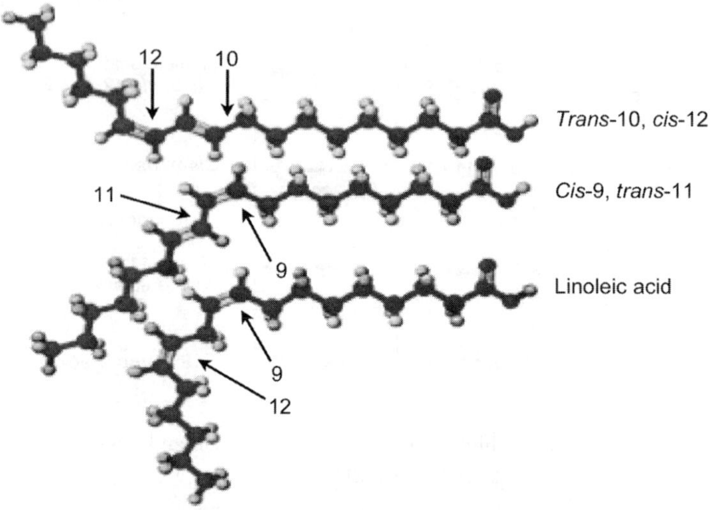

Fig. 8.2 Structures of linoleic acid, *cis*-9,*trans*-11 CLA and *trans*-10,*cis*-12 CLA. Adapted from Pariza *et al.* (2001), with permission.

appear to be less promising than was expected (Calder, 2002; Kelley & Erickson, 2003; Larsen *et al.*, 2003; Terpstra, 2004; Wahle *et al.*, 2004; Tricon *et al.*, 2005). Eight of these studies were conducted in subjects with normal body weight, whereas the other ten were conducted in overweight or obese subjects (Table 8.1). Although the majority of these studies used healthy subjects, three investigated a population of men with signs of the metabolic syndrome (Riserus *et al.*, 2001, 2002b, 2004a), while two used patients with type II diabetes (Belury *et al.*, 2003; Moloney *et al.*, 2004). Most of the studies were done in free-living subjects and were not strictly controlled for nutrient and energy intake. Only in the study by Zambell *et al.* (2000) were the subjects confined to a metabolic unit (for 94 days) and matched to controls for food intake. The amount of CLA consumed in the various studies ranged from 0.7 to 6.8 g/day and it was normally a 1:1 mixture of the *cis*-9,*trans*-11 and *trans*-10,*cis*-12 CLA isomers (Blankson *et al.*, 2000; Mougios *et al.*, 2001; Riserus *et al.*, 2001; Smedman & Vessby, 2001; Noone *et al.*, 2002; Belury *et al.*, 2003; Petridou *et al.*, 2003; Gaullier *et al.*, 2004; Moloney *et al.*, 2004), except for four studies that used a CLA preparation containing almost exclusively the *trans*-10,*cis*-12 isomer or the *cis*-9,*trans*-11 isomer (Riserus *et al.*, 2002b, 2004b; Malpuech-Brugere *et al.*, 2004; Tricon *et al.*, 2004a). However, the earliest studies employed Tonalin capsules, a mixture of small amounts of several different CLA isomers, in which *trans*-10,*cis*-12 and *cis*-9,*trans*-11 CLA isomers represented about 20% each (Berven *et al.*, 2000; Thom *et al.*, 2001; Zambell *et al.*, 2001; Kreider *et al.*, 2002). In all studies, CLA was administered in the form of capsules, except for the study of Malpuech-Brugere *et al.* (2004) which used a dairy-based drink with added synthetic CLA.

Table 8.1 Published studies investigating the effect of CLA on body weight and/or body composition in humans

Amount of CLA (g/day)	Form of CLA	Placebo	Duration	Subjects	Effect of CLA	Reference
3.4	*Tonalin	Olive oil	12 weeks	60 overweight or obese males and females age: >18 years	No effect on body weight or BMI	Berven *et al.* (2000)
1.7, 3.4, 5.1 and 6.8	50:50 *cis*-9,*trans*-11 and *trans*-10,*cis*-12	Olive oil	12 weeks	60 overweight or obese but healthy males and females	Decrease in body fat mass in 3.4 and 6.8 g/day groups No effect on body weight or BMI	Blankson *et al.* (2000)
3.9	*Tonalin	Sunflower oil	9 weeks in a metabolic suite suite	17 healthy females age: 20–41 years	No effect on body weight, body fat mass or body lean mass	Zambell *et al.* (2000)
0.7 then 1.4	50:50 *cis*-9,*trans*-11 and *trans*-10,*cis*-12	Soybean oil	4 weeks then 4 weeks	14 healthy males and 10 healthy females age: 19-24 years	Decrease in % body fat and fat mass during the high CLA intake compared with the low CLA intake	Mougios *et al.* (2001)
4.2	50:50 *cis*-9,*trans*-11 and *trans*-10,*cis*-12	Olive oil	4 weeks	24 abdominally obese males with signs of the metabolic syndrome age: 39–64 years	Decrease in SAD	Riserus *et al.* (2001)
4.2	50:50 *cis*-9,*trans*-11 and *trans*-10,*cis*-12	Olive oil	12 weeks	27 healthy males and 26 healthy females age: 23–63 years	Decrease in body fat No effect on body weight, BMI, waist/hip ratio or SAD	Smedman & Vessby (2001)
1.8	*Tonalin	Hydrogel	12 weeks	20 healthy exercising males and females age: 18–30 years	No effect on BMI or body weight Decrease in body fat	Thom *et al.* (2001)

Table 8.1 (continued)

3.0	50:50 *cis*-9,*trans*-11 and *trans*-10,*cis*-12 *vs* 80:20 *cis*-9,*trans*-11 and *trans*-10,*cis*-12	Linoleic acid	8 weeks	18 healthy males and 33 healthy females age: 31.6 years (mean)	No effect on body weight or BMI	Noone *et al.* (2002)
3.4	50:50 *cis*-9,*trans*-11 and *trans*-10,*cis*-12 *vs* *trans*-10,*cis*-12	Olive oil	12 weeks	60 abdominally obese males with signs of the metabolic syndrome age: 35–65 years	No effect on body composition Decrease in weight, BMI, waist circumference, SAD and body fat in the *trans*-10,*cis*-12 isomer group. Decrease in SAD and body fat in the CLA mixture group	Riserus *et al.* (2002b)
6.0	*Tonalin	Olive oil	28 days	23 experienced resistance-trained males age: 23 years (mean)	No effect on weight, body fat or lean mass	Kreider *et al.* (2002)
2.1	50:50 *cis*-9,*trans*-11 and *trans*-10,*cis*-12 CLA	Soybean oil	45 days	16 healthy females age: 19–24 years	No effect on body composition	Petridou *et al.* (2003)
6.0	50:50 *cis*-9,*trans*-11 and *trans*-10,*cis*-12	Safflower oil	8 weeks	21 subjects with type II diabetes	Levels of plasma *trans*-10,*cis*-12 CLA, but not *cis*-9,*trans*-11 CLA, were inversely associated with body weight	Belury *et al.* (2003)
1.8 and 3.6	*Tonalin	Oleic acid	13 weeks after a 3 weeks very low-calorie diet	54 overweight males and females age: 37.8 years (mean)	No effect on % body weight regain. Increased regain of fat free-mass.	Kamphuis *et al.* (2003a)

1.5 and 3.0	*cis*-9,*trans*-11 *vs* *trans*-10,*cis*-12	High oleic acid sunflower oil	18 weeks	81 healthy overweight males and females age: 35–65 years	No effect on weight, BMI or waist/hip ratio	Malpuech-Brugere *et al.* (2004)
4.5	50:50 *cis*-9,*trans*-11 and *trans*-10,*cis*-12 as FFA or TAG	Olive oil	1 year	180 healthy overweight males and females age: 18–65 years	Decrease in body fat mass in both CLA groups. Increase in lean body mass with CLA as FFA, but not as TAG	Gaullier *et al.* (2004)
3.0	*cis*-9,*trans*-11	Olive oil	12 weeks	25 abdominally obese males age: 35–65 years	No effect on weight, BMI, body fat, lean body mass, SAD or waist circumference	Riserus *et al.* (2004b)
0.59, 1.19, 2.38 (*cis*-9, *trans*-11); 0.63, 1.26, 2.52 (*trans*-10, *cis*12 CLA)	*cis*-9,*trans*-11 *vs* *trans*-10,*cis*12	None (crossover design)	8 weeks on each dose (doses increased sequentially; 6 week washout between isomers)	49 healthy males age: 20–47 years	No effect on weight, BMI, fat mass or fat-free mass	Tricon *et al.* (2004a)
3.0	50:50 *cis*-9,*trans*-11 and *trans*-10,*cis*-12	Palm oil + soybean oil	8 weeks	32 type 2 diabetics	No effect on BMI, waist-hip ratio or percent body fat	Moloney *et al.* (2004)

*Tonalin; 22.6% *trans*-10,*cis*-12, 23.6% *cis*-11,*trans*-13, 17.6% *cis*-9,*trans*-11, 16.6% *trans*-8,*cis*-10, 7.7% *trans*-9,*trans*-11 and *trans*-10,*trans*-12 and 11.9% other CLA isomers.

BMI, body mass index (kg/m^2); FFA, free fatty acid; SAD; sagittal abdominal diameter; TAG, triacylglycerol.

8.2.1 CLA and body weight

None of the studies demonstrated that CLA had a significant effect on body weight or body mass index (BMI) (Table 8.1), except for one study in which reductions in body weight were observed in patients with type II diabetes mellitus receiving a supplement containing 6 g/day of a 50:50 *cis*-9,*trans*-11 and *trans*-10,*cis*-12 CLA isomers for 8 weeks (Belury *et al.*, 2003). In addition, an inverse correlation was observed between body weight change and plasma concentration of *trans*-10,*cis*-12 CLA ($\Gamma = -0.4309$; $P < 0.05$) (Belury *et al.*, 2003) (Table 8.1). There was no correlation between body weight change and plasma concentration of the *cis*-9,*trans*-11 isomer (Belury *et al.*, 2003).

8.2.2 CLA and body composition in normal weight subjects

Four studies conducted in healthy, normal weight subjects have not demonstrated an effect of CLA on body fat mass (Zambell *et al.*, 2001; Kreider *et al.*, 2002; Petridou *et al.*, 2003; Tricon *et al.*, 2004b), while three studies have reported a modest reduction in fat mass after CLA supplementation (Mougios *et al.*, 2001; Smedman & Vessby, 2001; Thom *et al.*, 2001). However, although Mougios *et al.* (2001) reported that healthy volunteers receiving 1.4 g/day of CLA for 4 weeks had a significant decrease in fat mass and % body fat compared with a lower intake of CLA (0.7 g/day), fat mass and % body fat were not significantly different from the placebo group or from baseline values (Table 8.1). The overall conclusion from this study must be that CLA, at the doses used, has little effect on body fatness (Mougios *et al.*, 2001). Therefore, only two studies report a reduction in body fat in healthy subjects (Smedman & Vessby, 2001; Thom *et al.*, 2001).

It is of particular importance to address the effects of specific, highly purified isomers of CLA, rather than mixtures of CLA isomers, since it is possible that different isomers have different biological effects. Tricon *et al.* (2004a) examined the effects of highly enriched *cis*-9,*trans*-11 and *trans*-10,*cis*-12 preparations, each at three doses, on body composition in healthy males. Subjects provided a fasting blood sample at baseline and then every 8 weeks during CLA supplementation. They ($n = 49$) consumed one, two or four capsules (80–85% pure CLA in triacylglycerol form) per day for three consecutive 8-week periods. The capsules provided 0.59, 1.19 or 2.38 g/day *cis*-9,*trans*-11 CLA and 0.63, 1.26 or 2.52 g/day *trans*-10,*cis*-12 CLA, respectively (Fig. 8.3). The objective of the study was to identify the dose-response relationship of the two main CLA isomers on indices of body composition, measured by bioelectrical impedance analysis. There was no significant effect of either isomer of CLA at any dose on body weight, BMI, fat mass or fat-free mass (Tricon *et al.*, 2004a). The results are in general agreement with other studies conducted in healthy adults, where a mixture of CLA isomers had no effect on body weight or composition (Zambell *et al.*, 2000; Kreider *et al.*, 2002; Noone *et al.*, 2002; Petridou *et al.*, 2003). Animal studies have suggested that the *trans*-10,*cis*-12 isomer has the most potent body fat-reducing properties (Park *et al.*, 1999; Gavino *et al.*, 2000).

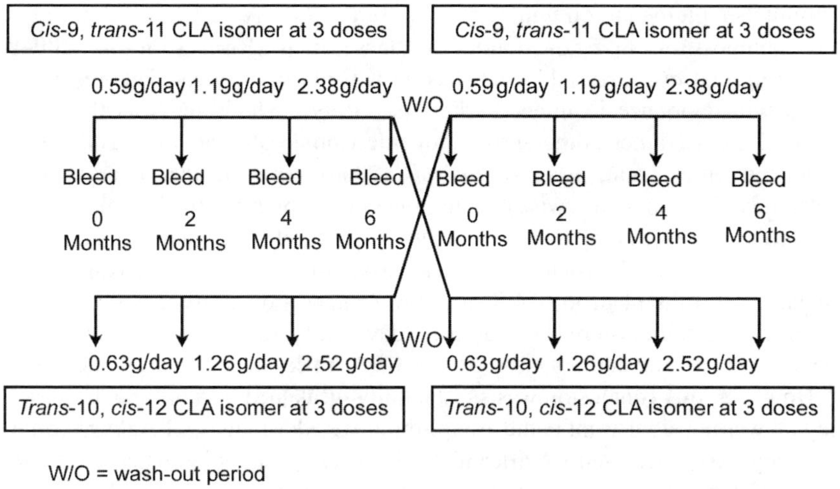

Fig. 8.3 Design of the study conducted by Burdge *et al.* (2004, 2005) and Tricon *et al.* (2004a,b). Reproduced with permission from the *American Journal of Clinical Nutrition*.

Consequently, the lack of effect of CLA supplementation on body composition in human trials has sometimes been explained by the fact that the CLA supplements used in most trials have contained a mixture of isomers and the *trans*-10,*cis*-12 isomer may have been present at a level below the threshold necessary to elicit body composition changes. However, the study by Tricon *et al.* (2004a) demonstrates that even a fairly high dose of *trans*-10,*cis*-12 CLA does not affect body composition in healthy subjects. Overall, therefore, there is no conclusive evidence to suggest that consumption of either a mixture of CLA isomers or of highly enriched preparations of single CLA isomers, results in a significant alteration in body composition in normal-weight subjects.

8.2.3 CLA and body composition in overweight and obese subjects

A summary of the studies looking at the effects of CLA on body composition in overweight and obese subjects is reported in Table 8.1. Four out of eight studies demonstrated that CLA supplementation had no effect on body composition in such subjects (Berven *et al.*, 2000; Malpuech-Brugere *et al.*, 2004; Moloney *et al.,* 2004; Riserus *et al.*, 2004b). There were no effects of pure *cis*-9,*trans*-11 CLA or *trans*-10,*cis*-12 CLA (given in a food matrix) on body fat mass in overweight humans after 18 weeks supplementation (Malpuech-Brugere *et al.*, 2004). Similarly, a 50:50 mixture of *cis*-9,*trans*-11 and *trans*-10,*cis*-12 CLA at a dose of 3 g/d did not alter body composition in overweight type 2 diabetics over an 8 week intervention period (Moloney *et al.,* 2004). In the study by Berven *et al.* (2000), 3.4 g/day CLA decreased mean body weight by 1.1 kg and mean BMI by 0.4 kg/m^2 after 12 weeks supplementation in overweight and obese participants. However, the overall treatment effect of CLA was not significant. Finally,

3 months supplementation with 3 g/day pure *cis*-9,*trans*-11 CLA did not affect body composition in 25 abdominally obese men (Riserus *et al.*, 2004b), suggesting that *cis*-9,*trans*-11 CLA has no anti-obesity effects. This result is in accord with evidence in mice (Park *et al.*, 1999), which suggests that *trans*-10,*cis*-12 CLA isomer is the anti-adipogenic isomer (Pariza *et al.*, 2001).

On the other hand, Blankson *et al.* (2000) reported that overweight or moderately obese, but otherwise healthy, subjects supplementing their diet with 3.4 or 6.8 g/day of a CLA preparation (Tonalin) for 12 weeks experienced significantly greater losses in DEXA-determined fat mass (−1.7 and −1.3 kg, respectively) compared with the placebo (+1.8 kg). However, no effects were observed when subjects were administered 1.7 or 5.1 g/day CLA, suggesting no clear dose–response effect. The authors claimed that CLA intake of 3.4 g/day reduced body fat. However, this conclusion was substantially weakened because the decrease in body fat was not significant in the group administered 5.1 g/day CLA. Furthermore, lean body mass increased significantly only in the group administered 6.8 g/day CLA, which was the group that reported maximum increase in the number of hours spent on intensive exercise (Blankson *et al.*, 2000).

In a second study, supplementation with 4.2 g/day CLA for 4 weeks to a group of abdominally obese men demonstrated a significant mean decrease in the sagittal abdominal diameter by 0.6 cm in the CLA group compared with the control group (Riserus *et al.*, 2001). There were also significant decreases in the waist/hip ratio and waist circumference within the CLA group, but these changes were not significantly different from those of the control group. Furthermore, in the studies by Riserus *et al.* (2001) and Blankson *et al.* (2000), the changes in body fat mass seen were within the prediction errors for the methods used (Kelley & Erickson, 2003).

In a third study, Gaullier *et al.* (2004) examined, for the first time, the long-term effect of 3 g/day CLA (in free fatty acid or triacylglycerol forms) in overweight humans (Table 8.1). They reported that 1 year supplementation of CLA (in either form) significantly lowered body fat mass, and that CLA (in the free fatty acid form) increased lean body mass compared with placebo (Gaullier *et al.*, 2004). However, the authors changed their techniques for measuring body composition halfway through the study and reported a reduction in calorie intake in all groups, which was greater in the two CLA groups. The authors also reported that the best responders to CLA (= 4.5% body fat mass reduction) were women and subjects with a higher BMI at baseline (Gaullier *et al.*, 2004). This is quite interesting since none of the studies looking at the effects of CLA on body composition stratified for gender or BMI.

Recently, Riserus *et al.* (2002b) reported that supplementation of the *trans*-10,*cis*-12 CLA isomer (~2 g/day) for 12 weeks was responsible for a significant trend towards a decrease in body fat, sagittal abdominal diameter, waist girth, BMI and weight in 60 obese men with signs of the metabolic syndrome, whereas only sagittal abdominal diameter and body fat decreased after a CLA mixture (50:50 mixture of *trans*-10,*cis*-12 and *cis*-9,*trans*-11 CLA isomers). This data would suggest that the *trans*-10,*cis*-12 CLA is the active isomer in terms of weight-loss (Riserus *et al.*, 2002b; Belury *et al.*, 2003), although this was not confirmed in the two studies looking at the effects of the pure CLA isomers (Malpuech-Brugere *et al.*, 2004; Tricon *et al.*, 2004a). Furthermore, there were no significant differences between groups (control *vs* CLA mixture *vs* *trans*-10,*cis*-12 CLA) in any of the body composition parameters measured after 12 weeks (Riserus *et al.*, 2002b).

Collectively, results from human studies regarding the effects of CLA on body composition in overweight and obese subjects are inconsistent. However, it is likely that the changes reported in at least some studies were the result of confounding variables such as food intake, exercise and the prediction errors for the methods used. In any case, the effects are much smaller than those observed in animals and the weight of evidence does not support a role for CLA in decreasing body fat in humans.

8.2.4 CLA and body weight regain

Most of the animal experiments in which CLA was found to decrease fat deposition were conducted in growing animals. It is important to emphasize that in many animal models dietary CLA induces a decrease in body fat without decreasing body weight (Park *et al.*, 1997). Thus, in most animal models the decrease in body fat appears to be due mostly to a reduction in body fat accretion (West *et al.*, 1998; Pariza, 2004). However, the published human trials described above were all designed to test the hypothesis that CLA ingestion will lower the amount of accumulated body fat in adult humans (Table 8.1). Only Kamphuis *et al.* (2003a,b) approached the issue differently, examining the effects of two doses of CLA administered after weight loss on body weight and body fat regain (Table 8.1). Overweight subjects were first submitted to a 3-week very-low-calorie weight loss diet and then supplemented with 1.8 or 3.6 g/day CLA (as Tonalin) or placebo for a 13-week intervention period during which they ate *ad libitum* (Kamphuis *et al.*, 2003a). Subjects taking CLA (at either dose) exhibited significantly greater regain of fat-free mass relative to control subjects, accompanied by an increase in resting metabolic rate. However, CLA did not affect percentage body weight regain (Kamphuis *et al.*, 2003a). Interestingly, measures of appetite (hunger, satiety and fullness) were also favourably and dose-dependently affected by CLA ingestion (Kamphuis *et al.*, 2003b). This study is in accordance with animal studies, suggesting that CLA might be most effective in controlling body fat accretion, rather than lowering the amount of accumulated body fat.

8.3 Incorporation of CLA into tissue lipids and CLA metabolism in humans

Despite the number of studies that have investigated the effects of increased CLA intake on health-related outcomes, there is relatively little information on the incorporation of CLA into blood and cellular lipids in humans consuming habitual diets or after receiving CLA supplements. This represents an important omission as it is not possible to relate the response of an outcome measure to the effectiveness of the supplementation regimen in raising the amount of CLA available within the body. In studies that do report CLA concentration, the *cis*-9,*trans*-11 isomer is readily detected (although at less than 0.5% of total fatty acids) in subjects consuming their habitual diet (Benito *et al.*, 2001; Masters *et al.*, 2002; Noone *et al.*, 2002; Petridou *et al.* 2003; Burdge *et al.* 2004). This reflects consumption of *cis*-9,*trans*-11 CLA in dairy products and meat from ruminants. The *trans*-10,*cis*-12 isomer which is a minor component of these foods is either absent (Benito *et al.*, 2001; Masters *et al.*, 2002; Burdge *et al.* 2004) or present at approximately ten-fold lower concentration than *cis*-9,*trans*-11 CLA (Petridou *et al.* 2003). The concentrations of *trans*-8,*cis*-10 CLA and *cis*-11,*trans*-13 CLA are approximately 0.2% plasma total fatty acids in individuals maintained on a non-CLA enriched diet (Benito *et al.*, 2001). CLA isomers are distributed differentially between plasma lipid classes. The relative concentrations of *cis*-9,*trans*-11 CLA in human plasma is triaclglycerols (TAG) > phospholipids ≡ cholesterol esters (CE) ≡ non-esterified fatty acids (Petridou *et al.* 2003; Burdge *et al.*, 2004). However, Petridou *et al.* (2003) reported similar concentrations of *trans*-10,*cis*-12 in plasma TAG, phospholipids and CE. The concentration of *cis*-9,*trans*-11 CLA in peripheral blood mononuclear cell total lipids in individuals consuming their habitual diets was 0.05 to 0.5% of total fatty acids (Kelley *et al.*, 2001; Albers *et al.*, 2003; Burdge *et al.*, 2004) and in erythrocytes it was 0.2% of total fatty acids (von Loeffelholz *et al.*, 2003; Burdge *et al.*, 2004b).

Increased consumption of *cis*-9,*trans*-11 CLA and *trans*-10,*cis*-12 CLA increases the concentrations of these isomers in plasma (Benito *et al.*, 2001; Masters *et al.*, 2002; Noone *et al.*, 2002; Petridou *et al.* 2003; Burdge *et al.*, 2004) and cellular lipids (von Loeffelholz *et al.* 2003; Burdge *et al.*, 2004, 2005). The level of incorporation is dependent upon the amount of CLA consumed (Burdge *et al.*, 2004). However, the incremental changes in the concentrations of individual CLA isomers in plasma lipids were typically less than 0.5% at intakes of 350 mg of a 50:50 mixture of *cis*-9,*trans*-11 CLA plus *trans*-10,*cis*-12 CLA (Petridou *et al.*, 2003), 1.5 g per day of mixed CLA isomers (Tonalin) (Masters *et al.*, 2002), 2.5 g per day of *cis*-9,*trans*-11 CLA or *trans*-10,*cis*-12 CLA (Burdge *et al.*, 2004a), 3.0 g per day of a 50:50 or 80:20 mix of *cis*-9,*trans*-11 CLA and *trans*-10,*cis*-12 CLA (Noone *et al.*, 2002) and 3.9 g per day total CLA (Benito *et al.*, 2001). Consumption of 1.5 g per day eicosapentaenoic acid and docosahexaenoic acid results in an increase in the concentrations of these fatty acids in plasma lipids of approximately 1 to 2.5% (for example see Finnegan *et al.*, 2003). This suggests that CLA may be incorporated less readily into plasma lipids than other polyunsaturated fatty acids, which may be a limiting factor in the efficacy of supplementation regimens in increasing the CLA content of tissue pools.

The concentration of CLA in plasma lipids is determined by bioavailability from the gut, and subsequent partitioning between β-oxidation, incorporation into tissue lipids, secretion from the gut and liver in lipoproteins, and turnover within the plasma compartment. There is only limited information available about the metabolic fate of CLA in humans. Using deuterated fatty acid ethyl esters, Emken *et al.* (2002) showed that the bioavailability of *cis*-9,*trans*-11 CLA and *trans*-10,*cis*-12 CLA after a bolus was lower than that of oleic acid. However, since the fatty acids were not ingested as TAG any effect of the conjugated double bonds on lipase activity would not have been detected. Incorporation of *cis*-9,*trans*-11 CLA and *trans*-10,*cis*-12 CLA into plasma CE and phospholipids was less than for linoleic and oleic acids, which suggests metabolic selection against incorporation into these lipid pools. Together these findings suggest that restricted bioavailability and negative metabolic selection may explain the limited impact of dietary supplementation studies on CLA concentrations in humans. There was some indication of conversion of CLA to 18:3 metabolites by Δ6-desaturase activity (Emken *et al.*, 2002).

Turpeinen *et al.* (2002) have shown that consuming 1.5, 3.0 or 4.5 g per day *trans*-vaccenic acid produced a dose-dependent increase in total serum *cis*-9,*trans*-11 CLA concentration, presumably by the action of hepatic delta-9-desaturase. While this indicates that humans possess some capacity for *cis*-9,*trans*-11 CLA biosynthesis, the increments in the concentration of this isomer were similar to those produced by ingesting equivalent doses of preformed *cis*-9,*trans*-11 CLA. This suggests that there is no major advantage of consuming *trans*-vaccenic acid as a source of *cis*-9, *trans*-11 CLA.

8.4 CLA and blood lipids

Several of the human studies described in Section 8.2 also reported the effects of CLA on plasma lipid concentrations. As for the reported body-fat lowering effect of CLA in humans, the results appear to be inconsistent and less promising than expected (Table 8.2). The studies by Berven *et al.* (2000), Benito *et al.* (2001), Riserus *et al.* (2001), Smedman & Vessby (2001) and Petridou *et al.* (2003) did not show any significant effect of CLA (a mixture of the *cis*-9,*trans*-11 and *trans*-10,*cis*-12) on plasma total cholesterol, low-density lipoprotein (LDL) and high-density lipoprotein (HDL) cholesterol or TAG concentrations.

Although these studies showed that CLA may not affect lipoprotein metabolism in humans, other reports suggest a detrimental HDL-lowering effect of CLA mixtures (Blankson *et al.*, 2000; Mougios *et al.*, 2001; Riserus *et al.*, 2002b; Gaullier *et al.*, 2004). This lowering of HDL cholesterol concentration by CLA appears to be more apparent in obese subjects (Blankson *et al.*, 2000; Riserus *et al.*, 2002b; Gaullier *et al.*, 2004), raising some safety concerns about CLA supplementation. In the study by Gaullier *et al.* (2004), a decrease in HDL cholesterol concentration was observed when CLA was supplemented in the TAG form (Table 8.2) and was not considered by the authors to be of clinical importance. However, Moloney *et al.* (2004) supplemented overweight type 2

Table 8.2 Published studies investigating the effect of CLA on plasma lipids in humans

Amount of CLA (g/day)	Form of CLA	Placebo	Duration	Subjects	Effect of CLA	Reference
3.4	*Tonalin	Olive oil	12 weeks	60 overweight or obese males and females age: >18 years	No effect on total cholesterol, LDL, HDL or TAG	Berven *et al.* (2000)
1.7, 3.4, 5.1 and 6.8	50:50 *cis*-9,*trans*-11 and *trans*-10,*cis*-12	Olive oil	12 weeks	60 overweight or obese but healthy males and females	Decrease in total cholesterol, LDL, HDL or TAG	Blankson *et al.* (2000)
3.9	*Tonalin	Sunflower oil	9 weeks in a metabolic suite	17 healthy females age: 20–41 years	No effect on total cholesterol, LDL, HDL or TAG	Benito *et al.* (2001)
0.7 then 1.4	50:50 *cis*-9,*trans*-11 and *trans*-10,*cis*-12	Soybean oil	4 weeks then 4 weeks	14 healthy males and 10 healthy females age: 19–24 years	Decrease in HDL during low dose. Tendency towards decrease in total cholesterol and TAG	Mougios *et al.* (2001)
4.2	50:50 *cis*-9,*trans*-11 and *trans*-10,*cis*-12	Olive oil	4 weeks	24 abdominally obese males with signs of the metabolic syndrome age: 39–64 years	No effect on total cholesterol, LDL, HDL or TAG	Riserus *et al.* (2001)
4.2	50:50 *cis*-9,*trans*-11 and *trans*-10,*cis*-12	Olive oil	12 weeks	27 healthy males and 26 healthy females age: 23–63 years	No effect on total cholesterol, LDL, HDL, TAG or NEFA	Smedman & Vessby (2001)
3.0	50:50 *cis*-9,*trans*-11 and *trans*-10,*cis*-12 *vs* 80:20 *cis*-9,*trans*-11 and *trans*-10,*cis*-12	Linoleic acid-rich vegetable oil	8 weeks	18 healthy males and 33 healthy females age: 31.6 years (mean)	Decrease in TAG with the 50:50 isomer mix. Decrease in VLDL with the 80:20 isomer mix	Noone *et al.* (2002)

3.4	50:50 *cis*-9,*trans*-11 and *trans*-10,*cis*-12 CLA *vs* *trans*-10,*cis*-12	Olive oil	12 weeks	60 abdominally obese males with signs of the metabolic syndrome age: 35–65 years	Decrease in HDL with *trans*-10,*cis*-12 CLA Tendency to decreased HDL with the CLA mix	Riserus *et al.* (2002b)
2.1	50:50 *cis*-9,*trans*-11 and *trans*-10,*cis*-12	Soybean oil	45 days	16 healthy females age: 19–24 years	No effect on total cholesterol, HDL, total cholesterol/HDL or TAG	Petridou *et al.* (2003)
4.5	50:50 *cis*-9,*trans*-11 and *trans*-10,*cis*-12 as FFA or TAG	Olive oil	1 year	180 healthy overweight males and females age: 18–65 years	No effect on total cholesterol or TAG. Decrease in HDL with CLA as TAG. Increase in LDL with CLA as FFA	Gaullier *et al.* (2004)
3.0	*cis*-9,*trans*-11 CLA	Olive oil	12 weeks	25 abdominally obese males age: 35–65 years	No effect on total cholesterol, LDL, HDL, VLDL or TAG	Riserus *et al.* (2004b)
0.59, 1.19, 2.38 (*cis*-9, *trans*-11); 0.63, 1.26, 2.52 (*trans*-10, *cis*12)	*cis*-9,*trans*-11 *vs* *trans*-10,*cis*12	None (crossover design)	8 weeks on each dose (doses increased sequentially; 6 week wash-out between isomers)	49 healthy males age: 20–47 years	Increased cholesterol/HDL-C, LDL-/HDL-c and TAG with *trans*-10,*cis*-12 CLA relative to *cis*-9,*trans*-11 CLA	Tricon *et al.* (2004b)
3.0	50:50 *cis*-9,*trans*-11 and *trans*-10,*cis*-12	Palm oil + soybean oil	8 weeks	32 type 2 diabetics	No effect on plasma TAG. CLA decreased LDL, increased HDL and decreased LDL:HDL ratio compared with baseline	Moloney *et al.* (2004)

*Tonalin; 22.6% *trans*-10,*cis*-12, 23.6% *cis*-11,*trans*-13, 17.6% *cis*-9,*trans*-11, 16.6% *trans*-8,*cis*-10, 7.7% *trans*-9,*trans*-11 and *trans*-10,*trans*-12 and 11.9% other CLA isomers.

FFA, free fatty acid; HDL, high-density lipoprotein; LDL, low-density lipoprotein; NEFA, non-esterified fatty acid; TAG, triacylglycerol; VLDL, very low-density lipoprotein.

diabetics with a 50:50 mixture of *cis*-9,*trans*-11 and *trans*-10,*cis*-12 CLA and reported favourable effects on the LDL:HDL ratio. The CLA mixture slightly decreased plasma LDL and increased HDL such that the ratio of LDL:HDL was significantly lower than at baseline (but not compared with the control group). In the study by Riserus *et al.* (2002b), a randomized, double-blind controlled trial, in which abdominally obese men were given 3.4 g/day CLA (isomer mixture), purified *trans*-10,*cis*-12 CLA, or placebo for 12 weeks, it was demonstrated that the *trans*-10,*cis*-12 isomer, but not the CLA mixture, was responsible for a significant decrease in HDL cholesterol concentration (−4%; $P < 0.01$) coupled with a non-significant tendency to increased very low-density lipoprotein (VLDL) TAG concentrations.

This last study would suggest that the *trans*-10,*cis*-12 CLA is the isomer responsible for impairment of the blood lipid profile. This was confirmed in a study investigating the specific effects of the two main CLA isomers at different doses on blood lipids in a double-blind, randomized, crossover study in healthy normolipidaemic males (Tricon *et al.*, 2004a). Dietary supplementation with highly enriched *cis*-9,*trans*-11 and *trans*-10,*cis*-12 CLA (0.59, 1.19 or 2.38 g/day and 0.63, 1.26 or 2.52 g/day for 8 weeks) resulted in divergent effects of the two isomers on the blood lipid profile in healthy humans (Tricon *et al.*, 2004a).

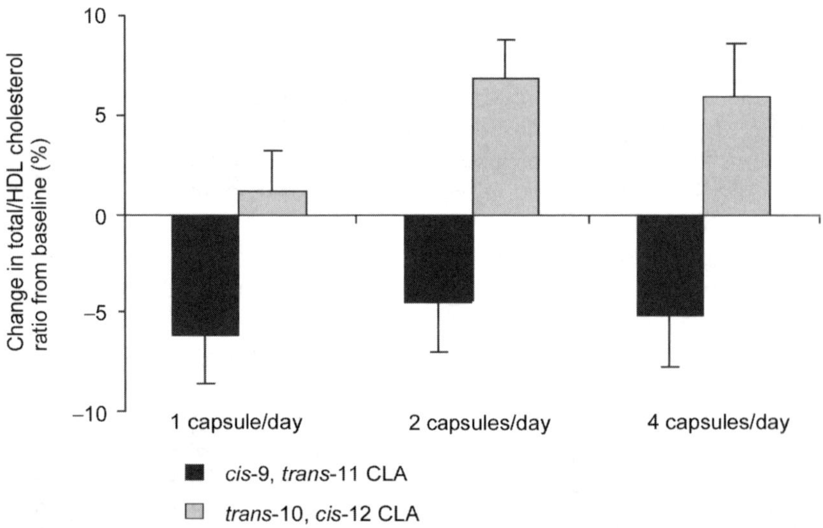

Fig. 8.4 Effects of *cis*-9,*trans*-11 CLA and *trans*-10,*cis*-12 CLA on percentage change in total-cholesterol/HDL-C ratio from baseline; 1 capsule/day, 0.59 g/day *cis*-9,*trans*-11 CLA or 0.63 g/day *trans*-10,*cis*-12 CLA; 2 capsules/day, 1.19 g/day *cis*-9,*trans*-11 CLA or 1.26 g/day *trans*-10,*cis*-12 CLA; 4 capsules/day, 2.38 g/day *cis*-9,*trans*-11 CLA or 2.52 g/day *trans*-10,*cis*-12 CLA. Reproduced with permission from the *American Journal of Clinical Nutrition*.

Mean plasma TAG concentration, the ratio of total to HDL-cholesterol (Fig. 8.4) and the ratio of LDL to HDL cholesterol were increased after supplementation with the *trans*-10,*cis*-12 CLA isomer (Tricon *et al.*, 2004a), demonstrating relative hyperlipidaemic properties of that isomer and hypolipidaemic properties of *cis*-9,*trans*-11 CLA. These results are in agreement with those of Riserus *et al.* (2002b), which suggest that the *trans*-10,*cis*-12 isomer may have some adverse effects on cardiovascular risk factors in obese and in healthy subjects. This is of concern because the *trans*-10,*cis*-12 CLA isomer is found in equal proportions with the *cis*-9,*trans*-11 CLA in weight-loss products, which are available in health food stores and over the Internet. However, the hypolipidaemic effects of the *cis*-9,*trans*-11 CLA observed by Tricon *et al.* (2004a) were not reported in the study by Riserus *et al.* (2004b) in abdominally obese men.

8.5 CLA and insulin sensitivity

Studies in animal models have reported antidiabetic effects of CLA (Houseknecht *et al.*, 1998; Ryder *et al.*, 2001; Evans *et al.*, 2002). Thus, on the basis of these reported findings it was speculated that CLA could potentially be useful for the treatment and prevention of type II diabetes and metabolic syndrome. However, of the studies published so far, most have reported no significant effect of CLA supplementation on fasting blood glucose or plasma insulin concentrations (Medina *et al.*, 2000; Smedman & Vessby, 2001; Noone *et al.*, 2002), although a few have reported detrimental effects (Riserus *et al.*, 2002b, 2004a; Moloney *et al.,* 2004). As a result, some researchers have raised concerns about the potential safety of CLA for humans in terms of insulin resistance (Riserus *et al.*, 2002b, 2004a; Moloney *et al.,* 2004; Larsen *et al.*, 2003).

Riserus *et al.* (2002b) conducted the only study to date that tested the effect of CLA using direct insulin sensitivity measurements. A group of 60 abdominally obese men with signs of the metabolic syndrome were randomly assigned to one of three supplements containing either 3.4 g/day of a CLA isomer mixture, the purified *trans*-10,*cis*-12 isomer, or a placebo for 12 weeks. The *trans*-10,*cis*-12 isomer significantly decreased insulin sensitivity (as determined by an intravenous glucose tolerance test) and increased fasting plasma glucose concentration compared with placebo. More recently, this group also conducted a randomized, double-blind, placebo-controlled study in 25 abdominally obese men who received 3 g/day of pure *cis*-9,*trans*-11 CLA or placebo (olive oil) for 3 months (Riserus *et al.*, 2004b). They observed that *cis*-9,*trans*-11 CLA also decreased insulin sensitivity by 15% ($P < 0.05$) compared with placebo (Riserus *et al.*, 2004b). However, it is perhaps surprising that both CLA isomers appear to decrease insulin sensitivity yet no effect is observed when a 50:50 CLA mix is supplemented (Riserus *et al.*, 2002b), particularly since Moloney *et al.* (2004) report a reduction in insulin sensitivity (calculated by surrogate measures) following supplementation with a 50:50 CLA mix in type 2 diabetics.

In another study (Fig. 8.1), Tricon *et al.* (2004a) suggested that the *trans*-10,*cis*-12 CLA increased fasting blood glucose concentration relative to the *cis*-9,*trans*-11 CLA isomer in healthy males. However, this was insufficient to modify the degree of insulin resistance or insulin sensitivity, calculated by the surrogate measures; the homeostasis model for insulin resistance (Matthews *et al.*, 1985) and the quantitative insulin-sensitivity check index (Katz *et al.*, 2000). In conclusion, it may be that the detrimental effect of the *trans*-10,*cis*-12 CLA isomer on insulin sensitivity observed by Riserus *et al.* (2002b) is only of significance in obese subjects with metabolic syndrome, but not in healthy subjects (Medina *et al.*, 2000; Smedman & Vessby, 2001; Noone *et al.*, 2002; Tricon *et al.*, 2004a). The issue of the effect of *cis*-9,*trans*-11 CLA, and of a 50:50 mixture of isomers, on insulin sensitivity remains unclear.

8.6 CLA, immune function and inflammation

8.6.1 CLA and immune function

There is very little information in relation to the effects of CLA on immune and inflammatory outcomes in human subjects. A placebo-controlled metabolic unit study was conducted in 17 healthy women supplemented with 3.9 g/day CLA (Tonalin capsules consisting of minor amounts of several different isomers, in which *trans*-10,*cis*-12 and *cis*-9,*trans*-11 CLA isomers represent ~20% each) for 9 weeks (Kelley *et al.*, 2000, 2001). None of the indices of immunity tested (number of circulating leukocytes, subsets within lymphocyte populations, T and B-cell proliferation, delayed hypersensitivity (DTH) skin response, and serum antibody titres after immunization with influenza vaccine) were affected by CLA supplementation (Kelley *et al.*, 2000). Fatty acid profiles of the peripheral blood mononuclear cells (PBMC) isolated demonstrated an eight-fold increase in CLA as a proportion of total fatty acids (0.12% total CLA to 0.97%); the largest increase was in the *cis*-11,*trans*-13 CLA isomer. CLA did not affect the production of eicosanoids (prostaglandin E_2 and leukotriene B_4) or cytokines (tumour necrosis factor [TNF]-α, interferon [IFN]-γ, interleukin [IL]-2, IL-1) by PBMCs after mitogen stimulation (Kelley *et al.*, 2001). There were also no changes in markers of immunity in experienced resistance-trained males receiving 6 g/day CLA (as Tonalin capsules) for 28 days versus placebo (olive oil) (Kreider *et al.*, 2002).

In contrast, the recently published results of a double-blinded intervention trial suggested that the individual isomers of CLA could have different effects on components of the immune system in humans. In that study, a 50:50 mixture of *cis*-9,*trans*-11 and *trans*-10,*cis*-12 CLA, at a dose of 1.7 g/day CLA resulted in a greater proportion of individuals producing a protective antibody titre (>10 IU/l) to hepatitis B vaccination, although the mean antibody titres did not differ between groups (Albers *et al.*, 2003). That study was the first in which CLA was shown to promote the humoral immune response in humans, as reflected by an increased seroprotection rate after vaccination. However, Kelley

& Erickson (2003) question the interpretation resulting from the use of arbitrary thresholds for seroprotective titres. Furthermore, in those healthy subjects, none of the other aspects of immune function measured (DTH response, natural killer cell activity, lymphocyte proliferation, and production of TNFα, IL-1β, IL-6, IFN-γ, IL-2, IL-4 and prostaglandin E_2) was affected (Albers *et al.*, 2003).

In a separate study of the two isomeric mixtures of CLA (50:50 and 80:20 of *cis*-9,*trans*-11 and *trans*-10,*cis*-12 CLA, respectively), the 80:20 mixture (3 g/day for 8 weeks) significantly enhanced peripheral blood lymphocyte proliferation in response to the T-cell mitogen phytohaemagglutinin, whereas treatment with the 50:50 mixture significantly decreased concanavalin (Con A)-induced proliferation (Roche *et al.*, 2001). This would suggest that the supplement providing more of the *cis*-9,*trans*-11 CLA isomer promoted the cell-mediated immune response, whereas the supplement which had a greater amount of the *trans*-10,*cis*-12 CLA isomer attenuated the immune response (Roche *et al.*, 2001).

A recent study described for the first time the effect of consuming increasing amounts of highly enriched preparations of *cis*-9,*trans*-11 and *trans*-10,*cis*-12 CLA on their incorporation into PBMCs (Burdge *et al.*, 2004) and on immune function (Tricon *et al.*, 2004b). Both *cis*-9,*trans*-11 and *trans*-10,*cis*-12 CLA isomers were incorporated in a dose-dependent manner into PBMC total lipids ($\Gamma = 0.285$ and $\Gamma = 0.273$, respectively; $P < 0.0005$) when consumed in the diet (Burdge *et al.*, 2004). There was no evidence for differential incorporation of these isomers into PBMCs, although the final concentration of each isomer was significantly lower than in plasma phosphatidylcholine and CE fractions at each dose (Burdge *et al.*, 2004). In terms of immune function, there were no effects of either isomer of CLA on PBMC subsets and on *ex vivo* cytokine production (Tricon *et al.*, 2004b). However, this study demonstrated for the first time a dose-dependent reduction in the activation of T lymphocytes, measured by cell surface expression of the early activation marker CD69, by both *cis*-9,*trans*-11 and *trans*-10,*cis*-12 CLA, which was inversely correlated with the proportions of both isomers in PBMC lipids (Tricon *et al.*, 2004b). However, since the function of CD69 has not been fully characterized, the implications and relevance of the effects of CLA on lymphocyte activation are not clear. Interestingly, CLA did not exhibit isomer-specific effects with respect to lymphocyte activation. This is in contrast to the differential effects of the two CLA isomers on blood lipids reported for the same subjects (Tricon *et al.*, 2004a).

To conclude from the few human studies published so far, CLA does not seem to be a strong modulator of immune function in humans. However, further studies are warranted looking at a larger number of measurements of immune function involved in both the adaptive and innate responses. Furthermore, until definitive molecular evidence on the mechanism(s) of action of CLA is available, it will be difficult to use CLA in possible preventive and therapeutic applications.

8.6.2 CLA and inflammation

C-reactive protein (CRP) is a marker of chronic subclinical inflammation, providing a sensitive indicator of underlying inflammation in the body, and levels are reported to be raised dramatically (up to 100-fold) in infection and inflammation (Tracy, 1998). Several large epidemiological studies have reported that a high serum level of CRP is a strong independent predictor of future myocardial infarction and stroke in individuals without known cardiovascular disease (Yudkin *et al.*, 1999; Ridker, 2001). Concern about CLA-induced elevations in serum CRP levels has arisen from a study by Riserus *et al.* (2002a), who investigated the effects of CLA in obese men with signs of the metabolic syndrome. They reported that a supplement highly enriched in *trans*-10,*cis*-12 CLA (3.4 g/day for 3 months) markedly increased CRP (+110%) compared with placebo (olive oil). CRP is an acute phase protein, synthesized and released from the liver, under the influence of IL-6.

Interestingly, the apparent *trans*-10,*cis*-12-CLA-induced serum CRP elevation was not accompanied by an increase in IL-6 levels (Riserus *et al.*, 2002a). In the study by Tricon *et al.* (2004a), there were no significant effects of either CLA isomer on serum CRP concentration. Moloney *et al.* (2004) demonstrated no effect of a 50:50 CLA mixture on serum CRP or IL-6 concentrations in overweight type 2 diabetics, but CLA did appear to lower plasma fibrinogen levels. Thus, the effects of CLA on inflammatory markers are inconsistent and the differences between studies cannot be explained by body weight or by the presence of metabolic syndrome.

8.7 CLA and breast cancer

There is compelling and consistent evidence from animal studies that CLA protects against the development of chemically induced mammary tumours (Ip *et al.*, 1991, 1995, 1999; Corl *et al.*, 2003; Thompson *et al.*, 1997). However, the minimum dose at which this effect is observed is approximately 0.1% (by weight) of the diet and a dose–response is observed between 0.1% and 1%. A dose of 0.1% CLA in animal studies equates to approximately 3–4 g/day in humans, which is clearly far greater than estimates of current consumption of this fatty acid. Nevertheless, there has been considerable interest in the potential anti-carcinogenic effects of CLA in humans, particularly with respect to breast cancer, which is the most commonly diagnosed cancer in women (Parkin, 2001). On the basis of epidemiological studies, established determinants of breast cancer include age, family history of breast cancer, body weight, change in weight over time, number and timing of reproductive events and lactation, exogenous and endogenous hormone concentrations, history of benign breast disease, exposure to radiation and alcohol consumption (Brekelmans, 2003). Striking geographical differences in breast cancer incidence have been suggested to be at least partly attributable to differences in exposure to lifestyle or environmental influences, including diet. Since dairy products are the major dietary source of CLA, the epidemiological literature on dairy product consumption and risk of breast cancer is relevant. However, the published epidemiological data do not provide consistent evidence for an association between consumption of dairy products and breast cancer risk (Moorman and Terry, 2004).

There are many explanations for this lack of association. First, dairy products are a diverse food group in terms of factors that could potentially influence cancer risk. For example, dairy products tend to have a relatively high saturated fat content, which may increase risk for breast cancer, but they are also rich in calcium and vitamin D, which may reduce breast cancer risk. Second, the assessment of dietary factors in relation to cancer risk is notoriously difficult and subject to may potential biases. Third, there may be confounding factors associated with high dairy intake; for example, individuals with a high consumption of butter, cheese or other high fat dairy products may be more likely to consume larger amounts of meat, which itself carries a higher risk for cancer.

Several studies have specifically addressed the hypothesis that dairy products affect breast cancer risk because they are sources of CLA (Aro *et al.,* 2000; Voorrips *et al.,* 2002; Chajes *et al*., 2002). A case-control study reported lower dietary intakes of CLA and lower serum CLA levels in breast cancer cases compared with controls, after adjustment for established breast cancer risk factors (Aro *et al*., 2000). However, this was not supported by two later studies (Voorrips *et al.,* 2002; Chajes *et al.,* 2002). Voorrips *et al.* (2002) reported a weak positive association between CLA intake and breast cancer incidence, which was not statistically significant. Furthermore, Chajes *et al.* (2002) reported that CLA concentrations in breast adipose tissue of breast cancer patients were not significantly higher than those in breast adipose tissue from women with benign breast conditions. Thus, human studies do not support the hypothesis that CLA is a protective factor in breast cancer. There is currently no data on CLA and other forms of cancer in humans.

8.8 Implications for food processors

A significant market for CLA supplements has developed in recent years. These supplements mainly consist of a 50:50 mixture of the *cis*-9,*trans*-11 and *trans*-10,*cis*-12 CLA isomers and are claimed to aid the loss of body fat. However, the evidence from studies in humans suggests that CLA supplementation (either as a mixture of isomers or as highly pure preparations) does not decrease body weight or body fat (Larsen *et al.,* 2003, Wahle *et al.,* 2004; Tricon *et al.,* 2005). Furthermore, there is accumulating evidence that the *trans*-10,*cis*-12 CLA isomer may adversely influence human health, in particular insulin sensitivity and blood lipids (Larsen *et al.,* 2003, Wahle *et al.,* 2004; Tricon *et al.,* 2005).

Despite the inconsistent data from CLA supplement studies, there has been increasing interest in the potential for naturally increasing the *cis*-9,*trans*-11

CLA content of milk and dairy products. Concentrations of CLA are higher in milk fat from cows offered fresh compared with conserved forages, and can also be enhanced using whole oilseeds or oil supplements (Lock and Bauman, 2004). Fish oil is more effective than plant oils for enhancing milk fat CLA content (Offer *et al.*, 1999; Chouinard *et al.*, 2001), and these responses can be further increased when fish oil is fed in combination with supplements rich in linoleic acid (Abu-Ghazaleh *et al.*, 2002, 2003). Several studies have indicated no adverse effects of CLA enrichment on the acceptability of milk (Baer *et al.*, 2001; Ramaswamy *et al.*, 2001; Avramis *et al.*, 2003; Jones *et al.*, 2005). However, nutritional strategies for the natural enhancement of the CLA content of milk also result in milk fat containing substantially increased *trans* C18:1 levels, particularly *trans*-11 18:1 (*trans* vaccenic acid; TVA), lowered saturated fatty acid concentrations, and a slightly higher *n*-3 polyunsaturated fatty acid content (Jones *et al.,* 2005). The increased levels of *trans* fatty acids could potentially have a detrimental influence on human health since increased intakes of the *trans* fatty acid elaidic acid (*trans*-9 18:1) are associated with greater risk of cardiovascular disease (Zock and Katan, 1992). On the other hand, the reduced saturated fatty acid content could act in concert with *cis*-9,*trans*-11 CLA in reducing the ratio of LDL to HDL cholesterol and of total to HDL cholesterol. There is clearly a need to determine the impact on human health of modified dairy products with this type of fatty acid profile and to determine whether the presence of TVA is indeed of concern. If the presence of TVA in CLA-enriched dairy products is demonstrated to have a detrimental effect on human health, alternative strategies would need to be devised to enrich milk with CLA without the associated increase in *trans* fatty acids. However, this would probably require feeding cattle with protected oils rich in CLA and the cost of this approach would be very high. The feeding of fish oils and seed oils to enrich milk with CLA are themselves expensive and may be unfeasible at a commercial level.

The study by Tricon *et al.* (2004a) would suggest that an intake of approximately 1.5 g/day *cis*-9,*trans*-11 CLA would be required for beneficial effects on blood lipids to occur (disregarding any potential effects of *trans* fatty acids). If this level of CLA intake were to be achieved without dramatically increasing the consumption of dairy products, a very high level of CLA enrichment of milk would be required (~5% of total fatty acids, representing a 10-fold increase in CLA). This level of enrichment may only be achieved transiently and may have a negative impact on the health of the dairy cow. Lower levels of enrichment of cow's milk with CLA (~3.5-fold) following feeding of fish meal and extruded soybean have, on the other hand, been shown to be maintained for an extended period of time, but it is unclear whether consumption at these levels would have any biological effects (Abu-Ghazaleh *et al.,* 2004). It is notable that the only study published to date which examines the effects of CLA-enriched dairy products on human body composition employed milk-based drinks to which synthetic CLA isomers were added post-production (Malpuech-Brugere *et al.*, 2004).

8.9 Future trends

More controlled studies in specific populations with purified isomers of CLA are needed and should be used to define the beneficial and detrimental effects of each individual CLA isomer in humans. The development of dairy products naturally enriched with CLA should be considered with caution, given the associated increase in *trans* fatty acids, which may counteract any beneficial effects to health. Therefore, strategies to enrich milk with *cis*-9,*trans*-11 CLA without the accompanying increase in TVA are likely to be important for the future development of CLA-enriched dairy products.

8.10 References

ABU-GHAZALEH AA, SCHINGOETHE DJ, HIPPEN AR & WHITLOCK LA (2002), Feeding fish meal and extruded soybeans enhances the conjugated linoleic acid (CLA) content of milk. *J. Dairy Sci.* **85**, 624–631.

ABU-GHAZALEH AA, SCHINGOETHE DJ, HIPPEN AR & KALSCHEUR KF (2003), Milk conjugated linoleic acid response to fish oil supplementation of diets differing in fatty acid profiles. *J. Dairy Sci.* **86**, 944–953.

ABU-GHAZALEH AA, SCHINGOETHE DJ, HIPPEN AR & KALSCHEUR KF (2004), Conjugated linoleic acid increases in milk when cows fed fish meal and extruded soybeans for an extended period of time. *J. Dairy Sci.* **87**, 1758–1766.

ALBERS R, VAN DER WIELEN RP, BRINK EJ, HENDRIKS HF, DOROVSKA-TARAN VN & MOHEDE IC (2003), Effects of *cis*-9,*trans*-11 and *trans*-10,*cis*-12 conjugated linoleic acid (CLA) isomers on immune function in healthy men. *Eur. J. Clin. Nutr.* **57**, 595–603.

ARO A, MANNISTO S, SALMINEN I, OVASKAINEN M-L, KATAJA V & UUSITUPA M (2000), Inverse association between dietary and serum conjugated linoleic acid and risk of breast cancer in postmenopausal women. *Nutr. Cancer* 38, 151–157.

AVRAMIS CA, WANG H, McBRIDE BW, WRIGHT TC & HILL AR (2003), Physical and processing properties of milk, butter and cheddar cheese from cows fed supplemental fish meal. *J. Dairy Sci.* **86**, 2568–2576.

AZAIN MJ, HAUSMAN DB, SISK MB, FLATT WP & JEWELL DE (2000), Dietary conjugated linoleic acid reduces rat adipose tissue cell size rather than cell number. *J. Nutr.* **130**, 1548–1554.

BAER RJ, RYALI J, SCHINGOETHE DJ, KASPERSON KM, DONOVAN DC, HIPPEN AR & FRANKLIN ST (2001), Composition and properties of milk and butter from cows fed fish oil. *J. Dairy Sci.* **84**, 345–352.

BASSAGANYA-RIERA J, HONTECILLAS R, ZIMMERMAN DR & WANNEMUEHLER MJ (2001), Dietary conjugated linoleic acid modulates phenotype and effector functions of porcine $CD8^+$ lymphocytes. *J. Nutr.* **131**, 2370–2377.

BASSAGANYA-RIERA J, HONTECILLAS R, ZIMMERMAN DR & WANNEMUEHLER MJ (2002), Long-term influence of lipid nutrition on the induction of $CD8^+$ responses to viral or bacterial antigens. *Vaccine* **20**, 1435–1444.

BELURY MA (2002), Inhibition of carcinogenesis by conjugated linoleic acid: potential mechanisms of action. *J. Nutr.* **132**, 2995–2998.

BELURY MA, MAHON A & BANNI S (2003), The conjugated linoleic acid (CLA) isomer, t10c12-CLA, is inversely associated with changes in body weight and serum leptin in subjects with type 2 diabetes mellitus. *J. Nutr.* **133**, 257S–260S.

BENITO P, NELSON GJ, KELLEY DS, BARTOLINI G, SCHMIDT PC & SIMON V (2001), The effect of conjugated linoleic acid on plasma lipoproteins and tissue fatty acid composition in humans. *Lipids* **36**, 229–236.

BERVEN G, BYE A, HALS O, BLANKSON H, FAGERTUN H, THOM E, WADSTEIN J & GUDMUNDSEN O (2000), Safety of conjugated linoleic acid (CLA) in overweight or obese human volunteers. *Eur. J. Lipid Sci. Technol.* **102**, 455–462.

BLANKSON H, STAKKESTAD JA, FAGERTUN H, THOM E, WADSTEIN J & GUDMUNDSEN O (2000), Conjugated linoleic acid reduces body fat mass in overweight and obese humans. *J. Nutr.* **130**, 2943–2948.

BREKELMANS CT (2003), Risk factors and risk reduction of breast and ovarian cancer. *Curr. Opin. Obstet. Gynecol.* **15**, 63–68.

BURDGE GC, LUPOLI B, RUSSELL JJ, TRICON S, KEW S, BANERJEE T, SHINGFIELD KJ, BEEVER DE, GRIMBLE RF, WILLIAMS CM, YAQOOB P & CALDER PC (2004), Incorporation of *cis*-9,*trans*-11 or *trans*-10,*cis*-12 conjugated linoleic acid into plasma and cellular lipids in healthy men. *J. Lipid Res.* **45**, 736–741.

BURDGE GC, DERRICK, PR, RUSSELL JJ, TRICON S, KEW S, BANERJEE T, GRIMBLE RF, WILLIAMS CM, YAQOOB P & CALDER PC (2005), Incorporation of *cis*-9, *trans*-11 or *trans*-10, *cis*-12 conjugated linoleic acid into human erythrocytes *in vivo. Nutr. Res.* **25**, 13–19.

CALDER PC (2002), Conjugated linoleic acid in humans – reasons to be cheerful? *Curr. Opin. Clin. Nutr. Metab. Care* **5**, 123–126.

CHAJES V, LAVILLONNIERE F, FERRARI P, JOURDAN ML, PINAULT M & MAILLARD V (2002), Conjugated linoleic acid content in breast adipose tissue is not associated with the relative risk of breast cancer in a population of French patients. *Cancer Epidemiol. Biomarkers Prev.* **11**, 672–673.

CHEW BP, WONG TS, SHULTZ TD & MAGNUSON NS (1997), Effects of conjugated dienoic derivatives of linoleic acid and beta-carotene in modulating lymphocyte and macrophage function. *Anticancer Res.* **17**, 1099–1106.

CHOUINARD PY, CORNEAU L, BUTLER WR, CHILLIARD Y, DRACKLEY JK & BAUMAN DE (2001) Effect of dietary lipid source on conjugated linoleic acid concentrations in milk fat. *J. Dairy Sci.* **84**, 680–690.

COOK ME, MILLER CC, PARK Y & PARIZA M (1993), Immune modulation by altered nutrient metabolism – nutritional control of immune-induced growth depression. *Poultry Sci.* **72**, 1301–1305.

CORL BA, BARBANO DM, BAUMAN DE & IP C (2003), *cis*-9,*trans*-11 CLA derived endogenously from *trans*-11 18:1 reduces cancer risk in rats. *J. Nutr.* **133**, 2893–2900.

DE DECKERE EAM, VAN AMELSVOORT JMM, McNEILL GP & JONES P (1999), Effects of conjugated linoleic acid (CLA) isomers on lipid levels and peroxisome proliferation in the hamster. *Br. J. Nutr.* **82**, 309–317.

DeLANY JP & WEST DB (2000), Changes in body composition with conjugated linoleic acid. *J. Am. Coll. Nutr.* **19**, 487S–493S.

DeLANY JP, BLOHM F, TRUETT AA, SCIMECA J & WEST DB (1999), Conjugated linoleic acid rapidly reduces body fat content in mice without affecting energy intake. *Am. J. Physiol. Reg. Integ. Comp. Physiol.* **276**, R1172–R1179.

EMKEN EA, ADLOF RO, DUVAL S, NELSON G & BENITO P (2002), Effect of dietary conjugated linoleic acid (CLA) on metabolism of isotope-labeled oleic, linoleic, and CLA isomers in women. *Lipids* **37**, 741–750.

EVANS M, BROWN J & MCINTOSH M (2002), Isomer-specific effects of conjugated linoleic acid (CLA) on adiposity and lipid metabolism. *J. Nutr. Biochem.* **13**, 508.

FINNEGAN YE, MINIHANE AM, LEIGH-FIRBANK EC, KEW S, MEIJER GW, MUGGLI R, CALDER PC & WILLIAMS CM (2003), Plant- and marine-derived n-3 polyunsaturated fatty acids have differential effects on fasting and postprandial blood lipid concentrations and on the susceptibility of LDL to oxidative modification in moderately hyperlipidemic subjects. *Am. J. Clin. Nutr.* **77**, 783–795.

GAULLIER JM, HALSE J, HOYE K, KRISTIANSEN K, FAGERTUN H, VIK H & GUDMUNDSEN O (2004), Conjugated linoleic acid supplementation for 1 y reduces body fat mass in healthy overweight humans. *Am. J. Clin. Nutr.* **79**, 1118–1125.

GAVINO VC, GAVINO G, LEBLANC MJ & TUCHWEBER B (2000), An isomeric mixture of conjugated linoleic acids but not pure *cis*-9,*trans*-11-octadecadienoic acid affects body weight gain and plasma lipids in hamsters. *J. Nutr.* **130**, 27–29.

HAYEK MG, HAN SN, WU DY, WATKINS BA, MEYDANI M, DORSEY JL, SMITH DE & MEYDANI SN (1999), Dietary conjugated linoleic acid influences the immune response of young and old C57BL/6NCrlBR mice. *J. Nutr.* **129**, 32–38.

HOUSEKNECHT KL, VANDEN HEUVEL JP, MOYA-CAMARENA SY, PORTOCARRERO CP, PECK LW, NICKEL KP & BELURY MA (1998), Dietary conjugated linoleic acid normalizes impaired glucose tolerance in the Zucker diabetic fatty fa/fa rat. *Biochem. Biophys. Res. Commun.* **247**, 911–911.

IP C, CHIN SF, SCIMECA JA & PARIZA MW (1991), Mammary cancer prevention by conjugated dienoic derivative of linoleic acid. *Cancer Res.* **51**, 6118–6124.

IP C, SINGH M, THOMPSON HJ & SCIMECA JA (1994), Conjugated linoleic acid suppresses mammary carcinogenesis and proliferative activity of the mammary gland in the rat. *Cancer Res.* **54**, 1212–1215.

IP C, SCIMECA JA & THOMPSON H (1995), Effect of timing and duration of dietary conjugated linoleic acid on mammary cancer prevention. *Nutr. Cancer* **24**, 241–247.

IP C, BANNI S, ANGIONI E, CARTA G, MCGINLEY J, THOMPSON HJ, BARBANO D & BAUMAN D (1999), Conjugated linoleic acid-enriched butter fat alters mammary gland morphogenesis and reduces cancer risk in rats. *J. Nutr.* **129**, 2135–2142.

JONES EL, SHINGFIELD KS, KOHEN C, JONES AK, LUPOLI B, GRANDISON AS, BEEVER DE, WILLIAMS CM, CALDER PC & YAQOOB P (2005), Chemical, physical and sensory properties of dairy products enriched with conjugated linoleic acid. *J. Dairy Sci.* **88**, 2923–2937.

KAMPHUIS MM, LEJEUNE MP, SARIS WH & WESTERTERP-PLANTENGA MS (2003a), The effect of conjugated linoleic acid supplementation after weight loss on body weight regain, body composition, and resting metabolic rate in overweight subjects. *Int. J. Obesity Related Metab. Disorders* **27**, 840–847.

KAMPHUIS MMJW, LEJEUNE MPGM, SARIS WHM & WESTERTERP-PLANTENGA MS (2003b), Effect of conjugated linoleic acid supplementation after weight loss on appetite and food intake in overweight subjects. *Eur. J. Clin. Nutr.* **57**, 1268–1274.

KATZ A, NAMBI SS, MATHER K, BARON AD, FOLLMANN DA, SULLIVAN G & QUON MJ (2000), Quantitative insulin sensitivity check index: a simple, accurate method for assessing insulin sensitivity in humans. *J. Clin. Endocrinol. Metab.* **85**, 2402–2410.

KELLEY DS & ERICKSON KL (2003), Modulation of body composition and immune cell functions by conjugated linoleic acid in humans and animal models: benefits vs. risks. *Lipids* **38**, 377–386.

KELLEY DS, TAYLOR PC, RUDOLPH IL, BENITO P, NELSON GJ, MACKEY BE & ERICKSON KL (2000), Dietary conjugated linoleic acid did not alter immune status in young healthy women. *Lipids* **35**, 1065–1071.

KELLEY DS, SIMON VA, TAYLOR PC, RUDOLPH IL, BENITO P, NELSON GJ, MACKEY BE & ERICKSON KL (2001), Dietary supplementation with conjugated linoleic acid increased its concentration in human peripheral blood mononuclear cells, but did not alter their function. *Lipids* **36**, 669–674.

KELLEY DS, WARREN JM, SIMON VA, BARTOLINI G, MACKEY BE & ERICKSON KL (2002), Similar effects of *c*9,*t*11-CLA and *t*10,*c*12-CLA on immune cell functions in mice. *Lipids* **37**, 725–728.

KREIDER RB, FERREIRA MP, GREENWOOD M, WILSON M & ALMADA AL (2002), Effects of conjugated linoleic acid supplementation during resistance training on body composition, bone density, strength, and selected hematological markers. *J. Strength Conditioning Res.* **16**, 325–334.

LARSEN TM, TOUBRO S & ASTRUP A (2003), Efficacy and safety of dietary supplements containing CLA for the treatment of obesity: evidence from animal and human studies. *J. Lipid Res.* **44**, 2234–2241.

LAWSON RE, MOSS AR & GIVENS DI (2001), The role of dairy products in supplying conjugated linoleic acid to man's diet: a review. *Nutr. Res. Rev.* **14**, 153–172.

LEE KN, KRITCHVESKY D & PARIZA MW (1994), Conjugated linoleic acid and atherosclerosis in rabbits. *Atherosclerosis* **108**, 19–25.

LOCK AL & BAUMAN DE (2004), Modifying milk fat composition of dairy cows to enhance fatty acids beneficial to human health. *Lipids* **39**, 1197–1206.

MALPUECH-BRUGERE C, VERBOEKET-VAN DE VENNE WP, MENSINK RP, ARNAL MA, MORIO B, BRANDOLINI M, SAEBO A, LASSEL TS, CHARDIGNY JM, SEBEDIO JL & BEAUFRERE B (2004), Effects of two conjugated linoleic acid isomers on body fat mass in overweight humans. *Obesity Res.* **12**, 591–598.

MASTERS, N, McGUIRE, MA, BEERMAN, KA, DASGUPTA N & McGUIRE M (2002), Maternal supplementation with CLA decreases milk fat in humans. *Lipids* **37**, 133–138.

MATTHEWS DR, HOSKER JP, RUDENSKI AS, NAYLOR BA, TREACHER DF & TURNER RC (1985), Homeostasis model assessment: insulin resistance and beta-cell function from fasting plasma glucose and insulin concentrations in man. *Diabetologia* **28**, 412–419.

McGUIRE MK, McGUIRE MA, RITZENTHALER KL & SCHULTZ TD (1999), Dietary sources and intakes of conjugated linoleic acid intake in humans. In *Advances in Conjugated Linoleic Acid research*, pp. 369–377 [MP Yurawecz, MM Mossoba, JKG Kramer, P M.W. and G Nelson, eds], Champaign: AOCS Press.

MEDINA EA, HORN WF, KEIM NL, HAVEL PJ, BENITO P, KELLEY DS, NELSON GJ & ERICKSON KL (2000), Conjugated linoleic acid supplementation in humans: effects on circulating leptin concentrations and appetite. *Lipids* **35**, 783–788.

MILLER CC, PARK Y, PARIZA MW & COOK ME (1994), Feeding conjugated linoleic-acid to animals partially overcomes catabolic responses due to endotoxin injection. *Biochem. Biophys. Res. Commun.* **198**, 1107–1112.

MOLONEY F, YEOW T-P, MULLEN A, NOLAN JJ & ROCHE HM (2004), Conjugated linoleic acid supplementation, insulin sensitivity and lipoprotein metabolism in patients with type 2 diabetes mellitus. *Am. J. Clin. Nutr.* **80**, 887–895.

MOORMAN PG & TERRY PD (2004), Consumption of dairy products and the risk of breast cancer: a review of the literature. *Am. J. Clin. Nutr.* **80**, 5–14.

MOUGIOS V, MATSAKAS A, PETRIDOU A, RING S, SAGREDOS A, MELISSOPOULOU A, TSIGILIS N & NIKOLAIDIS M (2001), Effect of supplementation with conjugated linoleic acid on human serum lipids and body fat. *J. Nutr. Biochem.* **12**, 585–594.

NICOLOSI RJ, ROGERS EJ, KRITCHEVSKY D, SCIMECA JA & HUTH PJ (1997), Dietary conjugated linoleic acid reduces plasma lipoproteins and early aortic atherosclerosis in hypercholesterolemic hamsters. *Artery* **22**, 266–277.

NOONE EJ, ROCHE HM, NUGENT AP & GIBNEY MJ (2002), The effect of dietary supplementation using isomeric blends of conjugated linoleic acid on lipid metabolism in healthy human subjects. *Br. J. Nutr.* **88**, 243–251.

OFFER NW, MARSDEN M, DIXON J, SPEAKE BK & THACKER FE (1999), Effect of dietary fat supplements on levels of n-3 poly-unsaturated fatty acids, *trans* acids and conjugated linoleic acid in bovine milk. *Animal Sci.* **69**, 613–625.

PARIZA MW (2004), Perspective on the safety and effectiveness of conjugated linoleic acid. *Am. J. Clin. Nutr.* **79**, 1132S–1136S.

PARIZA MW, PARK Y & COOK ME (2000), Mechanisms of action of conjugated linoleic acid: evidence and speculation. *Proc. Soc. Exp. Biol. Med.* **223**, 8–13.

PARIZA MW, PARK Y & COOK ME (2001), The biologically active isomers of conjugated linoleic acid. *Prog. Lipid Res.* **40**, 283–298.

PARK Y, ALBRIGHT KJ, LIU W, STORKSON JM, COOK ME & PARIZA MW (1997), Effect of conjugated linoleic acid on body composition in mice. *Lipids* **32**, 853–858.

PARK Y, STORKSON JM, ALBRIGHT KJ, LIU W & PARIZA MW (1999), Evidence that the *trans*-10,*cis*-12 isomer of conjugated linoleic acid induces body composition changes in mice. *Lipids* **34**, 235–241.

PARKIN DM (2001), Global cancer statistics in the year (2000) *Lancet Oncol.* **49**, 33–64.

PETRIDOU A, MOUGIOS V & SAGREDOS A (2003), Supplementation with CLA: isomer incorporation into serum lipids and effect on body fat of women. *Lipids* **38**, 805–811.

RAMASWAMY N, BAER RJ, SCHINGOETHE DJ, HIPPEN AR, KASPERSON KM & WHITLOCK LA (2001), Consumer evaluation of milk high in conjugated linoleic acid. *J. Dairy Sci.* **84**, 1607–1609.

RIDKER PM (2001), High-sensitivity C-reactive protein: potential adjunct for global risk assessment in the primary prevention of cardiovascular disease. *Circulation* **103**, 1813–1818.

RISERUS U, BERGLUND L & VESSBY B (2001), Conjugated linoleic acid (CLA) reduced abdominal adipose tissue in obese middle-aged men with signs of the metabolic syndrome: a randomised controlled trial. *Int. J. Obesity* **25**, 1129–1135.

RISERUS U, BASU S, JOVINGE S, FREDRIKSON GN, ARNOLV J & VESSBY B (2002a), Supplementation with conjugated linoleic acid causes isomer-dependent oxidative stress and elevated C-reactive protein. *Circulation* **106**, 1925–1929.

RISERUS U, BRISMAR K, ARNER P & VESSBY B (2002b), Treatment with dietary *trans*-10 *cis*-12 conjugated linoleic acid causes isomer-specific insulin resistance in obese men with the metabolic syndrome. *Diabetes Care* **25**, 1516–1521.

RISERUS U, SMEDMAN A, BASU S & VESSBY B (2004a), Metabolic effects of conjugated linoleic acid in humans: the Swedish experience. *Am. J. Clin. Nutr.* **79**, 1146S–1148S.

RISERUS U, VESSBY B, ARNLOV J & BASU S (2004b), Effects of *cis*-9,*trans*-11 conjugated linoleic acid supplementation on insulin sensitivity, lipid peroxidation, and proinflammatory markers in obese men. *Am. J. Clin. Nutr.* **80**, 279–283.

ROCHE HM, NOONE E, NUGENT AP & GIBNEY MJ (2001), Conjugated linoleic acid: a novel therapeutic nutrient? *Nutr. Res. Rev.* **14**, 173–187.

RYDER JW, PORTOCARRERO CP, SONG XM, CUI L, YU M, COMBATSIARIS T, GALUSKA D, BAUMAN DE, BARBANO DM, CHARRON MJ, ZIERATH JR & HOUSEKNECHT KL (2001), Isomer-specific antidiabetic properties of conjugated linoleic acid. Improved glucose tolerance, skeletal muscle insulin action, and *UCP-2* gene expression. *Diabetes* **50**, 1149–1157.

SEBEDIO J-L, GNAEDIG S & CHARDIGNY J-M (1999), Recent advances in conjugated linoleic acid research. *Curr. Opin. Clin. Nutr. Metab. Care* **2**, 499–506.

SMEDMAN A & VESSBY B (2001), Conjugated linoleic acid supplementation in humans – metabolic effects. *Lipids* **36**, 773–781.

STANGL GI (2000), Conjugated linoleic acid exhibits a strong fat-to-lean partitioning effect, reduces serum VLDL lipids and redistribute tissue lipids in food-restricted rats. *J. Nutr.* **130**, 1140–1146.

SUGANO M, TSUJITA A, YAMASAKI M, NOGUCHI M & YAMADA K (1998), Conjugated linoleic acid modulates tissue levels of chemical mediators and immunoglobulins in rats. *Lipids* **33**, 521–527.

TERPSTRA AH (2004), Effect of conjugated linoleic acid on body composition and plasma lipids in humans: an overview of the literature. *Am. J. Clin. Nutr.* **79**, 352–361.

THOM E, WADSTEIN J & GUDMUNDSEN O (2001), Conjugated linoleic acid reduces body fat in healthy exercising humans. *J. Int. Med. Res.* **29**, 392–396.

THOMPSON HJ, ZHU Z, BANNI S, DARCY K, LOFTUS T & IP C (1997), Morphological and biochemical status of the mammary gland as influenced by conjugated linoleic acid: implication for a reduction in mammary cancer risk. *Cancer Res.* **57**, 5067–5072.

TRACY RP (1998), Inflammation in cardiovascular disease, cat, horse, or both? *Circulation* **97**, 2000–2002.

TRICON S, BURDGE GC, RUSSELL JJ, JONES EL, GRIMBLE RF, WILLIAMS CM, YAQOOB P & CALDER PC (2004a), Opposing effects of *cis*-9,*trans*-11 and *trans*-10,*cis*-12 CLA on blood lipids in healthy humans. *Am. J. Clin. Nutr.* **80**, 614–620.

TRICON S, BURDGE GC, KEW S, BANERJEE T, RUSSELL JJ, GRIMBLE RF, WILLIAMS CM, CALDER PC & YAQOOB P (2004b), Effects of *cis*-9,*trans*-11 and *trans*-10,*cis*-12 conjugated linoleic acid on immune cell function in healthy humans. *Am. J. Clin. Nutr.* **80**, 1626–1633.

TRICON S, BURDGE GC, WILLIAMS CM, CALDER PC & YAQOOB P (2005), The effects of conjugated linoleic acid on human health related outcomes. *Proc. Nutr. Soc.* **64**, 171–182.

TSUBOYAMA-KASAOKA N, TAKAHASHI M, TANEMURA K, KIM HJ, TANGE T, OKUYAMA H, KASAI M, IKEMOTO S & EZAKI O (2000), Conjugated linoleic acid supplementation reduces adipose tissue by apoptosis and develops lipodystrophy in mice. *Diabetes* **49**, 1534–1542.

TUREK JJ, LI Y, SCHOENLEIN IA, ALLEN KGD & WATKINS BA (1997), Conjugated linoleic acid alters cytokine but not PGE(2) production in rats. *FASEB J.* **11**, 3755.

TUREK JJ, LI Y, SCHOENLEIN IA, ALLEN KGD & WATKINS BA (1998), Modulation of macrophage cytokine production by conjugated linoleic acids is influenced by the dietary n-6 : n-3 fatty acid ratio. *J. Nutr. Biochem.* **9**, 258–266.

TURPEINEN, AM, MUTANEN, M, ARO, A, SALMINEN, I, BASU, S, PALMQUIST, DL & GRIINARI, JM (2002), Bioconversion of vaccenic acid to conjugated linoleic acid in humans. *Am. J. Clin. Nutr.* **76**, 504–510.

VON LOEFFELHOLZ C, KRATZSCH J & JAHREIS G (2003), Influence of conjugated linoleic acids on body composition and selected serum and endocrine parameters in resistance-trained athletes. *Eur. J. Lipid Sci. Technol.* **105**, 251–259.

VOORRIPS LE, BRANTS HAM, KARDINAAL AFM, HIDDINK GJ, VAN DEN BRANDT PA & GOLDBOHM

RA (2002), Intake of conjugated linoleic acid, fat, and other fatty acids in relation to postmenopausal breast cancer: the Netherlands Cohort Study on Diet and Cancer. *Am. J. Clin. Nutr.* **76**, 873–882.

WAHLE KWJ, HEYS SD & ROTONDO D (2004), Conjugated linoleic acids: are they beneficial or detrimental to health? *Prog. Lip. Res.* **43**, 553–587.

WEST DB, DELANY JP, CAMET PM, BLOHM F, TRUETT AA & SCIMECA J (1998), Effects of conjugated linoleic acid on body fat and energy metabolism in the mouse. *Am. J. Physiol. Reg. Integ. Comp. Physiol.* **275**, R667–R672.

YAMASAKI M, CHUJO H, HIRAO A, KOYANAGI N, OKAMOTO T, TOJO N, OISHI A, IWATA T, YAMAUCHI-SATO Y, YAMAMOTO T, TSUTSUMI K, TACHIBANA H & YAMADA K (2003), Immunoglobulin and cytokine production from spleen lymphocytes is modulated in C57BL/6J mice by dietary *cis*-9,*trans*-11 and *trans*-10,*cis*-12 conjugated linoleic acid. *J. Nutr.* **133**, 784–788.

YUDKIN JS, STEHOUWER CDA, EMEIS JJ & COPPAK SW (1999), C-reactive protein in healthy subjects: Associations with obesity, insulin resistance, and endothelial dysfunction. *Arterioscler. Thromb. Vasc. Biol.* **19**, 972–978.

ZAMBELL KL, KEIM NL, VAN LOAN MD, GALE B, BENITO P, KELLEY DS & NELSON GJ (2000), Conjugated linoleic acid supplementation in humans: effects on body composition and energy expenditure. *Lipids* **35**, 777–782.

ZAMBELL KL, HORN WF & KEIM NL (2001), Conjugated linoleic acid supplementation in humans: Effects on fatty acid and glycerol kinetics. *Lipids* **36**, 767–772.

ZOCK PL & KATAN MB (1992), Hydrogenation alternatives: effects of trans fatty acids and stearic acid versus linoleic acid on serum lipids and lipoproteins in humans. *J. Lipid Res.* **33**, 399–410.

Part II

Reducing saturated fatty acids in food

9

The role of lipids in food quality

Z. E. Sikorski, Gdańsk University of Technology, Poland and G. Sikorska-Wiśniewska, Medical Academy of Gdańsk, Poland

9.1 Introduction

9.1.1 The contents, characteristics and distribution of lipids in major foods

Almost all food raw materials and products contain some quantities of lipids. A few types of foods are devoid of lipids, e.g. saccharose, clarified fruit juices, and wines. However, even an apparent saccharide commodity such as starch contains minute amounts of fatty acids (FAs) in its structure. In various vegetables and in most fruits the proportion of lipids is very low, usually not exceeding 0.3% wet weight. Lean beef and lean pork cuts, shellfish, white poultry meat, cow's milk, and grain contain 2–4% of lipids. Foods that are very rich in fats (30–35%) include fatty pork, fillets of fatty fish, and egg yolk (Table 9.1). The effect of selective breeding and of feeding practices on the content of fat in the carcasses of monogastric animals and ruminants is presented by Moloney in Chapter 13. Soybeans contain about 40% lipids, some sausages about 50%, and walnuts as much as 65% fat.

The lipids of plant and animal food raw materials are either structural lipids, i.e. components of cell and organelle membranes, or depot fat. Among the animal structural lipids are phospholipids and non-esterified cholesterol. The lipids of plant cell membranes are mainly phospholipids and glycolipids. Energy in plants and animals is generally stored in triacylglycerols (TAGs). Many fish, especially deep-water organisms, store energy in the form of wax esters that serve also as buoyancy regulators. The oil of some deep water fish, e.g. orange roughy, and of sperm whale comprises about 90% waxes.

The distribution of lipids in food raw materials is related to their role in the living plants and animal organisms. In an animal body they are accumulated

Table 9.1 Proximate contents of fat in fresh and processed foods, g/100 g wet weight (sources: Kramlich *et al.* 1973, Lushbough and Schweigert 1960, Nettleton 1985, Sikorski *et al.* 1990)

Food	Fat, percentage wet weight	Food	Fat, percentage wet weight
Meat and meat products		**Seafood, muscle, fresh**	
Beef		Cod	0.5
Chuck, medium[1]	16	Halibut	1.5
Loin, medium[1]	25	Herring, Atlantic	16
Loin, fat[1]	31	Redfish	5
Round, medium[1]	13	Saithe	0.7
Kidney[1]	8	Salmon, pink	5.5
Liver[1]	3	Sole	2
Tongue[1]	15	Spiny dogfish	5
Rib steak, lean portion[2]	5	Sturgeon, Russian	13
Tenderloin steak, lean[2]	9	Tuna, bluefin	4
		Walley pollock	1.5
Pork		Abalone	0.5
Ham, medium[1]	31	Clam	1.5
Loin, medium[1]	25	Crab	1
Shoulder butt, medium[1]	42	Lobster	1.3
Bacon, lean + marble + fat[2]	60	Oyster	1.5
Tenderloin, entire cut[2]	12	Scallop	0.7
Lamb		**Seafood products**	
Leg, medium[1]	18	Sockeye salmon, broiled	7.2
Rib, medium[1]	32	Sockeye salmon, canned	6.3
Shoulder, medium[1]	25	Shrimp, boiled	1.2
		Kippered herring	13
Sausages		Sild sardines, canned in oil	29
Bockwurst	24		
Bologna	23	**Milk and dairy products**	
Cervelat	38	Cow's milk, whole	3.9
Frankfurters	27	Goat's milk, whole	4.5
Liverwurst, smoked	27	Sheep's milk, whole	7.2
Mortadella	25	Cheeseburger	16
Salami, dry	38		

[1] raw, [2] cooked

primarily in the subcutaneous adipose tissue, furthermore as kidney, leaf, and groin fat, and as the intramuscular fat known as marbling, i.e. interspersing of fat within the lean tissue. The intramuscular fat is deposited in the loose networks of the perimysial connective tissue septa. Fat deposits are also located within the septa between individual muscles. They are known as intermuscular or seam fat. The adipose tissue serves as a structural, insulating, and contour-building material and as an energy-rich store of neutral fat. It consists of connective tissue with the cells almost entirely filled with fat. In a lean fish the concentration of lipids in the muscles is only about 0.7%, but the liver may contain up to 70% of oil. In fatty fish there is much fat both in the subcutaneous layer and in the muscles. In capelin about 40% and 25% of the total amount of fat are located in the lining of body cavity and in the skin, respectively, while in mackerel the skin and light muscle contain most of the fat, each about 35% of the total content (Mohr 1979).

In milk and many dairy products, mayonnaise, and comminuted meat and fish products the fat is dispersed in the form of globules. In fresh milk the globules are 0.5-10 μm in diameter. They are separated from each other in the aqueous medium by about 10 nm thick phospholipid–proteinaceous membranes that are covered by adsorbed lipoprotein particles. In fresh cheese the globules are surrounded by a protein shell and located in a protein network. In butter they are distributed in a matrix of free fat. The core of liquid fat of these globules is surrounded by fat crystals. In mayonnaise oil droplets are closely packed and form a honeycomb structure. In oilseeds the lipids are present in the form of lipid bodies, known also as spherosomes, 0.2-0.5 μm in diameter, which are embedded in a cytoplasmic protein network.

The content of fat in various food products depends on the recipe of the commodity. Contemporary formulae of processed foods are prepared such that both the sensory and nutritional properties of the produce are taken into consideration. In several cases the fat content is controlled within limits set by regulatory agencies. A typical example may be butter. According to EC regulations the minimum contents of milk fat in sweet cream salted, sweet cream unsalted, lactic unsalted, and concentrated butter are 80%, 82%, 82%, and 99.8%, respectively.

9.1.2 Stability of lipids in foods

Some lipids belong to the most labile components, liable to alterations under conditions of storage and processing of foods. The changes can be desirable or can lead to adverse effects on the quality of various commodities. Owing to the activity of endogenous, microbial, or purposely added enzymes, and as a result of chemical reactions, the lipids undergo hydrolysis and oxidation. While hydrolysis in foods is caused predominantly by enzymes, oxidative reactions may be enzymatic or chemical in nature. The sensitivity to changes depends on the accessibility of the lipid to enzyme attack and on the interactions with other food components. The interactions are restricted by the compartmentation of the structure of the food raw materials. Thus the rate of changes increases owing to disruption of the tissues, mincing, and mixing. The kinetics of the enzymatic and chemical interactions depends also on the pH of the food and on temperature. Generally the rate of lipid changes increases with temperature. Chemical reactions in fats during deep-frying have been recently described by Boskou (2003). Extensive accumulation of lipid degradation products may occur in many foods even at freezing temperatures, if the storage time extends over several months.

The chemical character of the lipids also has an effect on their stability. The susceptibility of various lipids to hydrolysis differs owing to the specificity of lipases and phospholipases towards the positional isomers of the acylglycerols. The rate of oxidative reactions depends primarily on the number and distribution of double bonds in the hydrocarbon chain – generally it increases with the increase in the degree of unsaturation of the FAs.

9.1.3 The impact of lipids on food quality

Lipids are important for the properties of foods by:

- contributing to the structure of various tissues and organelles;
- supplying substrates for synthesis of metabolites that are indispensable for the human organism;
- serving as the richest dietary source of energy;
- interacting with other components in creating the desirable, rheological properties of food commodities;
- yielding, as a result of enzymatic and chemical reactions, different products that affect the colour, flavour, texture, nutritive value, and safety of foods;
- carrying fat-soluble vitamins and other beneficial lipophilic compounds, e.g. β-carotene, as well as hydrophobic contaminants.

In this chapter the effect of lipids and their interactions on various attributes of sensory quality of some representative foods are presented, as well as concise information on the role of lipids in infant nutrition.

9.2 The contribution of lipids to the colour of foods

9.2.1 Lipid changes which influence the colour of red meats

The colour of meat of slaughter animals is affected by the contents and predominantly by the chemical state of haemoproteins – myoglobin (MbFe(II)) and to a lesser degree haemoglobin and the cytochromes (see also Section 13.6). The natural, cherry-red colour of beef meat on the fresh cut surface is due to the reduced forms of the muscle haemoproteins (Fig. 9.1). Oxygenation of the Fe(II)-containing pigments at high partial pressure of oxygen leads to formation of oxymyoglobin ($MbFe(II)O_2$) of light-red coloration. In beef meat the initial purplish-red colour turns to bright-red in about 30 min after exposing the cut surface to air. Oxidation results in a change of the colour to the undesirable brown. In beef muscle the brownish discoloration is perceptible when about 60% of the total amount of meat pigments is oxidized to metmyoglobin. In order to stabilize the desirable light-red colour of fresh meat it is necessary to avoid oxidation by using appropriate packaging of the cuts or by adding various antioxidants.

There is an interrelation between the undesirable changes in colour and the lipid oxidation in meat. Oxidation of $MbFe(II)O_2$ may be the first step in a chain of events leading to oxidative changes in lipids, and vice versa, oxidized muscle

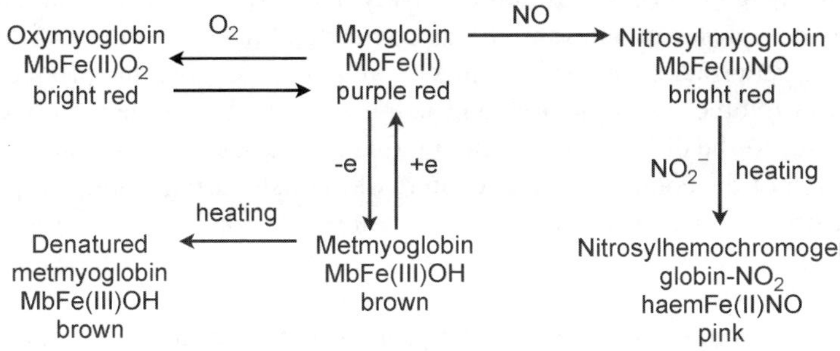

Fig. 9.1 The main changes in meat pigments.

lipids and liposomes can catalyse the browning of meat haemoproteins (Monahan 2000). Among the secondary lipid oxidation products found in meat are various aldehydes of different molecular weight and degree of unsaturation. The species present in highest concentrations are usually malonaldehyde, 4-hydroxy-2-nonenal, and hexanal. Many unsaturated aldehydes react readily with proteins. α, β-Unsaturated aldehydes may lead to colour changes by covalently binding to $MbFe(II)O_2$ and thus by changing the conformation of the molecule, that results in exposure of the haeme iron to oxidation (Faustman and Wang 2000).

Various carotenoids are able to decrease the rate of oxidation of $MbFe(II)O_2$ and to reduce oxidized forms of myoglobin, thus increasing the colour stability of meat (Mortensen and Skibsted 2000). Also α-tocopherol, although it is lipid soluble, is known to stabilize $MbFe(II)0_2$ in beef. It acts most probably by retarding the generation of primary lipid peroxides and the release of their water-soluble, pro-oxidative, free-radical breakdown products, predominantly unsaturated aldehydes or HO• radicals (Faustman and Wang 2000). Dietary supplementation of livestock with vitamin E is effective in delaying lipid oxidation and discoloration of fresh beef. The administration of antioxidants to the livestock in order to improve the colour stability of meat has been also treated by Moloney in Chapter 13.

The caselife of a beef cut, i.e. the time over which the meat retains the desirable bright-red colour and can be exhibited in retail display, prior to its being discounted in price, may reach from 1 to about 5 days. It depends on the reducing capacity of the muscles. The economic implications of undesirable colour changes in beef and the effectiveness of the applied counter-measures have been discussed by Smith *et al.* (2000).

9.2.2 Lipids and the colour of fish and crustaceans

The yellow, orange, red, purple, blue, silver, or green colours of the skin of many fish and of the shell of marine crustaceans, as well as the pink pigmentation of the flesh of salmonid fish, are an important quality asset of seafood. The vivid colours are a sign of prime freshness of many marine products. They are mainly caused by complexes of astaxanthin and canthaxanthin or their derivatives with proteins, glycoproteins, phosphorylated glycoproteins, glycolipoproteins, and lipoproteins. Numerous structures and colours of carotenoproteins are known. They are due to the diversity of the interacting molecules (Zagalsky *et al.* 1990). Dissociation of the complexes after capture of the fish during storage, especially in direct, bright light, causes fading of the colours. Oxidation of these pigments, especially in the presence of oxidized lipids results in loss in the appealing sight of the skin and flesh.

The reactions of oxidized lipids with proteins generate various compounds of similar colour as in Maillard or enzymic browning. Lipid peroxy radicals and lipid hydroperoxides or their decomposition products interact with amino acids, forming yellow to brown products. The browning rate is particularly high in reactions with cysteine, methionine, and tryptophan. Similar interactions occur between oxidizing lipids and proteins. The colour intensity increases with the increasing degree of unsaturation of the lipids. Therefore it is very intensive in fatty fish, rich in polyenoic fatty acids (PUFAs). The browning discoloration is objectionable especially in white fish muscle, where brown spots may occur even under refrigerated or frozen storage.

Most foods contain traces of heavy metals, especially Fe(II) or Fe (III) that are distributed between the lipid and aqueous phases. The ions present in the lipid phase are mainly bound to FA into complex salts or to phospholipids. This makes the lipid phase look orange brown. The ions remaining in the aqueous phase may react with different phenols, forming coloured complexes. The complexes of Fe(II) with pyrocatechol or pyrogallol derivatives are blue or violet, while those with Fe(III) are orange or brown.

9.2.3 Lipids as the carriers of food pigments

Natural fats and oils contain various lipochromes – lipid-soluble pigments that are responsible for the colour of the commodities. The content of the lipochromes in the natural oils depends on the species and degree of ripening of the oil-bearing plants. Most lipochromes are effectively removed during refining of oils.

Some natural oils are yellow or red owing to the presence of different carotenoids. The contents of these pigments in vegetable oils is usually about 50 μg/g, but in palm oil it is as high as 3 mg/g. Carotenes are present also in the flesh oil of redfish (*Sebastes marinus*). Carotenoid pigments impart the colour to many vegetables and fruits. In red pepper (*Capsicum annuum*, L.) the main red pigments are capsanthin and capsorubin. Capsanthin, which occurs in the free form and as monoesters and diesters of FAs, makes up about 50% of the total carotenoids in this vegetable. The oil-soluble extract is known as paprika oleoresin E-160 (c). The pericarp of the seed of *Bixa orellana* L. tree is a rich source of the orange-yellow diapocarotenoid bixin. The extract containing this pigment is used as a natural food colour. Furthermore, many hydroxycarotenoids (xanthophylls) are also present in plants in the form of esters of long chain FAs.

Some oils, especially olive oil, contain the green chlorophylls in concentrations up to several hundred micrograms per gram. The brown, toxic compound gossypol can be found in cottonseed oil.

Several natural pigments of plant origin are marketed in the form of solutions in oil, e.g. the turmeric colour (natural yellow 3) containing 20–40% of the pigment curcumin, extracted from *Curcuma domestica* (longa) L., luteine (natural yellow 29), and chlorophylls (natural green 3).

9.3 The role of lipids in the flavour of foods

9.3.1 Interactions of flavour compounds in foods

The perceived odour and aroma of food are related predominantly to the concentration of the volatile compounds in the vapour phase above the product. At any given temperature the vapour phase concentration depends on the contents of the respective compounds in the matrix, on their volatility, and on their affinity to other components of the food.

Flavour compounds in foods are entrapped by proteins, lipids, or polysaccharides. The binding may be due to hydrophobic interactions, as well as hydrogen, ionic, or covalent bonds, depending on the structure of the compounds and the interacting food constituent. Entrapment decreases the volatility of the molecules, thus reducing the rate of loss of flavour during storage of the products (Wu *et al.* 2002). The stability of the system depends on the pH and temperature of food.

Many aroma compounds are hydrophobic or at least have significant hydrophobic fragments. Thus in a food product they accumulate predominantly in the lipid phase, thereby greatly decreasing their partitioning into the aqueous and vapour phases. The air–lipid partition coefficient for any hydrophobic flavour compound that is present in the particular food system is affected at the given temperature by the FA composition of the fat phase and the degree of fat dispersion.

9.3.2 The effect of lipids on the flavour of meat products

The aroma of fresh raw meat of slaughter animals is only slight. Normally it has no real significance as a food quality criterion. Therefore the literature regarding the components responsible for the fresh meat aroma is very scarce, except for information regarding the species-specific flavour. However, meat stored too long under improper conditions may develop a rancid odour characteristic of fat oxidation – tallowy in beef, muttony in mutton, and cheesy, acrylic, or fishy in pork. Volatile aldehydes accumulating due to oxidation of PUFAs may contribute to the off-odour of poultry meat. Furthermore, a fishy off-flavour appears in turkey meat as a result of feeding the birds diets rich in PUFAs. This can be prevented by adding to the feed an appropriate amount of α-tocopherol.

The aroma characteristic of various processed meats and meaty dishes develops due to thermal degradation of precursors, predominantly nitrogenous compounds, the generation of volatiles in the Maillard reaction, and interactions of secondary lipid oxidation products. The odour developed by heating water-soluble precursors does not depend on the species of the slaughter animal. It is known as the meaty note. On the other hand, the species characteristics of cooked meat is contributed by the fat-soluble components that are transferred by heating into the vapour phase, as well as by volatiles generated due to changes in the lipids (Shahidi *et al.* 1986).

Several secondary lipid oxidation products are responsible for the rancid, fatty, pungent, and other undesirable off-flavour notes of cooked meats, especially of reheated dishes (warmed-over flavour). Hexanal may be regarded as the indicative compound, since its concentration in reheated meat may be about 10 times higher than in freshly cooked beef (Belitz *et al.* 2001). Cooking leads to liberation of phospholipids from the tissue membranes and of Fe(II) ions from myoglobin. The phospholipids are rich in PUFAs, while the inorganic Fe(II) is known for its catalytic effect on fat oxidation. The release of Fe(II) from myoglobin as a result of heat denaturation occurs in the same temperature range as the loss in oxidative stability of cooked muscle lipids (Decker and Xu 1998). The formation of the warmed-over flavour is less pronounced in cured cooked meats, since curing favours the binding of Fe(II) in the haemoproteins. Furthermore, the product of curing, MbFe(II)NO, has an antioxidant effect, and other volatile flavour compounds, characteristic for cured meats, are formed.

The off-flavours resulting from lipid oxidation are caused predominantly by carbonyl compounds. Pentanal and hexanal, if accumulated due to oxidation of PUFAs, contribute to the undesirable odour. Carbonyl compounds react with amino acids and proteins with formation of very objectionable off-flavours. The secondary products of oxidation of PUFAs, mainly 2,4-alkabienals and conjugated alkatrienals, react with amino acids producing typical fishy off-flavour. Hexanal and 2,4-decadienal may react with the Maillard reaction products, forming long chain alkylpyrazines and other odorous, heterocyclic compounds. Carbonyls and alcohols derived from lipids are also responsible for the characteristic odour that develops in meat sterilized by irradiation.

9.3.3 Lipids and seafood aroma

The mild, rather pleasant, plant-like, melon-like, seaweedy aroma of very fresh raw fish is chiefly caused by the presence of minute amounts of lipid degradation products. They are accompanied in the vapour phase above the fish by other volatiles, mainly trimethylamine, bromophenols, and several sulphur-containing compounds. In the very early post-harvest period the PUFAs of fish lipids are degraded in enzymatic reactions, catalysed by the endogenous lipoxygenases, hydroxyperoxide lyases, *Z,E*-enal izomerases, and alcohol dehydrogenases, to aldehydes, ketones, and alcohols with six, eight, and nine carbon atoms, respectively. Among these degradation products the following compounds have been identified: hexanal, 1-octen-3-ol, 1-octen-3-on, 1,5-octadien-3-ol, 1,5-octadien-3-on, 2,5-octadien-1-ol, 2,6-nonadienal, 2,6-nonadienol, and 3,6-nonadien-1-ol. The 8-carbon compounds carry the heavy, plant-like aroma, while the 9-carbon volatiles add the cucumber and melon-like note. The (*E*,*Z*)-2,6-nonadienal and 3,6-nonadien-1-ol are also responsible for the pronounced melon-like aroma of fresh Pacific oysters (Josephson *et al.* 1985). Microbial conversion of the carbonyl compounds into alcohols leads to gradual decrease in the intensity of the fresh fish aroma, since the odour threshold of the alcohols is higher than that of the carbonyl compounds. As a result of random autoxidation of the lipids accompanying the enzymatic processes, the very fresh green aroma is replaced with fishy aromas that are associated with oxidized fish oils (Lindsay 1990).

Long-term frozen storage of fish not protected from lipid oxidation causes rancid odour. In fatty fish the rate of oxidation is the highest in the subcutaneous fat layer, if this layer is exposed by skinning of the fillets. The presence of (*Z*)-4-heptenal, generated by the oxidation of the PUFA of phospholipids, is characteristic for the flavour of frozen stored, cooked cod. This compound has the ability to potentiate the stale, burned/fishy odour of oxidizing fish oils that is caused mainly by decatrienals (Lindsay 1990). The typical cooked shrimp aroma is in part due to the isomers of 5,8,11-tetradecatrien-one, derived from lipids in the presence of lipoxygenase (Kuo and Pan 1991). The undesirable odour caused by lipid oxidation in different cooked, ground fish products can be effectively prevented by various spices.

The aroma of the cooked muscle is characteristic for various groups of fish species, owing to different impact of the volatile compounds originating in lipid changes. The aroma notes and intensity, in a three-point scale, for three representative species are as follows (Prell and Sawyer 1988):

- Cod: briny 1–1.5, fresh fish 1.5, sweet 0.5–1, sour 0.5–1, shellfish (clam, scallop) 0.5
- Striped bass: gamey fish 1.5, fresh fish 1.5, sweet 1, sour 1
- Atlantic mackerel: gamey fish 2, fresh fish 2, sweet 0.5–1, briny 1, fish oil 1–1.5.

Fish oils rich in eicosapentaenoic acid (EPA) and docosahexaenoic acid (DHA) are used commercially for enriching many food products for health reasons. Since they are very susceptible to autoxidation even under ambient conditions, they must be protected against oxidizing conditions in order to prevent off-flavour development. Stabilization of fish oils enriched in DHA can be achieved by encapsulation. The oil is entrapped in partially enzyme-degraded starch and the microgranules are coated with a protein film, that has very low oxygen permeability (Ohshima 1998).

9.3.4 The role of lipids in the flavour of cheese and butter

The flavour of unripe cheese is caused by the olfactory action of a large number of volatile compounds present in the fresh milk in different, small

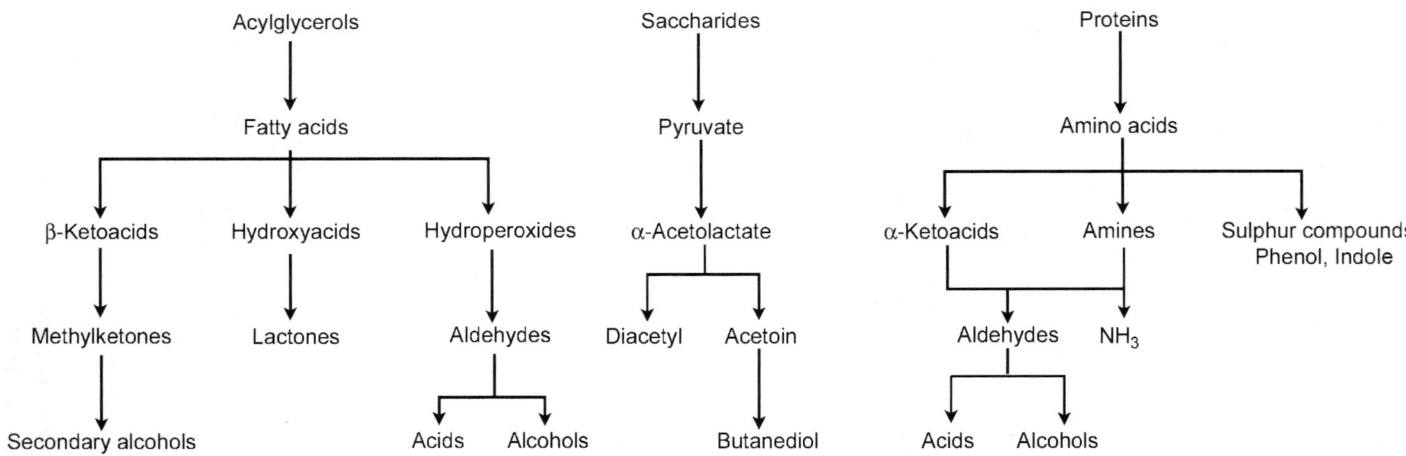

Fig. 9.2 Flavour compounds which may be derived from the main milk constituents in cheeses.

concentrations, predominantly dimethylsulphide, diacetyl, 2-methylbutanol, (*Z*)-4-heptenal, 3-buthenylisothiocyanate, and (*E*)-2-nonenal. The milk flavour may be affected by the cow's diet. If the cow's feed contains too large a proportion of soybeans in the winter, which are rich in linoleic acid, an oxidation off-flavour may occur early in the distribution chain and is correlated with high content of *n*-hexanal in the milk.

In the course of ripening, the typical flavour of ripe cheeses develops as a result of mainly enzymatic changes in the major components of the raw material – lactose, nitrogenous compounds, and lipids (Fig. 9.2). The reactions are catalysed by various enzymes – those present in the milk, added as clotting agents, and contributed by the microflora that participate in cheese making. In soft and mould-ripened cheeses the most important role is played by the enzymes of *Penicillium camemberti, Geotrichum candidum*, and *Brevibacterium linens* (Molimard and Spinnler 1996). Among the large number of at least 400 compounds affecting the flavour of cheeses there are some that can originate from different precursors and interact with each other. Therefore it is hardly possible to disclose what is the precise contribution of specific lipid degradation products to the flavour of different products.

Among the volatile flavour compounds of cheeses generated directly from lipids are FAs, methyl ketones and ketones, alcohols, and lactones. They differ in flavour perception thresholds and appear in cheeses in various concentrations and at different stages of ripening (Table 9.2). The FAs, C_4 to $C_{20,}$ originate from TAGs by way of hydrolysis catalysed by endogenous milk lipases and microbial enzymes. Some low molecular weight acids can be derived from lactose, amino acids, ketones, aldehydes, and esters. Only the short and medium chain FAs (MCFAs) have a sufficiently low perception threshold to affect significantly the flavour of cheeses in the given concentrations. However, the other acids are important precursors of a variety of volatile compounds. β-Oxidation leads to the formation of methyl ketones by moulds. The methyl ketones, among them heptan-2-one and nonan-2-one, are the most abundant volatile compounds in Camembert cheese. Diacetyl and acetoine are derived from lactose via pyruvate. Primary and secondary alcohols are important contributors to the flavour of mould-ripened cheeses by imparting the characteristic alcoholic, floral, and mushroom notes. They also serve as substrates in synthesis of esters. Alcohols are generated in lactose metabolism and can result from degradation of ketones. Lactones appear as derivatives of hydroxylated FAs. Lipids may participate in the formation of other volatile compounds contributing to cheese flavour via the reactions of their degradation products. These interactions have been described by Molimard and Spinnler (1996) and Belitz *et al.* (2001).

In cheeses of various varieties different compounds give the characteristic flavour notes. In Camembert and buffalo Mozzarella it is oct-1-en-3-ol, in bovine Mozzarella the 2-methylpropanoic acid ethyl ester, in Cheddar and Limburger it is methanethiol, in Roquefort and Blue cheese the methyl ketones, in Parmesan, Provolone, and Romano the butanoic, hexanoic, and octanoic acids, and in Brie the 2-methylpropanoic and 3-methylbutanoic acids.

Table 9.2 Selected flavour compounds in Camembert cheese (based on data compiled by Molimard and Spinnler 1996 and Belitz *et al.* 2001)

Compound	Flavour note	Perception threshold in water (μg/g)	Contents in cheese (μg/g)
Propionic acid	Vinegar, pungent	22–54	13–66
Butyric acid	Rancid, cheesy	0.3–7	35–205
Isovaleric acid	Rotten fruit, mild, fruity	0.07	100
Hexanoic acid	Pungent, blue cheese	5–15	25–145
Heptan-2-one	Roquefort cheese, blue cheese	0.0009–3	7–17.5 in fatty matter
Octan-2-one	Fruity, musty	0.15–1	Traces
Octan-3-one	Mushroom, fruity	0.05	Traces
Octa-1,5-dien-3-one	Geranium leaf, soil	0.001×10^{-3}	Traces
Octan-2-ol	Green	0.018	
Octanoic acid	Wax, soapy, goaty, musty, rancid, fruity	5.8–19	14
Oct-1-en-3-ol	Mushroom	0.01	0.07–0.13
Oct-1,5-dien-3-ol	Soil, geranium	0.01	
δ-Octalactone	Coconut, wine	0.57	
γ-Octalactone	Coconut, fruity	0.09–0.4	
Decan-2-one	Fruity, musty	0.19	Traces
δ-Decalactone	Coconut, peach	0.14–0.16	0.9–1.1
γ-Decalactone	Apricot, peach	0.09	
δ-Dodecalactone	Fresh fruit, peach	0.1–1	
Undecan-2-one	Floral, herbaceous	54	Traces
Ethylpropanoate	Pineapple	0.0099	Traces
Ethylhexanoate	Pineapple, banana	0.001	Traces
Isoamylacetate	Pear, banana	0.002	Traces
Diacetyl	Buttery	2.5	Traces
Methanethiol	Cooked cabbage	0.002	0.26
Dimethyldisulphide	Cauliflower, garlic, very ripe cheese	0.12	

The flavour of butter is due to the volatile components of the fat phase, which are complemented by the compounds of the watery phase. In fresh butter the largest contribution is made by short chain FAs, (*Z*)-4-heptenal, lactones, diacetyl, and dimethyl sulphide. On heating the concentration of lactones increases as a result of conversion of lactone precursors present in the fresh butter, also further methyl ketones are generated. Furthermore, the flavour is enriched by the contribution of different Maillard reaction products. The resulting flavour of heated butter depends on the temperature of heating. This knowledge is extensively utilized in different cuisines. Synergistic interactions of various compounds, even present in subthreshold concentrations, contribute to the perceived flavour of products containing butter as an ingredient. Butter is also a good carrier of flavourings, e.g. vanilla and sweet spices, that are used in confectionery, cakes, biscuits, croissants, and muffins. The flavourings are readily released on melting of chocolate. Butter serves also as a carrier of garlic aroma, herbs, and culinary spices in various sauces, gravies, and fillings, as well as in different ready meals.

9.4 Lipids and the texture of foods

9.4.1 The role of lipids in the texture of meat and meat products

The amount and distribution of intramuscular fat have been regarded as important characteristics of meat quality and are recognized as one of several criteria in establishing beef carcass quality grades. The degree of marbling is determined visually in cross-sections of the *longissimus dorsi* muscle. Among some professionals there is a belief that marbling contributes to meat tenderness. However, no unequivocal published evidence has been found showing high positive correlation between the contents of intramuscular fat and meat tenderness. The beneficial effect of marbling on meat quality may be due to the lubricating action of the fat layers during chewing and swallowing, which may be perceived as increased tenderness of tough meat samples. Intramuscular fat uniformly distributed on the cross-section of the meat cut, in limited amount, improves the flavour and juiciness, while meat with almost no marbling may be dry and deficient in flavour. The effect of fat on the tenderness of meat is also treated by Moloney in Chapter 13.

The consistency of the fatty tissues in meats depends on the FA composition of the fat, which in turn is affected by the characteristics of the fats contained in the feed given to the slaughter animals. This is especially pronounced in pork. Owing to solidification caused by chilling, the subcutaneous fat and marbling increase the firmness of the carcass and retail cuts and contribute to retaining the characteristic shape during handling and processing of meat.

9.4.2 The effect of lipids on the texture of fish and fish products

The texture of fish is generally more tender than that of mammalian and poultry meat. It varies significantly between species, depending on the composition and structure of the muscle. Within species it is affected mainly by pH, but in fish of some species also by the protein and fat content related to the feeding status (Howgate 1977).

In fish belonging to the fatty category the texture of meat is significantly affected by the presence of intramuscular fat. The liquid neutral lipids immobilized in the musculature 'dilute' the arrangement of the proteinaceous structures, thereby decreasing the overall mechanical strength of the meat. Thus the fillets of fish of fatty species containing much fat are more tender than those of specimens of the same species with depleted lipid reserves. The seasonal variability in the content of fat in the muscles of many fish belonging to fatty species may be very high. Fillets of Atlantic mackerel caught in April may contain from about 2% to about 22% fat, whereas in August the figures are 8% to 36% (Karl and Oehlenschläger 1986). It is well known by the processors that fish of many fatty species caught out of the feeding period, when the muscles are poor in fat, is not suitable for producing high-quality pasteurized, sterilized, salted, or smoked products. Baltic sprats caught during summer, containing less than 4% fat, are not used for hot smoking or canning. The highest sensory quality of hot smoked Atlantic mackerel can be guaranteed only if the raw material contains very much fat, even up to about 30% of muscle wet weight. Lightly salted, fatty sturgeon, salmon, herring, and anchovy have very tender texture, described as a visco-elastic body. A typical example may be the maatjes, i. e. mild salted, immature, fatty herring. The renowned German fish technologist Peter Biegler praised the high quality of mild salted, fatty fish by writing '*Ein mild gesalzener Lachs dürfte schon den Göttern gut gemundet haben*' (Biegler 1960).

In fish of many species a severe quality deterioration may occur during prolonged frozen storage due to crosslinking of myofibrillar proteins, which leads to so-called freezing denaturation. This is manifested in undesirable toughness of the meat after cooking and loss in water holding, fat emulsifying, and gel-forming capacity. The extent of these deteriorative changes increases with the time and temperature of frozen storage. Several mechanisms of freezing denaturation have been proposed. One of them may be the crosslinking reactions of amino acid residues with secondary products of lipid oxidation. Oxidizing lipids may participate in free radical polymerization, and the dialdehydes in protein–amine condensation. The freezing denaturation is especially severe in minced fish, because damaging of the muscle structures increases oxidation of lipids, especially if the mince contains also dark meat, rich in haematin compounds. Different measures that restrict lipid oxidation in frozen fish minces are effective in inhibiting the undesirable quality changes (Matsumoto and Noguchi 1992).

9.4.3 Lipids and the texture of emulsion type products

Lipids, in different forms, and their interactions with other food constituents, contribute to the rheological properties of food emulsions, including dairy products. Interactions of lipids with polysaccharides can be utilized in manufacturing low-calorie emulsion-type food commodities. An emulsion of 20% soybean oil in a water solution containing 1 to 1.5% microcrystalline cellulose can simulate a 65% pure oil emulsion as regards viscosity, yield value, flow properties, and stability (Phillips and Williams 1995).

Lipid droplets play a structure-forming role in oil-in-water emulsion-type products like milk, cream, ice cream, cheese, dressing, mayonnaise, and various comminuted meat commodities. These droplets are stabilized by interactions with proteins, lecithins, or different synthetic surfactants. In chilled, natural milk the lipoprotein membranes of fat globules interact on standing with a serum protein, thereby forming clusters of globules and leading to creaming. Clustering of the fat globules around the air bubbles contributes to the desirable characteristics of ice cream. The churning process used in making butter leads to concentration of the fat globules and spreading of the oil at the air–water interface, suppression of the foam, and formation of clumps of the water-in-oil emulsion.

9.4.4 The role of lipids and their interactions on the texture of baked goods

Lipids contribute to the texture of baked products by interacting with proteins and polysaccharides. Wheat flour contains about 1.5–2.5% lipids. One part of these lipids is free, extractable by petroleum ether. The other one, called bond lipids, can be extracted only with a polar solvent, e.g. water-saturated *n*-butanol. There is also a fraction of lipids, about 0.25% of the total content, firmly associated with starch. All fractions contain neutral lipids, glycolipids, and phospholipids, although in different proportions, and contribute to the behaviour of the dough. The neutral lipids are present in the flour in the form of spherosomes covered with membranes which contain phospholipids. The polar lipids are assembled into hexagonal micelles. On mixing of the flour with water they turn into lamellar liquid crystalline phases by stacking of stretched lipid bilayers separated by water lamellae (Marion *et al.* 1998). These lamellar phases stabilize the micro-emulsion of the neutral lipids in the dough and are together embedded in the network of the gluten proteins. The shortening effect of the lipids is due to disruption of the structure of the gluten network and contributes to increase in loaf volume and the formation of soft, even-textured crumb grain. Lipid monomers may probably form bridges between the gliadins and glutenins, thus affecting the dough elasticity and extensibility. Furthermore, the polar lipids stabilize the gas bubbles thanks to their surface-active properties and fill the gaps in proteinaceous films, thus preventing the escape of gas. This role is performed not only by the endogenous lipids of the flour, but also by shortenings or butter added to the dough. In pastry doughs and flaky crusts the added butter melts during baking to form impervious layers that prevent steam and carbon dioxide to escape. After cooling, the products have the characteristic flaky texture.

Wheat flour contains several low molecular weight proteins that in the non-denatured state have the ability to spontaneously bind lipids or lipid aggregates. These proteins, the thionins, ligoline, lipid transfer proteins, and puroindolines, rich in cysteine and basic amino acid residues, are very efficient foam stabilizers. They facilitate the spreading of lipids as a monolayer at air–water interfaces. Interactions of puroindoline-a with lysophosphatidylcholine have a synergistic effect on the foam stability of the system (Marion *et al.* 1998). Breads made with defatted flour have poor gas retention and low loaf volume.

Lipid interactions with polysaccharides in aqueous systems are due to hydrophobic effects. A typical example is binding of a monoacylglycerol molecule by amylose via accommodating the hydrophobic FA residue inside the amylose helix. As the result of this interaction, an amylose–lipid complex is formed that has a structure similar to that of the amylose–iodine complex. In a dough the heating applied in the baking process increases the degree of binding of lipids by amylose. The amylose–lipid complexes are able to form gels, thus affecting the texture of baked goods. The rheological properties of these gels depend on the concentration and type of the lipids and on the crystalline form of the complexes. Addition of lipids to starch gels may retard retrogradation. Another mechanism is the interaction of lipidic surfactant micelles, formed due to aggregation of the hydrocarbon chains, with their polar heads directed towards appropriate segments of the polysaccharides. These interactions also contribute to the gelling of many systems (Eliasson 1998).

9.5 Lipids and the nutritional value of infant foods

9.5.1 Lipid composition in human milk

Human milk is the best source of nutrients for infants, especially during the first 4–6 months of life. It contains the proper amount of lipids, proteins, saccharides, minerals, and vitamins required by the fast-growing organism, as well as immunological factors. The milk lipids originate from three main sources: mobilization of the mother's body fat stores, the diet, and the FA synthesis by the mammary gland (Ortiz-Olaya *et al.* 1996). The fat is present in milk in the form of globules, 1–10 mm in diameter, that are formed in the mammary gland. The globules are composed of a hydrophobic core covered by a membrane. The core is rich in TAGs and contains a small amount of cholesterol esters. The TAGs account for 98–99% of total fat. The membrane, made of phospholipids and structural proteins, contains some cholesterol and several enzymes. Cholesterol constitutes about 0.5% of total fat, diacyloglycerols 0.01%, phospholipids 0.8%, and free FAs 0.08% (Koletzko *et al.* 2001). The fat content of human milk is about 3.8–3.9 g/100 ml; it delivers 40–55% of total energy. The total lipid content varies in a small degree due to the ethnic differences, duration of lactation, and duration of pregnancy. Some infections, drugs, and metabolic disorders of the lactating women may cause a depletion of the fat amount.

The diet of lactating women plays a significant role in determining the FA composition of milk lipids (Fig. 9.3). The content of EPA and DHA can be increased by consumption of fatty sea fish, such as mackerel, herring, and salmon. The milk of vegetarian women contains more linoleic acid (LA) and less DHA than that of omnivorous mothers (Sanders *et al.* 1978). The predominant fraction of FAs are the saturated ones (about 45%), mainly palmitic acid, and the monoenoic acids, mostly oleic acid (about 39%); the rest is made up of PUFAs. Saturated acids play the main role as the energy source for the developing baby. Cholesterol is the major human milk sterol contributing approximately 90% of the total sterol content. A relatively large amount of cholesterol is consumed by the infant as compared with that taken by the adult. It has been proposed that its high consumption in the early life may control cholesterol and lipoprotein metabolism in adults (Reiser *et al.* 1979). Monoenoic

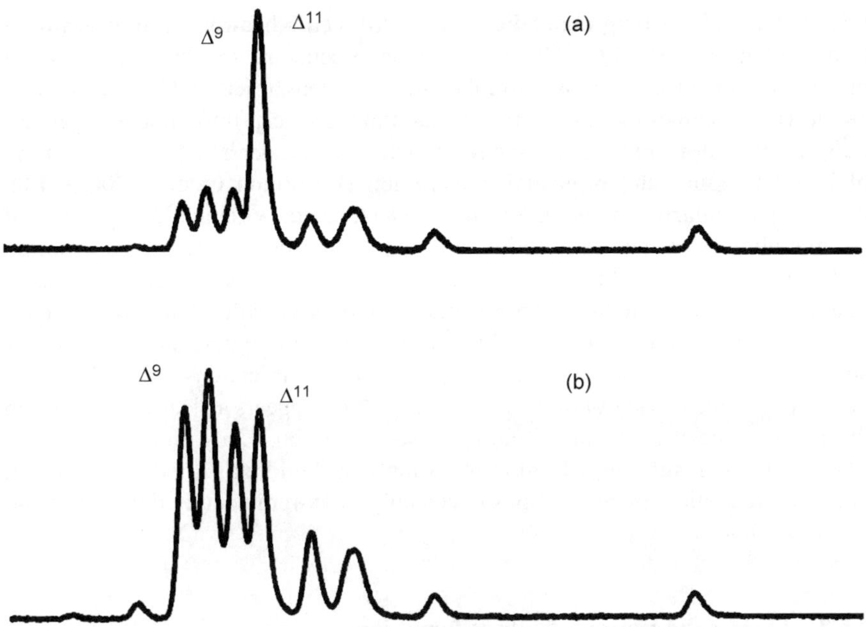

Fig. 9.3 The effect of diet on the C18:1 trans fatty acids in the lipids of human milk; Chromatograms (HR-GC) of FA methyl esters; (a) diet rich in cow's milk, (b) diet rich in hydrogenated vegetable oil (Courtesy of A. Stolyhwo).

FAs affect cholesterol metabolism, leading to decreased LDL fraction serum concentration. PUFAs include both the dietary essential LA and α-linolenic acid (ALA), as well as small amounts of ten other acids of the n-6 and n-3 series, which usually represent about 1–1.5% of total milk FAs (Table 9.3).

Table 9.3 The contents of fatty acids in mature human milk in Europe (source: Stolarczyk 1999)

Fatty acids	Mean value (% of total fatty acids)	Range (% of total fatty acids)
Saturated	45.2	39.0–51.3
Monoenoic	38.8	34.2–44.9
Polyenoic	13.6	8.5–19.6
LA	11.0	6.9–16.4
ALA	0.9	0.7–1.3
Arachidonic acid	0.5	0.2–1.2
DHA	0.3	0.1–0.6
n-6 Long chain PUFAs, total	1.2	0.4–2.2
n-3 Long chain PUFAs, total	0.6	0.3–1.8
LA/ALA	12.1	8.6–16.9
n-6/n-3	2.7	0.3–3.7

9.5.2 The role of long chain PUFAs in children's health and development

Long chain PUFAs (LC-PUFAs) serve as precursors for the formation of prostaglandins, prostacyclins, thromboxanes and leukotrienes. These mediators are powerful regulators of numerous tissue functions, e.g. thrombocyte aggregation, inflammatory reactions, immune functions, vascular reactivity, regulation of blood pressure and bronchial constriction (Uauy and Castillo 2003). LC-PUFAs, particularly arachidonic acid and DHA are the essential components of cell membranes in the brain, retina, and other nervous system tissues (Lanting and Boersma, 1996). Thus, the deficiency of LC-PUFAs is of great importance in a child's health. The lack of n-6 is manifested by growth retardation, desquamation, and thickening of the skin, decreased skin pigmentation, muscular contraction disorders, and increased susceptibility to infections. n-3 LC-PUFAs deficiency is the cause of brain dysfunction, which appears as learning and sleep disorders, paraesthesias, and abnormal visual function (Uauy and Mena 2001). The extent of insufficient LC-PUFAs supply in children's food is unknown, because the clinical manifestations occur only in extreme deficiency (Uauy and Castillo 2003).

9.5.3 Lipid composition of infant formulas

The composition of infant formulas and follow-up formulas is designed to mimic breast milk as much as possible. The fat in infant formulas is usually a blend of several vegetable oils. The choice is based on availability, nutritional properties, and relative costs. Usually soybean oil is used as a rich source of ALA (6–9%), in mixtures with corn, sunflower, rape, palm, and coconut oils. The coconut oil is valuable because of the large content of MCFAs; however, it contains large amounts of lauric and miristic acids that have atherogenic properties. Some formulas are supplemented with cow's milk fat.

According to the guidelines of ESPGAN Committee on Nutrition (Com. Directive 1996) the total fat content in starting formulas should range from 4.4 to 6.5 g/100 kcal and 3.3 to 6.5 g/100 kcal in follow-up formulas. This means, that lipids should contribute respectively 40–55% and 35–55% to the total energy supply. The detailed demands regarding FA in infant formulas are shown in Table 9.4. The directive does not recommend any proportions of the saturated to mono- and polyenoic FAs, despite the fact, that clinical research indicates worse absorption of long chain saturated FAs than unsaturated FAs. This reduced absorption contributes to the formation of insoluble calcium soaps and decreased calcium absorption. Monoenoic FAs seem to be the most advantageous owing to their highest intestinal absorption and resistance to oxidation. Further recommendations regard supplementation in LC-PUFA and permission for use of MCFA in amounts not higher than 40% of total fat.

The conversion rate of parent essential FAs into LC-PUFAs in both preterm and term infants is low owing to limited activity of the endogenous enzymatic LC-PUFAs synthesis from the precursor FAs. Pre-term infants have especially high demand for LC-PUFAs because of rapid use of these acids in fast-growing

Table 9.4 The contents of fatty acids in infant formulas (source: Com. Directive 96/4/EC)

Fatty acids	Contents in formulas (% of total fat)
Lauric	Maximum 15
Mirystic	Maximum 15
Linoleic	300–1200 mg/100 kcal
α-Linoleic	Minimum 50 mg/100 kcal
LA/ALA	5 : 1 to 15 : 1
Trans fatty acids	Maximum 1
Erucic	Maximum 1
LC-PUFA (C20–22)	
Total n-3	Maximum 4
Total n-6	Maximum 2
Arachidonic	Maximum 1
EPA	<DHA

Sesame and cotton oil – not permitted.

tissues, especially the brain, and inefficiency in the system of elongase and saturase. Therefore the enrichment of infant formulas with LC-PUFAs comparatively to human milk lipids (1% for n-6 LC-PUFAs and 0.5% for n-3 LC-PUFAs) is considered to improve the nutrient supply and to have beneficial effects on the early growth and development of formula-fed babies, especially as regards the visual acuity and development of cognitive functions during the first year of life (Birch *et al.* 2000; Markides *et al.* 1995). At present there is no requirement for supplementation of the formulas with LC-PUFAs. However, it is recommended for pre-term infants. Investigations regarding the development of cognitive and motor functions, as well as growth rate, in children up to 18 months-old have not shown any need for supplementing the milk formulations with LC PUFAs for healthy, term infants (Lucas *et al.* 1999).

Regarding the human milk as a standard, the ESPGAN Committee has recommended the contents of LA and ALA in infant formulas. LA should supply 4.5–10.8% of total energy. Taking into consideration the competitive antagonism of the n-3 and n-6 acids for the same enzymes, the proportion of the concentrations of LA : ALA has been set from 5 : 1 to 15 : 1 (Aggett *et al.* 1991).

LC-PUFAs used for supplementation of milk for babies are obtained from marine fish oils and from egg yolk lipids. Formula milk enriched by addition of n-3 FAs concentrates from fish oil or marine algae is commercially produced in Japan and USA (Ohshima 1998). In egg yolk the proportion of n-6 to n-3 FAs is similar to those in the human milk fat. Marine microalgae sources of EPA and DHA are treated by Jacobsen and Let in Chapter 19.

The ESPGAN recommendations do not deal with cholesterol. According to the present state of knowledge, rationally justified suggestions regarding the contents of cholesterol in infant formulas cannot be made.

9.5.4 Safety of the fats used in children's food

An important safety issue is the stability of oils in terms of lipid peroxidation; the high degree of unsaturation makes n-3 and n-6 PUFAs susceptible to oxidation and to generate pro-oxidants, leading to an oxidative stress (Cichon 2003). Because of the high content of LC-PUFAs in oils used in children's food, substantial amounts of antioxidants are required to preserve their structure. Unfortunately no international standards have yet been adopted regarding the maximum levels of secondary lipid oxidation products in infant formulas.

Trans FAs formed during industrial hydrogenation processes may contribute to decreased LC-PUFAs synthesis. The European Union has limited the contents of trans FAs at 4% of total fat of foods for infants and young children.

EC Directives on the fat content in infant formulas also placed limits on the content of lauric and myristic acids to prevent adverse long-term effects; these intermediate chain length FAs contribute to raising LDL cholesterol and thus may increase the risk of cardiovascular diseases in adults.

9.6 Future trends

Lipids of various composition and properties are in many aspects very important components which impart desirable features to many foods. However, their degradation, predominantly of oxidative nature, and interactions with other food constituents, especially in the form of secondary oxidation products, may lead to significant deterioration in quality. A better insight into the mechanisms of their degradation and interactions, particularly in conditions of food storage and processing, would enhance the beneficial role of lipids in creating the sensory quality of many commodities and in preventing undesirable effects.

Effective approaches to increasing the beneficial role of fat in foods may include:

- improvements in the formulation of processed products by fully utilizing the functional properties of lipids and the possible interactions with other food components in conditions of storage and processing;
- use of antioxidant treatments in various stages of food production to avoid undesirable oxidative changes of lipids;
- enzymatic modification of lipids to be used in food formulations to obtain 'tailor-made' fats most suitable for different food applications;
- better utilization of enzymatic lipid modifications for generating desirable flavour components suitable for improving the sensory quality of many processed foods;
- better utilization of fundamental knowledge on dispersed systems to be able to use most efficiently different fats in creating the desirable, rheological properties of emulsion-type products;
- use of mild processing parameters to avoid drastic thermal and oxidative changes in the lipid components of foods;

- use of additives, microencapsulation, and packaging systems that efficiently prevent deteriorative changes of fats in foods;
- use of rational food storage parameters and control of time–temperature conditions of storage;
- use of new developments in logistics to shorten the exposure time of food in retail systems.

9.7 References

AGGETT P, HASCHKE F, HEINE W, HARNELL O, KOLETZKO B, LAUNIALA K, REY J, RUBINO A, SCOCH G, SENTERRE J and TORMO R (1991), 'Committee Report: Comment on the content and composition of lipids in infant formulas: ESPGAN Committee on Nutrition', *Acta Paediatr Scand*, **80**, 887–896.

BELITZ H D, GROSCH W and SCHIEBERLE P (2001), *Lehrbuch der Lebensmittelchemie*, Berlin, Springer.

BIEGLER P (1960), 'Fischwaren-Technologie. Theorie und Praxis der Fabrikationsmethoden zur Konservierung von Fischen', in Baader K, *Der Fisch. Mitteilungen für die Fischindustrie*, Vol. V, Lübeck, Verlag Der Fisch – Clara Baader, p. 81.

BIRCH E E, GARFIELD S, HOFFMAN D R, UAUY R and BIRCH D G (2000), 'A randomised controlled trial of early dietary supply of long-chain polyunsaturated fatty acid and mental development in term infants', *Dev Mec Child Neurol*, **42**, 174–181.

BOSKOU D (2003), 'Frying fats', in Sikorski Z E and Kołakowska A, *Chemical and Functional Properties of Food Lipids*, Boca Raton, CRC Press, pp. 325–343.

CICHON R M (2003), 'Lipids in food structures', in Sikorski Z E and Kołakowska A, *Chemical and Functional Properties of Food Lipids*, Boca Raton, CRC Press, pp. 189–204.

COM. DIRECTIVE 96/4/EC, *Official Journal of the European Communities*, No. L49/13.

DECKER E A and XU Z (1998), 'Minimizing rancidity in muscle foods', *Food Technology*, **52**(10), 54–59.

ELIASSON A CH (1998), 'Lipid-carbohydrate interactions', in Hammer R J and Hoseney R C, *Interactions: the keys to cereal quality*. St Paul, American Association of Cereal Chemists, Inc., pp. 47–80.

FAUSTMAN C and WANG K W (2000), 'Potential mechanisms by which vitamin E improves oxidative stability of myoglobin', in Decker E, Faustman C and Lopez-Bote C J, *Antioxidants in Muscle Foods. Nutritional Strategies to Improve Quality*, New York, Wiley-Interscience, pp. 135–152.

HOWGATE P (1977), 'Aspects of fish texture', in Birch D C, Brennan J G, and Parker K J, *Sensory Properties of Foods,* London, Applied Science Publishers, pp. 240–269.

JOSEPHSON D B, LINDSAY R C and STUIBER D A (1985), 'Volatile compounds characterizing the aroma of fresh Atlantic and Pacific oysters', *J. Food Sci.,* **50**(1), 5–9.

KARL H and OEHLENSCHLÄGER J (1986), 'Zusammenhang zwischen Wasser- und Fettgehalt von Makrelenfilets aus dem Seegebiet westlich der Britischen Inseln', *Informationen für die Fischwirtschaft*, **33**(4), 184–187.

KOLETZKO B, RODRIGUEZ-PALMERO M, DEMMELMAIR H, FIDLER N, JENSEN R and SAUERWALD T (2001), 'Physiological aspects of human milk lipids', *Early Hum Dev*, **65** Suppl, S3–S18.

KRAMLICH W E, PEARSON A M and TAUBER F W (1973), *Processed Meats,* Westport, AVI

Publishing Company.

KUO J M and PAN B S (1991), 'Effects of lipoxygenase on formation of the cooked shrimp flavor compound – 5,8,11-tetradecatrien-2-one', *Agric Biol Chem*, **55**(3), 847–848.

LANTING C I and BOERSMA E R (1996), 'Lipids in infant nutrition and their impact on later development', *Curr Opin Lipidol*, **7**, 43–47.

LINDSAY R C (1990), 'Fish flavours', *Food Reviews International*, **6**(4), 437–455.

LUCAS A, STAFFORD M, MORLEY R, ABBOTT R, STEPHENSON T, MACFADYEN U, ELIAS-JONES A, AND CLEMENTS H (1999), 'Efficacy and safety of long-chain polyunsaturated fatty acid supplementation of infant-formula milk: a randomized trial', *Lancet*, **354**, 1948–1954.

LUSHBOUGH C H and SCHWEIGERT B S (1960), 'The nutritive content and the nutritional value of meat and meat products', in American Meat Institute Foundation, *The Science of Meat and Meat Products*, San Francisco and London, Freeman and Company, pp. 185–211.

MARION D, DUBREIL L, WILDE P J and CLARK D C (1998), 'Lipids, lipid-protein interactions and the quality of baked cereal products', in Hammer R J and Hoseney R C, *Interactions: The Keys to Cereal Quality*. St. Paul, Minnesota, American Association of Cereal Chemists, Inc., pp. 131–158.

MARKIDES M, NEUMANN M, SIMMER K, PATER J and GIBSON R (1995), 'Are long polyunsaturated fatty acids nutrients in infancy?', *Lancet*, **345**, 1463–1468.

MOHR V (1979), 'Nature of fat deposits in fish and principles of fat liberation', in *Proceedings of the Third Symposium on the Processing of Fish Meat and Oil*, London, International Association of Fish Meat Manufacturers, pp. 55–66.

MATSUMOTO J J and NOGUCHI S F (1992), 'Cryostabilization of protein in surimi', in Lanier T C and Lee C M, *Surimi Technology*. New York, Basel, Hong Kong, Marcel Dekker, Inc., pp. 357–388.

MOLIMARD P and SPINNLER H E (1996), 'Review: Compounds involved in the flavor of surface mold-ripened cheeses: origin and properties', *J Dairy Sci*, **79**, 169–184.

MONAHAN F J (2000), 'Oxidation of lipids in muscle foods: fundamental and applied concerns' , in Decker E, Faustman C, and Lopez-Bote C J, *Antioxidants in Muscle Foods. Nutritional Strategies to Improve Quality*, New York, Wiley-Interscience, pp. 3–23.

MORTENSEN A and SKIBSTED L H (2000), 'Antioxidant activity of carotenoids in muscle foods', in Decker E, Faustman C, and Lopez-Bote C J, *Antioxidants in Muscle Foods. Nutritional Strategies to Improve Quality*, New York, Wiley-Interscience, pp. 61–82.

NETTLETON J (1985), *Seafood Nutrition: Facts, Issues and Marketing of Nutrition in Fish and Shellfish*, Huntington, Osprey Books.

ORTIZ-OLAYA N, FLORES M E and DE SANTIAGO S (1996), 'Significance of lipid consumption during lactation', *Revista de Investigacion Clinica*, **46**(6), 473–478.

OHSHIMA T (1998), 'Recovery and use of nutraceutical products from marine resources', *Food Technol*, **52**(6), 50–53.

PHILLIPS G O and WILLIAMS P A (1995), 'Interaction of hydrocolloids in food systems', in Gaonkar A G, *Ingredient Interactions. Effect on Food Quality*, New York, Marcel Dekker, pp. 131–169.

PRELL P A and SAWYER F M (1988), 'Flavor profiles of 17 species of North Atlantic fish', *J Food Sci*, **53**(4), 1036–1042.

REISER R B, O'BRIEN C, HENDERSON G R and MORROE R (1979), 'Studies on a possible function for cholesterol in milk', *Nutr Rep Intl*, **19**, 835–849.

SANDERS T A B, ELLIS F R and DICKERSON J W T (1978), 'Studies of vegans: the fatty acid composition of plasma choline phosphoglycerides, erythrocytes, adipose tissue, and breast milk and some indicators of susceptibility to ischemic heart disease in vegans and omnivore controls', *Am J Clin Nutr*, **120**, S805–813.

SHAHIDI F, RUBIN L and D'SOUZA L A (1986), 'Meat flavor volatiles. A review on the composition, techniques of analysis, and sensory evaluation', *CRC Critical Rev Food Sci Nutr*, **24**(2), 141–243.

SIKORSKI Z E, KOŁAKOWSKA A and PAN B S (1990), 'The nutritive composition of the major groups of marine food organisms', in Sikorski Z E, *Seafood: Resources, Nutritional Composition, and Preservation*, Boca Raton, CRC Press, pp. 29–54.

SMITH G C, BELK K E, SOFOS J N, TATUM J D and WILLIAMS S N (2000), 'Economic implications of improved color stability in beef', in Decker E, Faustman C, and Lopez-Bote C J, *Antioxidants in Muscle Foods. Nutritional Strategies to Improve Quality*, New York, Wiley-Interscience, 397–426.

STOLARCZYK A (1999), 'Fats in infant formulas and special formulas'. *Pediatria Współczesna. Gastroenterologia, Hepatologia i Żywienie Dziecka*, **1**(2/3), 155–160.

STOLYHWO A (2005), Unpublished results.

UAUY R and CASTILLO C (2003), 'Lipid requirements of infants: implications for nutrient composition of fortified complementary foods', *J Nutr*, **133**, 2962S–2972S.

UAUY R and MENA P (2001), 'Lipids and neurodevelopment', *Nutr Rev*, **59**, 34–48.

WU CH M, KUO J M and PAN B S (2002), 'Flavor compounds', in Sikorski Z E, *Chemical and Functional Properties of Food Components*, Second Edition, Boca Raton, CRC Press, pp. 231–257.

ZAGALSKY P F, ELIOPAULOS E E and FINDLAY J B C (1990), 'The architecture of invertebrate carotenoproteins', *Comp. Biochem. Physiol.*, **97B**(1), 1–18.

10

Gaining consumer acceptance of low-fat foods

L. Lähteenmäki, VTT Biotechnology, Finland

10.1 Introduction

Lowering the fat content of diets has been a major target for nutrition education in developed countries in recent decades. Dietary fat causes two concerns that are often tied together in foods and dishes. An ample amount of fat in foods means that the energy density of the diet is high and this may contribute to weight gain. Overweight and obesity are known as crucial risk factors in developing several lifestyle-related diseases. Furthermore, the quality of fat is also important. The saturated fat in our diet is a major risk factor for heart diseases and has a negative impact on our blood lipid levels (see Chapter 1).

When people were asked about reasons behind their food choices the most commonly mentioned ones in a European cross-country survey were quality, price, taste, health and family concerns (Lappalainen *et al.*, 1998). The importance of these reasons varied among EU countries, but there is also a problem of interpreting the role and relevance of these different choice criteria. Taste is an experience-based characteristic describing the sensory pleasure derived from eating, whereas health mostly has to be conveyed through information about the nutrient content or the fat content. However, these results show that in general health is among the most important concerns when choices among food products are made.

In the same European study, respondents were asked what they regard as important in a healthy diet. Healthy eating meant a low-fat diet for 48% of respondents but there were differences among the European countries (Margetts *et al.*, 1997). People know that healthiness means a low-fat diet, but still this knowledge does not always translate itself into dietary choices. The reasons for this may be many.

Although vegetable oils, butter and fat spreads are not mentioned among best preferred foods, often foods that contain a high amount of fat tend to be among those that are well liked. Confectionery, desserts, pastry and biscuits are typically sweet products eaten as a reward or enjoyed in social events. Many dairy and meat products contain a considerable amount of fat. Sauces and dressings eaten with main courses, salads and desserts tend to be high in fat. All these foods have different roles in our daily eating and their choices are reasoned in different ways: choices among some alternatives within the product category may be more under cognitive reasoning whereas others are purely driven by hedonic, affect-based pleasure seeking. Even when the motivation to monitor one's own fat intake is high the task may prove to be too difficult. The fat comes from several sources and the calculation of total fat intake requires knowledge and processing of several factors: how much of different foods are eaten, what is their fat content and how to conclude the cumulative total intake from these various sources.

There are several ways of trying to lower the fat intake in our diets. The first is to avoid those foods that contain high amounts of fat and replace them with other foods that contain less or no fat at all; the second to favour those foods that are naturally low in fat, such as vegetables and fruit, assuming that the foods they replace contained more fat. Both of these approaches require considerable changes in the diet and food habits. The third option is to choose low-fat or non-fat alternatives of those products that are typically high in fat content. This means less pressure on changing diet-related practices and habits, but there are several factors that may hinder the acceptance of low-fat products. Lowering fat content in a product influences the sensory quality of the product and thus the hedonic pleasure derived from low-fat products may be lower than from their regular fat counterparts. The perceived healthiness of low-fat products may vary also among product categories. Although developing low-fat options has been one of the major trends in recent years, there are very few studies that have examined their significance in lowering the overall fat or energy content in the diet.

In this chapter the factors either promoting or obstructing the lowering of fat content in the diet are discussed with the focus on low-fat products. These aspects can be roughly divided into three groups: those related to food itself, those related to the individual and thirdly, those related to the nutritional advice (Fig. 10.1). In food products the sensory quality and direct pleasure derived from eating is known as the crucial factor for repeated choices. Modern consumers are used to good tasting products and are not ready to compromise taste for health. Societal norms and factors related to an individual should be mediated through individual attitudes towards health in general, and especially attitudes towards fat. Nutritional guidelines, whether official or unofficial, establish the social norms on fat and fat consumption and they are translated into a number of publicly supported educational advisory materials and campaigns. Finally the factors important for gaining acceptance of low-fat products are drawn together.

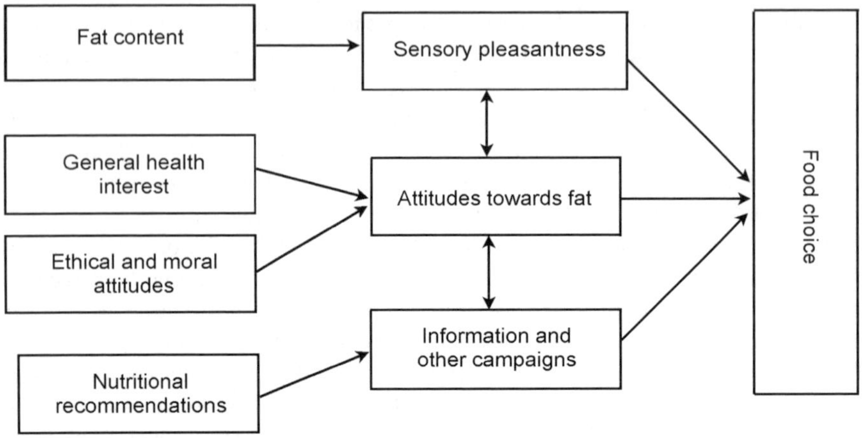

Fig. 10.1 Choices of low-fat options are related to product, individual and environmental factors.

10.2 Consumer preferences for fat in food products

10.2.1 Sensory characteristics and preferences for low-fat products

Fat is a crucial contributor to several texture attributes, such as creaminess, softness, melting in the mouth, juiciness and thickness (Drewnowski *et al.*, 1998; Mela, 1990). Most of these attributes are desired attributes and hence positively regarded qualities in food products (Elmore *et al.*, 1999). Perceived creaminess contributes to the liking for liquid dairy products (Richardson-Harman *et al.*, 2000). Therefore, changing fat content has an impact on the sensory quality of foods and thereby in the acceptability of products. As fat is a major component in many different types of foods from liquid to solid products, the effects in the sensory quality depend on the type of food and reducing fat from products needs to be tailored on a product-by-product basis.

Although we have some innate preferences, such as positive responses to sweetness and negative to bitterness and sourness, liking for a food is predominantly learned through various mechanisms. These mechanisms include exposure effects, conditioning, associative learning and learning from models. There has been some discussion about whether we have an inherent tendency to prefer high-fat foods. The arguments have revolved round the ideas that fat-related sensory perceptions, such as carrying aroma compounds or creamy and smooth texture attributes may be innately appealing. In many fat-containing foods both innately positive sweetness and high fat content are combined to create highly palatable products. Yet, the most likely reason for preference for fat-containing foods is the high energy content of fat which produces satiety. The preferences for flavours can be acquired with pairing a flavour with energy content. This may be a mechanism that also enhances our liking for high-fat foods (e.g. Mela, 1990). With the large amount of good-tasting food constantly available, this mechanism may have become maladaptive and may contribute to the increasing problem of overweight and obesity in developed countries. The relationship between preferences and fat intake is not explicit. In a study by Mela and Sacchetti (1991) no positive relationship between preference for fat in products and fat intake could be established, although moderate correlation was found between fat preferences and amount of body fat. Drewnowski and Hann (1999) in their study of young women found positive correlations among liking, use frequency and percentage of energy coming from fat.

The acceptability of low-fat products has been under intensive research, as one of the trends in the food industry is to develop new low-fat or non-fat product options. Fat can be reduced from products by replacing it with various components. The impact of fat reduction on the nutritional content depends on what has been used as the fat replacement: e.g. water, fibre-based ingredients or digestible carbohydrates. However, typically lowering fat content reduces energy density of a product. There are a number of studies that have compared the sensory quality and consumer responses to low-fat and regular fat products, but comparing the studies is very hard as they have all used different target products or at least different recipes for products; the methods of reducing and replacing fat have also varied.

On the whole, regular fat products are perceived as more acceptable when only the sensory quality is taken into account (e.g. Bowen *et al.*, 2003; Devereux *et al.*, 2003; Engell *et al.*, 1998; Folkenberg and Martens, 2003; Hamilton *et al.*, 2000; Vickers and Mullan, 1997), but there are also exceptions (Helgesen *et al.*, 1998). Although the regular fat products are used as the reference points for comparisons, the objective in many of these studies has been to find out how much fat can be reduced without major changes in acceptability and also the sensory impact of fat reduction.

The amount of fat that can be reduced without a considerable negative influence on acceptability varies among product types. Tailoring the sensory quality of low-fat products is mostly carried out within food companies and remains unpublished, but a number of studies have also been published. These studies try to define how much fat can be reduced in a specific type of product without major impact on sensory quality (Drewnowski *et al.*, 1998; Malinski *et al.*, 2003) or what kind of components can be used to replace fat (Devereux *et al.*, 2003; Murphy *et al.*, 2004). There are a large number of raw materials and technologies that can be used to produce low-fat products with high sensory quality, but all these have to be customised to the target product.

10.2.2 Effect of information on liking for products

Liking ratings measure the hedonic responses to foods, and in most blind tests the regular or normal fat options are rated as more pleasant, as described above. Yet, our liking responses are influenced by all the cues that are available in the evaluation context. Ability to make low-fat choices requires information about the product, and the basic assumption has been that knowledge about the low-fat content, e.g. labelling products as reduced fat options, would evoke the positive attitudes and thus increase the perceived pleasantness of these products. Although the information is a necessary option for promoting low-fat products it may not be sufficient, and the results about the impact of information on the hedonic responses have been somewhat contradictory.

In some studies no effect of information has been observed (Aaron *et al.*, 1995; Kähkönen *et al.*, 1997) or the effect has depended on the positive attitude towards low-fat options (Aaron *et al.*, 1994). The results have also depended on the type of product in question. Biscuits with a higher fat content were preferred when no information was provided (Engell *et al.*, 1998), but with labelling, low-fat options became more liked. Similar results were obtained with yoghurts (Folkenberg and Martens, 2003). Labelling did not switch the order of liking, but when the products were presented as labelled the difference in preference was more narrowly in favour for the regular fat options of cheese and biscuits, but for crisps there was no difference between the two fat levels (Hamilton *et al.*, 2000). When high-fat milkshakes were labelled as low-fat they received higher hedonic ratings than when they were correctly labelled in a laboratory setting with women over 50 years old (Bowen *et al.*, 2003). Sometimes a low-fat label can even reduce liking for the product. Westcombe and Wardle (1997) found that the low-fat label reduced the perceived pleasantness in cheese, but not in yoghurt. Yet, the reported likelihood of buying did not differ among cheese samples, but yoghurt with lower fat content had higher likelihood for buying than its normal or higher-fat counterpart (Westcombe and Wardle, 1997). Describing frankfurters as low-fat decreased their pleasantness ratings among men, but not in women (Kähkönen and Tuorila, 1999).

The varying label effects among product types, consumer attitudes and gender illustrate the challenges in promoting choices of low-fat foods by merely using information. Product categories carry diverse health images so that adding a low-fat label that implies increased healthfulness may have different merits depending on the product it is attached to. For some products with a negative health image, it may even be seen as inappropriate. Furthermore, foods are used in different use contexts. Some are part of meals or components in energy-providing snacks whereas others are foods eaten in social situations or used for pure pleasure-seeking. Also consumers' own attitudes and beliefs are crucial in processing label information and assessing its value.

10.2.3 Exposure to reduced fat products

People tend to like the foods they eat and choose the foods they like. Food preferences develop and are learned throughout the lifespan. Frequent exposure to foods is a mechanism that promotes the development of preferences, and those foods that are served during childhood create the basis for hedonic responses. Several studies have investigated how the exposure to low-fat products affects their preferences over time. Some studies have perceived no impact on preferences while others have observed some shifts in preferences.

In a study by Stubenitsky *et al.* (1999) participants used reduced fat sausages and chocolate bars over a period of 12 weeks. The weekly portion included two packages of eight sausages for the household and three chocolate bars for the participants' own use, adding up to roughly 24 exposures to sausages and 36 to chocolate bars. The acceptance of reduced fat products did not alter during the frequent exposure to them, regardless of whether participants knew that products were reduced fat or not. This implies that exposure as such had little impact on liking, but this may be due to the fact that pleasantness of reduced and regular fat sausages was almost identical in the beginning and only slightly lower for reduced fat option in chocolate bars. The sustained pleasantness indicates that the reduced fat products were acceptable enough for regular consumption. Pleasantness of low-fat spread increased during a week's use period, but only among those consumers who were informed about the low-fat content and had high health concern (Kähkönen *et al.*, 1996).

The perceived pleasantness of reduced fat products has to be sufficient to endorse the second choices that lead to frequent use. Exposure to reduced-fat and fat-free cream cheese did not lower the liking ratings if the switch was done gradually first from full-fat option to reduced-fat and then to fat-free, whereas a direct shift from full-fat to fat-free alternative lowered the consumption (Levis *et al.*, 2000). Gradual changes in sensory quality may be easier to accomplish than very abrupt modification to the diet. The same principle is observed in lowering salt content of products. As small changes in sodium content are difficult to perceive as lowered saltiness, reducing salt intake is easier to achieve in small steps over time.

10.2.4 Low-fat choices and their barriers in diet practices

Lack of knowledge is a factor that is frequently mentioned as a barrier against healthy eating. Europeans mentioned fat content among the most important aspects in defining the wholesomeness of a diet (Margetts *et al.*, 1997). In a study among British students, participants could recognise animal fat as a risk factor for heart disease (Wardle and Steptoe, 1991), but knowledge as such about the link between fat content and its health effects was not related to health-related dietary behaviours. In most cases the level of knowledge has not been related to dietary choices, but according to Wardle *et al.* (2000a) those whose nutritional knowledge was in the lowest quintile had higher fat intake than those whose knowledge score was in the higher quintiles. The lack of a linear relationship between knowledge and healthy choices is not surprising as food choices have many motivations. On the other hand, actual lack of knowledge on fat content hinders choices of low fat options, but most likely reasons are conflicting motivations.

The main barrier for not choosing healthy options in Norway was that liking was considered as a more important motivation for choices. Taking into account a partner's wishes was also a factor for women, and men listed the fact that others choose the foods as a barrier (Fagerli and Wandel, 1999). Similarly,

Tuorila *et al.* (2001) found that choices between fat-free and full-fat products were driven by hedonic responses. In an experimental study by Lloyd *et al.* (1995) where participants tried to reduce their fat intake according to dietary recommendations, the barriers for being able to carry out the low-fat choices was the reduced sensory pleasure, higher cost, lower convenience and lack of support from other family members. Furthermore, the ability to judge the fat content in the diet rose as a problem in making healthy choices.

Ability to make low-fat choices between product categories appear to differ because products vary in their roles in the diet and food system. In the USA (Goldberg and Strycker, 2002) the various practices for lowering fat content differed in their popularity. Trimming fat from red meat or using low-fat milk were done usually by over 50% of respondents, whereas the reported frequency for eating baked potatoes without butter or margarine, or eating low-fat cheese was 'rarely' for 56% and 48% of respondents, respectively. In Norway, the dietary changes people reported to have made during the past three years included changing to milk with lower fat content and using less fat on bread (Fagerli and Wandel, 1999). Using reduced fat products as a strategy to lower fat intake was tried by 30% of respondents in a study carried out by Lloyd *et al.* (1995). Of these only about half were happy with the change. The most tried and best liked changes were increasing fruit and vegetable intake, using reduced fat spread and reducing red meat. Strategies often tried, but proved to be hard to follow, were reducing the consumption of cakes and biscuits, snacks or cheese. Similarly, in a Dutch study, eating fewer high-fat foods was considered to be difficult to implement in dietary practices, while changes in preparation practices were more easy to accomplish (Assema *et al.*, 1999).

10.3 Fat and health: awareness among consumers

10.3.1 Role of healthiness in food choices

Foods can be categorised in many ways in relation to their assumed health effects (Fig. 10.2). Ordinary foods that contain little or no fat, an ample amount of fibre and vitamins can be considered as wholesome. Products enriched with vitamins or minerals, functional foods, organic foods or vegetarian foods all carry a health-related connotation. These foods do not necessarily differ from each other in their appearance, taste or any other directly observable product characteristics. Instead, consumers need to see the labels and get the information about the products. This means that low-fat products need to compete for consumer attention with all the other health-related messages. Healthiness is a multidimensional concept in consumers' minds and can be expressed in several ways in dietary practices, and following nutritional recommendations and making low-fat choices is only one possible path for consumers to take.

To be able to make healthy choices, consumers need information about the nutrient content or about the existence of any other beneficial compounds in the food product. Although information is a prerequisite for choosing a wholesome

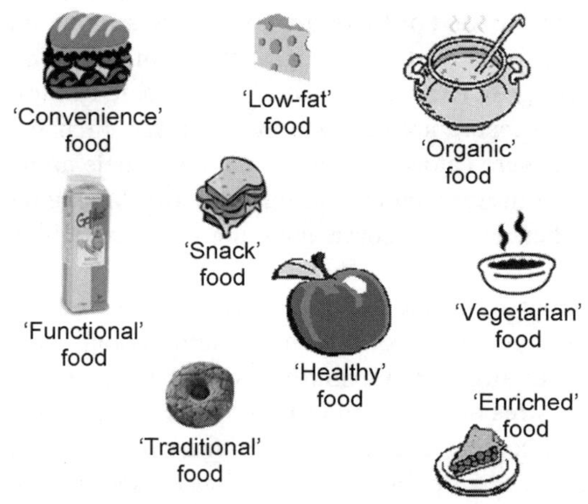

Fig. 10.2 Food products carry a number of labels that have a health-related associations.

option, it is not always a sufficient one. Healthiness is strongly a cognitive factor in food choices and those individuals who have a positive attitude towards healthiness in general tend to attach more weight to the nutritional content of food products. Roininen *et al.* (1999) developed an attitude scale to measure general health orientation. This scale has proved to be a useful tool to measure respondents health orientation among the British, Finnish and Dutch populations with the higher scores associated with choices of low-fat products (Roininen *et al.*, 2001; Zandstra *et al.*, 2001). This supports the notion that general health interest measures willingness to follow nutritional guidelines in food choices. In the study of Westcombe and Wardle (1997), higher concern for health was related to rating higher-fat labelled options of three products less pleasant, whereas positive attitude towards fat increased perceived pleasantness.

Women are more health conscious and regard avoiding fat as more important than men (Goldberg and Strycker, 2002; Roininen *et al.*, 1999; Rozin *et al.*, 1999; Wardle and Steptoe, 1991). About half of female students reported that they avoid fat and cholesterol in their diet whereas only one-third of male students did the same (Wardle and Steptoe, 1991).

10.3.2 Attitudes towards fat in food

Consumers in developed countries tend to have negative attitudes towards fat in food and fat gives a product a negative health image (Oakes and Slotterback, 2001; Oakes and Slotterback, 2002). Even 9–11-year-old children categorise healthiness of foods according to whether they contain fat or not (Noble *et al.*, 2000). When respondents were asked in a free word association task to give responses to the word 'food', American females responded more often with fat-related words, thus displaying higher concern for fat in their food compared to respondents from France or India (Rozin *et al.*, 2002). When consumers in

Finland were asked what kind of foods are considered as good for them and what as bad for them, the foods containing high amount of fat were categorised into the 'bad for me' category (Roininen *et al.*, 2000). Some of these high-fat foods were considered as pleasure giving, such as ice cream, French fries and chocolate, whereas others were categorised by some individuals not healthful and not pleasurable, such as sausages, butter and full-fat milk. Among the latter products preferences vary whereas most people unanimously report a liking for sweet fat-containing foods.

Fat can even contaminate other foods. In a study by Oakes (2005), the vitamin and mineral contents of the new combinations were perceived to decrease when fat- or sugar-containing items were added to food descriptions. Interpretation of this result is to some extent difficult since, while the absolute vitamin and mineral content does not change, the value per energy unit in food does decrease. From that point of view, consumers' comprehension is in harmony with nutritional relevance.

The negative image of fat-containing foods can be reflected on the users of these products. People judge other people according to what they eat, and healthy eating has social desirability and a moral dimension that can be reflected on the impressions we make of other people. These judgements are often subconscious and we are not fully aware of categorising people according to their dietary behaviour. Individuals consuming low-fat foods have been rated as more intelligent (Barker *et al.*, 1999; Fries and Croyle, 1993; Mooney *et al.*, 1994) and more attractive (Fries and Croyle, 1993; Mooney *et al.*, 1994) than those eating foods considered as unhealthy, fatty or fattening. On the other hand, healthy eating inserts its own negative burden in impressions: those who follow low-fat diets are also seen as more picky, self-centred (Fries and Croyle, 1993) and highly strung, and less happy (Barker *et al.*, 1999) than high-fat eaters. As could be expected, one's own fat intake influences the impressions strongly. High-fat eaters were described solely in negative terms by those who ate low-fat diets, whereas those with high-fat diets used both positive and negative terms (Barker *et al.*, 1999).

10.4 Promoting low-fat food products and diets

Several publicly supported campaigns have been launched to support low-fat choices in the diet. The two most widely used approaches have been either promoting the reduction in using high-fat foods by avoiding them or switching to low-fat options, or promoting the use of vegetables and fruits. The approach in these two messages has been very different: reducing fat intake is mostly a restrictive and negative message indicating what should not be eaten, while increasing fruit and vegetable use is a positive message, giving advice on desired behaviour. The basic assumption has been that positive messages would be easier to follow, but no difference in personal relevance or other motivational factors were found when these approaches were compared in a series of experimental studies (Brug *et al.*, 2003).

Very few of these campaigns have been evaluated in a systematic manner. Brug *et al.* (1999) have reviewed those nutrition education programmes that have used computer-generated feedback for participants on their fat intake. Those studies that aimed at the reduction of fat intake succeeded in their target. Correspondingly, when adults with elevated blood cholesterol levels participated in a guided dietary intervention, a low-fat diet was successful in lowering the fat intake and cholesterol, but had no impact on mood (Wardle *et al.*, 2000b). This suggests that following a low-fat diet does not reduce perceived well-being.

Pignone *et al.* (2003) have reviewed the effectiveness of counselling in reducing saturated fat intake or increasing fruit and vegetable consumption. Most of the controlled studies with at least three months follow-up period could be regarded as effective. From the 17 studies examining the saturated fat intake, 6 had reduced the saturated fat intake with over 3% units and 5 over 1.3% units. Similarly, seven out of ten studies on promoting vegetable consumption showed an increase of at least 0.3 servings or more per day, although very few studies clearly define how a portion was defined and what was included in the vegetable category. The more intense the counselling intervention was, the more effective it seemed to be in getting desired results, but even with less intense allocation of resources, such as newsletters mailed to home, the results were positive. Although the counselling seems to lower overall fat intake the role of single actions such as switching into low-fat or modified fat options was not assessed in the review.

Tailoring the message according to respondent's own behaviour has proved to be more effective in reducing fat intake than general information. Brug *et al.* (1999) concludes that personalised messages and information that is relevant to the respondent may be especially important in lowering the intake of fat because the sources of fat are so many. Hence, picking up those pieces that are relevant for oneself from the general messages is hard for an individual person. Furthermore, providing personalised suggestions and information about the better options may further improve the efficacy and relevance of the feedback.

Even basic information about one's own fat intake may modify the reception of health education material (Armitage and Conner, 2001). Those participants ($n = 272$) who were given an estimate of their fat intake reduced their intake of saturated fat more than those ($n = 244$) who did not receive any information when studied 5 months after the intervention. When the feedback group was further divided by the level of fat intake, the high-fat subgroup had decreased their intake more, whereas the low-fat subgroup had maintained their level of low intake. The authors argue that the personalised feedback on fat intake functioned for both of these groups as it guided those with high intake to reduce their fat consumption and supported those with low intake to maintain their consumption of fat. The original fat intake depended on participants' stage of change: those who had not even contemplated a low-fat diet had the highest fat intake (41% of the energy), whereas those who had started to restrict the fat intake or maintained a low-fat diet had the lowest intake (32% of the energy) (Armitage and Conner, 2001). However, the study population was recruited from a hospital and their motivation and awareness on health issues may be higher than in the population on average; the mean fat intake of participants was within the UK recommendation (<35% energy from fat) even at the beginning of the study.

Health promotion campaigns to targeted groups are relatively expensive to carry out. The more individual feedback they provide, the more effective they seem to be but at the same time more resources are required (Pignone *et al.*, 2003). If the individual approach is more effective than general information campaigns, the economical cost–benefit analysis should be carried out to evaluate the feasibility of these campaigns. In Brug *et al.*'s (1999) review the feedback was provided by personal letters and tailored newsletters, but the modern information technology provides Internet-based tools where immediate feedback can be constructed in a few seconds, if the tools for handling input information are appropriate and database on foods is sufficient. The computerised tools would also benefit health professionals in their counselling work. With computerised systems, large amounts of input data can not only be processed instantly but also be turned into comprehensible graphic visualisations that demonstrate the quality of diet and possible effects of changes in product choices. With these kind of tools the personal relevance of switching from a regular to low-fat option within one product category can be demonstrated; for example the contribution of milk into fat intake can be estimated in a person's diet, as it depends both on the fat content and amount consumed. The feedback systems provide instruments to motivate further changes.

10.5 Strategies to gain consumer acceptance of low-fat products

Consumers are well aware that excessive fat should be avoided in their diets, and also know that fat intake may contribute to weight gain and is a risk factor for cardiovascular diseases. In Western societies public concern supports the favourable attitude towards accepting low-fat products. Although there is a positive atmosphere for lowering fat content in the diet, there are several points that need to be taken into account when promoting the acceptance of low-fat options (Fig. 10.3).

The wide availability of low-fat options is crucial for their growing acceptability. Consumers vary in their food habits and therefore there is a need for a wide range of reduced-fat products within different product categories. The range of modified products is increasing and lowering fat is an ongoing trend in product development within companies. The challenge for these companies is to develop products with good sensory quality that has equal, or at least very close to equal, hedonic value for the consumers, as one of the major barriers against the use of low-fat options has been the reduced pleasantness (Fagerli and Wandel, 1999; Lloyd *et al.*, 1995; Tuorila *et al.*, 2001). Although people tend to like the options they are used to, switching to low-fat may be difficult if the gap in perceived pleasure is too wide (Levis *et al.*, 2000).

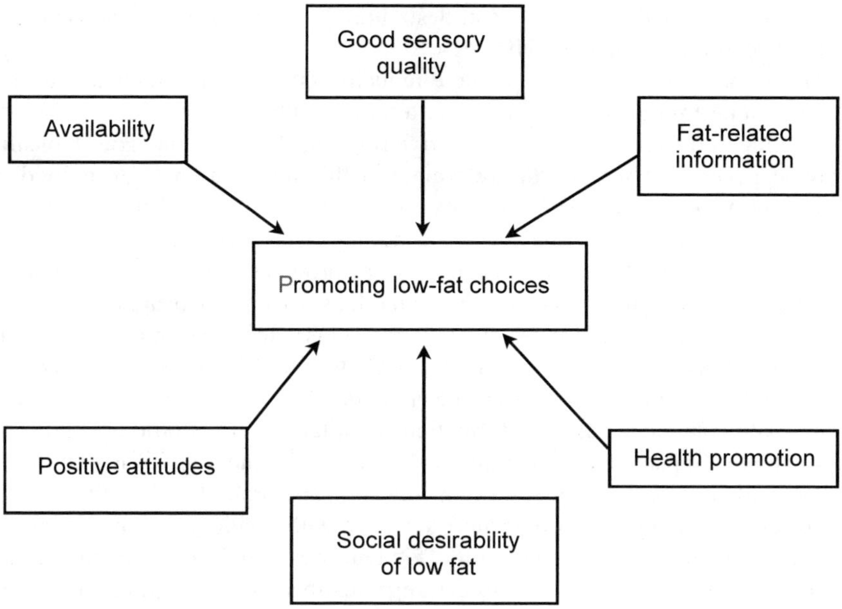

Fig. 10.3 The acceptance of low-fat products can be facilitated through several factors.

There also seem to be differences among product categories in how hard the change to low-fat options is. In general, the most challenging is to find low-fat options for high-fat foods and snacks that are used as delicacies (Assema *et al.*, 1999; Lloyd *et al.*, 1995). In these the hedonic value may have a higher role in food choices. The low-fat options tend to be more expensive than their regular counterparts, especially when new product alternatives are developed.

The attitude towards health and avoiding fat in food choices is a crucial factor in promoting low-fat choices. People pay attention to messages that are in accordance with their existing attitudes, and therefore any health-related messages are better perceived by those whose attitudes towards health in food choices are favourable. In general, both individual and societal attitudes towards fat are negative and should provide a good basis for promoting low-fat options. Although the overtly measured attitudes are negative towards fat, the conflict between pleasant taste properties of high-fat foods and subconscious impressions may interfere with attitudes (Barker *et al.*, 1999; Fagerli and Wandel, 1999; Tuorila *et al.*, 2001). Lowering fat intake is known to be beneficial, but the subconscious images of attaching low-fat eating with an impression of an unpleasant person may hinder the adoption of reduced-fat choices. This may be especially true for men, who are less health-conscious than women in general. There is a need to study these subconscious impressions that are related to food choices, in order to understand and overcome the obstacles for low-fat choices, especially among those population groups that are not openly positive towards low-fat choices and would most benefit from them. In addition to personal attitudes, social desirability has an impact on choosing and also on reporting on healthy choices.

Different campaigns try to promote reducing fat intake in the diet, and they are important for developing supportive attitudes, although their direct influence in guiding food choices may be short term. The health campaigns typically provide general advice and the relevance of this information to an individual consumer may be inadequate. The total fat intake comes from different types of products, and the role of them in contributing to the overall fat intake varies among individuals. The personal relevance of products also vary, so that some changes in diet are more easy to make than others. If consumers are not provided information that can be used to evaluate their own fat intake and recognise the products that contribute to it, the general messages may be received as such, but they are not integrated into dietary behaviours.

Providing the personalised information about fat content of products and what would be the impact of using certain low-fat options to the individual's fat intake is the challenge for the future nutrition education and promoting low-fat choices. Food-related behaviours become more scattered with smaller consumer segments that are time and context-dependent. This tendency should be responded to by developing new systems of processing health-related information where individuals could get not only feedback on their own fat-related choices, but also recommendations for desired changes and further information about the impact any changes made have had in the fat intake. The seemingly simple task of reducing fat intake in the diet requires a lot of information and the actual success relies on the correct understanding of portion sizes and the fat content of substitute foods. Novel tools to aid this process should be welcomed, and one possibility is to further develop the computer-aided feedback mechanisms into more individualised advice systems with immediate response mechanisms.

The acceptance of low-fat alternatives is increasing and consumers know they should reduce their fat intake, and mostly even feel positive about making these changes. To be able to practise low-fat choices the availability of good tasting fat-reduced alternatives is crucial. Health education promotes the positive attitude towards reducing fat, but making health-related messages more relevant for individuals together with providing better tools to monitoring one's own dietary practices would support the low-fat choices (Brug *et al.*, 1999).

10.6 Future trends

Official nutritional guidelines emphasise that fat should be consumed in moderation with special stress on the quality of fat. For those who wish to follow nutritional recommendations the low-fat options will become as standards, and the traditional regular fat options become the modifications.

There will also be alternative approaches that gain popularity, at least temporarily. The recent interest in the Atkins diet with its apparent success in weight reduction has given a different status to fat-containing foods. Another emerging trend has been the low-carbohydrate diet with special attention in avoiding carbohydrates that give high glycaemic responses. As many delicacies contain both fat and are high in sugar and thus have a high glycaemic index, the low glycaemic index diet also means reduction in fat intake. The different views and attitudes about fat will create a challenge for health promoters as individually relevant messages need to be tailored with more specificity.

10.7 References

AARON JI, MELA DJ, EVANS RE (1994), 'The influences of attitudes, beliefs and label information on perceptions of reduced fat spread.' *Appetite* **22**, 25–37.

AARON JI, EVANS RE, MELA DJ (1995), 'Paradoxical effect of a nutritional labelling scheme in a student cafeteria.' *Nutr Res* **15**, 1251–1261.

ARMITAGE CJ, CONNER M (2001), 'Efficacy of a minimal intervention to reduce fat intake.' *Soc Sci Med* **52**, 1517–1524.

ASSEMA P VAN, KEMPERS B, BRUG J, GLANZ K (1999), 'An exploratory study into Dutch consumers' experiences with implementing dietary recommendations to reduce fat intake.' *J Human Nutr Diet* **12**, 103–112.

BARKER ME, TANDY M, STOOKEY JD (1999), 'How are consumers of low-fat and high-fat diets perceived by those with lower and higher fat intake?' *Appetite* **33**, 309–317.

BOWEN D, GREEN P, VIZENOR N, VU C, KREUTER P, ROLLS B (2003), 'Effects of fat content on fat hedonics: cognition or taste.' *Phys Beh* **78**, 247–253.

BRUG J, CAMPBELL M, VAN ASSEMA P (1999), 'The application and impact of computer-generated personalized nutrition education: A review of the literature.' *Patient Educ Couns* **36**, 145–156.

BRUG J, RUITER RAC, VAN ASSEMA P (2003), 'The (ir)relevance of framing nutrition education messages.' *Nutr Health* **17**, 9–20.

DEVEREUX HM, JONES GP, MCCORMACK L, HUNTER WC (2003), 'Consumer acceptability of low fat foods containing inulin and oligofructose.' *J Food Sci* **68**, 1850–1854.

DREWNOWSKI A, HANN C (1999), 'Food preferences and reported frequencies of food consumption as predictors of current diet in young women.' *Am J Clin Nutr* **70**, 28–36.

DREWNOWSKI A, NORDENSTEN K, DWYER J (1998), 'Replacing sugar and fat in cookies: impact on product quality and preference.' *Food Qual Pref* **9**, 13–20.

ELMORE JR, HEYMANN H, JOHNSON J, HEWETT JE (1999), 'Preference mapping: relating acceptance of "creaminess" to a descriptive sensory map of a semisolid.' *Food Qual Pref* **10**, 465–475.

ENGELL D, BORDI P, BORJA M, LAMBERT C, ROLLS B (1998), 'Effects of information about fat content of food preferences in pre-adolescent children.' *Appetite* **30**, 269–282.

FAGERLI RAA, WANDEL M (1999), 'Gender differences in opinions and practices with regards to a 'healthy diet'.' *Appetite* **32**, 171–190

FOLKENBERG DM, MARTENS M (2003), 'Sensory properties of low fat yoghurts. Part B: hedonic evaluations of plain yoghurts by consumers correlated to fat content, sensory profile and consumer attitudes.' *Milchwissenschaft* **58**, 154–157.

FRIES E, CROYLE RT (1993), 'Stereotypes associated with a low-fat diet and their relevance to nutrition education.' *J Am Diet Assoc* **93**, 551–555.

GOLDBERG LR, STRYCKER LA (2002), 'Personality traits and eating habits: the assessment of food preferences in a large community sample.' *Pers Ind Diff* **32,** 49–65.

HAMILTON J, KNOX B, HILL D, PARR H (2000), 'Reduced fat products. Consumer perceptions and preferences.' *Br Food J* **102**, 494–504.

HELGESEN H, SOLHEIM R, NAES T (1998), 'Consumer purchase probability of dry fermented lamb sausages.' *Food Qual Pref* **9**, 295–301.

KÄHKÖNEN P, TUORILA H (1999), 'Consumer responses to reduced and regular fat content in different products: effects of gender, involvement and health concern.' *Food Qual Pref* **10**, 83–91.

KÄHKÖNEN P, TUORILA H, RITA H (1996), 'How information enhances acceptability of a low-fat spread.' *Food Qual Pref* **7**, 87–94.

KÄHKÖNEN P, TUORILA H, LAWLESS H (1997), 'Lack of effect of taste and nutrition claims on sensory and hedonic responses to a fat-free yoghurt'. *Food Qual Pref 8*, 125–130.

LAPPALAINEN R, KEARNEY J, GIBNEY M (1998), 'A Pan EU survey of consumer attitudes to food, nutrition and health: an overview.' *Food Qual Pref* **9**, 467–478.

LEVIS PA, CHAMBERS EIV, JOHNSON DE (2000), 'Consumption and liking of a fat modified product using short trials.' *Nutr Res* **20**, 791–804.

LLOYD HM, PAISLEY CM, MELA DJ (1995), 'Barriers to the adoption of reduced-fat diets in a UK population.' *J Am Diet Assoc* **95**, 316-322.

MALINSKI E, DANIEL JR, ZHANG XX, WHISTLER RL (2003), 'Isolation of small starch granules and determination of their fat mimic characteristics.' *Cereal Chem* **80**, 1–4.

MARGETTS B M, MARTINEZ J A, SABA A, HOLM L, KEARNEY M (1997), 'Definitions of 'healthy' eating: a pan-EU survey of consumer attitudes to food, nutrition and health.' *Eur J Clin Nutr* **51** (Suppl. 2), S23–S29.

MELA DJ (1990), 'The basis of dietary fat preferences.' *Trends Food Sci Tech* **1**, 71–73.

MELA DJ, SACCHETTI DA (1991), 'Sensory preferences for fats: relationships with diet and body composition.' *Am J Clin Nutr* **53**, 908–915.

MOONEY KM, DETORE J, MALLOY KA (1994), 'Perceptions of women related to food choice.' *Sex Roles* **31**, 433–442.

MURPHY SC, GILROY D, KERRY JF, BUCKLEY DJ, KERRY JP (2004), 'Evaluation of surimi, fat and water content in a low/no added pork sausage formulation using response surface methodology.' *Meat Sci* **66**, 689–701.

NOBLE C, CORNEY M, EVES A, KIPPS M, LUMBERS M (2000), 'Food choice and school meals: primary schoolchilren's perceptions of the healthiness of foods and nutritional implications of food choices.' *Hospitability Man* **19**, 413–432.

OAKES M (2005), 'Bad company: the addition of sugar, fat, or salt reduces the perceived vitamin and mineral content of foods.' *Food Qual Pref* **16**, 111–119.

OAKES ME, SLOTTERBACK CS (2001), 'Judgements of food healthfulness: food name stereotypes in adults over age 25.' *Appetite* **37**, 1–8.

OAKES ME, SLOTTERBACK CS (2002), 'The good, the bad, and the ugly: characteristics used by young, middle-aged, and older men and women, dieters and non-dieters to judge healthfulness of foods.' *Appetite* **38**, 91–97.

PIGNONE MP, AMMERMAN A, FERNANDEZ L, ORLEANS CT, PENDER N, WOOLF S, LOHR KN, SUTTON S (2003) 'Counseling to promote a healthy diet in adults.' *Am J Prev Med* **24**, 75–92.

RICHARDSON-HARMAN NJ, STEVENS R, WALKER S, GAMBLE J. MILLER M, WONG M, MCPHERSON A (2000), 'Mapping consumer perceptions of creaminess and liking for liquid dairy products.' *Food Qual Pref* **11**, 239–246.

ROININEN K, LÄHTEENMÄKI L, TUORILA H (1999), 'Quantification of consumer attitudes to health and hedonic characteristics of foods.' *Appetite,* **33**, 71–88.

ROININEN K, LÄHTEENMÄKI L, TUORILA H (2000), 'An application of means-end chain approach to consumers' orientation to health and hedonic characteristics of foods.' *Ecology Food Nutr* **39**, 61–81.

ROININEN K, TUORILA H, ZANDSTRA E H, DE GRAAF C, VEHKALAHTI K, STUBENITSKY K, MELA D J (2001), 'Differences in health and taste attitudes and reported behavior among Finnish, Dutch and British consumers: a cross-national validation of the health and taste attitude scales (HTAS)', *Appetite* **37**, 33–45.

ROZIN P, FISCHLER C, IMADA S, SARUBIN A, WRZESNIEWSKI A (1999), 'Atttiudes to food and the role of food in life in the USA, Japan, Flemish Belgium and France: possible implications to diet-health debate.' *Appetite* **33**, 163–180.

ROZIN P, KURZER N, COHEN AB (2002), 'Free associations to "food": the effects of gender, generation and culture.' *J Res Pers* **36**, 419–441.

STUBENITSKY K, AARON JI, CATT SL, MELA DJ (1999), 'Effect of information and extended use on the acceptance of reduced fat products.' *Food Qual Pref* **10**, 367–376.

TUORILA H, KRAMER FM, ENGELL D (2001), 'The choice of fat free vs. regular-fat fudge: the effects of liking for the alternative and the restraint status.' *Appetite* **37**, 27–32.

VICKERS Z, MULLAN L (1997), 'Liking and consumption of fat-free and full-fat cheese.' *Food Qual Pref* **8**, 91–95.

WARDLE J, STEPTOE A (1991), 'The European health and behaviour survey: rationale, methods and initial results from the United Kingdom.' *Soc Sci Med* **33,** 925-936.

WARDLE J, PARMENTER K, WALLER J (2000a), 'Nutrition knowledge and food intake.' *Appetite* **34**, 269–275.

WARDLE J, ROGERS P, JUDD P, TAYLOR MA, RAPOPORT L, GREEN M, NICHOLSON PERRY K (2000b), 'Randomized trial of the effects of cholesterol-lowering dietary treatment on physiological function.' *Am J Med* **108**, 547–553.

WESTCOMBE A, WARDLE J (1997), 'Influence of relative fat content information on responses to three foods.' *Appetite* **28**, 49–62.

ZANDSTRA EH, DE GRAAF C, VAN STAVEREN WA (2001), 'Influence of health and taste attitudes on consumption of low- and high-fat foods.' *Food Qual Pref* **12**, 75–82.

11

Optimising dairy milk fatty acid composition

D. I. Givens, University of Reading, UK and K. J. Shingfield, MTT AgriFood Research Finland, Finland

11.1 Introduction

Milk is a very complex food of great interest, not least since it is intended to be complete food for young animals. The key role of cow's milk in the human diet as a supplier of fats, amino acids and other key nutrients such as calcium has been recognised for a long time. Milk is essentially a complex colloidal system comprising globules of milk fat suspended in an aqueous medium containing lactose, a range of proteins, mineral salts and water-soluble vitamins. Typical milk from Holstein/Friesian cows will contain about 40, 36 and 45 g/kg of fat, protein and lactose, respectively, with an energy content of approximately 2.8 MJ/kg. The fat content of milk can vary considerably depending on the breed and nutrition of the cow. The effect of breed is reflected in the higher fat content of milk from Channel Island breeds (typically about 65 g/kg) compared with the Friesian/Holstein (typically about 35 g/kg). Overall in the UK, liquid milk, milk and dairy-derived foods contribute about 15% of the total energy intake (Givens and Shingfield, 2004) but a concern is that a high proportion (>0.5) of this energy is derived from fat.

Globally the demand for animal-derived foods in general is growing at a fast rate driven by a combination of population growth, urbanisation and rising income. Table 11.1 shows the trends in milk consumption over the past 40 years for various parts of the world. Although the historical and projected trend is upward, in the UK consumption of whole milk has halved between 1990 (mean 1232 ml/person/day) and 2000 (mean 664 ml/person/day), but consumption of semi-skimmed milk has almost doubled during this period (mean 975 ml/person/day in 2000) (DEFRA, 2001). At present, milk and dairy-derived foods are

Table 11.1 Trends in consumption of milk (from WHO/FAO, 2003)

Region	Milk (kg/person/year) 1964–66	1977–99	2030[1]
World	73.9	78.1	89.5
Developing countries	28.0	44.6	65.8
Transition countries	156.7	159.1	178.7
Industrialised countries	185.5	212.2	221.0

[1]Projected.

available in many forms and the contribution of the major dairy foods to nutrient and energy intakes of the UK population during 2000 is shown in Table 11.2. Milk and dairy food products are clearly major sources of calcium but contribute about 24% of the total fat consumed if butter is included (about 18% excluding butter).

Since the lipids in milk and dairy food products contain relatively large amounts of saturated fatty acids compared with other animal-derived lipids and notably more than lipids in chicken meat for example (Table 11.3), milk and dairy products make a major contribution to saturated fatty acid intake. A study on fatty acid intake across Europe (Hulshof *et al.*, 1999) showed that milk and milk-derived foods (including cheese and butter) were consistently the largest source of saturated fatty acids with the highest values seen in Germany and France where almost 60% of saturates came from this source. In the UK the contribution was almost 40% (Fig. 11.1). Interestingly, the contribution of butter to saturated fatty acid intake varied widely. In Greece, Spain, The Netherlands and Norway butter provided less than 5%, whereas high contributions were recorded in France (30%) and Germany (39%) with the UK being intermediate (10%). Also of note was the fact that across the countries studied, milk and milk derived foods contributed on average almost 40% of all *trans* fatty acids consumed. The contribution in Germany and France was particularly high at approximately 70 and 60% respectively although in the UK this was lower (24%). In all countries the predominant *trans* fatty acids were *trans* C18:1.

11.2 Milk fat synthesis

Milk fat comprises a complex mixture of lipids, most of which are present as triacylglycerides (about 98%), in addition to small amounts of di- and mono-acylglycerides, phospholipids, cholesterol and non-esterified fatty acids (Christie, 1995). Fatty acids secreted in milk originate from two sources, direct incorporation from the peripheral circulation and *de novo* synthesis in the mammary gland. *De novo* synthesis accounts for all C4:0 to C12:0, most of the C14:0 and about 50% of the C16:0 fatty acids in milk, whereas all C18:0 and longer chain fatty acids are derived entirely from circulating plasma lipids

Table 11.2 Energy and selected nutrients provided by milk and dairy products in the UK during 2000[1]

Nutrient	Liquid whole milk	Semi-skimmed milk	Full skimmed milk	Yoghurt and fromage frais	Cream	Butter	Cheese	Total
Energy								
Intake (MJ/day)	0.27	0.28	0.033	0.081	0.021	0.17	0.26	1.12
% of MDI[2]	3.7	3.8	0.45	1.1	0.28	2.3	3.6	15.3
Protein								
Intake (g/day)	3.2	4.9	0.82	1.2	0.08	0.03	3.8	14.0
% of MDI	4.9	7.4	1.2	1.8	0.1	0.1	5.7	21.1
Fat								
Intake (g/day)	3.8	2.4	0.05	1.1	0.49	4.6	5.3	17.8
% of MDI	5.1	3.3	0.1	1.5	0.7	6.2	7.2	24.1
Calcium								
Intake (mg/day)	115	173	29.4	31.2	2.3	1.0	113	465
% of MDI	13.4	20.0	3.4	3.6	0.3	0.1	13.1	54.0
Phosphorus								
Intake (mg/day)	90.9	135	23.2	29.5	2.0	0.1	85.7	366
% of ARDA[3]	16.5	24.5	4.2	5.4	0.36	0.02	15.6	66.5
Magnesium								
Intake (mg/day)	10.7	15.8	2.7	3.0	0.2	0.1	4.51	37.0
% of ARDA	3.8	5.5	0.95	1.1	0.07	0.04	1.6	13.0

[1]Data derived from a combination of the National Food Survey (DEFRA, 2001) and Food Standards Agency (2003).
[2]MDI, mean daily intake from the National Food Survey (DEFRA, 2001).
[3]ARDA, adult recommended daily allowance from Department of Health (1991).

Table 11.3 Typical fatty acid composition of milk and white chicken meat (adapted from McCance & Widdowson, 1998)

Fatty acid (g/100 g total fatty acids)	Cow's milk	Chicken meat (white)
C4:0	3.88	0
C6:0	2.49	0
C8:0	1.39	0
C10:0	3.05	0
C10:1	0.28	0
C11:0	1.39	0
C12:0	4.16	0
C14:0	11.36	0.99
C14:1 *cis*-9	1.11	0.00
C15:0	1.11	1.98
C16:0	29.36	21.78
C16:1 *cis*-9	1.94	3.96
C17:0	0.55	0.99
C17:1 *cis*-10	0.28	0.99
C18:0	11.36	6.93
C18:1 *cis*-9	21.88	39.60
C18:1 *trans*-11	0.28	2.97
C18:2 (n-6)	1.94	15.84
C18:3 (n-3)	0.55	1.98
C20:0	0.00	0.00
C20:5 (n-3)	0.00	0.99
C22:5 (n-3)	0.83	0.99
Summary		
Total saturates	70.08	32.67
Total MUFA	25.76	47.52
Total PUFA	3.32	19.80
n-6 PUFA	1.94	15.84
n-3 PUFA	1.39	3.96

(Hawke and Taylor, 1995). In most situations, direct uptake from plasma accounts for about 60% of the total amount of fatty acids secreted in milk (Chilliard *et al*., 2000).

De novo fatty acid synthesis in the mammary gland has an absolute requirement for carbon in the form of acetyl-CoA, the activity of two key enzymes (acetyl-CoA carboxylase and fatty acid synthetase) and a supply of NADPH-reducing equivalents (Hawke and Taylor, 1995). Acetate, and to a lesser extent β-hydroxybutyrate, contribute to the initial four carbon units required for fatty acid synthesis. Acetate is converted to acetyl Co A in the cytosol and incorporated into fatty acids via the malonyl-Co A pathway, whereas β-hydroxybutyrate is incorporated directly following activation to butyl Co A (Murphy, 2000). Acetyl, butyl and malonyl-Co A condense within the fatty acid synthetase complex with malonyl-Co A groups being continually added, thus promoting chain elongation. A distinctive feature of the bovine mammary gland is the

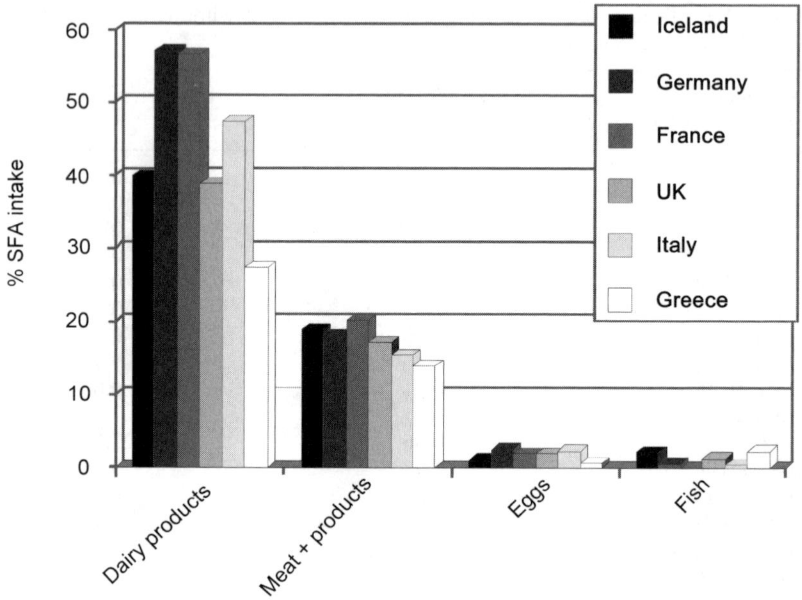

Fig. 11.1 Contribution of animal products to saturated fatty acid (SFA) intake in some European countries (from Hulsof *et al.*, 1999).

ability to release fatty acids from the synthetase complex at various stages, resulting in the secretion of a wide range of short and medium chain fatty acids.

Following intestinal absorption, long chain fatty acids are transported to the mammary gland in plasma in the form of non-esterified fatty acids and triacylglyceride-rich chylomicrons and very low-density lipoproteins (Chilliard *et al.*, 2000). Mammary uptake of low and high-density lipoproteins is fairly limited (Offer *et al.*, 2001b), which accounts, in part at least, for the low transfer efficiency of absorbed very long chain fatty acids into milk (Chilliard *et al.*, 2001; Rymer *et al.*, 2003).

Owing to extensive biohydrogenation of dietary unsaturated fatty acids in the rumen, C18:0 is normally the predominant long chain fatty acid available for absorption. However, *cis*-9 C18:1 output in milk exceeds that taken up from plasma due to the activity of stearoyl Co A (Δ-9) desaturase in mammary secretory cells (Kinsella, 1972). The insertion of the *cis*-9 double bond is believed to occur to ensure milk fluidity which is necessary for efficient ejection from the mammary gland (Grummer, 1991). Desaturation of C18:0 to *cis*-9 C18:1 is the main precursor product of the Δ-9 desaturase system and about 40% of C18:0 taken up by the gland can be converted (Chilliard *et al.*, 2000). Desaturation of C14:0 and C16:0 also occurs and more recent studies have shown that *trans*-11 C18:1, *trans*-12 C18:1 (Griinari *et al.*, 2000) and *trans*-7 C18:1 (Corl *et al.*, 2002; Piperova *et al.*, 2002) are also converted to *cis*-9,*trans*-11 C18:2, cis-9,*trans*-12 C18:2 and *trans*-7,*cis*-9 C18:2, respectively.

The *cis*-9,*trans*-11 C18:2 in milk is derived from two sources: formation in the rumen during metabolism of C18:2 n-6 in the diet and by endogenous synthesis in the mammary gland. Several studies have been conducted to assess the relative importance of these sources, based on measurements of milk fatty acid composition in response to post-ruminal infusions of sterculic acid that inhibits the activity of Δ-9 desaturase in the mammary gland or from the comparison of ruminal outflow and secretion of *cis*-9,*trans*-11 C18:2 in milk. Even though different approaches have been used, these suggest that proportionately between 70 and 90% of *cis*-9,*trans*-11 C18:2 in milk originates from endogenous conversion of *trans*-11 C18:1 in the mammary gland (Bauman *et al.*, 2003, Palmquist *et al.*, 2005). Typically, *trans*-7,*cis*-9 C18:2 is the second most abundant conjugated C18:2 isomer in milk fat (Sehat *et al.*, 1998; Yurawecz *et al.*, 1998). Ruminal formation of *trans*-7,*cis*-9 C18:2 is negligible (Corl *et al.*, 2002; Piperova *et al.*, 2002; Shingfield *et al.*, 2003) and therefore its appearance in milk is essentially derived from *trans*-7 C18:1 produced in the rumen. In contrast to *trans*-7,*cis*-9 and *cis*-9,*trans*-11, other conjugated C18:2 isomers in milk appear to be derived exclusively from metabolism of polyunsaturated C18 fatty acids in the rumen (Piperova *et al.*, 2002; Shingfield *et al.*, 2003).

Preformed and *de novo* synthesised fatty acids are incorporated into triacylglycerides via the glycerol-3-phosphate pathway (Hawke and Taylor, 1995). Proportionately between 0.50 and 0.60 of glycerol-3-phosphate is estimated to be derived from glucose, while the remainder comes from the glycerol released during lipolysis of plasma triacylglycerides (Bauman and Davis, 1974). In spite of sequential addition to the glycerol backbone, fatty acids are not randomly distributed within triacylglycerides. Saturated fatty acids are inserted mainly in the sn-1 position with shorter chain and unsaturated fatty acids in the sn-2 position, while C18 and long chain fatty acids are located in the sn-3 position (Demeyer and Doreau, 1999). In situations where short chain fatty acids are in short supply, such as in early lactation, the shortfall is thought to be compensated for by the provision of C18:1 fatty acids at the sn-3 position of the milk fat triacylglyceride (Hawke and Taylor, 1995).

11.3 The need to change the fatty acid composition of milk fat

11.3.1 Effects on plasma lipids

The relationship between dietary fat type and intake and cardiovascular disease (particularly coronary heart disease) has been extensively reported with strong and consistent associations seen from a wide body of data (Kris-Etherton *et al.*, 2001). While in general, saturated fatty acids raise total and low-density lipoprotein (LDL) cholesterol, individual fatty acids have markedly different effects. In particular myristic (C14:0) and palmitic (C16:0) acids have been associated with elevated plasma LDL cholesterol concentrations in human subjects (Katan *et al.*, 1995; Temme *et al.*, 1996) while the other major saturated fatty acid in foods, stearic acid (C18:0), has been shown to be essentially neutral (Bonanome and Grundy, 1988). Some studies suggest that lauric acid (C12:0) and C14:0 have more potent effects on plasma cholesterol than C16:0, while others suggest that C14:0 and C16:0 are more potent than C12:0. In any event, palmitic acid is quantitatively the most important saturated fatty acid in milk fat (Table 11.3).

Most of the C12:0 and C14:0 in the human diet is derived from milk fat (Gunstone *et al.*, 1994), and therefore the consumption of milk and dairy foods would be expected to have adverse effects on plasma cholesterol levels. The results from a large longitudinal cohort study of 2778 black and white men and women initially aged 18–30-years-old appear to support this (Steffen and Jacobs, 2003). In this study diet was assessed over a 7-year period and the various plasma cholesterol fractions measured. Plasma LDL cholesterol increased by 0.078 mmol/l across all quintiles of high-fat dairy intake ($P < 0.05$) although the authors proposed that the true mean increase was likely to be three to six times greater (0.26–0.47 mmol/l) after correction for within-subject errors in dietary assessment. However, it was evident from this study that volunteers consuming low-fat milk produced lower plasma concentrations of total and high-density lipoprotein (HDL) cholesterol, while those who consumed cream and butter produced higher levels of of total and HDL cholesterol.

The replacement of saturated fatty acids by both monounsaturated fatty acids (MUFAs) and polyunsaturated fatty acids (PUFAs) results in lower plasma total and LDL cholesterol and may have other beneficial outcomes. Recent work has for example shown that, *in vitro* at least, oleic acid may have an important role to play in inhibiting the growth of breast cancer cells (Menendez *et al.*, 2005). Although the cholesterol-lowering response to PUFA is greater than that of MUFA there has been some caution in recommending high-PUFA diets because of potentially adverse health effects of their lipoperoxidation products (Williams, 2000). Three important n-3 PUFAs are eicosapentaenoic acid (EPA C20:5 n-3), docosahexaenoic acids (DHA C22:6 n-3) and α-linolenic acid (C18:3 n-3). A substantial body of epidemiological data supports the cardioprotective actions of EPA/DHA as do intervention studies in populations at risk of cardiovascular disease (CVD). These data have led to a widespread belief that there should be small increases in n-3 PUFA intake (see Williams, 2000, for details). In general, fats in animal-derived foods are very poor sources of n-3 PUFA.

11.3.2 Effects on insulin sensitivity

Most attention has focused on the hypercholesterolaemic effect of saturated fatty acids and associated increases in CVD risk; however, there is now some evidence that high intakes of saturated fatty acids may also be related to reduced insulin sensitivity, which is a key factor in the development of the metabolic syndrome (Nugent, 2004). In epidemiological studies, high intakes of saturated fats have been associated with a higher risk of impaired glucose tolerance and higher fasting plasma glucose and insulin concentrations (Feskens and

Table 11.4 Effect of challenge with saturated fatty acids (SFA) or monounsaturated fatty acids (MUFA) on insulin parameters, plasma glucose and serum lipids in healthy men and women (from Vessby *et al.*, 2001)

	SFA diet			MUFA diet		
Measurement	Change[1]	Change (%)	P value	Change[1]	Change (%)	P value
Insulin sensitivity index (Si)	−4.2	−10.3	0.032	+0.10	+12.1	0.518
Serum insulin (mU/l)	+0.25	+3.5	0.466	−0.35	−5.8	0.049
Plasma glucose (mmol/l)	0.00	±0	0.995	−0.03	−0.60	0.413
Total cholesterol (mmol/l)	+0.14	+2.5	0.018	−0.15	−2.7	0.012
LDL cholesterol (mmol/l)	+0.15	+4.1	0.006	−0.19	−5.2	0.006

[1]Mean change during treatment expressed as least square mean.

Kromhout, 1990; Parker *et al.*, 1993; Feskens *et al.*, 1995). Notably, in a recent 3-month intervention study involving 162 healthy subjects (Vessby *et al.*, 2001) given diets rich in saturated fatty acids (from butter and margarine) or MUFA (from high oleic sunflower oil) showed that those on the saturated fatty acid diet had significantly impaired insulin sensitivity (−10%) while those on the MUFA diet showed no change (Table 11.4). Also of note in this study was that additional dietary inclusion of n-3 fatty acids from fish oil had no effect on insulin sensitivity or insulin secretion and the favourable effects of the MUFA diet were not seen in individuals with a high fat intake (>37% of energy intake).

The evidence summarised above clearly points to the need to reduce the intake of saturated fatty acids and the potential benefits from replacing them with MUFA and PUFA. Given the current contribution of milk and dairy-derived foods to the consumption of saturated fatty acids it is highly questionable as to whether the present situation is sustainable with respect to long-term human health.

Milk and dairy products are the main source of conjugated C18:2 in the human diet (Ritzenthaler *et al.*, 2001; Parodi, 2003) and there is evidence from studies with mice, hamsters and pigs to suggest that conjugated C18:2, the *trans*-10,*cis*-12 isomer in particular, causes hyperinsulinaemia and insulin resistance, which may be related to the inhibitory effects of this isomer on Δ-9 desaturase activity (Terpstra, 2004). However, a recent controlled intervention study with healthy men consuming relatively pure supplements of *cis*-9, *trans*-11 or *trans*-10,*cis*-12 C18:2 across a wide range of intakes (0.59–2.38 and 0.63–2.52 g/day) indicated no significant effects on plasma insulin concentrations, the homeostasis model for insulin resistance or on indices of insulin sensitivity (Tricon *et al.*, 2004). Furthermore, the concentration of *trans*-10,*cis*-12 C18:2 in milk fat is extremely low across a wide range of dairy cow diets (Sehat *et al.*, 1998; Piperova *et al.*, 2002; Shingfield *et al.*, 2003, 2005a), indicating that the contribution of milk and dairy products to *trans*-10,*cis*-12 C18:2 consumption in the human population would be extremely small.

11.4 Factors affecting milk fatty acid composition

Milk fatty acid composition can be manipulated by nutritional means or through exploitation of naturally occurring genetic variation. Even though changes in milk fatty acid composition have typically been realised by inclusion of lipid supplements in the diet, genotype is also an important factor. Milk from Jersey cows contains more fat than that from Holsteins (Drackley *et al.*, 2001; White *et al.*, 2001) and the proportion of C6:0 to C14:0 of total fatty acids, has, irrespective of diet, been reported to be lower in milk from Holstein than Jersey cows (Beaulieu and Palmquist, 1995). Comparisons of milk fatty acid composition of milk from cows of different breeds (Table 11.5) are consistent with the activity of Δ^9-desaturase being lower and the proportion of fatty acids in milk synthesised *de novo* being greater for the Channel Island breeds than the Holstein (Beaulieu and Palmquist, 1995). In a comparison of the Irish Holstein–Friesian, Dutch Holstein–Friesian, Montbeliardes and Normandes cows grazing the same pasture, Lawless *et al.* (1999) concluded that while there were differences between these breeds in the concentrations of C16:0, C18:0 and C18:1, it is questionable if these are sufficiently large to be of practical importance. Genetic selection for increased milk fat content also results in altered milk fatty acid composition, causing an increase in the proportion of short-chain fatty acids and a concomitant reduction in the amount of long-chained fatty acids (Palmquist *et al.*, 1993).

During the onset of lactation, the energy requirements for milk production exceed nutrient intake, and cows experience a period of negative energy balance, causing the mobilisation of long-chained fatty acids from adipose tissue and incorporation into milk fat. Irrespective of diet, the proportion of C6:0 to C12:0 is lower, and that of C18:0 and *cis*-9 C18:1 are higher in milk produced from cows in early lactation (< 30 days in milk) compared with mid (120 days) or late (210 days) lactation (Palmquist *et al.*, 1993; Auldist *et al.*, 1998). The distinctive changes in milk fatty acid composition associated during advances in the stage of lactation appear to reflect the contribution of mobilised adipose tissue to mammary fatty acid supply and the inhibitory effects of high mammary uptakes of long-chained fatty acids on *de novo* fatty acid synthesis.

It might be expected that the effect of diet during early lactation when substantial amounts of tissue lipids are being mobilised would be relatively small, but there is considerable evidence to indicate that nutrition has a greater effect on milk fatty acid composition in early than mid or late lactation (Chilliard, 1993; Palmquist *et al.*, 1993). Early studies demonstrated that the transfer efficiency of intravenously infused labelled triacylglycerides to milk declined from 30% in early lactation to 5% in late lactation, changes that have been attributed to a higher proportion of absorbed fatty acids being partitioned towards the mammary tissue during negative energy balance, an effect that declines as lactation progresses (Grummer, 1991). Even though it is clear that the stage of lactation, as related to the mobilisation of body fat stores, is an important determinant of milk fatty acid composition, these effects are relatively

Table 11.5 Effect of genotype on the fatty acid composition of bovine milk

Breed	Diet	C4:0	C6:0	C8:0	C10:0	C12:0	C14:0	C16:0	C18:0	*cis*-C18:1	*trans*-C18:1	Total C18:1	C18:2 (n-6)	CLA	C18:3 (n-3)	Reference
		Milk fatty acid composition (g/100g total fatty acids)														
Jersey	a	NR	0.9	0.9	2.9	4.0	10.9	32.4	14.4	NR	NR	22.1	3.5	NR	0.65	Stull and Brown (1964)
Guernsey	a	NR	1.0	0.9	2.5	3.1	10.5	32.9	14.9	NR	NR	22.6	3.5	NR	0.77	
Holstein	a	NR	0.8	0.8	2.2	2.9	9.9	30.7	14.2	NR	NR	25.4	3.7	NR	0.96	
Jersey	b	4.1	2.4	1.3	3.0	3.5	11.6	32.4	7.2	17.3	NR	NR	2.2	NR	0.48	Beaulieu and Palmquist
Holstein	b	4.0	2.8	1.8	4.3	5.0	12.6	30.2	8.1	15.1	NR	NR	2.2	NR	0.40	(1995)
Irish Holstein–Friesian	c	1.0	1.2	1.1	2.9	3.7	10.9	24.1	11.2	20.3	5.8	26.1	1.1	1.84	0.84	Lawless *et al.* (1999)
Dutch Holstein–Friesian	c	1.1	1.2	1.0	2.6	3.3	10.7	25.8	10.4	20.9	5.3	26.2	1.0	1.76	0.82	
Montbeliardes	c	1.0	1.2	1.0	2.8	3.5	11.0	22.8	11.5	21.8	5.8	27.6	1.1	1.99	0.83	
Normandes	c	1.1	1.2	1.0	2.8	3.6	10.9	23.7	11.9	21.1	5.5	26.6	1.1	1.67	0.77	
Jersey	d	1.1	1.7	1.2	2.7	3.1	10.4	31.3	15.5	NR	NR	20.9	2.5	0.32	0.37	White *et al.* (2001)
Holstein	d	1.1	1.5	0.9	2.0	2.3	9.4	31.7	15.4	NR	NR	23.3	2.5	0.41	0.38	
Brown Swiss	e	5.2	2.1	1.1	2.4	2.6	8.5	28.3	11.9	24.5	3.4	27.9	3.4	0.41	0.38	Kelsey *et al.* (2003)
Holstein	e	4.6	1.9	1.0	2.1	2.3	8.2	28.1	12.3	25.0	4.0	29.0	3.6	0.44	0.39	

[a] Lucerne hay and concentrates.
[b] Total mixed ration containing (g/kg dry matter) maize silage (300), Lucerne hay (250) and concentrates (450) supplemented with 750 g/day of calcium salts of palm oil distillate.
[c] Grazed grass.
[d] Total mixed ration containing (g/kg dry matter) maize silage (293), Lucerne silage (297) and concentrates (410).
[e] Total mixed ration containing (g/kg dry matter) Lucerne hay (369), steam flaked maize (282) and concentrates (349).
NR: not reported.
CLA refers to *cis*-9, *trans*-11 C18:2.

short term and are essentially complete within the first 4 to 6 weeks of lactation (Palmquist *et al.*, 1993).

Milk fat content and fatty acid composition can be significantly altered through nutrition, offering the opportunity to respond to changes in consumer requirements and provide foods more in line with recommendations for improving human health. The effect of nutrition on milk fatty acid composition has been extensively reviewed (Grummer, 1991; Palmquist *et al.*, 1993; Doreau *et al.*, 1999; Chilliard *et al.*, 2000, 2001; Jensen, 2002; Chilliard and Ferlay, 2004; Lock and Shingfield, 2004) and it is clear that within certain biological constraints, diets can be formulated to effect relatively large changes in milk fatty acid composition. However, the extent of changes in milk fatty acid composition that can be achieved through diet is significantly affected by lipid metabolism in the rumen, which serves to substantially alter the profile of fatty acids available for absorption.

Dairy cow diets typically contain low amounts of lipid (20–50 g/kg dry matter), but high proportions of PUFA as a result of C18:3 n-3 predominating in grasses and legumes and cereal grains and maize silage being rich in C18:2 n-6. Despite consuming diets rich in PUFA, C18:0 is the major C18 fatty acid absorbed in ruminant animals, owing to extensive metabolism of dietary lipids in the rumen. On entering the rumen, dietary lipids are exposed to microbial lipases that catalyse the hydrolysis of ester bonds in glycolipids, triacylglycerides and phospholipids, resulting in the release of non-esterified fatty acids (NEFA). The extent of hydrolysis is generally high (>85%), being higher for diets rich in protein, but decreased when high concentrate diets or mature forages are fed (Harfoot and Hazlewood, 1988; Doreau and Ferlay, 1994; Palmquist *et al.*, 2005). The NEFA released during hydrolysis are adsorbed onto feed particles and can be exposed to further metabolism, in a process generally referred to as biohydrogenation, or directly incorporated into bacterial lipids (Demeyer and Doreau, 1999). The presence of a free carboxyl group is an absolute requirement for the biohydrogenation of unsaturated NEFA, and as a result the rate of biohydrogenation is lower than that of hydrolysis, such that factors affecting lipolysis of dietary lipids in the rumen also impact on biohydrogenation. A wide range of rumen bacteria have lipolytic activity, but few species capable of biohydrogenation have been identified. Biohydrogenation of dietary fatty acids is extensive and for most diets proportionately 0.50–0.70, 0.70–0.95 and 0.85–1.00 of *cis*-9 C18:1, C18:2 n-6 and C18:3 n-3, respectively, is metabolised in the rumen (Harfoot and Hazlewood, 1988; Doreau and Ferlay, 1994; Demeyer and Doreau, 1999). The final reduction appears to be the rate-limiting step of biohydrogenation, and therefore *trans* C18:1 intermediates can accumulate in the rumen (Harfoot and Hazlewood, 1988; Griinari and Bauman, 1999).

Numerous *in vitro* and *in vivo* studies have allowed the major pathways of ruminal biohydrogenation to be elucidated (Harfoot and Hazlewood, 1988). Several rumen bacterial species capable of performing certain steps of the biohydrogenation process have been identified and classified based on the profile of biohydrogenation intermediates produced into two groups, with Group A bacteria converting PUFA to *trans* C18:1 and Group B catalysing the reduction of C18:1 to C18:0. It is generally considered that no single bacterium can catalyse all of the reactions required to convert C18:2 n-6 or C18:3 n-3 to C18:0. A more detailed appraisal of ruminal biohydrogenation of dietary fatty acids is provided by Harfoot and Hazlewood (1988) and Palmquist *et al.* (2005).

Fatty acids available for absorption are also derived from rumen microbes, primarily in the form of structural lipids. Bacterial and protozoal lipids make a considerable contribution to the total flow of lipid into the duodenum and estimated to be about 9 g fatty acids per kg dry matter intake. Microbial lipids are rich in C16:0 and C18:0, but also contain significant amounts of branched chain fatty acids and fatty acids with odd numbers of carbon atoms. For high forage diets, the flow of lipids entering the duodenum can be as much as 40% higher than dietary intake (Doreau and Ferlay, 1994). Fatty acids in the duodenum are mainly adsorbed onto feed particles and bacteria, with approximately 80% of lipids being in the form of NEFA (refer to Lock and Shingfield, 2004).

11.5 Strategies for improving the fatty acid content of raw milk

Feeding a wide range of lipid supplements in dairy cow rations is the most common nutritional means for manipulating milk fatty acid composition. However, both the type and source of fat influence the extent of changes that can be achieved. Often, attempts to enhance the concentration of one or more fatty acids causes changes in other fatty acids, which may serve to offset or negate potential beneficial effects. For example, feeding diets for enriching milk fat *cis*-9,*trans*-11 C18:2, C20:5 n-3 or C22:6 n-3 content also results in an unavoidable increase in *trans* C18:1 concentrations, changes that are generally perceived negatively by consumers and health professionals because of concerns over increased cardiovascular disease risk. In addition to putative benefits to long-term human health, there is also interest in altering fatty acid composition to improve the physical or processing properties of milk fat, but these changes have to be made without compromising the storage characteristics and shelf-life of the dairy-derived foods produced.

11.5.1 Decreasing the saturated fatty acid content of bovine milk

Supplements of plant oils or oilseeds rich in unsaturated C18 fatty acids can be used to reduce the proportion of short and medium chain fatty acids (C6:0–C16:0) and increase the concentrations of long-chain fatty acids in milk (Grummer, 1991; Doreau *et al.*, 1999). These changes are thought to occur due to long fatty acids (C16 and above) inhibiting *de novo* fatty acid synthesis in the mammary gland and because lipid supplements increase the amount of circulating long chain fatty acids available for incorporation into milk fat. In general, feeding plant oil lipid (other than palm oil rich in C16:0) has no effect on milk fat content of C4:0 or long chain (C16 and above), but consistently increases C18:0 concentrations at the expense of C16:0 (Palmquist *et al.*, 1993; Chilliard *et al.*, 2000). Furthermore, comparison of milk fatty acid responses when oils are fed in the diet compared with rumen-protected sources or duodenal infusions of these lipids has indicated that the proportion of C6 and C8 fatty acids are lowered when dietary fats are exposed to ruminal metabolism, whereas the increase in milk C18 content during early lactation or in response to duodenal infusions is associated with a reduction in C10–C16 content (Chilliard *et al.*, 2000). In all cases, inclusion of plant oils and oilseeds in the diet results in an unavoidable increase in milk *trans* C18:1 content in milk due to extensive lipolysis and biohydrogenation of C18 PUFA in the rumen (Table 11.6).

11.5.2 Increasing the *cis* monounsaturated fatty acid content of bovine milk

Owing to extensive metabolism of dietary unsaturated fatty acids, C18:0 is the predominant long chain fatty acid available for incorporation into milk fat. However, *cis*-9 C18:1 secretion in milk exceeds mammary C18:0 uptake due to the activity of stearoyl CoA (Δ-9) desaturase activity in mammary secretory cells. Conversion of C18:0 to *cis*-9 C18:1 is the predominant precursor product of the Δ-9 desaturase, transforming proportionately 40% of C18:0 uptake by the mammary gland (Chilliard *et al.*, 2000). It is therefore possible to exploit the endogenous conversion in the mammary gland to enhance milk fat *cis*-9 C18:1 by supplementing diets with lipids rich in C18:0 such as tallow or hydrogenated oils, but this strategy does not alter the *cis*-9 C18:1: C18:0 ratio in milk fat, and the feeding of tallow to dairy cows is not permitted within the European Union (Chilliard *et al.*, 2000). Feeding plant oils or oilseed rich in *cis*-9 C18:1 can be used to enhance milk fat *cis*-9 C18:1 content, but unless these sources are effectively protected from ruminal metabolism, this nutritional strategy will also increase the concentrations of *trans* C18:1 in milk (Table 11.6). Supplements of *cis*-9 C18:1 acyl amides (Jenkins, 1998; Loor *et al.*, 2002) or high levels of whole cracked rapeseeds in the diet (Givens *et al.*, 2003) have been shown to dramatically increase milk fat *cis*-9 C18:1 content (Table 11.6), but both approaches cause significant reductions in feed intake that can result in lowered milk production. As noted by Givens *et al.* (2003), reductions in milk production associated with feeding high levels of oilseeds or rumen protected lipid supplements would not be feasible in practice unless a considerable premium was paid for milk of altered fatty acid composition.

11.5.3 Increasing the polyunsaturated fatty acid content of bovine milk

Owing to extensive biohydrogenation in the rumen and the inability of ruminant tissue to synthesise PUFA, typical levels of C18:2 n-6 and C18:3 n-3 in milk fat are extremely low (Table 11.6). Even when high amounts of PUFA from plant

Table 11.6 Effect of plant-based lipids in the diet on the fatty acid composition of bovine milk

Lipid source	Intake (g/d)	Milk fatty acid composition (g/100 g total fatty acids)														Reference
		C4:0	C6:0	C8:0	C10:0	C12:0	C14:0	C16:0	C18:0	*cis*-9 C18:1	*trans*- C18:1	C18:1	C18:2 n-6	C18:3 n-3	CLA	
Control	0	2.9	2.5	1.6	3.7	4.2	12.5	30.1	11.2	19.4	1.6	21.7	1.3	0.40	0.46	Ryhanen *et al.* (2005)
Rapeseed oil	500	2.6	1.9	1.2	2.5	2.7	10.1	22.6	14.3	25.8	4.3	31.4	1.4	0.50	1.02	
Control	0	4.6	2.5	1.3	2.9	3.2	12.4	31.4	15.4	13.0	4.1	17.1	0.9	0.43	0.31	Shingfield *et al.*
Rapeseed oil	500	4.7	2.2	1.1	2.1	2.3	10.0	23.4	21.0	17.6	6.8	24.4	0.8	0.40	0.42	unpublished
Control	0	5.0	2.3	1.3	3.1	4.0	11.6	30.7	8.3	18.1	2.0	20.1	2.1	0.45	0.60	Givens *et al.* (2003)
Whole cracked	2530	3.2	1.1	0.6	1.3	1.9	7.9	19.8	14.1	34.7	2.6	37.3	2.4	0.48	1.02	
rapeseeds	4100	2.7	1.0	0.4	1.0	1.4	6.0	18.0	15.8	39.3	2.0	41.3	2.8	0.60	0.74	
Control	0	3.5	2.3	1.5	3.2	3.5	10.0	25.9	9.9	NR	NR	18.5	1.8	0.20	0.35	Chouinard *et al.* (2001)
Ca-salts of rapeseed oil	924	3.0	1.5	0.8	1.6	2.0	7.6	16.4	12.9	NR	NR	32.5	1.9	0.16	1.32	
Control	0	1.9	1.9	1.4	3.6	4.4	13.5	33.9	9.5	NR	NR	23.2	2.6	0.25		Jenkins (1998)
Oleamide[a]	350	1.4	1.0	0.5	1.3	1.7	7.8	20.4	9.4	NR	NR	48.2	3.8	0.12		
Control	0	5.1	3.7	1.8	5.3	4.7	14.0	32.1	7.9	15.8	1.5	17.3	2.6	0.50	0.50	Loor *et al.* (2002)
Canolamide[a]	300	5.4	3.3	1.4	3.4	2.9	10.7	21.4	13.0	27.5	2.9	30.4	2.7	0.70	0.7	
Control	0	4.6	2.5	1.3	2.9	3.2	12.4	31.4	15.4	13.0	4.1	17.1	0.9	0.43	0.31	Shingfield *et al.*
Soyabean oil	500	4.8	2.2	1.1	2.2	2.4	9.8	24.3	20.0	15.8	7.7	23.5	1.1	0.55	0.53	unpublished
Control	0	4.0	2.4	1.2	2.8	3.0	11.9	38.2	13.4	11.1	2.4	14.1	0.9	0.41	0.36	Shingfield *et al.*
Sunflower oil	500	4.4	2.2	1.1	2.1	2.8	9.3	25.5	23.0	13.8	7.0	21.8	1.3	0.26	0.71	upublished
Control	0	3.9	2.5	1.5	3.5	4.0	12.1	29.4	10.4	16.1	1.8	18.3	2.6	0.54	0.40	AbuGhazaleh *et al.* (2002)
Extruded soyabeans	454	3.9	2.3	1.3	2.8	3.0	10.1	24.0	12.1	18.9	3.8	23.1	4.5	0.87	0.87	

Table 11.6 Continued

Lipid source	Intake (g/d)	Milk fatty acid composition (g/100 g total fatty acids)														Reference
		C4:0	C6:0	C8:0	C10:0	C12:0	C14:0	C16:0	C18:0	*cis*-9 C18:1	*trans*- C18:1	C18:1	C18:2 n-6	C18:3 n-3	CLA	
Control	0	3.5	2.3	1.5	3.2	3.5	10.0	25.9	9.9	NR	NR	18.5	1.8	0.20	0.35	Chouinard *et al.* (2001)
Ca-salts of soyabean oil	848	3.4	1.6	0.9	1.6	1.8	6.9	16.4	13.3	NR	NR	31.8	2.2	0.16	2.25	
Control	0	1.1	1.0	0.8	2.7	5.0	14.4	37.5	9.8	20.4	1.7	22.1	3.6	NR	NR	Jenkins *et al.* (1996)
Butylsoyamide[b]	350	1.3	1.1	0.8	2.5	4.5	13.5	35.5	10.2	19.6	2.7	22.3	6.3	NR	NR	
Control	0	1.8	1.0	0.6	1.8	2.7	9.9	40.2	12.3	NR	1.1	21.0	2.0	0.72	0.16	Offer *et al.* (1999)
Linseed oil	250	1.8	1.0	0.6	1.5	2.1	8.8	34.0	15.6	NR	2.1	27.2	1.8	0.84	0.28	
Control	0	4.6	2.5	1.3	2.9	3.2	12.4	31.4	15.4	13.0	4.1	17.1	0.9	0.43	0.31	Shingfield *et al.*
Linseed oil	500	4.5	2.2	1.1	2.3	2.4	10.0	22.2	20.2	17.3	7.7	25.0	0.7	0.57	0.49	unpublished
Control	0	3.9	2.3	1.6	3.0	3.7	11.3	28.9	10.2	21.4	2.9	25.8	2.2	0.32	0.51	Offer *et al.* (2001a)
Crushed linseeds	1500	3.9	2.0	1.3	2.4	2.9	9.9	23.9	12.6	26.1	3.4	31.2	2.8	0.87	0.62	
Control	0	3.5	2.3	1.5	3.2	3.5	10.0	25.9	9.9	NR	NR	18.5	1.8	0.20	0.35	Chouinard *et al.* (2001)
Ca-salts of linseed oil	896	3.4	1.9	1.0	2.0	2.1	7.4	16.2	13.2	NR	NR	28.5	2.4	0.28	1.95	

[a] Prepared by reacting rapeseed oil with ethanolamine.
[b] Prepared by reacting soyabean oil with butylamine.
NR: not reported.
CLA refers to *cis*-9, *trans*-11 C18:2.

oils and oilseeds are included in the diet, absolute increases in C18:2 n-6 and C18:3 n-3 are relatively small (Table 11.6). It has often been considered that feeding oilseeds rather than the corresponding oil would enhance milk fat PUFA concentrations to a greater extent, owing to the seed coat protecting lipids from lipolysis and biohydrogenation in the rumen. Thus far, few direct comparisons have been made, and there is little consensus in the literature to suggest that oilseeds offer significant advantages over plant oils for enhancing milk fat PUFA concentrations (Chilliard and Ferlay, 2004).

In addition to increasing milk fat concentrations of C18 PUFA, there is also interest in enhancing the levels of C20:5 n-3 and C22:6 n-3 due to putative positive effects of these fatty acids on cardiovascular disease risk, type II diabetes, hypertension and certain types of carcinomas in human subjects (Williams, 2000; Wijendran and Hayes, 2004). For cows fed conventional diets based on forages and cereal-based concentrates, the level of C20:5 n-3 and C22:6 n-3 in milk fat is extremely low (typically less than 0.1 g/100 g fatty acids; Table 11.7). It is possible to increase levels of C20:5 n-3 and C22:6 n-3 in milk by feeding various sources of these fatty acids such as fish oil and marine alga lipids as illustrated in Table 11.7, but the level of enrichment in milk fat is very low with a typical efficiency of transfer of C20:5 n-3 and C22:6 n-3 from the diet into milk of 0.026 ($\pm$2.2) and 0.041 ($\pm$5.7), respectively (Chilliard *et al.*, 2001). These values are much lower than transfer efficiencies of 0.18–0.33 and 0.16–0.25, for C20:5 n-3 and C22:6 n-3, respectively, when fish oil is infused post-ruminally (Chilliard *et al.*, 2001). The poor transfer of C20:5 n-3 and C22:6 n-3 into milk when marine lipids are fed arises from extensive (between 74 and 100%) metabolism in the rumen (Doreau and Chilliard, 1997; Scollan *et al.*, 2001; Shingfield *et al.*, 2003) and preferential partitioning of these fatty acids into plasma phospholipids and cholesteryl esters that are poor substrates for mammary lipoprotein lipase (Offer *et al.*, 1999, 2001b; Rymer *et al.*, 2003).

Various technological approaches have been developed to protect plant or marine lipids from metabolism in the rumen, which include encapsulation of oils and oilseeds with a formaldehyde casein complex, calcium salts of fatty acids or fatty acyl amides. Most of these technologies have been developed to overcome the negative effects on animal performance of feeding high levels of lipid, but also allow significant and strategic changes in milk fatty acid composition, depending on the level of protection from metabolism in the rumen (Tables 11.6 and 11.7).

11.5.4 Increasing the conjugated linoleic acid content of bovine milk fat

In light of the potential beneficial effects on human health, numerous studies have examined the impact of nutrition, feeding management and physiological factors on milk fat CLA concentrations, and this area of research has been extensively reviewed in recent years (Griinari and Bauman, 1999; Bauman *et al.*, 2001, 2003; Chilliard *et al.*, 2001; Chilliard and Ferlay, 2004). Diet is the main determinant of milk fat CLA content, as compared with the effect of breed,

Table 11.7 Effect of marine lipids in the diet on the fatty acid composition of bovine milk

Lipid source	Intake (g/d)	Milk fatty acid composition (g/100 g total fatty acids)																Reference
		C4:0	C6:0	C8:0	C10:0	C12:0	C14:0	C16:0	C18:0	*cis*-9 C18:1	*trans*- C18:1	C18:1	C18:2 n-6	C18:3 n-3	CLA	C20:5 n-3	C22:6 n-3	
Control	0	1.8	1.0	0.6	1.8	2.7	9.9	40.2	12.3	NR	1.1	21.0	2.0	0.72	0.16	0.09	0.04	Offer *et al.* (1999)
Tuna orbital oil	95	1.8	1.0	0.6	1.7	2.5	9.9	39.5	10.5		3.5	23.7	1.8	0.71	0.52	0.11	0.07	
Fish oil	250	1.8	0.9	0.6	1.6	2.4	10.3	39.6	6.7		9.8	25.3	2.5	0.74	1.55	0.11	0.08	
Control	0	3.2	2.0	1.3	3.1	3.7	11.3	27.1	9.4	16.5	2.4	22.5	3.1	0.18	0.60	0.05	0.02	Donovan *et* al. (2000)
Menhaden fish oil	290	2.9	1.7	1.0	2.4	3.0	10.4	25.2	7.0	14.5	6.1	24.2	2.4	0.36	1.58	0.22	0.06	
	470	2.6	1.4	0.8	1.8	2.3	9.3	26.1	4.4	11.4	12.9	28.0	2.0	0.24	2.23	0.32	0.26	
	612	2.9	1.5	0.8	1.9	2.3	9.3	26.6	4.0	10.9	12.1	29.0	2.4	0.22	1.90	0.40	0.20	
Control	0	4.0	2.3	1.4	3.0	3.3	10.4	27.8	6.5	NR	NR	18.3	2.0	0.23	0.60	0.05	0.04	Chouinard *et al.* (2001)
Menhaden fish oil	184	3.3	1.7	1.0	2.4	2.9	10.9	26.6	3.5	NR	NR	21.0	1.9	0.23	1.75	0.15	0.54	
	368	3.1	1.6	0.9	2.1	2.6	9.8	24.9	2.5	NR	NR	22.8	1.6	0.28	1.70	0.35	0.64	
Control	0	3.9	2.5	1.5	3.5	4.0	12.1	29.4	10.4	16.1	1.8	18.3	2.6	0.54	0.40	0.05	0.04	AbuGhazaleh *et al.* (2002)
Menhaden fish oil	432	3.9	2.3	1.3	2.8	3.2	11.4	27.6	8.1	15.1	3.8	19.5	2.2	0.85	0.88	0.24	0.26	
Control	0	4.6	2.2	1.1	2.2	2.4	10.2	24.7	19.5	18.1	4.5	23.5	0.9	0.42	0.39	0.05	0.00	Shingfield *et al.* (2003)
Herring and mackerel oil	250	2.4	1.7	1.1	2.8	3.4	13.3	33.3	4.4	4.8	14.4	20.6	1.2	0.45	1.66	0.11	0.10	

Control	0	3.5	2.2	1.3	2.9	3.2	10.5	28.4	12.2	23.2	2.4	25.6	2.8	0.54	0.37		0.00	Franklin *et al.* (1999)
Xylose-treated algae	910	3.5	2.0	1.2	2.6	3.1	12.2	31.0	5.0	14.6	11.7	26.3	2.5	0.49	2.31		0.76	
Marine algae	910	3.6	2.0	1.1	2.5	3.0	11.8	33.0	4.3	13.0	12.8	25.8	2.7	0.47	2.62		0.46	
Control	0	3.9	2.3	1.6	3.0	3.7	11.3	28.9	10.2	21.4	2.9	25.8	2.2	0.32	0.51	0.05	0.04	Offer *et al.* (2001a)
Marine algae	600	3.5	1.9	1.2	2.4	3.2	11.2	28.4	7.7	18.1	8.8	29.4	2.4	0.36	0.92	0.09	0.30	
Control	0			1.2	2.2	2.2	9.2	31.6	13.5	21.2	4.1	25.3	3.6	0.60	1.60	0.00	0.00	Gulati *et al.* (2003)
Protected HIDHA fish oil[a]	3000			1.2	2.8	2.8	8.8	23.1	3.6	15.0	13.7	28.7	8.6	1.20	2.90	1.30	2.20	
Protected Max-EPA fish oil [a]	3000			1.1	2.3	2.4	8.9	23.6	2.8	11.9	17.0	28.9	6.1	0.80	5.10	1.40	0.70	
Control	0			1.4	2.3	2.4	9.0	25.6	14.7	23.7	4.5	28.2	2.7	0.9		0.00	0.00	Kitessa *et al.* (2004)
Protected tuna oil[a]	2000			1.7	2.8	2.9	8.8	23.0	11.4	19.7	5.8	25.5	6.5	1.3		0.61	1.09	

[a] Prepared by mixing full fat soyabeans and using formaldehyde as a tanning reagent.
NR: not reported.
CLA refers to *cis*-9, *trans*-11 C18:2.

stage of lactation or parity, but there is considerable variation (approximately three-fold) between individual animals fed the same diet (Peterson *et al.*, 2002; Lock and Garnsworthy, 2003; Kelsey *et al.*, 2003). Concentrations of CLA in milk can be enhanced using whole oilseeds or plant oils (Table 11.6), but greater increases have been reported when marine lipids are fed (Offer *et al.*, 1999, 2001a; Chouinard *et al.*, 2001; Table 11.7).

The reasons for the higher increases in milk fat CLA content, when fish oil or marine algae are included in the diet compared with an equivalent amount of plant oil, appear to be related to the inhibitory effects of marine lipids on the final reduction of *trans* C18:1 in the rumen. Feeding as little as 250 g of fish oil has no effect on *cis*-9,*trans*-11 C18:2 synthesised in the rumen, but dramatically increases the amount of *trans*-11 C18:1 leaving the rumen from 17.1 to 121.1 g/day, and thereby significantly increasing the supply of substrate for endogenous *cis*-9,*trans*-11 C18:2 synthesis in the mammary gland (Shingfield *et al.*, 2003). Plant oils rich in C18:2 n-6 and C18:3 n-3 also cause *trans*-11 C18:1 to accumulate in the rumen, but between two to three times as much vegetable lipid needs to be fed to elicit the same response reported for fish oil (Loor *et al.*, 2004; Shingfield *et al.*, 2004). Concentrations of CLA are also known to be higher in milk from pasture compared with dried grass, maize, grass or legume silages (Kelly *et al.*, 1998; Stanton *et al.*, 2003; Table 11.8). Under UK conditions, milk fat CLA content is higher during the spring and summer months as a result of higher intakes of fresh grass (Lock and Garnsworthy, 2003).

11.5.5 Implications for milk production systems (e.g. grazing *vs* housed cows)

Higher potential yields associated with lower production risks have tended to favour the use of forages rather than cereals to meet the energy and protein requirements of dairy cows. Owing to a year-round demand for dairy products and climatic constraints on grazing, milk production in most European countries is dependent on the production of high-quality conserved forages. Even though grasses and legumes contain relatively low amounts of lipid, forages in the basal ration can often be the main source of fatty acids in the diet (Harfoot and Hazlewood, 1988; Lock and Shingfield, 2004). In reviewing the literature and based on indirect comparisons, Chilliard *et al.* (2001) concluded that milk from diets containing maize silage can be expected to contain higher proportions of short-chained fatty acids and C18:2 n-6 than grass silage, while feeding ensiled compared with fresh grass would increase levels of C14:0 and C16:0 and lower the concentrations of C18:1, C18:2 n-6, C18:3 n-3 and CLA.

In recent years a number of studies have been conducted that generally affirm these changes in milk fatty acid composition in response to changes in the basal forage in the diet (Table 11.8). The reasons for the lowered levels of CLA in milk from ensiled compared with fresh herbage are intriguing and not readily apparent. Ensiling or drying reduces the fatty acid content of conserved forages, depending on the exposure to solar radiation and duration of wilting or drying.

Table 11.8 Effect of dietary forage on the fatty acid composition of bovine milk

Basal forage	Milk fatty acid composition (g/100 g total fatty acids)														Reference
	C4:0	C6:0	C8:0	C10:0	C12:0	C14:0	C16:0	C18:0	*cis*-9 C18:1	*trans*-C18:1	C18:1	C18:2 n-6	C18:3 n-3	CLA	
Fresh pasture (ryegrass + white clover)	NR	1.8	0.9	1.7	1.7	6.7	24.2	13.2	NR	NR	34.7	2.3	0.95	1.09	Kelly *et al.* (1998)
Maize and legume silages	NR	2.1	1.2	2.3	2.6	9.4	30.7	15.0	NR	NR	26.6	2.6	0.25	0.46	
Fresh pasture (crabgrass + white clover)	1.1	1.6	1.0	2.3	2.7	9.9	31.5	15.4	NR	NR	22.1	2.5	0.38	0.37	White *et al.* (2001)
Lucerne and maize silages	1.1	1.7	1.1	2.6	3.1	10.8	31.4	13.4	NR	NR	21.3	1.8	0.73	0.66	
Mixed grass swards	NR	NR	NR	NR	NR	8.9	22.6	11.0	23.8	4.9	28.7	1.0	1.0	2.43	Elgersma *et al.*
Grass and maize silages	NR	NR	NR	NR	NR	11.7	34.8	8.8	17.0	0.9	17.9	1.1	1.1	0.44	(2004)
Grass and legume swards	NR	NR	NR	1.8	2.3	9.1	25.1	12.1	NR	NR	32.6	1.4	2.02	2.21	Dhiman *et al.* (1999)
Lucerne hay and concentrates	NR	NR	NR	2.1	2.6	9.4	24.7	15.2	NR	NR	31.4	4.3	0.81	0.89	
Fresh Lucerne	5.8	2.3	1.2	NR	NR	9.8	29.6	8.9	NR	NR	21.5	1.6	1.13	NR	Whiting *et al.*
Lucerne silage	5.6	2.4	1.2	NR	NR	11.0	35.8	6.6	NR	NR	16.7	1.1	0.83	NR	(2004)
Perennial ryegrass silage	4.9	2.7	1.4	3.0	3.5	11.7	32.5	11.0	20.7	1.1	21.8	1.1	0.40	0.36	Dewhurst *et al.*
Red clover silage	5.8	3.0	1.4	2.8	3.3	11.3	30.6	11.6	20.2	1.3	21.5	1.6	1.28	0.41	(2003a)
White clover silage	5.2	3.0	1.6	3.5	4.2	12.7	32.9	9.7	17.9	1.1	19.0	1.5	0.96	0.34	
Grass hay	2.5	2.2	1.5	3.4	4.0	13.3	34.5	9.2	15.2	3.8	18.6	1.2	0.50	0.45	Shingfield *et al.*
Grass silage untreated	2.9	2.2	1.5	3.3	3.8	12.9	34.7	9.8	15.1	3.6	18.4	1.0	0.35	0.41	(2005b)
Grass silage + inoculant ensiling additive	2.9	2.3	1.5	3.4	3.9	13.1	33.8	10.0	15.3	3.7	18.7	1.0	0.43	0.41	
Grass silage + formic acid based ensiling additive	2.6	2.2	1.5	3.4	4.0	13.2	34.2	10.0	14.5	4.3	18.4	0.9	0.29	0.49	
Grass silage	4.0	1.9	1.5	4.0	5.1	14.0	42.4	7.6	NR	NR	14.8	1.9	0.7	NR	Havemose *et al.*
Maize silage	3.8	1.8	1.3	3.4	4.2	13.5	40.8	8.1	NR	NR	18.6	2.1	0.2	NR	(2004)

NR: not reported.
CLA refers to *cis*-9, *trans*-11 C18:2.

Conservation by drying generally results in more extensive oxidative losses of PUFA compared with ensiling, but the concentrations of CLA, as well as C18:2 n-6 and C18:3 n-3 are often higher in milk from hay than silage (Chilliard *et al.*, 2001; Shingfield *et al.*, 2005b). One possible explanation may be related to the differences in the extent of lipolysis of grass lipids prior to ingestion. Ensiling is known to cause substantial hydrolysis of the ester linkages of grass phospholipids and glycolipids in chloroplastic membranes, leading to a high proportion of PUFA being non-esterified and therefore immediately exposed to metabolism on entering the rumen, whereas complex lipids in dried forages may require further lipolysis on ingestion before ruminal biohydrogenation can take place.

11.5.6 Implications/applications for the food processor

Development of milk and dairy food products containing higher proportions of unsaturated fatty acids is desirable with respect to improving long-term human health, but it may also be advantageous in terms of improving product quality, such as increasing the spreadability of butter from cold or altering the textural properties of cheeses. For example, the ratio of C16:0 to *cis*-9 C18:1 in milk fat is considered to be the most accurate predictor of butter firmness, and an increase in milk fat C16:0 content coupled with lowered short chain fatty acid concentrations reduces the spreadability of butter (Chilliard and Ferlay, 2004). Production of milk fat containing higher levels of PUFAs has marked effects on the physical and processing properties of milk and dairy food products, and generally results in the manufacture of a softer butter or cheese (Palmquist *et al.*, 1993; Chilliard and Ferlay, 2004; Ryhänen *et al.*, 2005).

The sensory attributes of cheese and butter are defined by the physical structure and texture as well as inherent organoleptic properties. However, the shelf-life of milk and dairy food products and development of off-flavours is dependent on complex interactions between pro- and anti-oxidative processes that are influenced by the degree of fatty acid unsaturation, concentration of transition metal cations and levels of antioxidants (Barrefors *et al.*, 1995; Granelli *et al.*, 1998; Timmons *et al.*, 2001; Havemose *et al.*, 2004). Enriching milk fat C18:2 n-6 and C18:3 n-3 concentrations are known to increase the susceptibility of milk to oxidation and development of spontaneous off-flavours which can to some extent be controlled by increasing the levels of anti-oxidants in milk (Palmquist *et al.*, 1993; Barrefors *et al.*, 1995; Granelli *et al.*, 1998) using dietary supplements.

In spite of these potential problems, a number of studies have shown that it is possible to manufacture butter or cheese from milk produced from cows fed plant oils and oilseeds containing increased levels of *cis*-9 C18:1 and CLA and reduced concentrations of C12:0, C14:0 and C16:0 (Dhiman *et al.*, 1999; Ramaswamy *et al.*, 2001; Ryhänen *et al.*, 2005) without compromising the overall acceptability of these foods. Similarly, the organoleptic properties of milk and butter from diets containing (10 g/kg DM) low levels of fish oil (Ramaswamy *et al.*, 2001) or milk from cows fed rumen protected tuna oil

(Kitessa *et al.*, 2004) have been shown to be comparable to that of non-lipid supplemented diets.

11.6 Future trends

It seems likely that concerns about the relationship between diet and chronic disease will continue to increase, not least because of increasing cost to national health services for treating such conditions. This will increase the urgency to improve the health-related aspects of staple foods such as milk. Thus the future role of animal nutrition in creating foods closer to the optimum composition for long-term human health will become increasingly important. This, however, needs to be done with caution as there is increasing evidence that milk contains compounds which may actively promote long-term health. For example, a recent prospective study (Ness *et al.*, 2001) over 25 years, indicated that increased consumption of milk was associated with a substantially reduced risk of death from CVD and coronary heart disease (CHD) in particular (Fig. 11.2). Research is urgently required to identify and fully characterise the benefits associated with the consumption of these compounds and to understand how the levels in milk can be enhanced while also reducing the concentration of the less desirable fractions.

There is currently interest in the possibility of improved fatty acid composition of milk when produced from organic systems. Such improvements are likely to stem mainly from the increased use of fresh forages and legumes in diets for cows on organic systems since these forages have been shown to

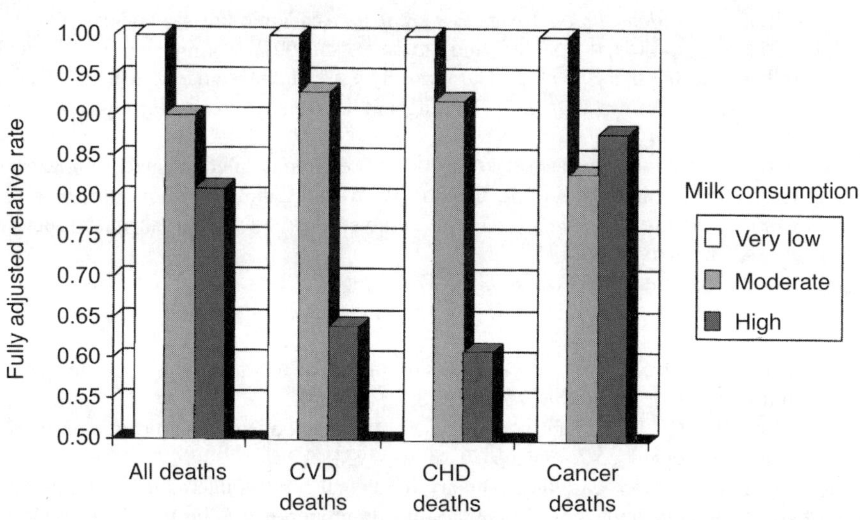

Fig. 11.2 Twenty five year relative mortality rate in 5765 men according to level of milk consumption (from Ness *et al.*, 2001).

increase the concentrations of C18:3 n-3 and CLA in milk fat (Dewhurst *et al.*, 2003b). Arguably, this has little to do with the adoption of organic production standards and the impact on the national diet over the year is likely to be very small. However, it is true that the production of improved milk and milk-derived foods by whatever approach, on a scale that will substantially affect national diets, will require both substantial political and financial incentives and large changes with animal husbandry and associated industries.

11.7 Acknowledgements

The preparation of this review was supported by LIPGENE, an Integrated Project within the EU funded Sixth Framework Research programme (see www.lipgene.tcd.ie).

11.8 References

ABUGHAZALEH A A, SCHINGOETHE D J, HIPPEN A R and WHITLOCK L A (2002), 'Feeding fish meal and extruded soybeans enhances the conjugated linoleic acid (CLA) content of milk', *J Dairy Sci*, **85**, 624–631.

AULDIST M J, WALSH B J and THOMSON N A (1998), 'Seasonal and lactational influences on bovine milk composition in New Zealand', *J Dairy Res*, **65**, 401–411.

BARREFORS P, GRANELLI K, APPELQVIST L A and BJÖERCK L (1995), 'Chemical characterization of raw milk samples with and without oxidative off-flavor', *J Dairy Sci*, **78**, 2691–2699.

BAUMAN D E and DAVIS C L (1974), 'Biosynthesis of milk fat', in Larson B L and Smith V R, editors, *Lactation: A Comprehensive Treatise*, Academic Press, London, 31–75.

BAUMAN D E, BAUMGARD L H, CORL B A and GRIINARI J M (2001), 'Conjugated linoleic acid (CLA) and the dairy cow', in Garnsworthy P C, and Wiseman J, editors, *Recent Advances in Animal Nutrition*, Nottingham University Press, Nottingham, 221–250.

BAUMAN D E, CORL B A and PETERSON D G (2003), 'The biology of conjugated linoleic acid in ruminants', in Sebedio J-L, Christie W W and Adlof R, editors, *Advances in Conjugated Linoleic Acid Research*, Volume 2, American Oil Chemists Society Press, Champaign, IL, 146–173.

BEAULIEU A D and PALMQUIST D L (1995), 'Differential effects of high fat diets on fatty acid composition in milk of Jersey and Holstein cows', *J Dairy Sci*, **78**, 1336–1344.

BONANOME A and GRUNDY S M (1988), 'Effect of dietary stearic acid on plasma cholesterol and lipoprotein', *New Eng J Med*, **318**, 1244–1248.

CHILLIARD Y (1993), 'Dietary fat and adipose tissue metabolism in ruminants, pigs, and rodents: a review', *J Dairy Sci*, **76**, 3897–3931.

CHILLIARD Y and FERLAY A (2004), 'Dietary lipids and forages interactions on cow and goat milk fatty acid composition and sensory properties', *Repr Nutr Dev*, **44**, 467–492.

CHILLARD Y, FERLAY A, MANSBRIDGE R M and DOREAU M (2000), 'Ruminant milk fat plasticity: nutritional control of saturated, polyunsaturated, trans and conjugated fatty acids', *Ann Zootech*, **49**, 181–205.

CHILLIARD Y, FERLAY A and DOREAU M (2001), 'Effect of different types of forages, animal fat or marine oils in cow's diet on milk fat secretion and composition, especially conjugated linoleic acid (CLA) and polyunsaturated fatty acids', *Liv Prod Sci*, **70**, 31–48.

CHOUINARD P Y, CORNEAU L, BUTLER, W R, CHILLIARD Y, DRACKLEY J K and BAUMAN D E (2001), 'Effect of dietary lipid source on conjugated linoleic acid concentrations in milk fat', *J Dairy Sci*, **84**, 680–690.

CHRISTIE W W (1995), 'Composition and structure of milk lipids', in Fox P F, editor, *Advanced Dairy Chemistry, Volume 2: Lipids*, Chapman and Hall, London, 1–36.

CORL B A, BAUMGARD L H , GRIINARI J M, DELMONTE P, MOREHOUSE K M, YURAWECZC M P and BAUMAN D E (2002), '*Trans*-7, *cis*-9 CLA is synthesized endogenously by delta 9-desaturase in dairy cows', *Lipids*, **37**, 681–688.

DEFRA (2001), 'The National Food Survey'. *Her Majesty's Stationary Office*, London. Available at: www.defra.gov.uk/esg/m_natstats.htm

DEMEYER D and DOREAU M (1999), 'Targets and procedures for altering ruminant meat and milk lipids', *Proc Nutr Soc*, **58**, 593–607.

DEPARTMENT OF HEALTH (1991), 'Report on Health and Social Subjects: No. 41, Dietary Reference Values for Food Energy and Nutrients for the United Kingdom, Report of the Panel on Dietary Reference Values of the Committee on Medical Aspects of Food Policy', *Her Majesty's Stationery Office*, London.

DEWHURST R J, FISHER, W J, TWEED J K S and WILKINS R J (2003a), 'Comparison of grass and legume silages for milk production 1. Production responses with different levels of concentrate', *J Dairy Sci*, **86**, 2598–2611.

DEWHURST R J, SCOLLAN N D, LEE M R F, OUGHAM H J and HUMPHREYS M O (2003b), 'Forage breeding and management to increase the beneficial fatty acid content of ruminant products', *Proc Nutr Soc*, **62**, 329–336.

DHIMAN T R, HELMINK E D, McMAHON D J, FIFE R L and PARIZA W (1999), 'Conjugated linoleic acid content of milk and cheese from cows fed extruded oilseeds', *J Dairy Sci*, **82**, 412–419.

DONOVAN D C, SCHINGOETHE D J, BAER R J, RYALI J, HIPPEN A R and FRANKLIN S T (2000), 'Influence of dietary fish oil on conjugated linoleic acid and other fatty acids in milk fat from lactating dairy cows', *J Dairy Sci*, **83**, 2620–2628.

DOREAU M and CHILLIARD Y (1997), 'Effects of ruminal or post-ruminal fish oil supplementation on intake and digestion in dairy cows', *Rep Nut Dev*, **37**, 113–124.

DOREAU M and FERLAY A (1994), 'Digestion and utilisation of fatty acids by ruminants', *Anim Feed Sci Technol*, **45**, 379–396.

DOREAU M, CHILLARD Y, RULQUIN H and DEMEYER D L (1999), 'Manipulation of milk fat in dairy cows', in Garnsworthy P C and Wiseman J, editors, *Recent Advances in Animal Nutrition*, Nottingham University Press, Nottingham, 81–109.

DRACKLEY J K, BEAULIEU A D and ELLIOTT J P (2001), 'Responses of milk fat composition to dietary fat or nonstructural carbohydrates in Holstein and Jersey cows', *J Dairy Sci*, **84**, 1231–1237.

ELGERSMA A, ELLEN G, VAN DER HORST H, BOER H, DEKKER P R and TAMMINGA S (2004), 'Quick changes in milk fat composition from cows after transition from fresh grass to a silage diet', *Anim Feed Sci Technol*, **117**, 13–27.

FESKENS E J M and KROMHOUT D (1990), 'Habitual dietary intake and glucose tolerance euglycaemic men: the Zutphen Study', *Int J Endocrinol*, **19**, 953–959.

FESKENS E J M, VIRTANEN S M, RASANEN L, TUOMILEHTO J, STENGARD J, PEKKANEN J, NISSINEN A and KROMHOUT D A (1995), '20-year follow-up of the Finnish and Dutch cohorts of the Seven Countries Study', *Diabetes Care*, **18**, 1104–1112.

FOOD STANDARDS AGENCY (2003), *National Diet and Nutrition Survey: Adults aged 16 to 64 years*, Volume 2. *Office for National Statistics*, Newport, 106 pp.

FRANKLIN S T, MARTIN K R, BAER R J, SCHINGOETHE D J and HIPPEN A R (1999), 'Dietary marine algae (*Schizochytrium* sp.) increases concentrations of conjugated linoleic, docosahexaenoic and transvaccenic acids in milk of dairy cows', *J Nutr*, **129**, 2048–2054.

GIVENS D I and SHINGFIELD K J (2004), 'Foods derived from animals: the impact of animal nutrition on their nutritive value and ability to sustain long term health', *Nutr Bull*, **29**, 325–332.

GIVENS D I, ALLISON R and BLAKE J S (2003), 'Enhancement of oleic acid and vitamin E concentrations of bovine milk using dietary supplements of whole rapeseed and vitamin E', *Anim Res*, **52**, 531–542.

GRANELLI K, BARREFORS P, BJÖERCK L and APPELQVIST L A (1998), 'Further studies on lipid composition of bovine milk in relation to spontaneous oxidative flavor', *J Sci Food Agr*, **77**, 161–171.

GRIINARI J M and BAUMAN D E (1999) 'Biosynthesis of conjugated linoleic acid and its incorporation into meat and milk in ruminants', in Yurawecz M P, Mossoba M M, Kramer J K G, Pariza M W and Nelson G J, editors, *Advances in Conjugated Linoleic Acid Research*, Volume 1, American Oil Chemists Society Press, Champaign, IL, 180–200.

GRIINARI J M, CORL B A, LACY S H, CHOUINARD P Y, NURMELAK V V and BAUMAN D E (2000), 'Conjugated linoleic acid is synthesized endogenously in lactating dairy cows by delta 9-Desaturase', *J Nutr*, **130**, 2285–2291.

GRUMMER R R (1991), 'Effect of feed on the composition of milk fat', *J Dairy Sci*, **74**, 3244–3257.

GULATI S K, MCGRATH S, WYNN P C and SCOTT T W (2003), 'Preliminary results on the relative incorporation of docosahexaenoic and eicosapentaenoic acids in cows milk from two types of rumen protected fish oil', *Int Dairy J*, **13**, 339–343.

GUNSTONE F D, HARWOOD J L and PADLEY F P (1994), 'Occurrence and characteristics of oils and fats', in Padley F D, Gunstone F D and Harwood J L, editors, *The Lipid Handbook*. Cambridge, The University Press, 47–224.

HARFOOT C G and HAZELWOOD G P (1988), 'Lipid metabolism in the rumen', in Hobson P N, editor, *The Rumen Microbial Ecosystem*, Elsevier Science Publishers, London, 285–322.

HAVEMOSE M S, WEISBJERG M R, WENDER L P and NIELSEN J H (2004), 'Influence of feeding different types of forage on the oxidative stability of milk', *Int Dairy J*, **14**, 563–570.

HAWKE T W and TAYLOR J C (1995), 'Influence of nutritional factors on the yield, composition and physical properties of milk fat', in Fox P F, editor, *Advanced Dairy Chemistry*, Volume 2: Lipids, Chapman and Hall, London, 37–88.

HULSOF K F A M, VAN ERP-BAART M A, ANTTOLAINEN M, BECKER W, CHURCH S M, COUET C, HERMANN-KUNZ E, KESTELOOT H, LETH T, MARTINS I, MOREIRAS O, MOSCHANDREAS J, PIZZOFERRATO L, RIMESTAD A H, THORGEIRSDOTTIR H, VAN AMELSVOORT J M M, ARO A, KAFATOS AG, LANZMANN-PETITHORY D and VAN POPPEL G (1999), 'Intake of fatty acids in Western Europe with emphasis on trans fatty acids: The TRANSFAIR study', *Eur J Clin Nutr*, **53**, 143–157.

JENKINS T C (1998), 'Fatty acid composition of milk from Holstein cows fed oleamide or canola oil', *J Dairy Sci*, **81**, 794–800.

JENKINS T C, BATEMAN H G and BLOCK S M (1996), 'Butylsoyamide increases unsaturation of fatty acids in plasma and milk of lactating dairy cows', *J Dairy Sci*, **79**, 585–590.

JENSEN R G (2002), 'The composition of bovine milk lipids: January 1995 to December 2000', *J Dairy Sci*, **85**, 295–350.

KATAN M B, ZOCK P L and MENSINK R P (1995), 'Dietary oils, serum lipoproteins, and coronary heart disease', *Amer J Clin Nutr*, **61**, 1368S–1373S.

KELLY M L, KOLVER E S, BAUMAN D E, AMBURGH VAN M E and MULLER L D (1998), 'Effect of intake of pasture on concentrations of conjugated linoleic acid in milk of lactating cows', *J Dairy Sci*, **81**, 1630–1636.

KELSEY J A, CORL B A, COLLIER R J and BAUMAN D E (2003), 'The effect of breed, parity, and stage of lactation on conjugated linoleic acid (CLA) in milk fat from dairy cows', *J Dairy Sci*, **86**, 2588–2597.

KINSELLA J E (1972), 'Stearyl CoA as a precursor of oleic acid and glycerolipids in mammary microsomes from lactating bovine: possible regulatory step in milk triglyceride synthesis', *Lipids*, **7**, 349–355.

KITESSA S M, GULATI S K, SIMOS G C, ASHES, J R, SCOTT T W, FLECK E and WYNN P C (2004), 'Supplementation of grazing cows with rumen-protected tuna oil enriches milk fat n-3 fatty acids without affecting milk production or sensory characteristics', *Brit J Nutr*, **91**, 271–277.

KRIS-ETHERTON P M, DANIELS S R, ECKEL R H, ENGLER M, HOWARD B V, KRAUSS R M, LICHTENSTEIN A H, SACKS F, ST. JEOR S and STAMPFER M (2001), 'Summary of the scientific conference on dietary fatty acids and cardiovascular health: *conference summary from the Nutrition Committee of the American Heart Association*', *Circulation*, **103**, 1034–1039.

LAWLESS F, STANTON C, L'ESCOP P, DEVERY R, DILLON P and MURPHY J J (1999), 'Influence of breed on bovine milk *cis*-9, *trans*-11 conjugated linoleic acid content', *Lives Prod Sci*, **62**, 43–49.

LOCK A L and GARNSWORTHY P C (2003), 'Seasonal variation in milk conjugated linoleic acid and delta(9)-desaturase activity in dairy cows', *Lives Prod Sci*, **79**, 47–59.

LOCK A L and SHINGFIELD K J (2004), 'Optimising milk composition' in Kebreab E, Mills J and Beever D E, editors, *Dairying – Using Science to Meet Consumers' Needs*, British Society of Animal Science, Publication 29, Nottingham University Press, Loughborough, UK, 107–188.

LOOR J J, HERBEIN J H and JENKINS T C (2002), 'Nutrient digestion, biohydrogenation, and fatty acid profiles in blood plasma and milk fat from lactating Holstein cows fed canola oil or canolamide', *Anim Feed Sci Technol*, **97**, 65–82.

LOOR J J, UEDA K, FERLAY A, CHILLIARD Y and DOREAU M (2004), 'Short communication: diurnal profiles of conjugated linoleic acids and trans fatty acids in ruminal fluid from cows fed a high concentrate diet supplemented with fish oil, linseed oil, or sunflower oil', *J Dairy Sci*, **87**, 2468–2471.

McCANCE R A and WIDDOWSON E M (1998), 'Fatty acids', Seventh Supplement to the 5th Edition of the *Composition of Foods*, Cambridge, The Royal Society of Chemistry and London, MAFF, 209.

MENENDEZ J A, VELLON L, COLOMER R and LUPU R (2005), 'Oleic acid, the main monounsaturated fatty acid of olive oil, suppresses Her-2/neu (erb B-2) expression and synergistically enhances the growth inhibitory effects of trastuzumab (Herceptine) in breast cancer cells with Her-2/neu oncogene amplification', *Ann Onc*, **16**, 359–371.

MURPHY J J (2000), *Synthesis of Milk Fat and Opportunities for Nutritional Manipulation*, British Society of Animal Science, Occasional Publication, no. 25, Penicuik, 201–222.

NESS A R, SMITH G D and HART C (2001) 'Milk, coronary heart disease and mortality', *J Epid Comm Health*, **55**, 379–382.

NUGENT A P (2004), 'The metabolic syndrome', *Nutr Bull*, **29**, 36–43.

OFFER N W, MARSDEN M, DIXON J, SPEAKE B K and THACKER F E (1999), 'Effect of dietary fat supplements on levels of n-3 polyunsaturated fatty acids, trans acids and conjugated linoleic acid in bovine milk', *Anim Sci*, **69**, 613–625.

OFFER N W, MARSDEN M and PHIPPS R H E (2001a), 'Effect of oil supplementation of a diet containing a high concentration of starch on levels of *trans* fatty acids and conjugated linoleic acids in bovine milk', *Anim Sci*, **73**, 533–540.

OFFER N W, SPEAKE B K, DIXON J and MARSDEN M (2001b), 'Effect of fish-oil supplementation on levels of (n-3) poly-unsaturated fatty acids in the lipoprotein fractions of bovine plasma', *Anim Sci*, **73**, 523–531.

PALMQUIST D L, BEAULIEU D A and BARBANO D M (1993), 'Feed and animal factors influencing milk fat composition', *J Dairy Sci*, **76**, 1753–1771.

PALMQUIST D L, LOCK A L, SHINGFIELD K J and BAUMAN D E (2005), 'Biosynthesis of conjugated linoleic acid in ruminants and Humans', in Taylor S L, editor, *Advances in Food and Nutrition Research 50*, Elsevier Inc., San Diego, CA, 336 pp.

PARKER D R, WEISS S T, TROISI R, CASSANO PA, VOKONAS P S and LANDSBERG L (1993), 'Relationship of dietary saturated fatty acids and body habitus to serum insulin concentrations: the Normative Aging Study', *Amer J Clin Nutr*, **58**, 129–136.

PARODI P W (2003), 'Conjugated linoleic acid in food', in Sebedio, J-L, Christie, W W and Adlof, R O, editors, *Advances in Conjugated Linoleic Acid Research*, Volume 2, American Oil Chemists Society Press, Champaign, IL, 101–122.

PETERSON D G, KELSEY J A and BAUMAN D E (2002), 'Analysis of variation in *cis*-9, *trans*-11 conjugated linoleic acid (CLA) in milk fat of dairy cows', *J Dairy Sci*, **85**, 2164–2172.

PIPEROVA L S, SAMPUGNA L, TETER B B, KALSCHEUR K F, YURAWECZ, M P, KU Y, MOREHOUSE K M and ERDMAN R A (2002), 'Duodenal and milk *trans* octadecanoic acid and conjugated linoleic acid (CLA) isomers indicate that postabsorptive synthesis is the predominant source of *cis*-9-containing CLA in lactating dairy cows', *J Nutr*, **132**, 1235–1241.

RAMASWAMY N, BAER R J, SCHINGOETHE D J, HIPPEN A R, KASPERSON K M and WHITLOCK L A (2001), 'Composition and flavor of milk and butter from cows fed fish oil, extruded soybeans, or their combination', *J Dairy Sci*, **84**, 2144–2151.

RITZENTHALER K L, MCGUIRE M K, FALEN R, SHULTZ T D, DASGUPTA N and McGUIRE M A (2001), 'Estimation of conjugated linoleic acid intake by written dietary assessment methodologies underestimates actual intake evaluated by food duplicate methodology', *J Nutr*, **131**, 1548–1554.

RYHÄNEN E-L, TALLAVAARA K, GRIINARI J M, JAAKKOLA S, MANTERE-ALHONEN S and SHINGFIELD K J (2005), 'Production of conjugated linoleic acid enriched milk and dairy products from cows receiving grass silage supplemented with a cereal-based concentrate containing rapeseed oil', *Int Dairy J*, **15**, 207–217.

RYMER C, GIVENS D I and WAHLE K W J (2003), 'Dietary strategies for increasing docosahexaenoic acid (DHA) and eicosapentaenoic acid (EPA) concentrations in bovine milk: a review', *Nutr Abs Rev, Series B*, **73**, 9R–25R.

SCOLLAN N D, DHANOA M S, CHOI, N J, MAENG W J, ENSER M and WOOD J D (2001), 'Biohydrogenation and digestion of long chain fatty acids in steers fed on different sources of lipid', *J Agric Sci, Camb*, **136**, 345–355.

SEHAT N, YURAWECZ M P, ROACH, J A G, MOSSOBA, M M, KRAMER J K G and KU Y (1998), 'Silver-ion high-performance liquid chromatographic separation and identification of conjugated linoleic acid isomers', *Lipids*, **33**, 217–221.

SHINGFIELD K J, AHVENJÄRVI S, TOIVONEN V, ÄRÖLÄ A, NURMELA K V V, HUHTANEN P and GRIINARI J M (2003), 'Effect of fish oil on biohydrogenation of fatty acids and milk fatty acid content in cows', *Anim Sci*, 77, 165–179.

SHINGFIELD K J, AHVENJÄRVI S, TOIVONEN V, HUHTANEN P and GRIINARI J M (2004), 'Synthesis of trans fatty acids and isomers of conjugated linoleic acid in the rumen of cows fed grass silage based diets supplemented with incremental levels of sunflower oil', *J Dairy Sci*, **87**, Supplement 1, 335.

SHINGFIELD K J, REYNOLDS C K, LUPOLI B, TOIVONEN V, YURAWECZ M P, DELMONTE P, GRIINARI J M, GRANDISON A S and BEEVER D E (2005a), 'Effect of forage type and proportion of concentrate in the diet on milk fatty acid composition in cows fed sunflower oil and fish oil', *Anim Sci*, **80**, 225–238.

SHINGFIELD K J, SALO-VÄÄNÄNEN P, PAHKALA E, TOIVONEN V, JAAKKOLA S, PIIRONEN V and HUHTANEN P (2005b), 'Effect of forage conservation method, concentrate level and propylene glycol on the fatty acid composition and vitamin content of milk', *J Dairy Res*, **72**, 349–361.

STANTON C, MURPHY J, McGRATH E and DEVERY R (2003), 'Animal feeding strategies for conjugated linoleic acid enrichment of milk', in Sébédio, J L, Christie W W and Adlof R, editors, *Advances in Conjugated Linoleic Acid Research*, Volume 2, American Oil Chemists Society Press, Champaign, IL, 123–145.

STEFFEN L M and JACOBS D R (2003), 'Relation between dairy food intake and plasma lipid levels: the CARDIA Study', *Austr J Dairy Technol*, **58**, 92–97.

STULL J W and BROWN W H (1964), 'Fatty acid composition of milk. II. Some differences in common dairy breeds', *J Dairy Sci*, **47**, 1412.

TEMME E H M, MENSINK R P and HORNSTRA G (1996), 'Comparison of the effects of diets enriched in lauric, palmitic, or oleic acids on serum lipids and lipoproteins in healthy women and men', *Amer J Clin Nutr*, **63**, 897–903.

TERPSTRA A H M (2004), 'Effect of conjugated linoleic acid on body composition and plasma lipids in humans: an overview of the literature', *Amer J Clin Nutr*, **79**, 352–361.

TIMMONS J S, WEISS W P, PALMQUIST D L and HARPER W J (2001), 'Relationships among dietary roasted soybeans, milk components, and spontaneous oxidized flavor of milk', *J Dairy Sci*, **84**, 2440–2449.

TRICON S, BURDGE G C, KEW S, BANERJEE T, RUSSELL J J, JONES E L, GRIMBLE R F, WILLIAMS C M, YAQOOB P and CALDER P C (2004), 'Opposing effects of *cis*-9,*trans*-11 and *trans*-10,*cis*-12 conjugated linoleic acid on blood lipids in healthy humans', *Amer J Clin Nutr*, **80**, 614–620.

VESSBY B, UUSITUPA M, HERMANSEN K, RICCARDI G, RIVELLESE A A, TAPSELL L C, NÄLSÉN C, BERGLUND L, LOUHERANTA A, RASMUSSEN B M, CALVERT G D, MAFFETONE A, PEDERSEN E, GUSTAFSSON L-B and STORLIEN L H (2001), 'Substituting dietary saturated for monounsaturated fat impairs insulin sensitivity in healthy men and women', *Diabetologia*, **44**, 312–319.

WHITE S L, BERTRAND J A, WADE M R, WASHBURN S P, GREEN J T and JENKINS T C (2001), 'Comparison of fatty acid content of milk from Jersey and Holstein cows consuming pasture or a total mixed ration', *J Dairy Sci*, **84**, 2295–2301.

WHITING C M, MUTSVANGWA T, WALTON J P, CANT J P and MCBRIDE B W (2004), 'Effects of feeding either fresh alfalfa or alfalfa silage on milk fatty acid content in Holstein dairy cows', *Anim Feed Sci Technol*, **113**, 27–37.

WHO/FAO (2003), *Diet, Nutrition and the Prevention of Chronic Diseases*, WHO, Report of a Joint WHO/FAO Expert Consultation, Geneva, 148.

WIJENDRAN V and HAYES K C (2004), 'Dietary n-6 and n-3 fatty acid balance and cardiovascular health', *Ann Rev Nutr*, **24**, 597–615.

WILLIAMS C M (2000), 'Dietary fatty acids and human health', *Ann Zootech*, **49**, 165–180.

YURAWECZ M P, ROACH J A G, SEHAT N, MOSSOBA M M, KRAMER J K G, FRITSCHE J, STEINHART H and KU Y (1998), 'A new conjugated linoleic acid isomer, 7 *trans*, 9 *cis*-octadecadienoic acid, in cow milk, cheese, beef and human milk and adipose tissue', *Lipids*, **33**, 803–809.

12

Optimising goat's milk and cheese fatty acid composition

Y. Chilliard, J. Rouel, A. Ferlay and L. Bernard, INRA, France, P. Gaborit, K. Raynal-Ljutovac and A. Lauret, ITPLC, France, and C. Leroux, INRA, France

12.1 Introduction

Lipid composition is one of the most important components of the technological and nutritional quality of goat milk. Lipids are involved in cheese yield (per kg of milk) and firmness, as well as in the flavour of caprine dairy products (Delacroix-Buchet and Lamberet, 2000). Furthermore, besides their quantitative contribution to the amount of dietary energy, the different lipid and fatty acid (FA) compounds (cholesterol, short and medium chain saturated, branched, mono- and polyunsaturated, *cis* and *trans*, conjugated FA, etc.) are potentially involved as positive or negative predisposing factors for the health of human consumers (Sébédio *et al.*, 1999; Williams, 2000; Jensen, 2002).

Dairy (including goat) products provide 25–60% of the overall saturated fat consumed by people in Europe, which makes them the preferential target of dieticians' criticisms (see Chapter 11). The deleterious reputation of saturated FAs should however be weighted with the fact that stearic acid has no atherogenic effect, that C12–C16 saturated FA should be atherogenic only when consumed in excessive amounts, and that saturated fat could even be protective when compared to a low-fat, high-carbohydrate diet (Legrand, 2001; Knopp and Retzlaff, 2004). The allegedly atherogenic effect of certain *trans* mono-unsaturated FA has not been confirmed as regards vaccenic acid (*trans*11-18:1), the main isomer present in milk (Lock *et al.*, 2004a). Furthermore, recent studies in humans showed that consumption of dairy products (Ness *et al.*, 2001; Pereira *et al.*, 2002) or milk fat (Warensjö *et al.*, 2004) sometimes decreases cardio-vascular and/or metabolic syndrome risk factors. The benefit of increasing the n-3/n-6 ratio of polyunsaturated FA (PUFA) has been confirmed (Williams, 2000). Lastly, rumenic acid (*cis*9,*trans*11-18:2), the main natural isomer of conjugated linoleic acids (CLA), exhibits interesting features, as demonstrated in animal models, for the prevention of certain forms of cancer in particular (Banni *et al.*, 2001; Ip *et al.*, 2003; Lock *et al.*, 2004b; see Chapter 8 for more information).

These new facts together underline, however, the interest of modulating milk FA composition. Mammals' milk FA composition is linked to intrinsic (animal species, breed, genotype, lactation and pregnancy stages) or extrinsic (environmental) factors. In a given animal species, the effects linked to breed or genotype are significant but restricted (Chilliard and Ferlay, 2004) and they can be achieved only in the mid-term. However, goats present a remarkable polymorphism at the alpha-s1 casein (CSN1S1) locus which is linked to large differences in milk protein and fat content (Grosclaude *et al.*, 1994). Recent results on the effect of this polymorphism on milk FA composition are therefore presented in the present chapter.

The lactation stage effect on milk fat content and FA composition is marked and mainly linked to lipid store mobilisation in early lactating goats (Chilliard *et al.*, 2003a), but it lasts only a few weeks each year. In contrast, seasonal effects are quantitatively very important, and mainly due to variations in feeding factors (Schmidely and Sauvant, 2001; Chilliard *et al.*, 2003a). Nutrition therefore constitutes a natural and economical way for farmers to sharply and rapidly modulate milk FA composition, in particular by adding lipid supplements to the diet. In goats, in contrast to cows, nearly all types of lipid supplements induce a sharp increase in milk fat content without modifying milk yield or protein content (Chilliard *et al.*, 2003a). This chapter summarises present knowledge in goats, and gives particular attention to the peculiarities of caprine species in relation to the impact of different diets on the main FA classes: saturated and *cis*-monounsaturated, PUFA and lastly CLA and *trans*-monounsaturated. The effects of nutrition in interaction with cheese-making technology on FA composition and sensory characteristics of goat cheese are presented in parallel in this chapter, because almost all goat's milk is consumed in cheese form.

12.1.1 Production and consumption of caprine dairy fat

France

France is the primary country in Europe for goat's milk production and its transformation into cheese. It has numerous and reliable data in this domain. In 2003, by taking into account the milk collected by companies and transformed on the farm, as well as the imports and exports, it is possible to estimate the consumption in France at 490 million litres of goat's milk, of which 3 million litres is consumed as UHT milk and the rest as cheese (that is to say 78 100 tonnes).

In 2003 this corresponds to 17 800 t of pure goat's milk fat consumed (Table 12.1), or 300 grams of fat per inhabitant per annum. If one takes into account the

Table 12.1 Consumption of caprine dairy fat in France in 2003 according to products

Type of consumed caprine dairy product	Quantity consumed in France	Equivalent consumed as dairy goat fat
UHT milk	3 Ml	100 t
Fresh lactic cheese and spread	13 100 t	2 650 t
Ripened lactic cheese	59 000 t	13 900 t
Camembert-type soft cheese	3 400 t	750 t
Cheese made from a mixture of cow and goat milk	2 600 t	400 t
Total		**17 800 t**

Sources: ITPLC estimation, according to ONILAIT, SCEES and IE.

fact that 78% of French households (results of SECODIP consumer sample group, 2003) consume some goat's milk cheese, one ends up with 380 g of caprine dairy fat in 2003 for actual consumers. That is a very small ingested annual quantity in itself, and notably in comparison with the French annual consumption of cow's milk fat which is estimated at 16.5 kg per inhabitant (in 2004, according to F. Chausson, CNIEL), the amount of dairy fat consumed represents only 2% of that resulting from cow's milk. Furthermore, it is advisable to take into account the structure of the consumption of goat's cheeses (SECODIP, 2003), which shows a markedly higher consumption by consumers in the 50–64 year age bracket (index 124 in volume, with regard to 100 for all the consumers) compared with the under 35-year-old age group of consumers (index 67) or single persons (index 60).

Europe

In the 25 countries of the European Union, only a few are significant producers of goat's milk and consumers of caprine dairy products: France, Spain, Greece, the Netherlands, Italy and Portugal. The milk is transformed almost exclusively into cheeses which are primarily consumed in the countries of production (with the exception of the Netherlands which exports two-thirds of its production).

The few available data are unclear and rather unreliable. Nevertheless it is possible to estimate the caprine dairy fat consumed per inhabitant and per annum (Table 12.2). Average annual consumption per inhabitant is low in the main consumer countries of caprine dairy products. It would be interesting, however, to be able to take into account the likely uneven distribution of consumption according to the inhabitants of a country. This would doubtless show that certain categories of person, notably in Greece where auto-consumption (as estimated in Table 12.2) accentuates the phenomenon, consume quantities of caprine dairy fat which become relatively important at individual level (several kg per annum).

Even though the fat content of goat's milk has increased in recent years (+0.3 g/kg a year in France, according to data of the LILCO) because of genetic

Table 12.2 Estimation of the annual consumption in 2003 of caprine dairy fat in the six main producing and consumer countries of the European Union

	Italy	Portugal	Netherlands	Greece	Spain	France
Goat's milk equivalent commercialised and consumed in the country (in Ml)[1]	30	30	40	240	370	490
Caprine dairy fat consumed by the total population (t)	1200	1200	1300	11 300	20 200	17 800
Average caprine dairy fat consumed per inhabitant (g)	20	110	80	1100	510	300

[1]The estimation takes into account imports and exports, but not the auto-consumption of the producing countries, which can be significant (in Spain, for example), and even considerable (in Greece, sometimes estimated to 160 Ml, i.e. 40% of total yield).
Sources: ITPLC estimation, according to (except France) Eurostat, Spanish Ministry of Agriculture, Greek Ministry.

selection and of improvement of feeding techniques especially, it is likely that the consumption of caprine dairy fat in the European Union is not going to vary largely in the near future.

12.2 Biochemical characteristics and origin of goat milk lipids

12.2.1 Milk fat globules and lipid classes

Dry matter and fat contents are of the same order of size in milks from dairy caprine or bovine species (Jarrige *et al.*, 1978), and in human milk (Hambraeus, 1984). However, within each species, fat content can change considerably according to animal breed or genotype, lactation stage, season, dietary factors, etc.

Milk fat is secreted by mammary epithelial secretory cells, as a finely dispersed emulsion of lipids: the milk fat globules. Processes of formation and secretion were extensively reviewed by Mather and Keenan (1998). Milk fat globules are derived from intracellular newly synthesised lipid micro-droplets, and surrounded by a presecretory monolayer membrane consisting of polar lipids and proteins. These droplets may repeatedly grow in size by fusing with each other to form cytoplasmic lipid droplets as they move from the basal to the apical part of the cell. For secretion into the alveolar lumen, they are enveloped in a bilayer membrane, which originates from the apical part of the secretory cell, and/or from secretory vesicles, which surround them in the cytoplasm, before releasing milk fat globules from the surface by exocytosis. Occasionally, cytoplasmic crescents are included between fat droplets and the last membrane. The proportion of globules with such crescents is species-dependent: 1% or less in cow milk, from 1 to 5% in goat milk, 1–8% and up to 29% in human milk; it seems to be genetically determined in human milk, in relation to coat-protein (butyrophilin and xanthine oxidase) composition and concentration (Huston and Patton, 1990). Once in the alveolar lumen, the surrounding membrane may undergo more or less extended loss and structural modifications (Mather and Keenan, 1998) which lead to a very stable lipid emulsion in milk.

Goat's and cow's milk fat globules have a similar mean diameter, but the percentage of small globules seems to be higher in goat's milk (Jenness, 1980; Jensen *et al.*, 1990; Mehaia, 1995). Furthermore, goat's milk lacks agglutinin, a factor involved in the creaming ability of cow's milk. These peculiarities could explain the low creaming ability of cold goat's milk. This ability is also related to the CSN1S1 genotype. Milk from goats with different alleles has different protein and fat contents (Grosclaude *et al.*, 1994; Table 12.3). Furthermore, the fat content of the cream from goats with the *FF*-CSN1S1 genotype (i.e. defective homozygous goats with low concentration of CSN1S1 in milk) was 49% lower than that of *AA* genotype goats (Pitel and Delacroix-Buchet, 1994). This could be related to differences in the size and/or structure of milk fat globules or to other factors linked to differences in secretory mechanisms between *AA* and *FF* goats (Neveu *et al.*, 2002), such as the presence of cytoplasmic crescents.

The distribution of total lipids in different lipid classes is similar between goat, cow and human milk (review by Chilliard and Lamberet, 2001). Triglycerides constitute 95–98% of total lipids. The apparently higher content in partial glycerides in caprine milk could reflect either a specificity of goats or between-laboratory differences in milk handling and conservation, or differences in methodology used for the measurement. Milk cholesterol is mainly in free form, and its content is lower in ruminant than in human milk. Goat's milk is poor in tocopherol and carotene, consistent with its white colour (Jenness, 1980).

12.2.2 Metabolic pathways and nutrient fluxes involved in milk fat synthesis

Milk FA have a dual origin: they are either taken up from plasma lipids (60% of the milk FA) or they are synthesised *de novo* (C4–C16) in the mammary gland from acetate and 3-hydroxybutyrate. Preformed FAs (mainly C16–C18) are transported in plasma as non-esterified FA (NEFA) or mainly as triglyceride-rich lipoproteins. The mammary gland uses plasma NEFA released by adipose tissue, which in ruminants are mainly 16:0, 18:0 and *cis*9-18:1. For this reason, lipid mobilization, which occurs in early lactation and/or when the energy balance is negative, induces a sharp increase in milk stearic and oleic acids (Chilliard *et al.*, 2003a). Lipoprotein lipase permits triglyceride hydrolysis and thus the uptake by the mammary gland of dietary FAs. Secretory mammary cells exhibit high delta-9 desaturase activity, which converts stearic acid (18:0) into oleic acid (*cis*9-18:1) and so contributes more than 50% of oleic acid secretion (Chilliard *et al.*, 2000). In addition, approximately 30% of the vaccenic acid originated in the rumen can be desaturated to form rumenic acid (Griinari and Bauman, 1999).

In the rumen, dietary lipids undergo high-intensity metabolism linked to microbial activity (see Chapter 11). Linoleic acid (*cis*9,*cis*12-18:2) is isomerized into rumenic acid, then the latter is hydrogenated into vaccenic acid and

Table 12.3 Effects of genotype at the alpha-s1 casein locus and of diet composition on goat dairy performances and milk fatty acid composition (Chilliard Y, Rouel J, Bruneteau E, Leroux C, unpublished)

	Genotype	Diet composition				Cow data[7]
	Low[1]% High[2]	C+MS+AH[3]	C+AH+MS[4]	C+GS+AH[5]	AH+C[6]	GH+C[8]
No. goats	–	18	18	17	18	
Milk yield (kg/day)	105	3.39[ab]	3.72[bc]	3.20[a]	3.94[c]	24.2
Fat content (g/kg)	83**	35.8	36.3	37.8	35.5	33.0
Protein content (g/kg)	84**	30.7[b]	29.7[b]	28.3 [a]	30.4[b]	31.0
Lactose content (g/kg)	99	46.6[b]	44.8 [a]	46.5 [b]	47.1 [b]	45.0
Lipolysis[9]	113[+]	0.29	0.28	0.21	0.31	–
C4:0[10]	104	2.16[b]	1.84[a]	2.72[d]	2.54 [c]	3.36
C6:0	94*	2.36[a]	2.45 [a]	2.76 [b]	2.82[b]	2.62
C8:0	88**	2.72[a]	2.90[ab]	2.86[ab]	3.09[b]	1.71
C9:0	84*	0.09[b]	0.06[a]	0.07[a]	0.06[a]	–
C10:0	87**	10.28[ab]	10.73 [bc]	9.59[a]	11.21[c]	3.90
C10:1c9	105	0.20[a]	0.27[b]	0.22 [a]	0.26[b]	0.37
C11:0	83**	0.12 [b]	0.10[a]	0.08[a]	0.10[a]	0.08
C12:0	84**	4.58[b]	5.11[c]	4.17[a]	5.49[c]	4.42
C13:0	90[+]	0.14[b]	0.20[d]	0.17[c]	0.09[a]	0.27
iso14	100	0.13[a]	0.12[a]	0.14[ab]	0.16[b]	0.14
C14:0	98	11.73[a]	12.73[b]	11.44[a]	13.09[b]	12.97
iso15	95	0.21[a]	0.26[c]	0.24[bc]	0.23[b]	0.38
anteiso15	93[+]	0.41[a]	0.51[b]	0.42[a]	0.50[b]	0.80
C14:1c9	111[+]	0.14[a]	0.17[b]	0.16[ab]	0.17[b]	1.11
C15:0	99	1.16[ab]	1.07[a]	1.15[a]	1.25[b]	1.38
iso16	95	0.24[a]	0.37[b]	0.35[b]	0.32[b]	0.32
C16:0	106**	30.89 [b]	28.59[a]	28.72 [a]	29.96[ab]	29.06
iso17	99	0.00[a]	0.42[c]	0.44[c]	0.36[b]	0.53
C16:1c9	111**	0.99 [c]	0.55 [a]	0.74[b]	0.55[a]	1.40
C17:0	103	0.65[b]	0.58[a]	0.81[c]	0.91[d]	0.77
C17:1	112*	0.22[a]	0.25[ab]	0.42[c]	0.26[b]	0.22
C18:0	89**	7.53[bc]	7.72[c]	6.86[ab]	6.12[a]	6.86
C18:1t6t7t8	101	0.15[b]	0.09[a]	0.07[a]	0.08[a]	0.20

C18:1t9	106	0.19^{c}	0.13^{b}	0.13^{b}	0.10^{a}	0.15
C18:1t10	105	0.18^{c}	0.15^{b}	0.12^{a}	0.12^{a}	0.30
C18:1t11	94	0.71^{b}	0.46^{a}	0.38^{a}	0.46^{a}	1.20
C18:1t12	100	0.20^{c}	0.10^{a}	0.11^{a}	0.13^{b}	0.22
C18:1t13t14	101	0.17^{a}	0.19^{b}	0.16^{a}	0.17^{a}	0.37
C18:1c9	113**	15.44^{b}	16.40^{b}	18.05^{c}	13.68^{a}	16.35
C18:1c11	103	0.36^{b}	0.34^{ab}	0.38^{b}	0.30^{a}	0.72
C18:1c12	102	0.17^{b}	0.10^{a}	0.11^{a}	0.12^{a}	0.15
C18:2c9t13	121**	0.16^{c}	0.08^{a}	0.12^{b}	0.09^{a}	0.13
18:2n-6	108**	2.00^{ab}	1.94^{a}	2.02^{ab}	2.12^{b}	1.73
C20:0	96	0.14	0.13	0.13	0.12	0.12
C18:3n3	98	0.22^{a}	0.20^{a}	0.42^{b}	0.62^{c}	0.84
CLAc9t11	119*	0.43^{b}	0.29^{a}	0.25^{a}	0.23^{a}	0.66
C20:4n6	107	0.11^{a}	0.12^{a}	0.16^{b}	0.14^{ab}	0.13
C20:5n3	73	0.04	0.04	0.07	0.05	0.07
C22:6n3	105	0.004^{a}	0.008^{ab}	0.006^{a}	0.016^{b}	0.01
C6:0 C13:0	87**	20.29^{ab}	21.56^{bc}	19.70^{a}	22.85^{c}	13.01
Total *trans*-C18:1	99	1.61^{b}	1.12^{a}	0.97^{a}	1.06^{a}	2.75
C10:1/C10:0	122**	0.020^{a}	0.025^{b}	0.024^{b}	0.023^{b}	0.096
C14:1/C14:0	113*	0.012	0.013	0.014	0.013	0.086
C16:1/C16:0	106	0.032^{c}	0.019^{a}	0.026^{b}	0.019^{a}	0.048
C17:1/C17:0	108**	0.34^{b}	0.43^{c}	0.52^{d}	0.28^{a}	0.28
C18:1c9/C18:0	124**	2.09^{a}	2.18^{a}	2.67^{b}	2.28^{a}	2.38
CLA/*trans*11-C18:1	126**	0.63^{b}	0.63^{b}	0.68^{b}	0.52^{a}	0.55

[1]33 goats (16*EF*, 13*FF*, 3*EO* and 1*FO*).
[2]38 goats (31 *AA*, 4*AB* and 3*AC*). Lactation number, days in milk (67–73) and body weight were the same for High and Low genotype. High and Low genotypes were balanced within each studied diet.
[3]Concentrate/Maize Silage/Alfalfa Hay, 58/27/15 (year 2001).
[4]Concentrate/Alfalfa Hay/Maize Silage, 60/28/12 (year 2004).
[5]Concentrate/Grass Silage/Alfalfa Hay, 60/24/16 (year 2002).
[6]Alfalfa Hay/Concentrate, 58/42 (year 2003).
[7]Adapted from Loor *et al.* (2005), using same analytical conditions.
[8]Grass Hay/Concentrate, 65/35.
[9]Lipolysis: g of oleic acid/100 g milk fat/34 hours post-milking at 4 °C.
[10]g/100 g total fatty acids.
+, *, ** = genotype effect ($P < 0.10$, 0.05, 0.01, respectively). $^{a, b, c, d}$ = significant diet (year) effect ($P < 0.05$).

eventually into stearic acid. Linolenic acid (*cis*9,*cis*12,*cis*15-18:3) induces a larger number of intermediates, including vaccenic acid, but rumenic acid production has not been reported. In dairy cows hydrogenation in the rumen averages 80% for linoleic acid and 92% for linolenic acid (Doreau and Ferlay, 1994), and decreases when the proportion of concentrate increases in the diet. The hydrogenation of *trans*-18:1 classically constitutes the limiting step for the full hydrogenation of unsaturated C18, and *trans*-C18:1 accumulation frequently occurs in the rumen, contrary to CLA (Griinari and Bauman, 1999). As a consequence, rumenic acid synthesis mainly occurs (probably more than 75%) in the udder (Bauman *et al.*, 2003), in proportion to the amount of vaccenic acid formed in the rumen (Chilliard *et al.*, 2003a; Loor *et al.*, 2003).

12.2.3 Mean fatty acid composition

The FA composition of milk triglycerides differs widely between ruminant and human species (Glass *et al.*, 1967), in particular because of the role of the rumen in lipid metabolism. Goat's milk is indeed richer in short and medium chain FAs (C4:0 to C10:0) as well as in myristic and stearic acids (C14:0 and C18:0). Conversely, it is poorer in C18:1 (mainly oleic acid) and C18:2 (mainly linoleic acid). Its low level of polyunsaturated FA is due to the high level of hydrogenation of dietary FA by ruminal microbes (review by Chilliard *et al.*, 2000). In comparison with milk of cows (Table 12.3 for animals receiving a similar hay-based diet non-supplemented with lipids), goat's milk is richer in medium chain FA (C6:0 to C12:0), particularly in C8:0 and C10:0, and poorer in butyric acid (C4). These differences suggest that the regulation of the elongation process of FAs (which are synthesised *de novo* by the 'fatty acid synthase' complex) differs between caprine and bovine mammary cell species.

Bovine milk is richer than goat's milk and particularly richer than human milk in FA with branched-chain FA with more than 10 carbons (2.1–3.1, 1.6–1.9 and 0.9% of total FA, respectively for the three animal species) (Massart-Leen *et al.*, 1981; Jensen, 1989; Alonso *et al.*, 1999; Table 12.3). This peculiarity of ruminant milk fat results from microbial metabolism of branched-chain amino acids in the rumen, since leucine and isoleucine give rise to iso-valeric and 2-methyl butyric acids; the corresponding acyl-CoA could be used as a primer in the elongating process to form the iso and anteiso series up to C17. Furthermore, goat milk contains minor volatile branched-chain FA with one methyl or ethyl group (Ha and Lindsay, 1990a; Lamberet *et al.*, 1996; Alonso *et al.*, 1999). These FA probably arise from tissue metabolism of propionate and butyrate absorbed from the rumen, such metabolism differing perhaps between bovine and caprine species. Interestingly, two of these minor FA (4-methyloctanoic acid which was first found with 4-methylnonanoic acid in mutton meat (Wong *et al.*, 1975), and 4-ethyloctanoic acid) are involved in goat flavour. Ha and Lindsay (1990b) proposed pathways for their formation in ruminant fat, by analogy with descriptions of fat from uropygial glands in waterfowl (e.g. Rainwater and Kolattukudy, 1982). But almost nothing is known of the way in which such a synthesis is regulated within the different tissues in ruminants. For example, according to Sugiyama *et al.* (1986), a homologous series of 4-ethyl branched-chain FA, in free and bound forms, is the main fat component from neck sebaceous glands of adult buck. This suggests that addition of ethylmalonyl-CoA at different stages of the FA elongation process takes place in the sebaceous gland cells.

The delta-9 desaturation ratios are lower in goat's than in cow's milk for C10:0, C14:0 and C16:0, but not for C17:0, C18:0 and *trans*11-C18:1 (Table 12.3), which could reflect a species peculiarity in the affinity of the delta-9 desaturase for FA with different chain-length.

Milk unsaturated FA may contain one or several *trans* double bonds. About 5–15% of total C18:1 are of *trans* configuration in goat (Bickerstaffe *et al.*, 1972; Calderon *et al.*, 1984; Alonso *et al.*, 1999; Table 12.3), cow (Storry and Rook, 1965; Selner and Schultz, 1980; Chilliard *et al.*, 2001; Loor *et al.*, 2005) and human species (Jensen, 1989; Guesnet et *al.*, 1993; Chen *et al.*, 1995). However, the proportion of different *trans* isomers varies between species: the main *trans*-FA (35–40%) is vaccenic acid (C18:1, n-7 or Δ11) in goat and cow milk, whereas human milk fat *trans*-C18:1 contains larger percentages of FA with the double bond located on carbons 6 to 14 (Bickerstaffe *et al.*, 1972; Alonso *et al.*, 1999; Precht and Molkentin, 1999; LeDoux *et al.*, 2002; Table 12.3). The profile of human milk fat is probably related to the consumption of a mixture of ruminant milk fat and of margarines, the latter being richer in Δ6 to Δ14 *trans*-C18:1, especially Δ6 to Δ10. When animals receive similar diets, goat's milk appears to be poorer in *trans*-C18:1 isomers than cow's milk (Table 12.3). Quantitatively, the *trans*-C16:1 isomers represent less than 0.2% of total FA, or 5% of all *trans*-C16:1 and C18:1 isomers in ruminant milk fat. The distribution patterns of *cis*- and *trans*-C16:1 isomers are very similar for goat's and cow's cheese fats (Destaillats *et al.*, 2000).

The *trans* FA of margarines originate from industrial hydrogenation of polyunsaturated FA from vegetable oils, whereas ruminant *trans* FA originate from ruminal hydrogenation of polyunsaturated FA of forages and concentrates. It is interesting to emphasise that milk fat from monogastric farm animals (that do not consume ruminant milk fat or margarines) is almost devoid of vaccenic acid and CLA, whereas human milk fat is of an intermediate composition. The mean milk CLA values from goat studies were in the range 0.2–0.9% of total FA (Alonso *et al.*, 1999; Gulati *et al.*, 2000; Chilliard *et al.*, 2003a), *i.e.* similar to observations in dairy cows receiving diets without added lipids (Griinari and Bauman, 1999; Chilliard *et al.*, 2000; Loor *et al.*, 2005).

The different FA are not esterified at random on the three carbons of the triglyceride glycerol skeleton. In ruminants, short and medium chain FA (C4 to C10) are mainly esterified on carbon 3, especially in the goat (Table 12.4). Human milk contains a higher proportion of C16:0 on carbon 2. This could explain the high digestibility of this FA in this milk, since 2-monoglycerides are more easily absorbed in the intestine. On the other hand, oleic and linoleic acids are largely esterified on carbon 3 in both goat and human milks.

Table 12.4 Distribution of fatty acids on the carbons of glycerol[1]

	Goat	Cow	Human
C4	3	3	–
C6	3	3–2	–
C8	3	3–2	–
C10	3–2	2–3	–
C12	2–1	2–1	–
C14	2	2	2–3
C16	1–2	1–2	2
C16:1	1–2	1–2	3
C18	1	1	1
C18:1	3–2	1–3	3–1
C18:2	3	2	3–1

[1]From Kuksis *et al.* (1973); Davies *et al.* (1983); Ha & Lindsay (1993).
The figures (1/2/3) indicate glycerol carbons on which each FA is more particularly esterified.

The peculiarities of mammary lipogenesis in ruminants contribute to decrease the melting point of milk fat, thus reversing the potential increase of this melting point that would result from FA hydrogenation in the rumen. Indeed, the lack of FA elongation above 16 carbons, and the presence of mechanisms for terminating elongation in the fatty acid synthase complex (Moore and Christie, 1981), both increase the percentage of short- and medium-chain FA. Furthermore, the presence of branched-chain FA, and the delta-9 desaturation of C10:0–C16:0, C18:0 and vaccenic acid also decrease the melting point of FA for a given chain length. Finally, the asymmetry of triglycerides further decreases their melting point, for a given FA composition. The maintenance of the melting point value within a range, allowing milk fat to be liquid at body temperature, is an obligatory homeostatic regulation inherited from the evolution of mammalian species. These adaptations obviously occurred in interaction with the digestive peculiarities of each species although other factors (or random adaptation) probably occurred, since significant differences exist within ruminant species (*e.g.* cows *vs* goat) and within monogastric species (*e.g.* human *vs* rodents, Jenness, 1974).

The peculiarities of goat's milk lipids (small fat globules, lack of agglutinin, high content in C8:0–C10:0, and high percentage of the short and medium chain FA esterified on the carbon 3 of the glycerol skeleton) probably explain that goat milk fat digestibility tends to be higher than that of cow milk in piglets (Février *et al.*, 1993) and humans (Hachelaf *et al.*, 1993).

12.3 Effect of alpha-s1 casein genotype on milk fatty acid composition

The comparison of two groups of goats with different CSN1S1 genotypes (Table 12.3) confirms the largely lower milk protein (+5.0 g/kg) and fat (+6.8 g/kg) contents (Grosclaude *et al.*, 1994) in the Low genotype group (carrying the defective alleles) whereas milk yield and milk lactose content are not changed. Furthermore, post-milking fat lipolysis was higher in the Low group, in agreement with previous results (Delacroix-Buchet and Lamberet, 2000; Chilliard *et al.*, 2003a).

There are significant differences in the contents of at least 17 milk FAs, with low CSN1S1 goats having less C6 to C13 saturated FA (−2.9 g/100 g FA), less stearic acid (−0.8 g/100 g FA), and more palmitic (+1.7 g/100 g/FA), oleic (+1.9 g/100 g FA), linoleic (+0.15 g/100 g FA) and rumenic (+0.05 g/100 g FA) acids than high CSN1S1 goats have. Furthermore the delta-9 desaturation ratios were significantly higher in low CSN1S1 goats for C10:0, C14:0, C17:0, C18:0, *trans*11-C18:1 and *trans*13-C18:1 (Table 12.3), which strongly suggests a higher mammary desaturase activity in these animals, specially for C18:0 and *trans*11-C18:1. This could partly explain the higher milk fat percentage of oleic and rumenic acids in low CSN1S1 goats.

Previous results on cheeses obtained in another laboratory on two groups of homozygous low and high CSN1S1 goats (Delacroix-Buchet *et al.*, 1996; Lamberet *et al.*, 1996) showed differences for C8:0, C10:0, C12:0, C16:0, C18:0 and total C18:1 percentages, but of smaller magnitude than observed in our study on individual goats in controlled feeding conditions. Interestingly, the between-group differences in the two studies published in 1996 for milk protein and fat contents (4.6 and 3.0 g/kg) were similar to our study for protein but less than half for fat content. Thus, a higher genotype effect on fat concentration seems to be linked to a higher effect on its FA profile. Interestingly, a comparison (Beaulieu and Palmquist, 1995) between Holstein and Jersey cow breeds (i.e. with low *vs* high milk fat content) showed differences in milk FA composition (C6-C14 and 18:0 decreased, and *cis*-18:1 increased) similar to those observed in Low *vs* High CSN1S1 genotype goats (present study). Thus, as in cows, there could be a positive correlation between goat's milk fat content and percentage of C6–C14. We hypothesise that the observed engorgement of endoplasmic reticulum in mammary secretory cells of low CSN1S1 genotype goats (Chanat *et al.*, 1999), and the resulting impairment in milk fat secretion process (Neveu *et al.*, 2002), could yield a negative feedback which impairs preferentially the malonyl-CoA dependent synthesis of medium chain FA.

The physiological significance of these changes is not obvious, since in individual FA arising from *de novo* synthesis (*e.g.* C12:0, C14:0 and C16:0) are not modified similarly. The finding of a link between delta-9 desaturation ratio and CSN1S1 genotype is of interest and could support genetic selection in favour of low CSN1S1 genotype. Nevertheless, the occurrence of polymorphism in the delta-9 desaturase gene in goats (Bernard *et al.*, 2001) would open a complementary field of investigations. We did not find any significant differences between *AA* and *FF* goats in mammary mRNA levels of a few lipogenic enzymes involved in *de novo* FA synthesis or long chain FA uptake, although there was a trend for a higher delta-9 desaturase mRNA level in low CSN1S1 (*FF* genotype) compared to high CSN1S1 (*AA* genotype) goats (Leroux *et al.*, 2003). Anyway, it is likely that the opposite changes between short and medium chain FAs (C6–C13) on one hand, and delta-9 desaturation ratios from C10:0 to *trans*-C18:1 isomers on the other hand, could contribute to the control of the melting point of milk fat, which needs to remain liquid at the temperature occurring in mammary secretory cells. Finally, the higher lipoprotein lipase activity in native milk, the higher development of post-milking lipolysis and goat flavour in low CSN1S1 genotype goats could be related in part to their higher percentage of palmitic acid (review by Chilliard *et al.*, 2003a) and/or to peculiarities of milk fat globules (see Section 12.2.1). These results suggest that low (compared with high) CSN1S1 genotype goats may yield milk with more flavour typicity, although no major difference in the nutritional value of the fat fraction can be predicted on the basis of the present knowledge.

12.4 Controlling milk fatty acid composition by animal diet

The comparison of four different diets, commonly used in intensive goat dairy farms in France, shows numerous significant differences (Table 12.3). For example, concentrate + maize silage diet (compared to alfalfa hay + concentrate diet) increased several minor *cis*- and *trans*-isomers of C18:1 and decreased butyric and myristic acid percentages. Grass silage increased oleic acid at the expense of C10:0, C12:0 and C14:0, but this could have resulted indirectly from a lower feed intake (and consequently decreased milk yield and increased adipose tissue FA mobilisation) due to a low palatability of this particular grass silage. Altogether, the observed differences are of small extent, especially if compared with effects of lipid supplementation which are reviewed in Sections 12.4.1 to 12.4.3.

12.4.1 Saturated fatty acids and oleic acid

The potential to decrease medium chain saturated FAs (C10 to C16:0) is very large. For example, with hay-based diets, these FAs represented 59% of goat milk fat and fell to 38% after linseed oil supplementation, or to 33% if vitamin E was added with linseed oil (Table 12.5). The 'Saturated FA Atherogenic index' (SFAAI = C12% + 4C14% + C16%, from Ulbricht and Southgate, 1991), was 75–89% for 11 control diets and was decreased to 48–63% in 25 lipid-supplemented diets (Tables 12.5 and 12.6).

Most FA originating from mammary *de novo* lipogenesis are saturated (C4:0 to C16:0). Long-chain FAs (at least 18 carbon atoms) are powerful inhibitors of *de novo* lipogenesis. This effect is more marked when FAs have a longer chain, are more unsaturated and contain more *trans* double bonds (Bernard *et al.*, 2005a). Thus, when the bioavailability of C18 FAs increases (as a result of either increased dietary intake or body lipid mobilisation), C8:0 to C16:0 secretion decreases, and their concentration decreases even more through dilution in a larger quantity of long-chain FAs. Contrary to medium-chain FAs, short-chain FA concentrations (C4:0, C6:0 and C8:0 to a lesser extent) are classically either unchanged or only slightly reduced by increased lipid supplementation in the diet or body lipid mobilisation (Chilliard *et al.*, 2000, 2003a).

Stearic acid secretion in milk can be increased either by increasing stearic acid intake or by supplementation of C18 unsaturated FAs because they are partly hydrogenated into stearic acid in the rumen. The same applies to oleic acid either through the secretion of dietary oleic acid or from its synthesis through the action of mammary delta-9 desaturase on stearic acid. Thus, when unprotected vegetable oils or seeds rich in oleic, linoleic or linolenic acids are given to ruminants, the main response is an increase in the stearic acid produced in the rumen, which is then transformed in part into oleic acid in the udder. In goats, when comparing diets combining different forages, concentrate percentages and lipid sources, it appears that the highest milk oleic percentages (more than 24% of total FA) are obtained either with unprotected high-oleic sunflower oil (and more with rye-grass than with maize silage) (Table 12.6) or with oilseeds, in the rank lupin > soybean > linseed > sunflower (Chilliard and Ferlay, 2004; Bernard *et al.*, 2005c). Milk oleic percentage was only marginally increased by either linseed oil or sunflower oil supplementations (Tables 12.5 and 12.6) except when forage was natural grassland hay (trial 3). It can be observed that the *cis*9-18:1/18:0 ratio is decreased by lipid supplements: more markedly by raw or extruded oilseeds than oil, and more markedly by PUFA-rich oils than high-oleic oil (Chilliard and Ferlay, 2004). These results suggest that the desaturation ratio of stearic acid is decreased by diets which increase the availability of either PUFAs or *trans*-FAs (Tables 12.5 and 12.6), since these FAs are putative inhibitors of the mammary delta-9-desaturase (Bernard *et al.*, 2005a,d).

The case of lupin seeds is interesting because this seed, rich in 18:1 and 18:2, is the only one that did not decrease the desaturation ratio and which did not increase (or even decreased) goat milk PUFAs and vaccenic acid percentages (Chilliard *et al.*, 2003a), suggesting that its unsaturated FAs were totally hydrogenated, despite the fact that it was consumed as crude whole seed. Conversely, either linseed oil or linseed supplementations decreased strongly the desaturation ratio, simultaneously to the high increases in both 18:3n-3 and *trans*-FAs percentages in milk fat (Tables 12.5 and 12.6; Bernard *et al.*, 2005d).

12.4.2 Polyunsaturated fatty acids

PUFAs are not synthesised by tissues in ruminants, and therefore their concentration in milk is closely related to the quantities absorbed in the intestine – hence the quantities leaving the rumen. Those quantities may be increased by dietary PUFA intake and by factors which affect rumen hydrogenation, such as FA trapping in vegetable cells, high forage/concentrate ratio or the implementation of PUFA-rich oil encapsulation techniques. There are numerous results in cows concerning the effects of marine oils on milk fat in order to increase C20:5 n-3 and C22:6 n-3 (see Chilliard *et al.*, 2001 and Chapter 11 for reviews). However few data are available for goats (Kitessa *et al.*, 2001; Sanz

Table 12.5 Concentrate–oil–vitamin E interactions and effects of extruded oilseeds on dairy performances, milk fatty acid composition and goat cheese sensory quality[1] (adapted from Bernard *et al.*, 2005b; Chilliard *et al.*, 2004b, 2005b; Chilliard and Ferlay, 2004; Ferlay *et al.*, 2004; Rouel *et al.*, 2004, 2005)

	Trial 1							Trial2							Trial 3		
No. goats	12	12	12	12	12	12	12	11	12	12	12	12	12	12	14	14	14
F: C[2]	High	Medium	High	Medium	High	Medium	High	High	Low	High	Low	High	Low	High	High	LowS	LowR
Lipid suppl.[3]	–	–	LO	LO	LO+E	LO+E	EL	–	–	LO	LO	SO	SO	ELS	SO	SO	SO
E.E.% DM[4]	2.1	3.0	6.1	7.3	6.5	7.0	5.7	1.5	3.0	8.3	10.3	7.7	10.1	8.0	8.9	8.4	7.4
Cc. % DM[5]	32	56	27	53	30	52	29	33	67	25	69	24	68	31	43	63	69
Starch % DM	13.8	34.7	4.5	25.9	4.8	24.8	8.0	12.5	36.4	9.0	38.6	8.5	37.6	13.9	16.4	33.6	31.8
Milk (kg/day)	4.26^{a}	4.39^{ab}	4.25^{a}	4.28^{a}	4.19^{a}	4.74^{b}	4.26^{a}	3.40^{a}	4.33^{c}	3.29^{a}	3.96^{b}	3.52^{a}	4.14^{c}	3.51^{a}	2.75^{a}	3.21^{b}	3.34^{b}
Milk fat (g/kg)	28.1^{a}	27.0^{a}	33.2^{b}	33.3^{b}	34.9^{b}	34.8^{b}	35.4^{b}	28.6^{a}	25.3^{a}	34.4^{bc}	32.4^{b}	36.7^{c}	33.8^{bc}	39.6^{d}	36.8^{b}	33.3^{a}	32.6^{a}
SFAAI[6,7]	88.9^{e}	81.2^{d}	58.6^{bc}	62.1^{c}	54.5^{a}	62.6^{c}	55.9^{ab}	89.2^{c}	84.0^{c}	53.4^{a}	60.2^{b}	48.7^{a}	61.7^{b}	51.2^{a}	49.5^{a}	58.3^{b}	64.6^{c}
18:0[7]	6.3^{a}	6.1^{a}	9.7^{c}	8.6^{b}	10.9^{d}	9.3^{bc}	11.3^{d}	5.4^{a}	6.9^{b}	9.5^{c}	9.4^{b}	9.6^{c}	10.3^{c}	12.2^{d}	15.7^{b}	15.0^{b}	12.3^{a}
18:1 c9[7]	14.9^{b}	14.4^{ab}	15.0^{b}	13.3^{a}	14.9^{b}	13.3^{a}	14.6^{b}	13.0^{a}	14.8^{cd}	13.2^{ab}	14.3^{bc}	16.8^{e}	15.9^{e}	15.7^{de}	25.7^{c}	22.8^{b}	19.8^{a}
18:1 t11[7]	0.54^{a}	1.27^{a}	7.78^{c}	7.36^{bc}	9.52^{d}	8.15^{c}	6.48^{b}	0.51^{a}	0.89^{a}	10.27^{c}	6.19^{b}	12.72^{d}	6.82^{b}	9.12^{c}	3.23^{c}	1.98^{b}	0.96^{a}
Rumenic[7]	0.30^{a}	0.70^{a}	3.05^{c}	3.33^{c}	3.25^{c}	3.08^{c}	2.09^{b}	0.34^{a}	0.48^{a}	3.53^{c}	2.74^{b}	5.07^{d}	2.94^{bc}	3.23^{bc}	1.73^{c}	1.01^{b}	0.57^{a}
Other *trans*[7,8]	0.6^{a}	1.3^{b}	4.7^{c}	4.9^{c}	5.6^{de}	5.7^{e}	5.0^{cd}	0.7^{a}	1.1^{a}	6.3^{c}	6.8^{c}	4.0^{b}	3.6^{b}	4.6^{b}	3.3^{a}	3.3^{a}	4.2^{a}
18:1 t10[7]	0.12^{a}	0.33^{ab}	0.43^{ab}	1.00^{c}	0.57^{b}	1.06^{c}	0.59^{b}	0.17^{a}	0.18^{a}	0.41^{a}	1.42^{c}	0.95^{bc}	1.07^{bc}	0.65^{ab}	0.88^{a}	1.03^{a}	2.17^{b}
18:3 n-3[7]	0.78^{b}	0.43^{a}	1.69^{d}	1.08^{c}	1.74^{d}	1.19^{c}	2.66^{e}	0.49^{b}	0.24^{a}	1.29^{c}	0.50^{b}	0.39^{b}	0.13^{a}	1.32^{c}	0.32^{ab}	0.28^{a}	0.36^{b}
ALA/LA[9]	0.28^{b}	0.11^{a}	0.91^{d}	0.54^{c}	0.95^{d}	0.59^{cd}	1.26^{e}	0.27^{c}	0.10^{b}	0.87^{e}	0.28^{c}	0.10^{b}	0.06^{a}	0.45^{d}	0.15^{a}	0.14^{a}	0.14^{a}
Lipolysis[10]	0.36^{c}	0.24^{bc}	0.18^{ab}	0.20^{ab}	0.11^{a}	0.23^{bc}	0.18^{ab}	0.47^{d}	0.37^{cd}	0.11^{a}	0.23^{bc}	0.20^{a}	0.20^{a}	0.16^{a}	–	–	–
Cheese goaty flavour[11]	1.59^{b}	–	1.24^{a}	–	1.63^{b}	1.69^{b}	1.50^{b}	–	–	–	–	–	–	–	–	–	–
Hedonic evaluation[12]	4.9^{bc}	–	4.1^{a}	–	4.4^{ab}	–	5.1^{c}	–	–	1.7	–	2.3	–	–	–	–	–

[1]Trials 1 and 2 were on 7 groups of goats, with a treatment period of 5 weeks. Trial 3 was a 3×3 Latin Square design with 3-week periods.
[2]Forage: Concentrate ratio; Trial 1: Alfalfa Hay; Trial 2: Alfalfa Hay + Maize Silage, 0.35 kg DM/d; Trial 3: Natural grassland Hay; LowS, R = Low forage + Slowly or Rapidly degradable starch, respectively.
[3] – : Control, LO: Linseed Oil, SO: Sunflower Oil, EL: Extruded Linseed (70) and wheat (30); ELS: Extruded Linseeds (40), Sunflower seeds (30) and wheat (30); 130 or 180 g oil/day in trials 1, 3 or 2, respectively; E: Vitamin E (1250 IU/day) (a, b, c, d, e: means within a trial with different letters differ at $P < 0.05$).
[4]Ether Extract % diet Dry Matter.
[5]Concentrate, including lipids.
[6]Saturated FA Atherogenic Index: (C12:0% + (4 × C14:0%) + C16:0%).
[7]Fatty acids as w% of total FA.
[8]Others *trans* : *trans*-C18:1 and C18:2, except vaccenic and rumenic acids, but including 18:1*t*10.
[9]ALA: Alpha-Linolenic Acid, LA: Linoleic Acid.
[10]Lipolysis: g of oleic acid/100 g milk fat/34 hours post-milking at 4 °C.
[11]Spread lactic cheese made with pasteurised milk, evaluated by an expert panel, note 0 to 10.
[12]Spread lactic cheese made with pasteurised milk. Hedonic evaluation, note 1 to 7, given by a consumer panel (60 people in trial 1; 8 people in trial 2).

Table 12.6 Forage–oil interactions on dairy performances, milk fatty acid composition and goat cheese sensory quality[1] (adapted from Chilliard *et al.*, 2003c, 2004a, 2005a; Ferlay *et al.*, 2003; Gaborit *et al.*, 2002, 2004; Rouel *et al.*, 2003)

	Trial 4						Trial 5							Trial 6			Trial 7		
No. goats	12	12	12	10	12	12	12	12	12	12	12	12	12	13	13	13	14	14	14
Forages[2]	MS	MS	MS	AH	AH	AH	AH	RH	RH	RH	FR	FR	FR	NH	NH	NH	MS	MS	MS
Lipid suppl.[3]	–	OSO	LO	–	OSO	LO	–	–	OSO	LO	–	OSO	LO	–	SO	LO	–	SO	LO
E.E.% DM[4]	2.3	9.3	9.0	1.8	6.3	6.3	1.4	1.7	7.2	7.0	1.8	8.4	7.6	2.3	8.0	8.1	2.0	8.2	8.4
Cc. % DM[5]	55	44	41	45	36	36	43	49	47	46	54	56	50	56	51	52	61	55	55
Starch % DM	16.5	19.9	20.4	18.0	15.6	15.6	16.5	17.0	10.0	9.7	18.8	11.9	10.7	11.9	6.7	6.7	26.5	20.6	20.6
Milk (kg/d)	3.40^{a}	3.44^{a}	3.93^{b}	3.77^{ab}	3.86^{b}	3.91^{b}	2.98^{ab}	2.98^{ab}	3.02^{ab}	3.25^{b}	2.59^{a}	2.83^{ab}	3.07^{ab}	3.34^{a}	3.32^{a}	3.30^{a}	3.37^{a}	3.62^{b}	3.47^{ab}
Milk fat (g/kg)	29.7^{ab}	34.5^{c}	31.3^{bc}	27.1^{a}	30.6^{ab}	33.0^{bc}	31.6^{c}	27.5^{ab}	30.0^{bc}	31.9^{cd}	26.7^{a}	31.6^{b}	34.5^{d}	32.3^{a}	37.9^{b}	37.4^{b}	31.4^{a}	31.6^{a}	35.3^{b}
SFAAI[6,7]	75.3^{b}	52.5^{a}	52.9^{a}	84.6^{c}	54.9^{a}	51.4^{a}	84.9^{b}	85.9^{b}	50.4^{a}	49.9^{a}	82.3^{b}	48.7^{a}	48.1^{a}	78.2^{b}	49.0^{a}	49.4^{a}	83.8^{b}	54.3^{a}	55.6^{a}
18:0[7]	7.4^{a}	15.3^{d}	9.8^{b}	6.3^{a}	12.2^{c}	9.3^{b}	6.0^{ab}	5.4^{a}	14.0^{d}	10.7^{c}	6.9^{b}	16.2^{e}	10.8^{c}	6.9^{a}	12.5^{b}	11.6^{b}	4.9^{a}	9.0^{c}	8.2^{b}
18:1 c9[7]	18.5^{b}	25.3^{c}	15.2^{a}	15.0^{a}	26.5^{c}	14.9^{a}	14.6^{a}	14.8^{ab}	28.8^{d}	17.2^{c}	16.4^{bc}	28.3^{d}	16.5^{bc}	16.9^{a}	20.6^{b}	18.0^{a}	13.7^{a}	15.7^{b}	15.3^{b}
18:1 t11[7]	1.25^{ab}	1.68^{ab}	5.56^{c}	0.57^{a}	2.14^{b}	8.68^{d}	0.43^{a}	0.91^{a}	1.82^{b}	8.33^{c}	0.70^{a}	1.95^{b}	9.34^{d}	1.51^{a}	9.02^{c}	8.14^{b}	1.17^{a}	8.50^{c}	5.36^{b}
Rumenic[7]	0.69^{ab}	0.72^{ab}	2.09^{c}	0.33^{a}	1.10^{b}	3.65^{d}	0.31^{a}	0.51^{ab}	0.84^{b}	3.92^{c}	0.51^{ab}	0.84^{b}	4.04^{c}	0.87^{a}	3.86^{b}	3.46^{b}	0.88^{a}	4.48^{c}	2.70^{b}
Other *trans*[7, 8]	1.4^{a}	6.3^{b}	11.3^{c}	0.4^{a}	5.7^{b}	6.5^{b}	0.9^{a}	0.9^{a}	5.2^{b}	6.5^{c}	0.9^{a}	5.2^{b}	6.3^{c}	1.3^{a}	2.9^{b}	5.3^{c}	1.6^{a}	6.7^{b}	9.2^{c}
18:1 t10[7]	0.28^{a}	2.46^{b}	3.55^{b}	0.07^{a}	0.98^{a}	0.22^{a}	0.15^{a}	0.13^{a}	1.08^{c}	0.59^{b}	0.13^{a}	1.17^{c}	0.42^{ab}	0.15	0.50	0.33	0.44^{a}	3.23^{c}	1.56^{b}
18:3 n-3[7]	0.41^{b}	0.20^{a}	0.75^{d}	0.73^{d}	0.55^{c}	1.53^{e}	0.46^{cd}	0.49^{d}	0.28^{b}	0.89^{e}	0.38^{c}	0.17^{a}	0.87^{e}	1.04^{b}	0.57^{a}	1.15^{b}	0.19^{a}	0.15^{a}	0.69^{b}
ALA/LA[9]	0.18^{a}	0.14^{a}	0.47^{c}	0.34^{b}	0.35^{b}	0.85^{d}	0.21^{b}	0.27^{c}	0.20^{b}	0.66^{d}	0.23^{b}	0.14^{a}	0.64^{d}	0.49^{b}	0.26^{a}	0.83^{c}	0.08^{a}	0.05^{a}	0.36^{b}
Lipolysis[10]	0.31^{b}	0.18^{ab}	0.18^{ab}	0.48^{c}	0.18^{ab}	0.15^{a}	0.29^{a}	0.35^{ab}	0.29^{a}	0.24^{a}	0.47^{b}	0.21^{a}	0.20^{a}	0.24^{a}	0.08^{b}	0.11^{b}	0.43^{a}	0.37^{a}	0.35^{a}
Cheese goaty flavour[11]	2.50	2.28	2.28	2.46	2.11	2.18	2.30	1.81	1.76	1.30	1.54	1.92	1.82	–	–	–	–	–	–
Cheese flavour defects[12]	0/7	0/7	1/7	0/7	0/7	1/7	0/7	0/7	1/7	2/7	0/7	1/7	0/7	–	–	–	–	–	–

[1]Trials 4 and 5 were on 6 and 7 groups of goats, respectively, with a treatment period of 10 weeks (or 5 and 10 weeks for flavour criteria). Trials 6 and 7 were 3x3 Latin Square design with 3-week periods.
[2]MS: Maize Silage, AH: Alfalfa Hay, RH: Rye-grass Hay, FR: Fresh Rye-grass, NH: Natural grassland Hay.
[3]–: Control, OSO: Oleic Sunflower Oil, LO: Linseed Oil, SO: Sunflower Oil (130 g oil/day). (a, b, c, d, e: means within a trial with different letters differ at $P < 0.05$).
[4]Ether Extract % diet Dry Matter.
[5]Concentrate, including lipids.
[6]Saturated FA Atherogenic Index: (C12:0% + (4 × C14:0%) + C16:0%).
[7]Fatty acids as w% of total FA.
[8]Others *trans* : *trans*-C18:1 and C18:2, except vaccenic and rumenic acids, but including 18:1*t*10.
[9]ALA: Alpha-Linolenic Acid, LA: Linoleic Acid.
[10]Lipolysis: g of oleic acid/100 g milk fat/34 hours post-milking at 4 °C.
[11]Fresh lactic cheese made with raw milk, evaluated by an expert panel, note 0 to 10.
[12]Ripened lactic cheese made with pasteurised milk. Flavour criterion is a defect when score > predetermined level. 7 potential flavour defects (acid/bitter/metallic oxidised/pungent/rancid/salted/soapy).

Sampelayo *et al.*, 2004) on this topic, and thus the present chapter is focused on C18-PUFAs.

Linoleic acid

With most non-lipid-supplemented diets, the proportion of linoleic acid (C18:2n-6) in cow's or goat's milk FA is classically between 2 and 3%. When rations are supplemented with linoleic acid-rich seeds or oils like soybean or sunflower, that proportion rarely exceeds control values by more than 1.5% (Chilliard and Ferlay, 2004; Bernard *et al.*, 2005c; Schmidely *et al.*, 2005). It has often been suggested that giving lipids in the form of seeds rather than oil limits rumen hydrogenation because seed sheaths would restrict bacterial access to lipids. Comparing the effects of sunflower oil and seeds in goats revealed that seed C18:2 was, paradoxically, more strongly hydrogenated to stearic acid than oil C18:2, found either intact or in the form of *trans* FA and CLA in milk (Chilliard *et al.*, 2003a). It may therefore be supposed that the slow release of seed lipids enhances their total hydrogenation. A similar observation was made with C18:2-rich lupin seed, which strongly increased stearic and oleic acids while reducing milk C18:2n-6 and CLA.

The addition of linseed oil (18:3-rich) to a cow's or goat's diet decreased specifically milk linoleic acid percentage, probably because it increased linolenic percentage. Opposite responses between these two PUFAs were also observed when sunflower oil (18:2-rich) was added (Table 12.6). This illustrates that the different PUFAs are not secreted independently from each other. Lastly, it is worth remembering that increasing the linoleic acid proportion in dairy products is not a target in itself, insofar as improving the nutritional value of those products first requires an increase in the linolenic/linoleic ratio. This ratio tended to be higher with hay than maize silage diets, and was sharply increased by linseed oil supplementation (Tables 12.5 and 12.6).

Linolenic acid

Fresh green grass is the main source of alpha-linolenic acid, which explains why milk produced from grass-based diets contains more C18:3 n-3 than maize silage-based or concentrate-rich ones (Tables 12.5 and 12.6). Apart from forage, only linseed provides very high linolenic acid levels, representing more than 50% of FAs present. Few trials have been conducted where goats' diets were supplemented with linseed oil or seeds. It has been observed that C18:3 from whole crude linseeds was more widely hydrogenated to C18:0 than C18:3 from free oil (Chilliard *et al.*, 2003a) as previously observed with sunflower C18:2. In other respects, linseed oil C18:3 seems to be less hydrogenated when given to goats receiving hay-based diets than either diets rich in concentrates or maize silage-based diets (Table 12.6, trial 4; Table 12.5; trials 1 and 2). The response to extruded linseeds was high in the goat, where linolenic acid increased more (+19 mg/g) than after linseed oil supplementation (+9 mg/g) (Table 12.5). Mere formaldehyde treatment of linseed increased goat milk C18:3 concentration more than untanned seed (+11 *vs* +6 mg/g) but not beyond the effect of a similar dose of unprotected oil (+13 mg/g) (Chilliard *et al.*, 2003a; Bernard *et al.*, 2005d). The milk C18:3 concentration increased more with linseeds or linseed oil supplementation in the goat than in the cow (Chilliard and Ferlay, 2004).

12.4.3 *Trans* fatty acids and CLA

Regulation of milk fat content and secretion

Cow's milk fat content is decreased by low-fibre and high-starch diets, and more markedly with the simultaneous administration of unprotected, unsaturated vegetable oils, which sharply reduced mammary lipid secretion and strongly increased the proportions of *trans*10-18:1 and to a certain extent, of *trans*10, *cis*12-18:2 (a minor CLA isomer) (reviews in Griinari and Bauman, 2003; Loor *et al.*, 2005). It is worth noting that under such conditions, vaccenic and rumenic acid syntheses increased only slightly compared with high-fibre diets supplemented with oil (Griinari and Bauman, 2003). Those new results revived the theory of FA biohydrogenation as the central mechanism of milk fat depression with certain diets. *Trans*10,*cis*12-CLA and *trans*10-18:1 are, however, not the only candidates to induce milk fat depression, and other C18:1, C18:2 or C18:3 isomers produced in the rumen and/or in the udder might be involved (Griinari and Bauman, 2003; Shingfield *et al.*, 2003; Loor *et al.*, 2005).

Although milk fat depression in cows seems to be related to the increase of specific *trans* FA, the situation is less clear in goats. In that species, milk fat content and yield are not reduced, but are almost always increased by vegetable oil supplementation (Chilliard *et al.*, 2003a), even when added to low-fibre (Table 12.5 and Schmidely *et al.*, 2005) or maize silage-based (Table 12.6) diets. Milk fat content increase after lipid supplementation was however less marked when goats were given maize silage (Fig. 12.1), reflecting either the high milk fat content ensured by this basal diet, or a negative effect of the *trans*10-18:1 increase which was specifically induced by the maize silage-oil interaction, thus limiting the positive effect of oils on milk fat content and on CLA secretion which was otherwise observed with the hay diets (Tables 12.5 and 12.6). In the range of the concentrate percentages (35–70%) of the 36 diets that were studied, high concentrations of *trans*10-18:1 (1.1–3.2%) were indeed always observed with either high-concentrate (>50%) diets or maize silage or fresh rye-grass diets supplemented with oleic-, linoleic- or linolenic-rich oil. For hay-based diets, high *trans*10-18:1 and low milk fat content responses were observed only with high-oleic sunflower oil supplementation (Fig. 12.1), consistently with a possible *cis*9-18:1 isomerisation into *trans*10-18:1 in the rumen (Mosley *et al.*, 2002).

Thus, in our database, the milk fat yield response of 22 lipid-supplemented groups of goats was always positive, but its extent was negatively correlated ($r = -0.71$) to the concentration in milk of *trans*10-18:1 (Fig. 12.1). Increasing dietary concentrate% without lipid supplementation increased milk yield, decreased slightly goat's milk fat content (−1 to −3 g/kg) but did not change or

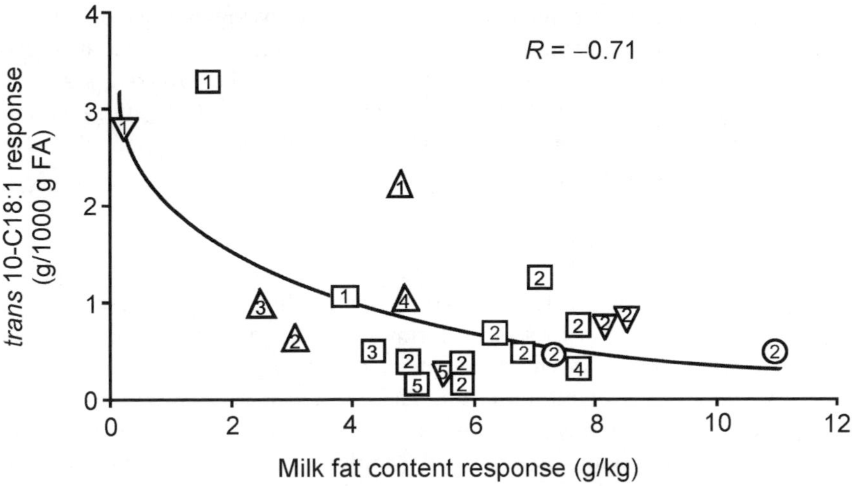

Fig. 12.1 Relationship between milk fat content and *trans*10-C18:1 responses to lipid supplementation in dairy goats (adapted from data in Tables 12.5 and 12.6: 22 'lipid-supplemented groups *minus* corresponding control group' in trials 1, 2, 4, 5, 6, 7). △, ▽, □, ○ = high-oleic sunflower oil, high-linoleic sunflower oil, linseed oil, extruded oilseeds, respectively. 1, 2, 3, 4, 5 = maize silage, alfalfa hay, rye-grass hay, fresh rye-grass, natural grassland hay, respectively.

increased slightly milk fat *trans*10-18:1 (+0.01 to 0.21 g/100 g, Table 12.5; Schmidely and Sauvant, 2001; LeDoux *et al.*, 2002), which is much less than the *trans*10-18:1 increase observed with lipid supplementation of medium- or high-concentrate diets (Tables 12.5 and 12.6). In diets containing sunflower oil and supplemented rapidly degradable starch (trial 3, Table 12.5), milk fat yield and C8–C16 secretion, as well as mammary acetyl-CoA carboxylase activity, increased despite the simultaneous increase in *trans*10-18:1 secretion (Bernard *et al.*, 2005e). Thus, other factors than *trans*10-18:1 are likely to be involved in the regulation of mammary lipogenesis in goats.

In trial 5 (84 goats, Table 12.6), there was no correlation between the milk fat content and the proportions of the various *trans*-18:1 or CLA isomers (including *trans*10-18:1 and *trans*10,*cis*12 CLA) (Chilliard *et al.*, 2003b), contrary to what was observed in dairy cows (see above). This could be related to the fact that *trans*10,*cis*12 CLA, (i) did not increase in goat milk, even when *trans*10-18:1 increased (Tables 12.5 and 12.6) and (ii) that this CLA isomer did not inhibit milk fat secretion when infused post-ruminally in goats (P. Andrade and P. Schmidely, personal communication), contrary to cows (Griinari and Bauman, 2003). However, goat's milk fat content was negatively correlated with several saturated and monounsaturated C14 to C16 FAs and n-6 PUFAs, and positively with stearic acid (Chilliard *et al.*, 2003b; Bernard *et al.*, 2005a), which confirmed that this substrate is a major regulating factor of mammary lipid secretion in that species, as suggested in earlier studies with lipid-poor diets (Delage and Fehr, 1967). Contrary to what was observed in the cow (Focant *et* *al.*, 2001), vitamin E supplementation to goats receiving linseed oil did not interact with forage: concentrate ratio, and did not change either milk fat content or *trans*10-18:1 percentage, although it increased the other *trans*-FAs and the 18:0, and decreased the C10–C16:0 percentages and the 18:0 desaturation ratio (Table 12.5). Thus vitamin E tended to increase further the main effects of linseed oil addition to the goat's diet.

Effects of feeding factors on milk trans *and conjugated fatty acids*
The dietary factors that influence the milk CLA and *trans*11-18:1 concentration are included in two main categories: (i) diets providing lipid precursors (C18:2 or C18:3) for CLA and/or *trans*-18:1 formation in the rumen, and (ii) diets that modify the microbial activity associated with PUFA hydrogenation in the rumen. Combinations of these various factors induce wide variations of goat milk CLA and *trans*-18:1 concentrations, and strong interactions occur between forages, starchy concentrates and lipid supplements (Tables 12.5 and 12.6). C18:2-rich vegetable oils (e.g. sunflower oil) highly increase milk rumenic acid content. Overall, vegetable oils increase milk rumenic acid more than extruded seeds, which in turn increase it more than raw seeds. This effect is indeed more or less marked according to plant oil presentation, because PUFAs from free oil, extruded seeds or raw seeds disrupt rumen metabolism more or less intensively. Increasing linseed oil (C18:3-rich) intake increased milk rumenic acid concentration. That could be explained by a ruminal conversion of C18:3 to *trans*11-18:1, which would be later desaturated by delta-9 desaturase to yield rumenic acid in mammary or other tissues.

There is indeed a strong linear correlation between milk rumenic acid and *trans*11-18:1 concentrations under a wide variety of diets, either in goats (Chilliard *et al.*, 2003a; Nudda *et al.*, 2003) or cows (Griinari and Bauman, 1999, 2003). In the 36 diets studied in goats (Tables 12.5 and 12.6), the rumenic : vaccenic ratio was 0.6–0.7 for control diets, and 0.3–0.5 for lipid supplemented diets. With combinations of five different forages with either no oil addition or 18:1-, 18:2- or 18:3-rich oils, we observed a considerable range of rumenic acid, from 0.3 to 5.1% of total FAs. The main factor of variation was the nature of oil with sunflower (18:2-rich) $\geq$ linseed (18:3-rich) $\gg$ oleic sunflower (18:1-rich) > no oil addition. The response to oleic acid-rich oil, albeit much less than similar amount of either linseed or sunflower oil, is consistent with a possible *cis*9-18:1 isomerisation into *trans*11-18:1 in the rumen (Mosley *et al.*, 2002) or could be due to an inhibition of the last step of hydrogenation of dietary PUFA. For a given oil supplementation, the response to oil interacted strongly with the nature of forage. Thus the response to sunflower oil was highest with maize silage (trial 7 *vs* trial 6) and lowest with high-concentrate diet (68%, trial 2), whereas the response to linseed oil was lower with maize silage than with either hays or fresh grass (Tables 12.5 and 12.6). However, milk rumenic acid response to linseed oil supplementation was not changed when dietary concentrate increased from 30% to 54%, and this was not changed by vitamin E supplementation, but decreased with high-concentrate (69%) diet. The responses were lower with extruded linseeds or sunflower seeds than with the same doses of oils (Table 12.5).

Data in cows suggest that milk vaccenic and rumenic acid responses to lipid supplementation could be transient, with a maximum during the first 2 weeks after the beginning of lipid supplementation and that the decrease after 3 weeks was accompanied by a strong increase in milk fat *trans*10-18:1 percentage, that was more marked with high-concentrate + maize silage diets (Chilliard and Ferlay, 2004; Roy *et al.*, 2005). This raises the question of the sustainability of high CLA responses in dairy cattle, and further studies are needed on interactions between dietary fibre, starch, FAs and other components. We recently obtained data on the short-term kinetics of CLA response in goat's milk. Even with high-concentrate diets and with polyunsaturated oils, the response of rumenic acid reached a maximum 2 weeks after the beginning of oil supplementation, and then remained stable at very high levels (Fig. 12.2) despite *trans*10-18:1 percentage increasing 5–8 times above control values in diets without dietary oils (Table 12.5). Furthermore, high CLA levels were observed after 10 weeks of lipid supplementation (Table 12.6) without a decrease from what was observed in the same goats after 5 weeks (Chilliard *et al.*, 2003a, 2004a; Chilliard and Ferlay, 2004). This shows that the goat is a very good

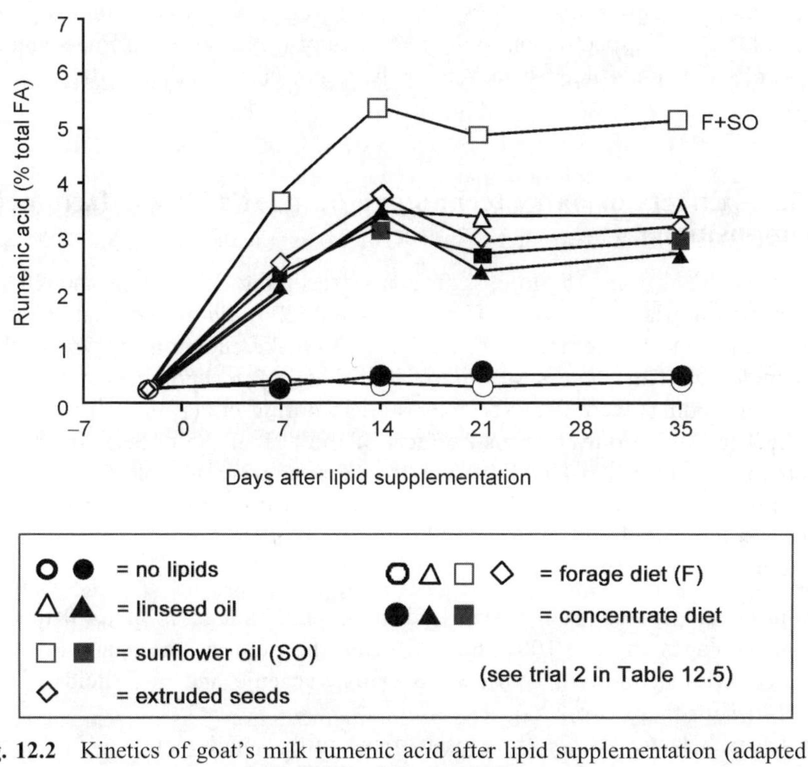

Fig. 12.2 Kinetics of goat's milk rumenic acid after lipid supplementation (adapted from Chilliard *et al.*, 2005b).

responder and that its milk rumenic acid response is stable during at least 2.5 months. In field conditions, goat milk CLA was 44% higher in a grazing system compared with a hay + grains diet (Di Trana *et al.*, 2003).

Few data are available on the influence of feeding on the various milk 18:1 and CLA isomers. Rumenic acid is classically the one whose concentration is the most variable because of the importance of its mammary synthesis by delta-9 desaturase. In addition, this enzyme synthesises *trans*7,*cis*9-CLA, quantitatively the second most abundant isomer present in milk. That isomer is increased in cows by low-fibre diets supplemented with soybean oil (Piperova *et al.*, 2000) and probably in goats by high-oleic sunflower oil supplementation (Ferlay *et al.*, 2003). Low-fibre diets increase *cis*11,*trans*13 and *cis*9,*cis*11-CLA isomers, whereas linseed oil increases *cis*9,*cis*11, *trans*11,*cis*13- and *trans*11,*trans*13 CLA, as well as *trans*13-18:1, *cis*9,*trans*13-18:2 and *trans*11,*cis*15-18:2, (Chilliard et *al.*, 2003c for goats; Loor *et al.*, 2005 for cows). *Trans*10,*cis*12-CLA always remained at trace levels in goats. It should be stressed that the achievement of high levels of rumenic acid (>2% of total FAs) with oil supplements is accompanied by high levels not only of vaccenic acid (6–13%) but also of other *trans*-isomers of C18:1 and conjugated or non-conjugated C18:2 (3–6% with grass-based diets, 9–11% with maize silage diets, and for a given forage, linseed oil> oleic sunflower oil >sunflower oil, Tables 12.5 and 12.6) and probably *trans* isomers of C18:3 as suggested by cow studies (Loor *et al.*, 2005). The respective physiological roles of these various isomers and their possible nutritional interest to humans have not been studied to date.

12.5 Effects of dairy technology on goat's cheese fatty acid composition

Pooled milks from 15 groups of goats (receiving 15 among the 20 diets described in trials 1, 4 and 5, Tables 12.5 and 12.6), with a very large scale of between-group FA composition, were used to make cheese using five different technologies. Thirty cheeses from trial 1 (5 diets × 3 technologies × 2 durations of lipid feeding) were analysed after storage during either 30 or 60 days at 2–4 °C. There were only marginal effects of the age of the cheeses on their FA composition (e.g. +0.4 and −0.2 g/100 g for palmitic and oleic acid, respectively). Independently of age, several significant differences were observed in cheeses compared with milks (Table 12.7), although they were of low extent. The more important are:

- in cheese spread from pasteurised lactic curd, increases in C4:0 to C14:0 percentages (+5.1 g/100 g total FA for the sum of these six FAs), and decreases in most of C18-FA, specially vaccenic and oleic acids (−2.3 g/100 g for these two FAs);
- in fresh lactic cheese from pasteurised milk, small increases in C10:0 to C14:0, and small decrease in C18:0;

Table 12.7 Effect of cheese-making technology on changes in goat dairy product fatty acid composition, g/100 g total FA (adapted from Ferlay *et al.*, 2005, and unpublished results)

Cheesemaking	Series A			Series B		Series C				
Products	Milks[1]	Spread[2]	RLP[3]	Milks[4]	SRP[5]	Milks[6]	FLP[7]	RLP[8]	RLR[9]	SRP[10]
No.	5	10	10	5	10	10	10	10	10	10
C4:0	2.85^{b}	3.31^{a}	1.82^{c}	2.60^{a}	1.94^{b}	2.65^{a}	2.47^{a}	2.04^{b}	2.25^{ab}	2.44^{a}
C6:0	2.54^{b}	2.84^{a}	1.85^{c}	2.46^{a}	1.95^{b}	2.55	2.45	2.19	2.36	2.49
C8:0	2.49^{b}	3.15^{a}	2.26^{b}	2.49^{a}	2.22^{b}	2.61	2.68	2.59	2.78	2.77
C10:0	7.61^{b}	9.86^{a}	7.93^{b}	8.04^{b}	8.67^{a}	8.80^{c}	9.37^{b}	9.55^{ab}	10.05^{a}	9.80^{ab}
C12:0	3.27^{c}	3.98^{a}	3.71^{b}	3.66^{b}	4.09^{a}	3.98^{c}	4.26^{b}	4.49^{ab}	4.70^{a}	4.48^{ab}
C14:0	9.13^{b}	9.83^{a}	10.03^{a}	9.60^{b}	10.64^{a}	10.10^{c}	10.67^{b}	11.26^{a}	11.45^{a}	11.37^{a}
C16:0	20.65	19.95	21.41	21.74^{b}	22.49^{a}	23.58	23.81	24.48	23.99	24.38
C18:0	9.60^{ab}	8.89^{b}	10.39^{a}	8.77^{b}	9.67^{a}	8.95^{a}	8.36^{b}	8.29^{b}	8.01^{b}	8.89^{a}
trans-C18:1	9.81^{ab}	8.66^{b}	9.55^{a}	9.22^{b}	8.78^{a}	5.99	5.82	5.84	5.62	5.53
*trans*10	0.55^{b}	0.86^{a}	0.75^{a}	0.44^{a}	0.71^{b}	0.78	0.78	0.81	0.79	0.80
*trans*11	6.51^{a}	5.25^{b}	5.89^{a}	6.13	5.21	3.10	3.10	2.95	2.81	2.58
*cis*9-C18:1	14.59^{a}	13.55^{b}	13.98^{ab}	14.45^{a}	12.95^{b}	16.87^{a}	16.86^{a}	15.88^{b}	15.59^{b}	15.36^{b}
c9t13-C18:2	0.44^{a}	0.40^{b}	0.41^{b}	0.44	0.43	0.28^{a}	0.26^{ab}	0.25^{ab}	0.24^{b}	0.26^{ab}
t11c15-C18:2	1.67^{a}	1.31^{b}	1.43^{a}	1.57	1.35	0.69	0.70	0.67	0.64	0.63
C18:2 n-6	1.96^{a}	1.80^{b}	2.00^{a}	1.93	1.80	1.69^{a}	1.66^{a}	1.60^{a}	1.60^{a}	1.50^{b}
C18:3 n-3	1.61	1.35	1.40	1.51^{a}	1.37^{b}	0.58	0.57	0.51	0.51	0.55
c9t11-CLA	2.37	2.05	2.15	2.41	2.05	1.33^{a}	1.35^{a}	1.30^{a}	1.18^{ab}	1.05^{b}

[1]Milks from 5 diets studied in Trial 1 (Table 12.5) after 5 weeks of lipid supplementation.
[2]Spread from pasteurised lactic curd, 30- ($n = 5$) or 60-day ($n = 5$) old.
[3]Ripened Lactic cheese, Pasteurised milk, St.-Maure type, 30- ($n = 5$) or 60-days ($n = 5$) old.
[4]Milks from 5 diets studied in Trial 1 (Table 12.5) after 9 weeks of lipid supplementation.
[5] Soft ripened cheese, Pasteurised milk, Camembert type, 30- ($n = 5$) or 60-day ($n = 5$) old.
[6]Milks from 10 diets studied in Trials 4 and 5 (Table 12.6) after 4–5 weeks of lipid supplementation.
[7]Fresh Lactic cheese, Pasteurised milk, St.-Maure type, 15 day-old.
[8]Ripened Lactic, Pasteurised milk, 30-days old.
[9]Ripened Lactic cheese, from Raw milk, 30-days old.
[10]Soft ripened cheese, Pasteurised milk, Camembert type, 30-day old.
[a,b,c] within a series, products with different letters differ at $P < 0.05$.

- in ripened lactic cheeses (from either pasteurised or raw milk), increases in C10:0 to C14:0 and decreases in oleic acid;
- in soft ripened cheeses from pasteurised milk, increases in C10:0 to C14:0, decrease in oleic acid, and (significantly or not) small decreases in butyric, caproic, linoleic, alpha-linolenic, rumenic acids and *trans*-C18:1 isomers (except *trans*10-C18:1).

Thus, the more constant effects across cheese technologies were clear increases in C10:0, C12:0 and C14:0 and, less markedly, a decrease in oleic acid. Very few changes were observed for PUFA, including rumenic acid (in agreement with data on bovine dairy products, e.g. Ferlay *et al.*, 2002; Gnädig *et al.*, 2004). A peculiarity was noted for spread technology, with small increases in C4:0 to C8:0. However, the effects of cheese-making on cheese FA profile (as compared to milks) are minor, and much lower (Table 12.7) than the very important effects of dietary factors (Tables 12.5 and 12.6). Thus cheese FA composition depends mainly on milk composition and its variation factors at the animal level.

12.6 Animal diet, processing and sensory quality of dairy products

Before recommending to farmers changes to their feeding strategies to modify milk FA composition, it has to be ascertained that such practices would not be detrimental to the milk cheese-making ability and sensory quality of dairy products (Chilliard and Ferlay, 2004). The experiments reviewed here have shown effects of forage and lipid supplements and their interactions on goat cheese flavour (Gaborit *et al.*, 2002, 2004, and Tables 12.5 and 12.6, for 166 cheese-makings using six different technologies): spread, fresh or ripened lactic cheeses (St.-Maure type) from raw or pasteurised milk, soft ripened cheese (Camembert type) from pasteurised milk.

Linseed oil or oleic sunflower oil supplementation (4–7% of the ration) increased flavour intensities but tended to reduce the 'goaty' taste in milk, fresh lactic cheese from raw milk or spread lactic cheese from pasteurised milk (but not in ripened lactic cheese). This effect on 'goaty' taste is partly linked to the lower secretion of lipoprotein lipase (Chilliard *et al.*, 2003a) and reduced post-milking lipolysis (Table 12.5 and 12.6). Also, minor defects such as bitter, piquant, oxidised or fishy flavours may occur, especially with linseed oil when added to alfalfa hay diets, which increased strongly milk C18:3 concentration (Table 12.6). Defects were more pronounced when oil supplementations were delivered at a high level (7% of total diet DM), which resulted in lower flavour scores by the consumer panel (Table 12.5). However, the supplementation with extruded linseeds at 4% oil in total diet DM maximised milk C18:3 concentration without decreasing the sensorial quality of cheese. Thus, the presence of natural antioxidants in the non-oil fraction of the extruded seeds could be hypothesised. Lipid supplementation did not alter cheese-making ability, and improved the cheese fondant texture (Gaborit *et al.*, 2004) and the cheese yield and fat recovery ratio due to the higher milk fat content.

12.7 Conclusions

The FA composition of caprine dairy products depends largely on animal factors, although the effect of technological factors are very low. The genotype for alpha-s1 casein has significant effects on milk fat and its FA composition. Feeding factors are, however, the most potent method to vary ruminant milk FA composition in many ways. Recent advances in the knowledge of FA synthesis mechanisms, and the putative physiological effects of these FAs in human consumers have significantly boosted ongoing research and potential applications. As regards goat nutrition, experimental results (Chilliard *et al.*, 2003a, and present review) show that lipid supplementation does not change net energy intake, milk yield and protein yield, strongly increases milk fat and lactose content and allows much less saturated FA, much more oleic and/or vaccenic + rumenic acids, and more linolenic acid and other *trans* FAs. The responses of goats are clearly different from cow's responses for many aspects of mammary lipid secretion (Bernard *et al.*, 2005a).

It is clear that the plasticity of milk fat composition is very large, with numerous interactions between forage, concentrates, oils and vitamins, on almost all major and minor FAs. It is emphasised that the addition of vegetable oils to maize silage diets increases sharply the *trans* FAs other than rumenic and vaccenic acids. The aim of future research is to better understand the effects of using grass-based diets, new combinations of feedstuffs and nutrients in concentrates, and oilseed technology and processing, in order to increase more selectively FAs of interest for human nutrition, without increasing less desired FAs and without decreasing the sensory quality of dairy products.

Insofar as human nutritional recommendations may still vary in the coming years, and as the putative effect of a large number of specific FAs (*trans* isomers of C18:1, C18:2, C18:3, etc.) on human health are not yet known, animal nutritionists have to keep exploring the response patterns of major and minor milk FA and to model their synthesis mechanisms. At the same time, the side effects of the various dietary practices on health safety (antinutritional factors, pro-oxidant effects, etc.), on technological and sensory quality as well as on the image of dairy products need to be better assessed.

12.8 Acknowledgements

The authors thank P. Capitan, E. Bruneteau, P. Caugnon, J.M. Chabosseau, P. Guillouet, G. Gandemer, G. Lamberet, A. Combeau, A. Ollier and D. Roux for their help and/or advice during goat experiments, and the secretarial assistance of P. Béraud. Experimental work was funded by the French Ministry of

Research (AQS-P204), the Poitou-Charentes Region and by BIOCLA Project QLK1-2002-02362 within the EU Fifth Framework Research programme (www.teagasc.ie/research/dprc/biocla/index.htm). The preparation of this review was supported by LIPGENE, an Integrated Project within the EU funded Sixth Framework Research programme (www.lipgene.tcd.ie).

12.9 References

ALONSO L, FONTECHA J, LOZADA L, FRAGA M J and JUAREZ M (1999), 'Fatty acid composition of caprine milk: major, branched-chain, and *trans* fatty acids', *J Dairy Sci*, **82**, 878–884.

BANNI S, ANGIONI E, MURRU E, CARTA G, MELIS M P, BAUMAN D, DONG Y and IP C (2001), 'Vaccenic adic feeding increases tissue levels of conjugated linoleic acid and suppresses development of premalignant lesions in rat mammary gland', *Nutr Cancer*, **41**, 91–97.

BAUMAN D E, CORL B A and PETERSON D G (2003), 'The biology of conjugated linoleic acids in ruminants', in Sébédio J L, Christie W W and Adlof R, (Editors), *Advances in Conjugated Linoleic Acid Research*, Vol.2. *Am Oil Chem Soc Press*. Champaign, Illinois, pp. 146–173.

BEAULIEU A D and PALMQUIST D L (1995), 'Differential effects of high fat diets on fatty acid composition in milk of Jersey and Holstein cows', *J Dairy Sci*, **78**, 1336–1344.

BERNARD L, LEROUX C, HAYES H, GAUTIER M, CHILLIARD Y and MARTIN P (2001) 'Characterization of the caprine stearoyl-CoA desaturase gene and mRNA showing an unusually long 3′-UTR sequence arising from a single exon', *Gene*, **281**, 53–61.

BERNARD L, LEROUX C and CHILLIARD Y (2005a), 'Characterisation and nutritional regulation of the main lipogenic genes in the ruminant lactating mammary gland', *10th International Symposium on Ruminant Physiology*, Copenhagen, Denmark, 30 Aug–4 Sept 2004, in Sejrsen K, Hvelplund T, Nielsen MO (eds), *Ruminant physiology: digestion, metabolism and impact of nutrition on gene expression, immunology and stress*, Wageningen Acad. Publ. (NL), in press.

BERNARD L, ROUEL J, FERLAY A and CHILLIARD Y (2005b), 'Effects of concentrate level and starch degradability on milk yield and fatty acid (FA) composition in goats receiving a diet supplemented in sunflower oil', in *Book of Abstracts, 56th Annual Meeting of European Association for Animal Production*, 5–8 June 2005, Uppsala, Sweden. Wageningen Acad. Publ. (NL), p. 161.

BERNARD L, LEROUX C, BONNET M, ROUEL J, MARTIN P and CHILLIARD Y (2005c), 'Expression and nutritional regulation of lipogenic genes in mammary gland and adipose tissues of lactating goats', *J Dairy Res*, **72**, 250–255.

BERNARD L, ROUEL J, LEROUX C, FERLAY A, FAULCONNIER Y, LEGRAND P and CHILLIARD Y (2005d), 'Mammary lipid metabolism and fatty acid secretion in Alpine goats fed vegetable lipids', *J Dairy Sci*, **88**, 1478–1489.

BERNARD L, LEROUX C, FAULCONNIER Y, DURAND D and CHILLIARD Y (2005e), 'Effects of concentrate level and starch degradability on expression of mammary lipogenic genes in goats receiving a diet supplemented in sunflower oil', in *Book of Abstracts, 56th Annual Meeting of European Association for Animal Production*, 5–8 June 2005, Uppsala, Sweden, Wageningen Acad. Publ. (NL), p. 161.

BICKERSTAFFE R, NOAKES D E and ANNISON E F (1972), 'Quantitative aspects of fatty acid biohydrogenation, absorption and transfer into milk fat in the lactating goat, with special reference to the *cis*- and *trans*-isomers of octadecenoate and linoleate', *Biochem J*, **130**, 607–617.

CALDERON I, DE PETERS E J, SMITH N E and FRANKE A A (1984), 'Composition of goat's milk: changes within milking and effects of a high concentrate diet', *J Dairy Sci*, **67**, 1905–1911.

CHANAT E, MARTIN P and OLLIVIER-BOUSQUET M (1999), 'α_{s1}-casein is required for the efficient transport of β- and κ-casein from the endoplasmic reticulum to the Golgi apparatus of mammary epithelial cells', *J Cell Sci*, **112**, 3399–3412.

CHEN Z Y, PELLETIER G, HOLLYWOOD R and RATNAYAKE W M N (1995), '*Trans* fatty acid isomers in Canadian human milk', *Lipids*, **30**, 15–21.

CHILLIARD Y and FERLAY A (2004), 'Dietary lipids and forages interactions on cow and goat milk fatty acid composition and sensory properties', *Reprod Nutr Dev*, **44**, 467–492.

CHILLIARD Y and LAMBERET G (2001), 'Biochemical characteristics of goat milk lipids and lipolytic system. A comparison with cow's and human milk. Effects of lipid supplementation', in Freund G, (ed.), *Recent Advances on Goat Milk Quality, Raw Material for Cheese-making* (ITPLC edn, ISBN 2-9514868-1-2), 71–114.

CHILLIARD Y, FERLAY A, MANSBRIDGE R M and DOREAU M (2000), 'Ruminant milk fat plasticity: nutritional control of saturated, polyunsaturated, *trans* and conjugated fatty acids', *Annales de Zootechnie*, **49**, 181–205.

CHILLIARD Y, FERLAY A and DOREAU M (2001), 'Effect of different types of forages, animal fat or marine oils in cow's diet on milk fat secretion and composition, especially conjugated linoleic acid (CLA) and polyunsaturated fatty acids', *Livet Prod Sci*, **70**, 31–48.

CHILLIARD Y, FERLAY A, ROUEL J and LAMBERET G (2003a), 'A review of nutritional and physiological factors affecting goat milk lipid synthesis and lipolysis', *J Dairy Sci*, **86**, 1751–1770.

CHILLIARD Y, ROUEL J, CAPITAN P, CHABOSSEAU J M, RAYNAL-LJUTOVAC K and FERLAY A (2003b), 'Correlations between milk fat content and fatty acid composition in goats receiving different combinations of forages and lipid supplements', in *Book of Abstracts, 54th Annual Meeting of European Association for Animal Production*, Rome, Italy, 31 Aug.–3 Sept., p. 343.

CHILLIARD Y, ROUEL J, CHABOSSEAU J M, CAPITAN P, GABORIT P and FERLAY A (2003c), 'Interactions between raygras preservation and linseed oil supplementation on goat milk yield and composition, including *trans* and conjugated fatty acids', in *Book of Abstracts, 54th Annual Meeting of European Association for Animal Production*, Rome, Italy, 31 Aug.–3 Sept., p. 343.

CHILLIARD Y, BERNARD L, ROUEL J, FERLAY A, GABORIT P, RAYNAL-LJUTOVAC K and LAURET A (2004a), 'Effet de l'alimentation et de sa composition en matière grasse sur la qualité du lait et des produits laitiers caprins (aptitude technologique, qualité sensorielle) et la production d'acides gras présentant un avantage pour la santé du consommateur', Compte rendu de fin de recherche financée par le ministère de la Recherche (AQS-P204). INRA-ITPLC, Clemont-Ferrand, pp. 1–39.

CHILLIARD Y, ROUEL J, LELOUTRE L, BRUNETEAU E, CAPITAN P, LAURET A and FERLAY A (2004b), 'Effects of extruded linseed substitution to linseed oil and/or soybean meal, on milk yield and fatty acid (FA) composition in goats receiving a high-forage diet', in *Book of Abstracts, 55th Annual Meeting of European Association for Animal Production*, Bled, Slovenia, 5–9 Sept., p. 135.

CHILLIARD Y, ROUEL J, FERLAY A, BERNARD L, GABORIT P, RAYNAL-LJUTOVAC K and LAURET A (2005a), 'Effects of type of forage and lipid supplementation on goat milk fatty acids and sensorial properties of cheeses', in *Future of the Sheep and Goat Dairy Sector*, Special issue of the International Dairy Federation No. 0501/part 5, pp. 297–304.

CHILLIARD Y, ROUEL J, GUILLOUET P, RAYNAL-LJUTOVAC K, LELOUTRE L and FERLAY A (2005b), 'Kinetics of responses of goat milk fatty acids to dietary forage: concentrate ratio and/or high doses of sunflower or linseed oil, or extruded mixture of seeds', in *Book of Abstracts, 56th Annual Meeting of European Association for Animal Production*, 5–8 June 2005, Uppsala, Sweden, Wageningen Acad. Publ. (NL), p. 268.

DAVIES D T, HOLT C and CHRISTIE W W (1983), 'The composition of milk', in T.B. Mepham (ed.), *Biochemistry of Lactation*, Elsevier Sci Publ, Amsterdam, pp. 71–117.

DELACROIX-BUCHET A and LAMBERET G (2000), 'Sensorial properties and typicity of goat dairy products', in *7th Int. Conf on Goats*, Tours, France. 15–21 May 2000. Vol. 2, pp. 559–563.

DELACROIX-BUCHET A, DEGAS C, LAMBERET G and VASSAL L (1996), 'Influence des variants AA et FF de la caséine αs1 caprine sur le rendement fromager et les caractéristiques des fromages', *Lait*, **76**, 217–241.

DELAGE J and FEHR P M (1967), 'Influence des lipides alimentaires sur la sécrétion des acides gras par la mamelle de chèvre. I. Influence de la teneur du régime en lipides sur le taux butyreux du lait et sa composition en acides gras', *Ann Biol Anim Biochim Biophys*, **7**, 437–444.

DESTAILLATS F, WOLFF R L, PRECHT D and MOLKENTIN J (2000), 'Study of individual *trans*- and *cis*-16:1 isomers in cow, goat, and ewe cheese fats by gas-liquid chromatography with emphasis on the *trans*-Δ3 isomer'; *Lipids*, **35**, 1027–1032.

DI TRANA A, CIFUNI G F, BRAGHIERI A, FEDELE V, CLAPS S and RUBINO R (2003) 'Influence of feeding system and season on CLA content in goat milk', in *Book of Abstract, 54th Annual Meeting of European Association for Animal Production*, Rome, Italy, 31 Aug.–3 Sept., p. 350.

DOREAU M and FERLAY A (1994), 'Digestion and utilisation of fatty acids by ruminants', *Anim Feed Sci Technol*, **45**, 379–396.

FERLAY A, VERDIER-METZ I, PRADEL PH, MARTIN B, VAN DER HORST H, BALLOT N and CHILLIARD Y (2002), 'Effets respectifs d'une alimentation à base d'herbe et de la transformation fromagère sur la composition en acides gras d'intérêt nutritionnel de fromage de type Saint-Nectaire ou Cantal', *Rencontres Recherches Ruminants*, **9**, 367.

FERLAY A, ROUEL J, CHABOSSEAU J M, CAPITAN P, RAYNAL-LJUTOVAC K and CHILLIARD Y (2003), 'Interactions between raygrass preservation and high-oleic sunflower oil supplementation on goat milk composition, including *trans* and conjugated fatty acids', in *Book of Abstracts, 54th Annual Meeting of European Association for Animal Production*, Rome, Italy, 31 Aug.–3 Sept, p. 350.

FERLAY A, ROUEL J, CAPITAN P, BRUNETEAU E, GABORIT P, LELOUTRE L and CHILLIARD Y (2004), 'Concentrate level and vitamin E supplementation do not interact on milk yield and fatty acid (FA) composition in goats receiving alfalfa hay and linseed oil', in *Book of Abstracts, 55th Annual Meeting of European Association for Animal Production*, Bled, Slovenia, 5–9 Sept., p. 119.

FERLAY A, GABORIT P, RAYNAL-LJUTOVAC K, ROUEL J, LAURET A and CHILLIARD Y (2005),

'Effets de différentes technologies fromagères sur la composition en acides gras d'intérêt nutritionnel de fromages caprins', *Rencontres Recherches Ruminants*, **12**, 408.

FÉVRIER C, MOUROT J, JAGUELIN Y, MOUNIER A and LEBRETON Y (1993), 'Utilisations digestives comparées des laits UHT de chèvre et de vache. Effets nutritionnels de la gélification. Utilisation du modèle porcin', *Le Lait*, **73**, 581–592.

FOCANT M, GRIINARI M, MIGNOLET E and LARONDELLE Y (2001), 'Effet de la supplémentation en vitamine E sur la production d'acides linoléiques conjugués par la vache laitière', in *Symp. 'Santé animale, santé humaine. Productions animales naturellement riches en oméga 3 et CLA favorables à la santé'*, Ciney, Belgique, 26 Oct., 2 pp.

GABORIT P, RAYNAL K, LAURET A, CHABOSSEAU J M, ROUEL J and CHILLIARD Y (2002), 'Flavour of goat milk and cheeses according to feeding : alfalfa hay or maize silage with oleic sunflower or linseed oil supplementation', *Grassland Science in Europe* Br. Grassland Soc., Reading, UK, Vol. 7, pp. 562–563.

GABORIT P, ROUEL J, BRUNETEAU E, RAYNAL-LJUTOVAC K, FERLAY A, LAURET A and CHILLIARD Y (2004), 'Impact of dietary lipid supplementation on goat milk fat and sensorial properties of cheeses', in Proc. 8th Int Conference on Goats. Pretoria, South Africa, 4–9 July, p. 41.

GLASS R L, TROOLIN H A and JENNESS R (1967), 'Comparative biochemical studies of milks. IV. Constituent fatty acids of milk fats', *Com Biochem Physiol*, **22**, 415–425.

GNÄDIG S, CHAMBA J F, PERREARD E, CHAPPAZ S, CHARDIGNY J M, RICKERT R, STEINHART H and SEBEDIO J L (2004) 'Influence of manufacturing conditions on the conjugated linoleic acid content and the isomer composition in ripened French Emmental cheese', *J Dairy Res*, **71**, 367–371.

GRIINARI J M and BAUMAN D E (1999), 'Biosynthesis of conjugated linoleic acid and its incorporation into meat and milk in ruminants', in Yurawecz M P, Mossoba M M, Kramer J K G, Pariza M W and Nelson G L (eds), *Advances in Conjugated Linoleic Acid Research*, Vol. 1. Am Oil Chem Soc Press, Champaign, Illinois, pp. 180–200.

GRIINARI J M and BAUMAN D E (2003), 'Update on theories of diet-induced milk fat depression and potential applications', *Rec Adv Anim Nutr*, **37**, 115–156.

GROSCLAUDE F, RICORDEAU G, MARTIN P, REMEUF F, VASSAL L and BOUILLON J (1994), 'Du gène au fromage: le polymorphisme de la caséine α-s1 caprine, ses effets, son évolution', *INRA Prod Anim*, **7**, 3–19.

GUESNET P, ANTOINE J M, ROCHETTE DE LEMPDES J B, GALENT A and DURAND G (1993), 'Polyunsaturated fatty acid composition of human milk in France: changes during the course of lactation and regional differences', *Eur J Clin Nutr*, **47**, 700–710.

GULATI S K, KITESSA S M, ASHES J R, FLECK E, BYERS E B, BYERS Y G and SCOTT T W (2000), 'Protection of conjugated linoleic acids from ruminal hydrogenation and their incorporation into milk fat', *Anim Feed Sc. Technol*, **86**, 139–148.

HA J K and LINDSAY R C (1990a), 'Method for the quantitative analysis of volatile free and total branched-chain fatty acid in cheese and milk fat', *J Dairy Sci*, **73**, 1988–1999.

HA J K and LINDSAY R C (1990b), 'Distribution of volatile branched-chain fatty acids in perinephric fats of various red meat species', *Lebensm-Wiss. u.-Technol*, **23**, 433–440.

HA J K and LINDSAY R C (1993), 'Release of volatile branched-chain and other fatty acids from ruminant milk fats by various lipases', *J Dairy Sci*, **76**, 677–690.

HACHELAF W, BOUKHRELDA M, BENBOUABDELLAH M, COQUIN P, DESJEUX J F, BOUDRAA G and

TOUHAMI M (1993), 'Digestibilité des graisses du lait de chèvre chez des enfants présentant une malnutrition d'origine digestive. Comparaison avec le lait de vache', *Lait*, **73**, 593–599.

HAMBRAEUS L (1984), 'Human milk composition', *Nutr Abstr Rev Clin Nutr*, Series A, **54**, 219–236.

HUSTON G E and PATTON S (1990), 'Factors related to the formation of cytoplasmic crescents on milk fat globules', *J Dairy Sci*, **73**, 2061–2066.

IP M M, MASSO-WELCH P A and IP C (2003), 'Prevention of mammary cancer with conjugated linoleic acid: role of the stroma and the epithelium', *J Mammary Gland Biol Neoplasia*, **8**, 103–118.

JARRIGE R, PETIT M and TISSIER M (1978), 'Reproduction, gestation, lactation', in Alimentation des Ruminants, INRA, Publ. 78000 Versailles (France), pp. 229–243.

JENNESS R (1974), 'The composition of milk', in Larson B L and Smith V R (eds). *Lactation: A Comprehensive Treatise*, Vol. III, Academic Press, New York, pp. 3–107.

JENNESS R (1980), 'Composition and characteristics of goat milk: Review 1968–1979', *J Dairy Sci*, **63**, 1505–1630.

JENSEN R G (1989), *The Lipids of Human Milk*, CRC Press, Inc., Boca Raton, Florida, USA.

JENSEN R G (2002), 'The composition of bovine milk lipids': January 1995 to December 2000. *J Dairy Sci*, **85**, 295–350.

JENSEN R G, FERRIS A, LAMMI-KEEFE C J and HENDERSON R A (1990), 'Lipids of bovine and human milks: a comparison', *J Dairy Sci*, **73**, 223–240.

KITESSA S M, GULATI S K, ASHES J R, FLECK E, SCOTT T W and NICHOLS P D (2001), 'Utilisation of fish oil in ruminants II. Transfer of fish oil fatty acids into goats' milk', *Anim Feed Sci Technol*, **89**, 201–208.

KNOPP R H and RETZLAFF B M (2004), 'Saturated fat prevents coronary artery disease? An American paradox', *Am J Clin Nutr*, **80**, 1102–1103.

KUKSIS A, MARAI L and MYHER J J (1973), 'Triglyceride structure of milk fats', *J Am Oil Chem Soc*, **50**, 193–201.

LAMBERET G, DEGAS C, DELACROIX-BUCHET A and VASSAL L (1996), 'Influence de caractères lies aux allèles A et F de la caséine αs1 caprine sur la flaveur chèvre: fabrications fromagères avec échange de protéines et de matières grasses', *Lait*, **76**, 349–361.

LEDOUX M, ROUZEAU A, BAS P and SAUVANT D (2002), 'Occurrence of *trans*-C18:1 fatty acid isomers in goat milk: effect of two dietary regimens', *J Dairy Sci*, **85**, 190–197.

LEGRAND P (2001), 'ANCs for fat', *Sciences des aliments*, **21**, 348–360.

LEROUX C, LE PROVOST F, PETIT E, BERNARD L, CHILLIARD Y and MARTIN P (2003), 'Real-time RT-PCR and cDNA macroarray to study the impact of the genetic polymorphism at the α_{s1}-casein locus on the expression of genes in the goat mammary gland during lactation', *Reprod Nutr Dev*, **43**, 459–469.

LOCK A L, J W PERFIELD II and BAUMAN D E (2004a), '*Trans* fatty acids in ruminant-derived foods: fact and fiction', *Proc Cornell Nutr Conf*, pp. 123–134.

LOCK A L, CORL B A, BARBANO D M, BAUMAN D E and IP C (2004b), 'The anticarcinogenic effect of *trans*-11 18:1 is dependent on its conversion to *cis*-9, *trans*-11 CLA by Δ9-desaturase in rats', *J Nutr*, **134**, 2698–2704.

LOOR J J, UEDA K, FERLAY A, DOREAU M and CHILLIARD Y (2003), 'Transfer of dietary fatty acids and hydrogenation intermediates from duodenum to milk in cows fed diets varying in forage : concentrate ratio and level of linseed, sunflower or fish oil', *J Dairy Sci*, **86** (Suppl. 1), 272.

LOOR J J, FERLAY A, OLLIER A, DOREAU M and CHILLIARD Y (2005), 'Relationship among *trans* and conjugated fatty acids and bovine milk fat yield due to dietary concentrate and linseed oil', *J Dairy Sci*, **88**, 726–740.

MASSART-LEEN A M, DE POTTER H and SCHAMP N (1981), 'Composition and variability of the branched chain fatty acid fraction in the milk of goats and cows', *Lipids*, **16**, 286–292.

MATHER I H and KEENAN T W (1998), 'Origin and secretion of milk lipids', *J Mammary Gland Biol Neoplasia*, **3**, 259–273.

MEHAIA M A (1995), 'The fat globule size distribution in camel, goat, ewe and cow milk', *Milchwissenschaft*, **50**, 260–263.

MOORE J H and CHRISTIE W W (1981), 'Lipid metabolism in the mammary gland of ruminant animals', in Christie W W (ed.), *Lipid Metabolism in Ruminant Animals*. Pergamon Press, Oxford, pp. 227–277.

MOSLEY E E, POWELL G L, RILEY M B and JENKINS T C (2002), 'Microbial biohydrogenation of oleic acid to *trans* isomers *in vitro*', *J Lipid Res*, **43**, 290–296.

NESS A R, SMITH G D and HART C (2001), 'Milk, coronary heart disease and mortality', *J Epid Comm Health*, **55**, 379–382.

NEVEU C, RIAUBLANC A, MIRANDA G, CHICH J F and MARTIN P (2002), 'Is the apocrine milk secretion process observed in the goat species rooted in the perturbation of the intracellular transport mechanism induced by defective alleles at the alpha(s1)-Cn locus?', *Reprod Nutr Dev*, **42**, 163–172.

NUDDA A, USAI M G, MULAS S and PULINA G (2003) 'Utilization of extruded linseed cakes to modify fatty acid composition and increase CLA contents in goat milk', in *Book of Abstract, 54th Annual Meeting of European Association for Animal Production*, Rome, Italy, 31 Aug.–3 Sept., p. 119.

PEREIRA M A, JACOBS D R, VAN HORN L, SLATTERY M L, KARTASHOV A I and LUDWIG DS (2002), 'Dairy consumption, obesity, and the insulin resistance syndrome in young adults. The CARDIA study', *JAMA*, **287**, 2081–2089.

PIPEROVA L S, TETER B B, BRUCKENTAL I, SAMPUGNA J, MILLS S E, YURAWECZ M P, FRITSCHE J, KU K and ERDMAN R A (2000), 'Mammary lipogenic enzyme activity, *trans* fatty acids and conjugated linoleic acids are altered in lactating dairy cows fed a milk fat-depressing diet', *J Nutr*, **130**, 2658–2674.

PITEL G and DELACROIX-BUCHET A (1994), *Compte-rendu d'activité, Station de Recherches Laitières*, INRA, Jouy-en-Josas (France).

PRECHT D and MOLKENTIN J (1999), 'C18:1, C18:2 and C18:3 *trans* and *cis* fatty acid isomers including conjugated *cis* Δ9, *trans* Δ11 linoleic acid (CLA) as well as total fat composition of German human milk lipids', *Nahrung*, **43**, 233–244.

RAINWATER D L and KOLATTUKUDY P E (1982), 'Purification and characterization of acyl-CoA carboxylase from uropygial gland which produces multimethyl-branched acids and evidence for its identity with avian acetyl-CoA carboxylase', *Arch Biochem Biophys*, **213**, 372–383.

ROUEL J, FERLAY A, CHABOSSEAU J M, CAPITAN P, GABORIT P and CHILLIARD Y (2003), 'Effects of fresh raygrass, raygrass hay or alfalfa hay on goat milk yield and composition, including *trans* and conjugated fatty acids', in *Book of Abstracts, 54th Annual Meeting of European Association for Animal Production*, Rome, Italy, 31 Aug.–3 Sept., p. 349.

ROUEL J, FERLAY A, BRUNETEAU E, CAPITAN P, RAYNAL-LJUTOVAC K and CHILLIARD Y (2004),

'Interactions between starchy concentrate and linseed oil supplementation on goat milk yield and composition, including *trans* and conjugated fatty acids (FA)', in *Book of Abstracts, 55th Annual Meeting of Euopean Association for Animal Production*, Bled, Slovenia, 5–9 Sept., p. 124.

ROUEL J, BRUNETEAU E, GUILLOUET P, FERLAY A, GABORIT P, LELOUTRE L and CHILLIARD Y (2005), 'Goat dairy performances according to dietary forage:concentrate ratio and/or high doses of sunflower or linseed oil, or extruded mixture of seeds', in *Book of Abstracts, 56th Annual Meeting of European Association for Animal Production*, 5–8 June 2005, Uppsala, Sweden, Wageningen Acad. Publ. (NL), p. 280.

ROY A, FERLAY A, OLLIER A and CHILLIARD Y (2005), 'Kinetics of *trans* and conjugated fatty acids (FA) concentrations in cow milk after addition of plant oils to different basal diets', in *Book of Abstracts, 56th Annual Meeting of European Association for Animal Production*, 5–8 June 2005, Uppsala, Sweden, Wageningen Acad. Publ. (NL), p. 136.

SANZ SAMPELAYO M R, MARTIN ALONSO J J, PEREZ L, GIL EXTREMERA F and BOZA J (2004), 'Dietary supplements for lactating goats by polyunsaturated fatty acid-rich protected fat. Effects after supplement withdrawal', *J Dairy Sci*, **87**, 1796–1802.

SCHMIDELY P and SAUVANT D (2001), 'Taux butyreux et composition de la matière grasse du lait chez les petits ruminants: effets de l'apport de matières grasses ou d'aliment concentré', *INRA Prod Anim*, **14**, 337–354.

SCHMIDELY P, MORAND-FEHR P and SAUVANT D (2005) 'Influence of extruded soybeans with or without bicarbonate on milk performance and fatty acid composition of goat milk', *J Dairy Sci*, **88**, 757–765.

SÉBÉDIO J L, GNÄDIG S and CHARDIGNY J M (1999), 'Recent advances in conjugated linoleic acid research', *Curr Opin Clin Nutr Metabolic Care*, **2**, 499–506.

SELNER D R and SCHULTZ L H (1980), 'Effects of feeding oleic acid or hydrogenated vegetable oils to lactating cows', *J Dairy Sci* **63**, 1235–1241.

SHINGFIELD K J, AHVENJÄRVI S, TOIVONEN V, ÄRÖLÄ A, NURMELA K V V, HUHTANEN P and GRIINARI J M (2003), 'Effect of fish oil on biohydrogenation of fatty acids and milk fatty acid content in cows', *Anim Sci*, **77**, 165–179.

STORRY J E and ROOK J A F (1965), 'The effects of a diet low in hay and high in flaked maize on milk fat secretion and on the concentrations of certain constituents in the blood plasma of the cow', *Br J Nutr*, **19**, 101–109.

SUGIYAMA T, MATSUURA H, SASADA H, MASAKI J and YAMASHITA K (1986), 'Characterization of fatty acids in the sebum of goats according to sex and age', *Agric Biol Chem*, **50**, 3049–3052.

ULBRICHT T L V AND SOUTHGATE D A T (1991), 'Coronary heart disease: seven dietary factors', *Lancet*, **338**, 985–992.

WARENSJÖ E, JANSSON J H, BERGLUND L, BOMAN K, AHRÉN B, WEINEHALL L, LINDAHL B, HALLMANS G and VESSBY B (2004), 'Estimated intake of milk fat is negatively associated with cardiovascular risk factors and does not increase the risk of a first acute myocardial infarction. A prospective case-control study', *Br J Nutr*, **91**, 635–642.

WILLIAMS C M (2000), 'Dietary fatty acids and human health', *Ann Zootech*, **49**, 165–180.

WONG E, JOHSON C B and NIXON LN (1975), 'The contribution of 4-methyloctanoic (hircinoic) acid to mutton and goat meat flavour', *N Z J Agric Res*, **18**, 261–266.

13

Reducing fats in raw meat

A. P. Moloney, Teagasc, Grange Research Centre, Ireland

13.1 Introduction

Fat is an essential component of meat for sensory perception of juiciness, flavour and texture. Fat in meat also supplies fatty acids that cannot be synthesised by humans and can act as a carrier of lipid-soluble vitamins and antioxidants. Healthiness and sensory expectation are important quality criteria that influence the decision of a consumer to purchase a particular food product. Negative perceptions of red meat, in particular, as an excessively fat food have contributed to beef and lamb losing market share to competing meats and other protein sources throughout the developed world. The range in fat content of muscle foods will be illustrated.

Loss of market share has provided impetus for the modification of traditional meat production systems. Fresh meat production systems represent the combined and interacting effects of genotype, sex, age at slaughter and nutrition before slaughter, all of which can contribute to differences in the fat concentration of fresh meat. These influences will be briefly reviewed and it will be demonstrated that modern lean red meat can have an intramuscular fat concentration of 25–50 g/kg and can be considered a low-fat food. The opportunities to alter the diet of animals to produce flavoursome meat that has a low fat concentration, an increased concentration of human health-enhancing compounds, and a fatty acid profile more compatible with current human dietary recommendations will be illustrated. The implications of such alterations in the composition of meat on characteristics important to the meat processor are reviewed. The chapter will end with a commentary on likely future trends in the fat content of meat and meat products including the possibility of meat being recognised as a functional food.

13.2 The fat content of meat

13.2.1 Total fat

The fat in meat supplies essential fatty acids and vitamins and plays an essential role in the sensory perception of juiciness, flavour and texture. Historically, animal products were considered to be wholesome, versatile foods for humans and important for human health. A briefing paper from the British Nutrition Foundation (1999) concluded that 'meat and meat products are an integral part of the UK diet and make a valuable contribution to nutritional intakes'. The fat content of meat varies with the choice of cut or meat product, the species of animal and the production system through which that animal has come. Fat is present in meat as structural components of the muscle membranes, as storage droplets of triacylglycerol between the muscles (intermuscular fat), as adipose

Table 13.1 Total fat and fatty acid concentration of raw meat and meat products (g/100 g) (adapted from MAFF, 1998)

	Fat	SFA*	MUFA*	PUFA*
Beef, average, lean	4.3	1.74	1.76	0.20
Fillet steak	7.0	3.04	2.54	0.36
Sirloin steak	7.7	3.30	3.03	0.26
Brisket	11.0	4.36	4.37	0.31
Minced beef, extra lean	9.6	4.02	3.58	0.25
Lamb, average, lean	8.0	3.46	2.58	0.36
Leg (83% lean, 17% fat)	12.3	5.36	4.05	0.63
Loin chops, lean	10.7	4.64	3.30	0.51
Bacon, back, fat trimmed, grilled	12.3	4.6	5.2	1.6
Pork, average, lean	4.0	1.36	1.50	0.51
Pork fillet strips	5.9	1.32	1.74	2.17
Leg (83% lean, 17% fat)	10.2	3.59	4.37	1.42
Pork steaks	3.7	1.29	1.42	0.58
Chicken, dark meat	2.8	0.74	1.28	0.55
Chicken, light meat	1.1	0.31	0.48	0.22
Chicken, skin	48.3	13.40	23.06	7.89
Turkey, dark meat	7.0	2.10	2.48	1.74
Turkey, light meat	1.9	0.62	0.67	0.43
Turkey, skin	30.7	9.97	11.51	6.64
Chicken korma	5.8	1.7	1.9	1.8
Chilli con carne, chilled/frozen, reheated	4.3	1.9	1.9	0.2
Ham, canned	4.5	1.6	2.0	0.4
Lamb kheema	14.5	3.8	5.3	4.2
Lamb kheema, reduced fat	9.7	3.4	3.6	1.8
Pork and beef sausages, grilled	20.3	7.5	9.1	2.2
Pork sausages, reduced fat, grilled	13.8	4.9	5.9	2.1
Salami	39.2	14.6	17.7	4.4
Steak and kidney pie, single crust	16.4	6.1	6.7	2.5
Turkey pie, single crust	10.3	4.5	3.7	1.5

*SFA = saturated fatty acids, MUFA = monounsaturated fatty acids, PUFA = polyunsaturated fatty acids.

Table 13.2 Fat composition of different muscles of beef cattle finished at pasture or in a feedlot (adapted from Rule *et al.*, 2002)

	Pasture	Feedlot
Total fatty acids (mg/g)		
Longissimus dorsi	10.7	28.8
Semitendinosus	8.2	22.9
Supraspinatus	13.8	26.6
SFA (% fatty acids)		
Longissimus dorsi	41.7	44.0
Semitendinosus	38.9	42.0
Supraspinatus	35.5	41.0
PUFA (% fatty acids)		
Longissimus dorsi	9.5	5.0
Semitendinosus	14.4	6.1
Supraspinatus	12.2	7.2
Cholesterol (mg/100 g)		
Longissimus dorsi	52.3	52.7
Semitendinosus	48.7	53.4
Supraspinatus	52.7	61.4

tissue within the muscles (intramuscular fat or marbling) and as subcutaneous fat (under the skin). Most of the fat in adipose tissue is present as glycerol esters, but the fat of muscle also contains a considerable quantity of phospholipids. In phospholipids one of the three hydroxyl groups of glycerol is combined with choline, ethanol-amine, serine, inositol or glucose. In the plasmalogens the second hydroxyl group of glycerol is esterified with a long-chain fatty aldehyde instead of with fatty acid; and in sphingomyelin the amino alcohol sphingosine is bound by an amide link to a fatty acid and by an ester link to phosphoryl-choline. Of the total phospholipids in beef muscle, lecithin accounts for about 62%, cephalins for 30% and sphingomyelin for less than 10% (Lawrie, 1998).

Data on the fat content of a range of meat products are compiled and published in food composition tables by several agencies, worldwide, so only selected examples are shown in Table 13.1. Within a carcass, there is considerable variation among muscles in total fat content and in fatty acid composition. This is illustrated in Table 13.2 which shows the longissimus dorsi (striploin) to be intermediate in fat content between the semitendinosus (outside round) and the supraspinatus muscle (chuck).

The fat content of meat products can vary considerably, depending on the proportion of lean and fat from the original meat as well as the level of inclusion of other ingredients. Traditional meat products such as sausages, pastry-covered pies and salami are high in fat (up to 50%) but modern products include ready meals and prepared meats that can be low in fat (5%). While reduced-fat meat products are now available, the potential for product development in this area has not been fully exploited.

13.2.2 Fatty acids

The fatty acid compositions of selected meat and meat products are also shown in Tables 13.1 and 13.2. Most meats provide similar proportions of saturated fatty acids (SFAs) and monounsaturated fatty acids (MUFAs), making them an important source of the latter. While the ratio of polyunsaturated fatty acids (PUFAs) to SFAs is lower in ruminant tissue than non-ruminant tissue, SFAs represent less than half the total fatty acids of beef and of SFA, 30% are represented by stearic acid, which has been shown to be neutral in its effect on plasma cholesterol in humans (Bonanome & Grundy, 1988). This indicates that the common reference to beef fat as very saturated is erroneous. Meat contributes to PUFA consumption, including docosahexaenoic acid and eicosapentaenoic acid for which there are few rich sources apart from oil-rich fish. Docosahexaenoic acid has an important role in the development of the central nervous system of the newborn while eicosapentaenoic acid is involved in blood clotting and the inflammatory response. Meat from ruminant animals in particular, but also monogastrics can be a source of conjugated linoleic acid (CLA) (Section 13.5.2).

13.2.3 Cholesterol

A review of the cholesterol content of meat indicates that levels of cholesterol are generally not high in fatty meat or meat products compared with other foods. The cholesterol content of a meat is related to the number of muscle fibres so tends to be higher in muscle that is more red than in whiter muscle. While many people believe that meat and dairy products are the foods that contribute most cholesterol, for most people the only significant source of cholesterol in the diet is eggs. Thus, a chicken egg can contain 380 mg of cholesterol/100 g compared with 60–70 mg/100 g for beef, pork and lamb (MAFF, 1998; Chizzolini *et al.*, 1999).

13.3 Breeding effects on the fat content and composition of meat

13.3.1 Fat content

An increase in fat deposition per se is generally accompanied by an increase in intramuscular fat concentration. The degree of fatness is determined by genotype, the weight of the carcass and how close the animal is to its ultimate mature size when slaughtered. In animal production systems that have evolved to optimise economic efficiency, several of these factors may vary. The impact of these factors will be illustrated separately but probable interactions with the other factors and nutrition (Section 13.4) should also be considered. Across genotype, breeds that have light mature bodyweights mature earlier than those with a heavier mature bodyweight. Therefore at a constant time relative to birth, earlier maturing animals will be fatter than late maturing animals. This is illustrated by the data of Keane (2000) shown in Table 13.3 for different breeds

Table 13.3 Fat concentration (g/kg) of beef carcass and longissimus dorsi (LD) muscle (adapted from Keane, 2000)

	Carcass weight (kg)					
	300		350		400	
Sire breed[a]	Fat[b]	LD[c]	Fat	LD	Fat	LD
Angus	220	45	300	80	380	115
Friesian	170	35	235	65	300	95
Hereford	210	40	285	75	360	110
MRI	175	35	240	65	310	100
Piedmontese	120	25	160	40	210	60
Limousin	135	25	180	45	235	65
Romagnola	130	25	175	45	230	65
Blonde	120	25	160	40	210	60
Simmental	135	25	180	45	235	65
Belgian Blue	120	25	160	40	210	60
Charolais	130	25	175	45	230	65

[a]Mated to Friesian cows.
[b]Total dissectable fat in the carcass.
[c]Lipid, rounded to nearest 5 g/kg.

of beef cattle. At 300 kg carcass weight, Friesians had 170 g fat/kg carcass. The corresponding proportions for Herefords and Angus, earlier maturing breeds, were 210 g/kg and 220 g/kg, respectively and for the later maturing Limousin, Charolais and Belgian Blue breeds was 135 g/kg, 130 g/kg and 120 g/kg, respectively. As carcass weight increased, the proportions of fat increased and proportions of muscle and bone decreased. Compared with a 300 kg animal a 400 kg Friesian carcass had 300 g fat/kg. Corresponding proportions for Angus and Charolais were 380 g/kg and 230 g/kg respectively. Intramuscular lipid proportion increased with increasing carcass weight and did so more rapidly for earlier-maturing breeds. For example, over the carcass weight range 300 to 400 kg, lipid concentration increased by 70 g/kg for Angus compared with an increase of only 35 g/kg for Belgian Blues. Similar lipid concentrations would be obtained from a Hereford carcass weighing 300 kg and a Charolais carcass weighing 350 kg. With respect to sex, heifers of the same breed grown together with steers achieved a similar carcass composition at a lighter carcass weight (267 vs 326 kg) i.e. heifers are earlier maturing than steers (Keane, 1993). Similarly, castration of intact male animals renders the resulting castrates more early maturing with respect to body composition.

In general for any particular ration, an increase in intake by a meat-producing animal will promote a higher growth rate and a fatter carcass (at a similar carcass weight), i.e. growth rate per se will increase fat deposition relative to protein deposition (Owens *et al.*, 1995). This seems to reflect some maximal rate of muscle growth which appears to be related to age as well as protein intake

(Bass *et al.*, 1990). However, there is some opportunity to decrease fatness by manipulating the growth path relatively close to slaughter. Thus Moloney *et al.* (2001a) reported that compared with cattle finished on a grass silage and concentrate ration, feeding unsupplemented silage for 56 days followed by the same amount of concentrates offered *ad libitum* decreased internal fat weight and longissimus dorsi lipid concentration. Practical methods of decreasing fatness in farm animals have been reviewed (Bass *et al.*, 1990).

13.3.2 Fatty acids

Many comparisons of animal factors are confounded by differences in fatness. In general, increasing fatness results in greater unsaturation of lipid with the MUFA proportion increasing and SFA proportion decreasing (Duckett *et al.*, 1993). In parallel, the relative proportion of PUFAs and the PUFA : SFA ratio decrease with increasing fatness. However, where corrections have been made for fatness, some differences in fatty acid composition due to genotype have been reported. Zembayashi *et al.* (1995) suggested that the Japanese Black breed of cattle has a genetic predisposition for producing lipids with higher MUFA concentrations than other breeds studied. The Wagyu beef breed is characterised by greater intramuscular than subcutaneous fat deposition and was found to have higher concentrations of MUFA and a higher MUFA : SFA ratio than other breeds in several studies (Xie *et al.*, 1996). Similarly for pigs, the Duroc breed, characterised by higher amounts of intramuscular fat relative to backfat, had higher intramuscular SFA and MUFA proportions and lower PUFA proportions than British Landrace pigs (Cameron and Enser, 1991). In both breeds, increasing intramuscular fat deposition caused a relatively greater increase in the MUFA proportion than the SFA proportion. Breed differences and effects of maturity or growth stage on the subcutaneous or intramuscular fatty acid composition of beef have been reviewed by de Smet *et al.* (2004). With regard to sex, fewer comparisons have been made but Malau-Aduli *et al.* (1998) reported phospholipid PUFA : SFA ratios of 0.27 and 0.54 for steers and heifers respectively, fed on pasture.

Specific breed differences in the n-6:n-3 PUFA ratio and in the concentration of longer chain n-3 PUFA that probably could not be attributed to differences in intramuscular fat concentration have also been reported. Choi *et al.* (2000) reported significantly higher proportions of C18:3n-3 in neutral lipids and phospholipids and higher proportions of C20:5n-3 and C22:5n-3 in phospholipids of Welsh Black compared with Holstein Friesian cattle, resulting in a lower n-6:n-3 ratio in Welsh Black. The preferential deposition of n-3 PUFA was maintained on diets containing supplemental n-3 PUFA, indicating no breed × diet interaction. Itoh *et al.* (1999) found significant differences between Angus and Simmental cattle in the deposition of C18:3n-3 and of the longer chain fatty acids, but breed × diet interactions were present for some of the fatty acids, making it difficult to interpret the breed effects.

Despite the above, de Smet *et al.* (2004) concluded that much of the differences in fatty acid composition apparently due to genotype could be explained by variation in intramuscular fat concentration and that effects of genotype were generally much smaller than effects due to diet.

13.4 Dietary effects on the fat content and composition of meat

13.4.1 Fat content

When examining the effects of diet on the fat content of meat it is important to separate the direct effects of dietary ingredients from indirect effects of possible differences in energy intake on carcass weight and fatness. Carcass fatness in monogastrics and ruminants can be influenced by the energy and protein concentration in the diet. However, the extent to which the lean-to-fat ratio in the carcass is altered by dietary manipulations is limited in the absence of a major impact on growth rate and feed efficiency. In pigs, restricting the energy intake by feeding a low-energy (low-fat and/or high-fibre) diet will reduce carcass fat deposition. Other nutrients must be supplied in sufficient amounts to support maximum lean tissue accretion or restriction in energy intake may result in protein being used for energy purposes. Feeding excess protein, i.e. excess essential amino acids, to pigs will result in a higher lean-to-fat ratio in the carcass but the effect is primarily a result of energy restriction relative to protein. Changes in intramuscular fat concentration can also be accomplished by varying the energy and protein composition of the diet.

Knowledge of energy and amino acid nutrition of ruminants is not as advanced as for monogastrics mainly because of pre-fermentation and transformation of dietary ingredients in the rumen of ruminants. Nevertheless, there is a body of evidence that unwilted, extensively fermented grass silage can increase fatness relative to wilted silage/hay or non-silage-based diets and that starchy ingredients promote greater fatness than digestible fibre-based ingredients. In a grass silage-based ration, protein supplied in excess of requirement increased carcass fatness (Steen and Robson, 1995). Increasing propionate supply from the rumen by addition of sodium propionate to the diet decreased fat deposition (Moloney, 1998, 2002). Many studies have compared the effects of forage-based diets with concentrate (usually grain)-based diets, but in a literature survey, Muir *et al.* (1998) found little difference in marbling between grain-fed and grass-fed beef at the same carcass weight. This conclusion is supported by French *et al.* (2000). Recently, Kruk *et al.* (2004) reported that a decrease in consumption of vitamin A by cattle resulted in an increase in intramuscular fat that was muscle dependent.

13.4.2 Fatty acids

Fatty acid deposition in monogastrics largely reflects dietary fatty acid composition (Wood and Enser, 1997). This is illustrated by data from Verbecke

Table 13.4 Influence of fat sources on fatty acid composition of pig muscle (adapted from Verbeke *et al.*, 1999; Leskanich *et al.*, 1997*)

	Fat source						
Fatty acids	Tallow	Rapeseed	Soybeans	Linseed	Safflower	*Tallow/ soybean	*Rapeseed/ fish oil
C18:1 (%)	44.06	46.55	38.75	38.17	48.8	33.72	36.47
C18:2 (%)	10.36	10.54	14.98	10.68	10.4	18.20	15.4
C18:3 (%)	0.52	1.11	1.04	4.41	1.40	0.78	1.00
PUFA/SFA	0.30	0.32	0.37	0.36	0.34	0.80	0.70
n-6:n-3	19.92	9.50	14.40	2.42	7.43	7.30	4.6
C20:5 (%)	–	–	–	–	–	0.68	1.13
C22:5 (%)	–	–	–	–	–	1.09	1.16
C22:6 (%)	–	–	–	–	–	0.77	0.99

et al. (1999) and Leskanich *et al.* (1997) in Table 13.4. Intramuscular fat in pigs had high MUFA, reflecting endogenous synthesis, but incorporation of oilseeds in the diet can increase the PUFA : SFA ratio and decrease the n-6:n-3 PUFA ratio while incorporation of fish oil can increase the long chain PUFA. An important difference between monogastrics and ruminants is that the long-chain n-3 PUFA, including eicosapentaenoic acid and docosahexaenoic acid, are not incorporated into triacylglycerols to any important extent in ruminants. They are incorporated mainly into membrane phospholipids and therefore, are found predominantly in muscle (Enser *et al.*, 1996). This provides the opportunity to manipulate intramuscular fatty acid composition of ruminant meat without large increases in fatness per se.

In ruminants, dietary PUFAs are hydrogenated to SFAs but a proportion of dietary unsaturated fatty acids bypasses the rumen intact and is absorbed and deposited in body fat (Wood and Enser, 1997). Increasing the dietary supply of PUFA, particularly n-3 PUFA, is one strategy to increase PUFA concentrations in ruminant meat. The main sources of fatty acids in ruminant rations are forages, oils and oilseeds, fish oil and marine algae and fat supplements. In Table 13.5, inclusion of bruised whole linseed, a rich source of linolenic acid, resulted in 100% increase in the concentration of linolenic acid in muscle while a linseed oil–fish oil treatment increased the marine n-3 PUFA concentrations (Scollan *et al.*, 2001). The fatty acid composition of beef and particularly the PUFA : SFA ratio can be more efficiently modified by including in the diet, fatty acids that are protected from ruminal hydrogenation (Scott *et al.*, 1971; Demeyer and Doreau, 1999). Scollan *et al.* (2003) showed that a protected lipid supplement markedly improved the PUFA : SFA ratio in muscle (Table 13.5).

Grass has higher PUFA and particularly higher n-3 PUFA, primarily as linolenic acid, than grain-based ruminant feeds. In general, grass-fed beef has higher concentrations of PUFA, particularly in the phospholipid fraction, than grain-fed beef (Griebenow *et al.*, 1997). An increase in the proportion of grass in

Table 13.5 Influence of fat sources on the fatty acid composition (mg/100 g tissue) of beef muscle (adapted from Scollan *et al.*, 2001, 2003)

(i) Different sources of oil

Fatty acids	Control	Linseed	Fish oil	Linseed/ fish oil	s.e.d.	Significance[1]
C16:0	1029	1089	1305	1171	206.0	NS
C18:0	528	581	543	490	104.0	NS
C18:1	1209	1471	1260	1225	279.0	NS
C18:2	81	78	66	64	9.2	NS
C18:3	22	43	26	30	5.6	**
C20:4	23	21	14	17	1.5	***
C20:5	11	16	23	15	1.9	***
C22:6	2.2	2.4	4.6	4.9	0.52	***
Total fatty acids	3529	4222	4292	3973	741.0	NS
P:S	0.07	0.07	0.05	0.05	0.011	NS
n-6:n-3	2.00	1.19	0.91	1.11	0.141	**

(ii) Oil protected from ruminal biohydrogenation

Fatty acids	Control	500 g PLS[2]	1000 g PLS[2]	s.e.d.	Significance[1]
C16:0	986	843	598	117.8	*
C18:0	508	421	331	61.6	*
C18:1	1195	1144	759	177.0	*
C18:2	100	195	215	9.5	**
C18:3	23	46	46	4.3	**
C20:4	28	27	28	2.0	NS
C20:5	10	10	9	1.2	NS
C22:6	2	2	2	0.4	NS
Total fatty acids	3505	3260	2421	430.8	*
P:S	0.06	0.19	0.28	0.029	**
n-6:n-3	4.6	4.4	4.7	0.48	NS

1 NS = not significant.
2 PLS = protected lipid supplement.
* = $P < 0.05$; ** = $P < 0.01$; *** = $P < 0.001$.

the diet of finishing steers decreased the SFA concentration, increased the PUFA : SFA ratio, increased the n-3 PUFA concentration and decreased the n-6:n-3 PUFA ratio (French *et al.*, 2000). These beneficial effects of grass are related to time at pasture (Table 13.6). The effects of forages *per se* on the fatty acid composition of beef have been recently reviewed (Scollan *et al.*, 2005). The n-3 PUFA detected in meat from the grass-fed cattle in these studies were predominantly linolenic acid. The health benefits of n-3 PUFA from plant and marine (i.e. longer chain fatty acids) sources appear to differ. An expert workshop on this issue (de Deckere *et al.*, 1998) concluded that

Table 13.6 Nutritionally important fatty acids of longissimus thoracis muscle in Friesian steers fed on grass for differing times (Noci *et al.*, 2005a)

	Days at grass				s.e.d.	P[1]
	0	40	99	158		
Percentage						
SFA	45.4	45.8	45.5	43.2	0.77	**L,Q
18:1 *trans-11*	1.35	1.93	2.27	3.01	0.18	**L
CLA *cis*-9,*trans*-11	0.50	0.50	0.57	0.71	0.06	***L
n-6 PUFA	3.25	3.20	2.97	3.31	0.23	NS
n-3 PUFA	1.79	2.06	1.91	2.43	0.17	**L
n-6/n-3 ratio	2.00	1.79	1.56	1.32	0.10	***L
P/S ratio	0.12	0.14	0.12	0.15	0.009	*
mg/100 g muscle						
SFA	1117	1060	1262	1090	80.8	*
18:1 *trans-11*	32.5	44.9	60.2	76.6	4.54	***L
CLA *cis*-9,*trans*-11	12.3	12.1	15.2	18.4	1.79	***L
n-6 PUFA	77.3	79.3	76.8	78.6	3.87	NS
n-3 PUFA	39.1	44.3	51.7	59.7	3.07	***L

[1]L and Q are significant linear and quadratic effects of days at grass, respectively.
SFA = saturated fatty acids, PUFA = polyunsaturated fatty acids.
$*P < 0.05$; $**P < 0.01$; $***P < 0.001$.

> there is incomplete but growing evidence that consumption of the plant n-3 PUFA, alpha-linolenic acid, reduces the risk of coronary heart disease. An intake of 2 g/d or 1% of energy of alpha-linolenic acid appears prudent. The ratio of total n-3 over n-6 PUFA (linoleic acid) is not useful for characterising foods or diets because plant and marine n-3 PUFA show different effects, and because a decrease in n-6 PUFA intake does not produce the same effects as an increase in n-3 PUFA intake. Separate recommendations for alpha-linolenic acid, marine n-3 PUFA and linoleic acid are preferred.

Grass-fed beef can contribute to diets designed to achieve an increased consumption of n-3 PUFA.

13.5 Strategies for improving the fat content and composition of meat

13.5.1 Fat content

Medical authorities worldwide recommend that population energy intake from fat should not exceed 30–35%, that energy intake from SFAs should not exceed 10% of total energy intake and that energy intake from MUFAs and PUFAs should be approximately 16% and 7%, respectively, of energy intake.

Furthermore, an increase in n-3 PUFA consumption such that the ratio of n-6:n-3 PUFA is <4:1 has also been recommended (Department of Health, 1994; Gibney, 1993; United States Department of Agriculture, 2000). Such recommendations have also provided impetus to develop strategies to alter the total fat concentration and the fatty acid composition of meat fat to be more compatible with consumer requirements. In the early 1980s, the red meat industry began to modify production systems to produce less fat in meat. The fat content of the carcass has decreased in Britain by over 30% for pork, making many pork cuts comparable with chicken, 15% for beef and 10% for lamb, with further reductions anticipated for beef and lamb over the next 5–10 years (Higgs, 2000). These achievements are due to selective breeding and feeding practices designed to increase the carcass lean to fat ratio; official carcass classification systems designed to favour leaner production; and modern butchery techniques (seaming out whole muscles, and trimming away all intermuscular fat). Beef produced during our research had a marbling fat concentration in the order of 20–50 g/kg reflecting current beef production systems. It is already possible therefore to produce beef that satisfies the definition of a low-fat food, i.e food with a fat concentration of 3 g/100 g or less. Such beef is considerably different from that represented in many tables of food composition (>70–100 g/kg).

It can be seen from the discussion in Section 13.3.1 that use of later maturing breeds, slaughtering at lighter weights, use of males rather than females or use of bulls rather than steers will all contribute to a decrease in fat content in the carcass and in muscle. Selection for leanness within a breed may also offer scope to decrease fatness. However, Maher *et al.* (2004) reported that while a Charolais sire selected for better conformation (muscling) produced offspring with a leaner carcass than an average Charolais sire, the intramuscular fat content of muscle was unchanged. New molecular biology tools will probably accelerate the selection of leaner animals and also allow identification of the 'fattening' potential of unselected animals. For example, polymorphisms in the leptin gene that correlate with fat deposition in cattle have been recently reported (Nkrumah *et al.*, 2004).

The possibilities of altering carcass composition by nutritional modification as mentioned in Section 13.4.1 are under active investigation. Exogenous agents such as somatotropin and beta-adrenergic agonists are not permitted in the European Union but are potent tools to decrease fatness and to increase leanness in most meat species. They are currently used in many countries (Beermann and Dunshea, 2004).

13.5.2 Fatty acids

Considerable effort is being expended on optimising the concentrations of fatty acids in meat for which there are nutritional guidelines such as SFA, MUFA, PUFA, n-6 PUFA and n-3 PUFA. The main strategy is to modify the diet of meat animals and to build on the possibilities outlined in Section 13.4.2. To this end, methods to control the transformation of dietary lipids by ruminal micro-organisms are being explored. The outcomes of a recently completed EU-funded project on this topic were summarised by Scollan *et al.* (2004a). For monogastric animals, the thrust of research is to protect meat with a high long-chain PUFA concentration from oxidation during display and processing (Section 13.6).

A more recent strategy is to enhance the concentrations of novel fatty acids, with putative human health benefits. One such compound is CLA. Conjugated linoleic acid refers to a mixture of positional and geometric isomers of linoleic acid (18:2 n-6). The *cis*-9,*trans*-11 form is believed to be the most common natural form of CLA with biological activity, representing 75–90% of total CLA in meat, but biological activity has been proposed for other isomers, especially the *trans*-10,*cis*-12 isomer. In experimental animals CLA has been shown to be an anticarcinogen, and to have anti-atherogenic, immunomodulating, growth-promoting, lean body mass-enhancing and antidiabetic properties. To date there is limited evidence of these beneficial effects in humans (see Chapter 8) but several human studies are in progress. CLA is found in highest concentrations in fat from ruminant animals, where it is produced in the rumen as the first intermediate in the biohydrogenation of dietary linoleic acid. In the second step of the pathway, the conjugated diene is hydrogenated to *trans*-11 octadecenoic acid (*trans*-vaccinic acid) which is now believed to be a substrate for tissue synthesis of CLA via an enzymatic desaturation reaction. The concentration of CLA in beef from a variety of sources is summarised in Table 13.7. Factors that affect CLA content of beef include pasture compared with feedlot-finished, the nature of the diet in the feedlot, whether the diet contained oil or oilseed, the fatty acid composition of the oil, and the other dietary components in the feed, such as proportion of grain and type of forage. Concentrations of CLA in Irish

Table 13.7 Conjugated linoleic acid (CLA) concentrations (mg/g fat) in uncooked beef (adapted from Moloney *et al.*, 2001b; Mir *et al.*, 2004)

Diet	Country	CLA concentration
Unknown	Canada	1.2–3.0
Barley (800 g/kg diet)	Canada	1.7–1.8
Grass silage and concentrate	United Kingdom	3.2–8.0
Maize (820 g/kg diet)	United States	3.9–4.9
Unknown	United States	2.9–4.3
Unknown	United States	1.7–5.5
Grain	United States	5.1
Concentrate	Japan	3.4
Grass	United States	7.4
Grass (?)	Australia	2.3-12.5
Grass	Ireland	3.7–10.8
Grass and sunflower oil	Ireland	17.6
Unknown	Germany	1.2–12.0
Corn + extruded soybeans	United States	6.6–7.8
Range	United States	3.5–5.6
Feedlot	United States	2.9–3.2
Feedlot + soybeans	United States	3.2–3.6

and Australian beef can be two to three times higher than those in United States beef. This presumably reflects the greater consumption of PUFA-rich pasture throughout the year by cattle in these countries. Thus, an increase in the proportion of grass in the diet caused a linear increase in CLA concentration, while a grass silage/concentrate diet resulted in a lower CLA concentration than a grass-based diet with a similar forage to concentrate ratio (French *et al.*, 2000). The CLA concentration in muscle was dependent on the time at pasture (Noci *et al.*, 2005a). Inclusion of sunflower oil in the supplementary concentrate to a silage-based diet also linearly increased muscle CLA (Noci *et al.*, 2005b). Dietary CLA is hydrogenated in the rumen so protection of dietary CLA from ruminal biohydrogenation is being examined with equivocal results. Gassman *et al.* (2000) reported a 2.4 and 3.0-fold increase in intramuscular CLA concentration in rib and round muscle, respectively, in response to inclusion of 2.5% protected CLA in the diet of cattle.

Dietary inclusion of CLA has been shown to markedly increase the CLA concentration of pig muscle (from 0.09 to 0.55% total fatty acids in the study of Eggert *et al.*, 2001) and chicken muscle with preferential incorporation of the *cis*-9,*trans*-11 CLA isomer. However, use of synthetic CLA appears to increase the proportion of SFA (and to decrease the proportion of MUFA) in muscle, an undesirable effect from a human health perspective.

Gläser *et al.* (2000) fed hydrogenated fat, rich in *trans* isomers of C18:1 resulting in a higher *cis*-9,*trans*-11 CLA content in the adipose tissue of pigs compared with the control diets (0.44 and <0.01 g CLA/100 g of total fatty acids, respectively). These results suggest that formation of *cis*-9,*trans*-11 CLA through the action of the Δ^9 desaturase on *trans*-11 C18:1 also occurs in non-ruminants, such as pigs.

13.6 Implications for the food processor

In addition to the perception of healthiness, characteristics important to consumer perception of the quality or experience of eating meat, such as colour, tenderness/texture, juiciness and flavour, may also be influenced by the amount and composition of fat in meat (cf. Chapter 9).

The appearance of fresh meat and products is a major influence on the purchase decision of the consumer. The colour of adipose tissue largely reflects the concentrations of dietary carotenoids, i.e. adipose tissue becomes more yellow with increasing consumption of β-carotene and lutein and the overall perception of meat colour is influenced by the amount of visible fat in meat. The colour of muscle largely reflects the concentration (and oxidation state) of myoglobin. When beef is exposed to air for a prolonged period, the bright red, oxidised myoglobin colour changes slowly to brown because of conversion of myoglobin to metmyoglobin. This loss of desirable colour is linked to the oxidation of meat lipids, the rate of which is a function of the concentration and degree of unsaturation of lipids. Thus, increasing the concentration of PUFA in meat increases the susceptibility of muscle lipid to oxidative breakdown during conditioning and retail display (Wood *et al.*, 2003). Wood *et al.* (2003) concluded, based on studies with monogastrics, that only when concentrations of linolenic acid approach 3% of lipids are there any adverse effects on lipid or colour stability, or flavour, in particular if processing conditions accelerate lipid oxidation. In support of this conclusion, when the concentration of C18:3 in beef was increased from 0.7% to 1.2% of total lipids by feeding linseeds (Vatansever *et al.*, 2000) or to 1.9% by use of a ruminally protected lipid supplement (Enser *et al.*, 2001; Scollan *et al.*, 2003), little effect on lipid stability or flavour characteristics was observed. When C18:3 was increased to 3.5% of total fatty acids (Scollan *et al.*, 2004b,c), the value of TBARS (a measure of lipid oxidation) after 10 days display increased considerably above the level of 2 mg malonaldehyde per kg of meat at which rancidity may be detected by consumers (Wood *et al.*, 2003). Colour saturation or intensity was also affected by feeding, declining fastest with higher levels of inclusion of the lipid supplement. Higher sensory scores for 'abnormal' and 'rancid' were also recorded (see below).

The extent of lipid oxidation in meat is limited by the presence of antioxidants such as vitamin E (either added to the diet of present naturally) and other phenolic compounds from the diet with antioxidant activity. Thus, while grass-fed beef generally has a higher PUFA concentration than grain-fed beef, and therefore greater potential for lipid oxidation, pasture-fed beef is generally more resistant to lipid oxidation than grain-fed beef (O'Sullivan *et al.*, 2003). This observation generally holds for fresh or aged meat (Yang *et al.*, 2002) and meat that has undergone long-term frozen storage (Farouk and Wieliczko, 2003). Indeed, Farouk and Wieliczko (2003) concluded that there is not much difference in the functional properties of beef finished on pasture or grain even in long-term frozen storage. This reflects higher deposition of plant-derived antioxidants, in particular vitamin E, in meat from pasture-fed cattle but also increased activity of some anti-oxidant enzymes (Gatellier *et al.*, 2004). However, Realini *et al.* (2004) reported that while fresh steaks from pasture-fed cattle had greater lipid stability than those from concentrate-fed cattle, when the meat was minced the opposite was the case. The authors suggest that mincing, by disrupting cellular integrity, exposes more PUFA to oxidation, i.e. it provides a greater test of antioxidative protection of the n-3 PUFA in grass-fed beef. This may also occur during freezing and cooking. Similarly, Yang *et al.* (2002) reported that at similar vitamin E concentrations, pasture-fed beef was less stable than concentrate beef, again highlighting the influence of the fatty acid composition of pasture-fed beef. The appropriate ratio of vitamin E (and other antioxidants) to n-3 PUFA in meat to ensure lipid and colour stability during processing remains to be determined and is clearly a challenge to the processor of meat enriched with PUFAs.

The possible impact of fatness on meat tenderness has been the subject of much discussion. As the animal matures, fat is deposited first in subcutaneous and intermuscular sites, which could provide extra insulation for muscles against the effects of refrigeration and so prevent 'cold-shortening' (induced toughness).

Fat subsequently accumulates in muscle (intramuscular or marbling fat) in the perimysial connective tissue. At high intramuscular fat concentration, e.g. in Kobe beef, when the intramuscular fat concentration can exceed 200 g/kg muscle, the dilution of fibrous protein by soft fat may decrease the resistance to shearing or chewing. Also, fat cell expansion in the perimysial connective tissue can open up the muscle structure. The consensus opinion now is that a decrease in intramuscular fat to 2–3% will not impair eating quality of meat (Wood, 1990; Miller, 2002). This has been observed with pork loin or lean chicken breast (Chizzolini *et al.*, 1999). A reduction in intramuscular fat content to 2–5% with a relatively greater reduction in 'waste' fat such as the subcutaneous and inter-muscular depots, would make a positive contribution to production efficiency and consumer health without negatively impacting on meat quality.

The compiled literature data of Owens and Gardner (1999) indicate that juiciness was negatively related to *longissimus* moisture and positively related to *longissimus* fat concentration. Savell and Cross (1988) stated that 'fat may affect juiciness by enhancing the water-holding capacity of meat, by lubricating the muscle fibres during cooking, by increasing the tenderness of meat and thus the apparent sensation of juiciness, or by stimulating salivary flow during mastication'.

As the fat content of meat increases, so does flavour. Thus, beef from fatter animals is more intense in flavour than meat from leaner animals. Flavour is an important component of the eating quality of all foods but the flavour or odour of raw meat is of minor importance compared with that generated by cooking meat.. Many of the flavour compounds of meat are contained in the fat component or are released due to chemical changes in the fat, alone and in interaction with the protein component, during ageing and cooking. Some oxidation is required for optimum flavour development in beef. The products of heat-induced oxidation of fatty acids, particularly PUFAs, such as aliphatic aldehydes, ketones and alcohols, may have intrinsic flavours and they may also react further with Maillard products to give other compounds that contribute to flavour (Elmore *et al.*, 1997; Chapter 9). Flavour is also influenced by the deposition of 'aromatic' compounds from the feed in the fat of the animal. This is characteristic of some, but not all, pasture/grass diets and some plants, particularly legumes, contain specific flavour-inducing components and their concentration in meat is directly related to the concentration of fat.

Increasing the content of n-3 PUFA increased sensory attributes such as 'greasy' and 'fishy' (for example with longer-term grass feeding). Elevating the levels of PUFA further through either the provision of a ruminally protected lipid supplement rich in PUFA or by infusing PUFA directly into the duodenum increased the sensory scores for factors such as 'abnormal' and 'rancid' (see Wood *et al.*, 2003; Scollan *et al.*, 2004a). While some of these notes such as 'fishy' or 'rancid' flavour may appear negative, they can contribute to the strength of an overall flavour and may increase the overall attractiveness of meat. Concentrated ingredients for perfumes often have unpleasant odours, which become pleasant when diluted and mixed with other fragrances.

Individual fatty acids have been associated with specific flavours. Myristic, palmitic and margaric acids have been related to 'cowey' and 'painty' flavours of beef, while Larick and Turner (1990) showed that as the concentration of linolenic acid in muscle phospholipids declined and that of linoleic acid increased, flavours identified as 'sweet' and 'gamey' declined, whereas 'sour', 'blood like' and 'cooked beef fat' increased. During post-mortem ageing, desirable flavours (beefy, brothy, browned-carmel and sweet) typically decrease while bitter and sour flavours increase. Besides altering the flavour of fresh beef, unsaturated fatty acids are susceptible to the development of 'off-flavours' or rancidity during ageing or with exposure to oxygen. Beef from grass-fed cattle developed off-flavours more quickly during ageing than beef from grain-fed cattle, while fishy flavours often are detected in beef from grass-fed cattle after several months of storage even if the beef is frozen during storage (Moore and Harbord, 1977; Xiong *et al.*, 1996). Dietary supplements of antioxidants may delay appearance of objectionable flavours, particularly for beef with higher concentrations of PUFAs.

Changes in the fatty acid composition of meat therefore provide challenges to processors and retailers to maintain the flavours required in existing markets. However, such changes also provide opportunities to develop new markets for beef with non-traditional flavours.

13.7 Future trends

In the UK between 1989 and 1999, consumption of primary poultry meat and other meat products increased while that of carcass meat (beef, meal, mutton, lamb and pork) declined (Robinson, 2001). Robinson (2001) considered this increase in consumption to be due mainly 'to increases in meat-based ready meals and takeaways eaten at home'. This clearly reflects consumer desire for convenience products and presents a major challenge to the non-poultry sector and to the prime red meat sector, in particular. To regain market share, this sector of the meat industry will have to develop a more diverse range of products.

The decline in carcass meat consumption probably also reflects consumer preference for low-fat meat and meat products, guided by medical advice. Recent developments in decreasing the total fat concentration of meat and manipulating the fatty acid concentration have been illustrated in earlier sections of this chapter. There are clear opportunities to manipulate the animal component of fatness by integrating the various contributing factors, i.e. breed selection, use of non-castrated male animals, slaughtered young and fed appropriately, etc. It is likely that the nutrient requirements to optimise protein accretion while minimising adipose tissue accretion will be defined more precisely than at present. Current and future research will then focus on optimising both the supply of nutrients and the time when they are supplied (both diurnally and during the lifetime of the animal) to allow the target animal to achieve its genetically determined body and muscle composition.

The data presented on factors affecting the fatty acid composition of the intramuscular fat of meat demonstrate that meat can be produced that has a fatty acid profile more compatible with current medical recommendations for human diet composition. In particular, red meats can now be produced that are low in fat, have a lower concentration of atherogenic SFA, higher MUFA and PUFA concentrations and a lower n-6:n-3 PUFA ratio than was possible previously. It is also being increasingly recognised that one MUFA, oleic acid which decreases serum cholesterol, can represent up to 45% of the fat in red meat and that one SFA, stearic acid, which can represent up to 30% of total SFA does not contribute to coronary heart disease. This indicates that the perception that all SFA are 'unhealthy' is incorrect. Since the n-6:n-3 PUFA ratio in meat is within the desirable range, future research will focus on enhancing the fatty acid profile of meat even further, in particular with the use of emerging rumen protection technology. Parallel research will be required to ensure adequate antioxidant protection in meat with an improved PUFA : SFA ratio.

The so-called 'lipid hypothesis' has guided medical advice for many years. This hypothesis is being increasingly refined, and is perceived as an overly simplistic means of explaining the relationship between diet and cardiovascular disease, particularly as on-going research on lipid metabolism in humans and its relationship to health and disease yields data inconsistent with this hypothesis. Moreover, the hypothesis that a low-fat, high-carbohydrate diet is best for preventing obesity, a disorder often considered to reflect fat consumption is also being increasingly rejected. It is to be hoped that future medical guidelines will reflect the findings of recent dietary intervention-type research rather than be based predominantly on correlations arising from epidemiological, retrospective-type studies. The discovery of CLA, together with the finding that ruminant fat is its primary natural source, is a potentially positive advance for red meat, in particular. Clarification of the health-enhancing and disease-preventing properties of CLA in humans is the subject of extensive research worldwide as is identification of strategies to increase CLA content in meat. At present, data on the health benefits of CLA in humans are equivocal but effects in humans do not seem to be as great as those observed in laboratory animals (see Chapter 8). The value of CLA, in particular the *cis*9,*trans*11 isomer, in contributing to a healthy image of meat is dependent on demonstration of a positive effect on human health. In this event, research should focus on maximising its concentration in meat. The recent report that CLA from beef could decrease lipid storage in rats at a lower level of dietary inclusion than synthetic CLA (Mir *et al.*, 2003) is most encouraging in this regard. Moreover, future meat could be considered a functional food, i.e. a food that has health benefits beyond basic nutrition. The American Dietetic Association has endorsed lean beef and lamb as functional foods (1999). Research on strategies to increase the CLA concentration in meat will continue and the observation that CLA is deposited in adipose tissue as well as in the intramuscular phospholipid fraction will provide high CLA fat as a functional ingredient for healthy processed meats (see Jimenez-Colmenero *et al.*, 2001; Murray *et al.*, 2004).

The positive contribution of meat to the human diet and recognition that, even at present, meat has a role in a healthy diet is not appreciated by consumers (Bruhn, 2000). Of consumers surveyed in the US, fish was perceived as very healthful by 57% and poultry by 55%, but meat such as beef, pork and lamb was seen as very healthful by only 13%; an additional 45% considered it somewhat healthful. Bruhn (2000) states that the potential for health-enhancing products is substantial. Enhanced nutritional components in animal products meet the preferences of consumers and health professionals. There is a need now and in the future for the meat industry to convey the positive nutritional contributions of meat products such as iron, zinc, 'healthy' fatty acids and CLA to both consumers and health professionals. The conclusion of Bruhn (2000) that 'communication is the key to correct consumer (and medical) myths and to increase awareness of new information or enhanced properties of healthful food' is most appropriate advice to all sectors of the meat industry for the future.

13.8 Sources of information

Gurr, M.I. *Lipids in Nutrition and Heath: A Reappraisal.* The Oily Press, Bridgewater, 221pp.

Dr. Atkins New Diet Revolution. Vermilion, London, 417pp.

Erasmus, U. *Fats that heal, fats that kill.* Alive Books Burnaby BC, Canada, 456pp.

'Meat in the Diet'. Briefing paper. The British Nutrition Foundation, London, 24pp.

McCance and Widdowson's The Composition of Foods. The Royal Society of Chemistry and Ministry of Agriculture, Fisheries and Food (and supplements).

Web sites:

Enhancing the content of beneficial fatty acids in beef and improving meat quality for the consumer: www.healthybeef.iger.bbsrc.ac.uk

Conjugated linoleic acid references: http://www.wisc.edu/fri/clarefs.htm

British Nutrition Foundation: http://www.nutrition.org.uk

Healthfinder – gateway to reliable consumer health information: www.healthfinder.gov

US Department of Agriculture, Nutrient data laboratory USDA. Nutrient database for standard reference, release 14: http://www.nal.usda.gov/fnic/foodcomp

13.9 References

AMERICAN DIETETIC ASSOCIATION (1999). Functional foods – position of ADA. *Journal of the American Dietetic Association* **99**, 1278–1285.

BASS, J.J., BUTLER-HOGG, B.W. and KIRTON, A.H. (1990). Practical methods of controlling fatness in farm animals, pp 145–200. In *Reducing Fat in Meat Animals* (J.D. Wood and A.V. Fisher, editors) Elsevier Applied Science, London and New York.

BEERMANN, D.M. and DUNSHEA, F.R. (2004) *Metabolic modifiers for use in animal production. Animal Agriculture's future through biotechnology, part 3*. Issue paper no. 23, Council for Agricultural Science and Technology, Ames, IA, USA.

BONANOME, A. and GRUNDY, S.M. (1988). Effect of dietary stearic acid on plasma cholesterol and lipoprotein levels. *New England Journal of Medicine* **318**, 1244–1248.

BRITISH NUTRITION FOUNDATION (1999). *Meat in the Diet.* London: British Nutrition Foundation.

BRUHN, C. (2000). Consumer reactions, popular fancies, and scientific facts related to the healthfulness of meat products. *Proceedings of the American Society of Animal Science 1999*. Available at http://www.asas.org/jas/symposia/proceedings/0910.pdf

CAMERON, N.D. and ENSER, M. (1991). Fatty acid composition of lipid in longissimus dorsi muscle of Duroc and British Landrace pigs and its relationship with lipid quality. *Meat Science* **29**, 295–307.

CHIZZOLINI, R., ZANARDI, E., DERIGONI, V. and GHIDINI, S. (1999). Calorific value and cholesterol content of normal and low-fat meat and meat products. *Trends in Food Science and Technology* **10**, 119–128.

CHOI, N.J., ENSER, M., WOOD, J.D. and SCOLLAN, N.D. (2000). Effect of breed on the deposition in beef muscle and adipose tissue of dietary n-3 polyunsaturated fatty acids. *Animal Science* **71**, 509–579.

DE DECKERE, E.A.M., KORVER, O., VERSCHUREN, P.M. and KATAN, M.B. (1998). Health aspects of fish and n-3 polyunsaturated fatty acids from plant and marine origin. *European Journal of Clinical Nutrition* **52**, 749–753.

DE SMET, S., RAES, K. and DEMEYER, D. (2004). Meat fatty acid composition as affected by genetic factors: a Review. *Animal Research* **53**, 81–98.

DEMEYER, D. and DOREAU, M. (1999). Targets and procedures for altering ruminant meat and milk lipids. *Proceedings of the Nutrition Society* **58**, 593–607.

DEPARTMENT OF HEALTH (1994). *Nutritional Aspects of Cardiovascular Disease*. Report on Health and Social Subjects no. 46. HMSO, London.

DUCKETT, S.K., WAGNER, D.G., YATES, L.D., DOLEZAL, M.G. and MAY, S.G. (1993). Effects of time on feed on beef nutrient composition. *Journal of Animal Science* **71**, 2079–2088.

EGGERT, J.M., BELURY, M.A., KEMPA-STECZKO, A., MILLS, S.E. and SCHINCKEL, A.P. (2001). Effects of conjugated linoleic acid on the belly firmness and fatty acid composition of genetically lean pigs. *Journal of Animal Science* **79**, 2866–2872.

ELMORE, J.S., MOTTRAM, D.S., ENSER, M. and WOOD, J.D. (1997). Thiazoles and 3-thiazolines in cooked beef aroma. *Journal of Agricultural and Food Chemistry* **45**, 3603–3607.

ENSER, M., HALLETT, K., HEWETT, B., FURSEY, G.A.J. and WOOD, J.D. (1996). Fatty acid content and composition of English beef, lamb and pork at retail. *Meat Science* **44**, 443–458.

ENSER, M., SCOLLAN, N., GULATI, S., RICHARDSON, I., NUTE, G. and WOOD, J. (2001). The effects of ruminally-protected dietary lipid on the lipid composition and quality of beef muscle. *Proceedings of the 47th International Congress of Meat Science of Technology*, 12–13.

FAROUK, M.M. and WIELICZKO, K.J. (2003). Effect of diet and fat content on the functional properties of thawed beef. *Meat Science* **64**, 451–458.

FRENCH, P., STANTON, C., LAWLESS, F., O'RIORDAN, E.G., MONAHAN, F.J., CAFFREY, P.J. and MOLONEY, A.P. (2000). Fatty acid composition, including conjugated linoleic acid, of intramuscular fat from steers offered grazed grass, grass silage or concentrate-based diets. *Journal of Animal Science* **78**, 2849–2855.

GASSMAN, K.J., BEITZ, D.C., PASSISH, F.C. and TRENKLE, A. (2000). Effects of feeding calcium salts of CLA to finishing steers. *Journal of Animal Science* **78** (Suppl 1), 275.

GATELLIER, P., MERCIER, Y. and RENERRE, M. (2004). Effect of diet finishing mode (pasture or mixed diet) on antioxidant status of Charolais bovine meat. *Meat Science* **67**, 385–394.

GIBNEY, M.J. (1993). Fat in animal products: facts and perceptions. In *Safety and Quality of Food from Animals*. British Society of Animal Production Occasional Publication no. 17, pp. 57–61 [JD. Wood and TLJ. Lawrence, editors]. BSAP, Edinburgh.

GLASER, K.R., SCHEEDER, M.R.L. and WENK J.C. (2000). Dietary C18:1 *trans* fatty acids increase conjugated linoleic acid in adipose tissue of pigs. *European Journal of Lipid Science and Technology* **102**, 684–686.

GRIEBENOW, R.L., MARTZ, F.A. and MORROW, R.E. (1997). Forage-based beef finishing systems: A review. *Journal of Production Agriculture* **10**, 84–91.

HIGGS, J.D. (2000). Leaner meat: an overview of the compositional changes in red meat over the last 20 years and how these have been achieved. *Food Science and Technology Today* **14**, 22–26.

ITOH, M., JOHNSON, C.B., COSGROVE, G.P., MUIR, P.D. and PURCHAS, R.W. (1999). Intramuscular fatty acid composition of neutral and polar lipids for heavy-weight Angus and Simmental steers finished on pasture or grain. *Journal of the Science of Food and Agriculture* **79**, 821-827.

JIMENEZ-COLMENERO, F., CARBALLO, J. and COFRADES, S. (2001). Healthier meat and meat products: their role as functional foods. *Meat Science* **59**, 5–13.

KEANE, M.G. (1993). Relative tissue growth patterns and carcass composition in beef cattle. *Irish Grassland and Animal Production Association Journal* **27**, 64–77.

KEANE, M.G. (2000). Productivity and carcass traits of various sire breeds. In: *Advisory in-service training*, Teagasc, Grange Research Centre, Ireland.

KRUK, Z.A., SIEBERT, B.D., PITCHFORD, W.S., DAVIS, J., HARPER, G.S. and BOTTEMA, C.D.K. (2004). The effect of vitamin A on fatness in lot-fed cattle 1. Fat quality. *Proceedings of the 50th International Congress of Meat Science on Technology.*

LARICK, D.K. and TURNER, B.E. (1990). Flavour characteristics of forage and grain-fed beef as influenced by phospholipid and fatty acid compositional differences. *Journal of Food Science* **55**, 312–368.

LAWRIE, R.A. (1998). Chemical and biochemical constituents of muscle. Chapter 4 in: *Lawrie's Meat Science*, Sixth Edition. Woodhead Publishing Limited, Cambridge.

LESKANICH, C.O., MATTHEWS, K.R., WARKUP, C.C., NOBLE, R.C. and HAZZLEDINE, M. (1997). The effect of dietary oil containing (n-3) fatty acids on the fatty acid, physicochemical, and organoleptic characteristics of pig meat and fat. *Journal of Animal Science* **75**, 673–683.

MAFF (MINISTRY OF AGRICULTURE, FISHERIES AND FOOD) (1998). Fatty acids. Supplement to McCance and Widdowsons *The Composition of Foods*. MAFF, London.

MAHER, S.C., MULLEN, A.M., MOLONEY, A.P., DRENNAN, M.J., BUCKLEY, D.J. and KERRY, J.P. (2004). Colour composition and eating quality of beef from the progeny of two Charolais sires. *Meat Science* **67**, 73–80.

MALAU-ADULI, A.E.O., SIEBERT, B.D., BOTTEMA, C.D.K. and PITCHFORD, W.S. (1998). Breed comparison of the fatty acid composition of muscle phospholipids in Jersey and Limousin cattle. *Journal of Animal Science* **76**, 766–773.

MILLER, R.K. (2002). Factors affecting the quality of raw meat. In: *Meat Processing,*

Improving Quality, (J. Kerry, J. Kerry and D. Ledward, editors), pp 27–63. Woodhood Publishing Limited, Cambridge.

MIR, P.S., OKINE, E.K., GOONEWARDENE, L., HE, M.L. and MIR, Z. (2003). Effects of synthetic conjugated linoleic acid (CLA) or bio-formed CLA as high CLA beef on rat growth and adipose tissue development. *Canadian Journal of Animal Science* **83**, 583–592.

MIR, P.S., McALLISTER, T.A., SCOTT, S., AALHUS, J., BARON, V., McCARTNEY, D., CHARMLEY, E., GOONEWORDENE, L., BASARAB, J., OKINE, E., WESELAKE, R.J. and MIR, Z. (2004). Conjugated linoleic acid-enriched beef production. *American Journal of Chemical Nutrition* **79** (Suppl), 12075–12115.

MOLONEY, A.P. (1998). Growth and carcass composition in sheep offered isoenergetic rations which resulted in different concentrations of ruminal metabolites. *Livestock Production Science* **56**, 157–164.

MOLONEY, A.P. (2002). Growth and carcass composition in sheep offered low or high metabolisable protein supplemented with sodium propionate. *Proceedings of the Agricultural Research Forum,* 20–21.

MOLONEY, A.P., KEANE, M.G., DUNNE, P.G., MOONEY, M.T. and TROY, D.J. (2001a). Delayed concentrate feeding in a grass silage/concentrate beef finishing system: Effects on fat colour and meat quality. *Proceedings of the 47th International Congress of Meat Science of Technology*, 188–189.

MOLONEY, A.P., MOONEY, M.T., KERRY, J.P. and TROY, D.J. (2001b) Producing tender and flavoursome beef with enhanced nutritional characteristics. *Proceedings of the Nutrition Society* **60**, 221–229.

MOORE, V.J. and HARBORD, M.W. (1977). Palatability of beef from cattle fed maize silage and pasture. *New Zealand Journal of Agriculture Research* **20**, 279–281.

MUIR, P.D., DEAKER, J.M. and BROWN, M.D. (1998). Effect of forage- and grain-based systems on beef quality: a review. *New Zealand Journal of Agricultural Research* **41**, 623–635.

MURRAY, B.E., SARRIES, V., DALTON, D., MOLONEY, A.P. and TROY, D.J. (2004). Development of beef burger meat patties enriched in CLA. *Proceedings of the 50th International Congress of Meat Science of Technology*, 921–923.

NKRUMAH, J.D., LI, C. BASARAB, J.B. GUERCIO S. MENG, Y. MURDOCH, B. HANSEN, C. and MOORE, S.S. (2004). Association of a single nucleotide polymorphism in the bovine leptin gene with feed intake, feed efficiency, growth, feeding behavior, carcass quality and body composition. *Canadian Journal of Animal Science* **84**, 211–219.

NOCI, F., FRENCH, P., MONAHAN, F.J. and MOLONEY, A.P. (2005a). The fatty acid composition of muscle fat and subcutaneous adipose tissue of pasture-fed beef heifers: Influence of duration of grazing. *Journal of Animal Science* **83**, 1167–1178.

NOCI, F., O'KIELY, P., MONAHAN, F.J., STANTON, C. and MOLONEY, A.P. (2005b). Conjugated linoleic acid concentration in M. Longissimus dorsi from heifers offered sunflower oil-based concentrates and conserved forages. *Meat Science* **69**, 509–518.

O'SULLIVAN, A., GALVIN, K., MOLONEY, A.P., TROY, D.J., O'SULLIVAN K. and KERRY, J.P. (2003). Effect of pre-slaughter ratios of forages and or concentrates on the composition and quality of retail packaged beef. *Meat Science* **63**, 279–286.

OWENS, F.N. and GARDNER, B.A. (1999). Ruminant nutrition and meat quality. *Proceedings of the Annual Reciprocal Meat Conference* **52**, 25–36.

OWENS, F.N., GILL, D.R., SECRIST, D.S. and COLEMAN, S.W. (1995). Review of some aspects of growth and development of feedlot cattle. *Journal of Animal Science* **73**, 3152–3172.

REALINI, C.E., DUCKETT, S.K., BRITO, G.W., DALLA RIZZA, M. and DE MATTOS, D. (2004). Effect of pasture vs. concentrate feeding with or without antioxidants on carcass characteristics, fatty acid composition, and quality of Uruguayan beef. *Meat Science* **66**, 567–577.

ROBINSON, F. (2001). The nutritional contribution of meat to the British diet: recent trends and analyses. *Nutrition Bulletin* **26**, 283–293.

RULE, D.C., BROUGHTAN, K.S., SHELLITO, S.M. and MAIORANO, G. (2002). Comparison of muscle fatty acid profiles and cholesterol concentrations of bison, beef cattle, elk and chicken. *Journal of Animal Science* **80**, 1202–1211.

SAVELL, J.W. and CROSS, H.R. (1988), 'The role of fat in the palatability of beef, pork, and lamb'. In: *Designing Foods*; *Animal Product Options in the Marketplace*. National Academy Press, Washington, DC.

SCOLLAN, N.D., CHOI, N.J., KURT, E., FISHER, A.V., ENSER, M. and WOOD, J.D. (2001). Manipulating the fatty acid composition of muscle and adipose tissue in beef cattle. *British Journal of Nutrition* **85**, 115–124.

SCOLLAN, N.D., ENSER, M., GULATI, S., RICHARDSON, R.I. and WOOD, J.D. (2003). Effect of including a ruminally protected lipid supplement in the diet on the fatty acid composition of beef muscle in Charolais steers. *British Journal of Nutrition* **90**, 709–716.

SCOLLAN, N.D., RICHARDSON, R.I., DE SMET, S., MOLONEY, A.P., DOREAU, M., BAUCHART, D. and NUERNBERG, K. (2004a). Enhancing the content of beneficial fatty acids in beef and consequences for meat quality. In: *Indicators of Milk and Beef Quality* (JF Hocquette and S Gigli, editors), pp. 151–162. Wageningen Academic Publishers, NL.

SCOLLAN, N.D., ENSER, M., RICHARDSON, R.I., GULATI, S., HALLET, K.G., NUTE, G.R. and WOOD, J.D. (2004b). The effects of ruminally protected dietary lipid on the fatty acid composition and quality of beef muscle. *Proceedings of the 50th International Congress of Meat Science and Technology*, 528–531.

SCOLLAN, N.D., ENSER, M., RICHARDSON, I., GULATI, S., HALLETT, K.G. and WOOD, J.D. (2004c). The effects of including ruminally protected lipid in the diet of Charolais steers on animal performance, carcass quality and the fatty acid composition of longissimus dorsi muscle. *Proceedings of the British Society of Animal Science Meeting,* York, UK, 87.

SCOLLAN, N.D., DEWHURST, R.J., MOLONEY, A.P. and MURPHY, J.J. (2005). Improving the quality of products from grassland. In: *Grassland: A global science* (D.A. McGilloway, editor), pp. 41–56. Wageningen Academic Publishers, The Netherlands.

SCOTT, T.W., COOK, L.J. and MILLS, S.C. (1971). Protection of dietary polyunsaturated fatty acids against microbial hydrogenation in ruminants. *Journal of the American Oil Chemists Society* **48***,* 358–364.

STEEN, R.V.J. and ROBSON, A. (1995). Effects of forage to concentrate ratio in the diet and protein intake on the performance and carcass composition of beef heifers. *Journal of Agricultural Science, Cambridge* **125**, 125–135.

UNITED STATES DEPARTMENT OF AGRICULTURE (USDA) (2000). *Dietary Guidelines Advisory Committee, Dietary Guidelines for Americans.*

VATANSEVER, L., KURT, E., ENSER, M., NUTE, G.R., SCOLLAN, N.D., WOOD, J.D. and RICHARDSON, R.I. (2000). Shelf life and eating quality of beef from cattle of different breeds given diets differing in n-3 polyunsaturated fatty acid composition. *Animal Science* **71**, 471–482.

VERBECKE, W., OECKEL, M.J. VAN, WARRANTS, N., VIAENE, J. and BOUCQUE, CH.V. (1999). Consumer perception, facts and possibilities to improve acceptability of health and sensory characteristics of pork. *Meat Science* **53**, 77–99.

WOOD J.D. (1990) Consequences for meat quality of reducing carcass fatness. In *Reducing Fat in Meat Animals* (JD Wood and AV Fisher, editors), pp. 344–397. Elsevier Applied Science, London.

WOOD, J.D. and ENSER, M. (1997). Factors influencing fatty acids in meat and the role of antioxidants in improving meat quality. *British Journal of Nutrition* **78**, S49–S60.

WOOD, J.D., RICHARDSON, R.I., NUTE, G.R., FISHER, A.V., CAMPO, M.M., KASAPIDOU, E., SHREAD, P.R. and ENSER, M. (2003). Effects of fatty acids on meat quality: a review. *Meat Science* **66**, 21–32.

XIE, Y.R., BUSBOOM, J.R., GASKINS, C.T., JOHNSON, K.A., REEVES, J.J., WRIGHT, R.W. and CRONRATH, J.D. (1996). Effects of breed and sire on carcass characteristics and fatty acid profiles and crossbred Wagyu and Angus steers. *Meat Science* **43**, 167–177.

XIONGYL, MOODY W.G., BLANCHARD S.P., LIU G. and BURRIS W.R. (1996). Postmortem proteolytic and organoleptic changes in hot-boned muscle from grass-and grain-fed and zeranol-implanted cattle. *Food Research International* **29**, 27–34.

YANG, A., LANARI, M.C, BREWSTER, M. and TUME, R.K. (2002). Lipid stability and meat colour of beef from pasture – and grain-fed cattle with or without vitamin E supplement. *Meat Science* **60**, 41–50.

ZAMBAYASHI, M., NISHIMURA, K., LUNT, D.K. and SMITH, S.B. (1995). Effect of breed type and sex on the fatty acid composition of subcutaneous and intramuscular lipids of finishing steers and heifers. *Journal of Animal Science* 73, 3325–3332.

14

Producing low-fat meat products

J. F. Kerry and J. P. Kerry, University College Cork, Ireland

14.1 Introduction

The House of Commons UK Health Committee Report (2004) recently raised concerns over the increasing burden of obesity within England, in terms of yearly deaths (30 000) and total costs to the economy estimated at £2 billion (inclusive of financial losses through sick leave), with approximately £0.5 billion of this economic loss being calculated as NHS treatment/medical costs. Moreover, the report determined that levels of obesity have nearly trebled in the past 20 years, with life expectancy being reduced on average by 9 years as a result of this form of malnutrition. These reported figures do not include the added cost of overweight, which naturally compounds the situation where the physical cost of obesity as it is currently measured arises from the exposure of individuals to this risk factor of overweight in past decades. Similar concerns have been raised within Ireland where a figure of approximately €30 million has been estimated for in-patient costs alone in 2003 for a number of Irish hospitals. This year about 2000 premature deaths in Ireland will be attributed to obesity and the numbers are growing relentlessly. Using the accepted EU environmental cost benefit method, these deaths alone may be costing the state as much as €4bn per year (National Taskforce on Obesity, 2005).

The logical and temporal relationship between the exposure to obesity and overweight and their costly sequelae makes the available estimates on the burden of obesity inappropriate for accurately predicting future increases or to effectively quantify how these conditions actually impinge upon one's overall quality of life (Hu *et al.*, 1999; Vass, 2002).

The World Health Organization (1998) estimated that there are more than 250 million prevalent cases of obesity worldwide, equivalent to 7% of the adult population. The actual costs of obesity within different countries have been further estimated to account for approximately 2 to 8% of total health care expenditure (Seidell, 1999).

Obesity is now acknowledged as being a worldwide problem and is fast reaching epidemic proportions particularly in more affluent Western societies and no country has yet developed an effective approach to deal with it. Although the reported prevalence of obesity in England and Ireland is still lower than estimates for the United States, there has been a significant net increase in obesity within Europe that parallels the trend in the United States.

The causes of obesity are varied including differences in: regions/areas, gender, ethnic group and socio-economic background (Marshall *et al.*, 2000; Whincup *et al.*, 2002). However, changes in lifestyle, increasingly sedentary populations, the increasing mechanisation of modern life combined with changes in eating patterns and the consumption of diets richer in energy-dense foods (high-fat, high-calorific diets) have been reported as being some of the most significant factors (Vass, 2002). Dietary guidelines issued by the WHO recommend that fat intake should ideally contribute between 15 and 30% of total calories (33 g/1000 kcal or 39 g/5000 kJ) with saturates providing less than 10% (11 g/1000 kcal or 13 g/5000 kJ) of the total, with cholesterol intake being further limited to 300 mg/day (Canadian Paediatric Society, 1994).

Dietary intervention studies support the concept that restricting saturates and cholesterol and increasing the intake of essential fatty acids, especially n-3 fatty acids, reduces coronary heart disease (CHD) risk (Law, 2000; Schaefer, 2002). Regular consumption of red meat has been associated in epidemiological studies with increased risks of CHD, as well as colon and other cancers; possible mechanisms may involve dietary cholesterol, saturates, haem iron, and the presence of carcinogens formed in cooking (Kushi *et al.*, 1995; Mann *et al.*, 2001).

Active promotion by health professionals of the Mediterranean diet pyramid based on food patterns typical of Greece and southern Italy in the early 1960s, where adult life expectancy was among the highest in the world and rates of CHD, certain cancers and other diet-related chronic diseases were among the lowest, has been employed as a way of trying to educate consumers about healthy eating patterns (Dixon *et al.*, 2001; Kushi *et al.*, 1995; Paneras *et al.*, 1996; Willett *et al.*, 1995). Thus the '*prudent pattern*' of food consumption endorsed by health professionals has been characterised by a higher intake of vegetables, fruit, legumes, whole grains, fish and poultry, with a shift away from the '*Western pattern*' of food consumption characterised by a higher intake of red meat, processed meat, refined grains, sweets and dessert, French fries and high-fat dairy products (Hu *et al.*, 2000; Slattery *et al.*, 1998). Reduction in portion size (i.e. mini size as well as single serve packs) has been proposed and adopted by several food companies in an attempt to reduce calorie content of foods (DiNardo *et al.*, 2004).

Perhaps the greatest challenges to confront the meat sector is being realised as a need for fundamental rationalisation (i.e. production, processing, marketing methods, etc.) based on the adverse publicity regarding the correlation between meat products and obesity together with certain dietary linked diseases. Current consumer-driven demands for consistent wholesome, safe and convenient meats, based on the increased growing awareness of the links between diet and health, will remain the challenge of this sector for the foreseeable future (Storer *et al.*, 1998). The requirement to successfully and consistently reformulate meat products in order to quantitatively and qualitatively modify the lipids they contain while maintaining all the desirable organoleptic traits of traditional full-fat products will naturally play a pivotal role in the continuing developments within this area of low-fat meat processing and forms the principal theme of this chapter.

14.2 Nutritional and health-promoting properties of fats

While nutritional concerns relating to the excessive levels of fat being consumed in Western cultures are warranted, it is also important to acknowledge the essential beneficial role that lipids and lipid-related compounds play in disease prevention and growth. Phospholipids, glycolipids and cholesterol play a structural role in cell membranes with lipids also having an important function in biochemical regulatory systems. These lipid fractions can serve as precursors for beneficial biologically active compounds such as prostaglandins, steroid hormones and bile acids (Dunford, 2001). Animal fat contribution to overall calorific intake and moreover the proportion of fat (and type) present within meat products is a further cause of dietary concern for consumers (Paniangvait *et al.*, 1995).

It is reported that in Western countries, approximately 36–40% of total calories are obtained from fat, with over 50% of this value being obtained via meat products (Sheard *et al.*, 1998). A breakdown of the composite analysis (protein, fat and moisture, etc.) of a range of meat cuts is presented in Table 14.1 in order to illustrate the typical fat levels (and calorific values) that may be obtained from select muscle cuts. However, further analysis of the fatty acid profiles of meats reveals that it contains less than 50% saturates and up to 70% unsaturated fatty acids (King *et al.*, 1996; Paniangvait *et al.*, 1995; Romans *et al.*, 1994). Thus, it is perhaps unfortunate that processed meats (and red meats) are described as nutritionally '*unhealthy*' when saturates are taken into consideration (Table 14.2).

In terms of cholesterol, it is interesting to note that meat contains less than 75 mg/100 g, with the exception of certain by-products such as brain (2000–3000 mg/100), liver (300–350 mg/100 g) and heart (140–260 mg/100 g), where levels are considerably elevated (Bender, 1998; Paniangvait *et al.*, 1995; Romans *et al.*, 1994). However, the application of such by-products in further meat processing is somewhat limited. Zubillaga and Maerker (1991), using chromatographic analysis, identified a number of cholesterol-based fractions including (i) 7-ketocholesterol, (ii) cholesterol 5-alpha, 6-alpha-epoxide, and

Table 14.1 Composition analysis of a range of different cuts of meat (from Sawyer, 1975)

Cut of meat	Protein	Moisture (%)	Fat (%)	Ash (%)	Cal/100 g (%)
Beef					
Chuck	18.6	65	16	0.9	220
Flank	19.9	61	18	0.9	250
Loin	16.7	57	25	0.8	290
Rib	17.4	59	23	0.8	280
Topside	19.5	69	11	1.0	180
Rump	16.2	55	28	0.8	320
Pork					
Ham	15.2	53	31	0.8	340
Loin	16.4	58	25	0.9	300
Shoulder	13.5	49	37	0.7	390
Spare rib	14.6	53	32	0.8	350
Poultry					
Breast	12.8	48	37	0.7	380
Leg	18.0	64	18	0.9	240
Lamb					
Loin	18.6	65	16	0.7	220
Rib	14.9	52	32	0.8	360
Shoulder	15.6	58	25	0.8	300

(iii) cholesterol 5-beta, 6-beta-epoxide in veal, beef, pork and chicken muscles. All muscle tissues were reported to contain the three cholesterol products in measurable quantities with 7-ketocholesterol constituting greater than 50% of the oxidation products detected. Confusion has arisen over the terms *blood cholesterol* and *dietary cholesterol*. For most individuals dietary cholesterol has little or no effect on blood cholesterol levels because reduced synthesis in the

Table 14.2 Composition of fat and lean (per 100 g wet weight) of selected fresh meat cuts (from McCance and Widdowson, 1991)

					Fat			
	Water (g)	Protein (g)	Fat (g)	Energy (MJ)	Saturates (g)	Mono-unsaturates (g)	Poly-unsaturates (g)	Cholesterol (mg)
Beef, fat	24	9	67	2.6	29	32	3	90
Beef lean	74	20	5	0.5	2	2	0.2	60
Lamb, fat	21	6	72	2.8	36	28	3	75
Lamb lean	70	21	9	0.7	4	3	0.4	80
Pork, fat	21	7	71	2.8	26	29	11	75
Pork lean	72	21	7	0.6	2.5	3	1	70

body compensates for increased dietary intake. However, there are individuals who are sensitive to dietary cholesterol (Reiser and Shorland, 1990) and most authorities advise a general reduction in cholesterol intake for total populations.

As consumer knowledge of the beneficial effects of fat fractions evolves, current negative attitudes towards fat will naturally shift. Moreover, technological advances in oil fractionation/separation and encapsulation technologies for the development of pure lipid-related bioactive compounds with health promoting properties (Dunford, 2001; Schaefer, 2002) will see the debate on fat and its relationship with diet and health continue (Table 14.3). In terms of fat reduction, perhaps it is more accurate to comment on the actual percentage of total calories obtained via a typical meat serving. Calorific values (per gram) of basic food components are reported as: fat 9 Kcal, protein 4 Kcal and carbohydrate 4 Kcal. In the calorie reduction of a food system, one usually reduces the fat fraction as its energy value contribution to the food product is twice that of protein or carbohydrate. In processed meat products containing 10–12% protein and 25–30% fat, approximately 80% of the total calorific value is sourced from fat. However, in meat derivatives containing 6% fat, as much as 50% of the total calories are obtained from fatty compounds suggesting that it is only possible to reduce the calorific contribution of fat to <30% by reducing fat levels within the product to 2% or less (Shand and Schmidt, 1990). This fat reduction is usually achieved in conjunction with addition of suitable replacers/substitutes that enhance the protein/carbohydrate balance (Lyons *et al.*, 1999). However, reduction/removal of fat and its subsequent replacement with alternative functional ingredients will naturally result in a net contribution to the total calorific content of the product. Perhaps it is this monitoring of total calories and the actual fat contribution to calorific value that will form the basis of future evaluation and development of reduced/low-fat meat products (Colmenero *et al.*, 2001).

14.3 Textural characteristics of meat products attributed to fat

The presence (or incorporation) of fat within food products (especially meats) naturally has a significant influence on their overall sensory properties as it builds texture, mouthfeel and accounts for a critical proportion of the overall physical food matrix (Mela and Marshall, 1992; Yackinous and Guinard, 2000). Moreover, the physico-chemical properties of fat allow it to actively contribute to the textural properties of: smoothness, viscosity, creaminess, mouthcoating, moistness, chewiness, cohesiveness, hardness and crispness within food systems (Drewnowski, 1997; Marshall, 1990).

During the preparation of meat and processed meat products, levels of fat can range between 5% and 30% with typical full-fat products containing fat levels of 20–25% (Berry, 1997; Claus *et al.*, 1990; Paneras *et al.*, 1996). Processed meats have traditionally contained higher fat concentrations than their fresh whole-

Table 14.3 Lipid-related bioactive compounds suitable for use in food applications (from Danford, 2001)

Ingredient	Source	Structure	Health benefits	Reference
Linoleic acid (long chain polyunsaturated fatty acids) (PUFAs)	Animal and plant sources.	18-carbon molecule that contains double bonds in the *cis*-9 and *cis*-12 configurations.	An essential fatty acid.	WHO/FAO (1977)
Conjugated linoleic acid (CLA)	Milkfat, natural and processed cheeses, meat products, and plant oils. Animal (ruminant) sources of CLA richer than plant forms.	Isomers of linoleic acid that possess conjugated double bonds in the *cis* or *trans* configurations at positions 9 and 11 or at positions 10 and 12.	Inhibits tumour growth, reduces atherosclerotic risk and reduces body fat.	Ha *et al.* (1989)
Gamma-linolenic acid (GLA)	Evening primrose oil, borage and Hempseed oils.		Reduces inflammation, use in diabetic treatments, neuropathy, atopic eczema and certain cancers. Effective in the treatment of age-related diseases, alcoholism, hyperactivity, cardiovascular disease, and gastrointestinal, gynaecological, neurological and immunological disorders.	McDonald and Fitzpatrick (1998); Broadhurst and Winther (2000)

Table 14.3 Continued

Ingredient	Source	Structure	Health benefits	Reference
Alpha-linolenic acid (ALA)	Flaxseed, rapeseed, and walnuts are rich in ALA.	Isomer of linolenic acid.	Reported to inhibit the production of eicosanoids, alters the production of several prostanoids, reduces blood pressure in hypertensives, and lowers TGs and cholesterol. Retards tumour growth.	Oomah and Mazza (1999); Johnston (1995)
Omega-3 fatty acids	Fish and microalgae.	Eicosapentaenoic acid (EPA).	Benefits, such as preventing coronary heart disease, hypertension, type 2 diabetes, renal disease, rheumatoid arthritis, ulcerative colitis, and chronic obstructive pulmonary disease and aiding brain development and growth.	Simopoulos (1999)
Tocopherols and ami-tocotrienols (vitamin E)	Germ and bran fraction of certain seeds and cereals.	Both consist of a chroman backbone (two rings: one phenolic and the other heterocyclic) and an isoprenoid C-16 side chain with 3 chiral centres. Tocopherols have a saturated side chain. Depending on the number and position of the methyl groups on the side chain, these compounds are designated as α, β, γ and δ tocopherols.	Strong evidence that they play a role in the prevention of some chronic diseases such as heart disease and some cancers. Antioxidative function.	Traber and Packer (1995)

Plant sterols	Minor components of all vegetable oils. Unsaponifiable fraction of oil.	Ferulic acid-esterified sterol commonly known as oryzanol.	Reported to have diverse health benefits, including antioxidant and hypolipidaemic effects and stimulation of growth and hypothalamus activity.	Nicolasi *et al.* (1992)
Squalene	Naturally occurring terpenoid hydrocarbons in fish liver and olive oils.	*shinkaizameekisu* (deep-sea shark liver oil).	South East Asian folk medicine for chronic skin and liver diseases.	Nakamura *et al.* (1997)
Phospholipids	Soybean lecithin.	Usually contain only two fatty acid groups per molecule, unlike triglycerides where all three OH groups of glycerol are esterified to fatty acids. The third OH group on the glycerol backbone is linked to aliphatic compounds containing phosphoric acid and nitrogen residues.	Essential constituents of all living cells.	
Phosphatidyl-choline (PC)			Various metabolic disorders, such as lowering cholesterol levels, treating neurological disorders, and improving learning and memory.	Hanin (1979)
Medium chain triglycerides (MCTs)	Sources include coconut and palm kernel oils.	Contain fatty acids of primarily 8- and 10-carbon chain length.	Have been used in the treatment of fat malabsorption-related diseases and as a significant source of energy for preterm infants	Willis and Marangoni (1999)

muscle retail counterparts, largely because of the range of processing methods employed and the homogeneous nature of the end-products produced (Colmenero, 1996). Lowering the fat content of processed meats to more nutritionally acceptable levels (especially <15% fat) in emulsified comminuted products, such as frankfurters, gives rise to a less palatable product with a poor flavour and increased toughness (Claus, 1991; Colmenero, 1996; Rust and Olsen, 1988; Sofos and Allen, 1977). Matulis *et al.* (1995a) reported that acceptable frankfurters could be successfully manufactured with a minimum fat content of 11.25% fat in combination with 1.3% sodium chloride using lean meat at pH 6.0. However, numerous studies have shown that total substitution of fat with water in low-fat meat processing can result in an unacceptable product texture (soft product) with increased purge loss due to the physical inability of lean meat to adequately bind this excess water (Ahmed *et al.*, 1990; Claus and Hunt, 1991; Claus *et al.*, 1989; Gregg *et al.*, 1993). Studies have also reported on the correlation between fat reduction in processed meats and negative changes in product yield, colour and product acceptability on cooking (Claus, 1991; Huffman *et al.*, 1991; Troutt *et al.*, 1992). Thus, removal of fat from a meat system without adequate physical manipulation and/or addition of fat substitutes will result in an unacceptable final product texture (Keeton, 1991, 1994).

Perhaps the most convincing argument relating to the physical and quality changes that usually occur on reduction/removal of fat from meat products is realised through the ever-expanding range of texturising aids and fat mimetics that are commercially available. Based on this observation it is reasonable to argue that there is unfortunately no panacea or single ingredient that can totally replace fat or successfully impart all the quality characteristics that lipids provide to a meat product. As a result, the contribution of fat to processed meat eating quality should not be taken for granted, especially where fat reduction in the formulation is being considered.

14.4 The role of fat in flavour development in meat products

While texture and mouthfeel properties are important determinants of perceived fattiness in low-fat (<10%) meat systems Drewnowski and Schwartz, 1990; Mela and Marshall, 1992), the more important role of fat and its role in the perception of fat flavour have only been recently highlighted (Chevance and Farmer, 1999a,b; Tepper and Kuang, 1996; Yackinous and Guinard, 2000). Many of today's low-fat and fat-free products are failing to meet the fatty sensation expectations of the consumer (Williams, 1992, 1994), with the flavour component of these food systems usually being held accountable (Drewnowski, 1990; Yackinous and Guinard, 2000). Natural fat flavour development in meat products may be influenced through several factors including: animal production methods (Melton, 1990; Moloney 1999), meat processing/manufacturing methods, storage conditions (McMillin *et al.*, 1991), packaging techniques (Ho *et al.*, 1995), as well as culinary issues and combinations thereof.

Animal production systems can indirectly influence final meat flavour where leanness is encouraged *via* genetic selection (Solomon *et al.*, 2000); muscle growth is manipulated through the use of metabolic modifiers (Anderson, 2000; Dikeman, 2000) and/or through the type of animal feeds employed (i.e. forage, silage, grain, polyunsaturated fats, edible oils, and other concentrates/supplements, etc.) (Ahn *et al.*, 1995; Maruri and Larick, 1992). The latter option directly influences the actual flavour and oxidative stability of animal fat, which functions as a natural reservoir for fat-soluble volatiles and antioxidants present within the feeds employed (Maruri and Larick, 1992; McMillin, *et al.*, 1991; Morrissey *et al.*, 1998). Moreover, metabolic compounds have also been linked with off-flavours in meat products. For example, boar taint in pigs has been attributed primarily to the presence of two compounds in boar fat, androstenone (5-alpha-androst-16-ene-3-one) and skatole (3-methyl indole) (Zabolotsky *et al.*, 1995).

The type of meat species utilised further influences the sensory perception based largely on flavour differences attributed to their fat fractions. Ha and Lindsay (1991) quantitatively assessed caprine, ovine, bovine, equine, swine and cervine perinephric fats for volatile alkylphenols, phenol and thiophenol compounds. Results showed that sheepy-muttony aromas in ovine fats were contributed by *p*-cresol, 2-isopropylphenol, 3,4-dimethylphenol, thymol, carvacrol, 3-isopropylphenol and 4-isopropylphenol. Cresols, especially *m*-cresol, appeared to contribute to beef flavours, with high concentrations of thiophenol producing the unpleasant mutton aromas of ram fat.

Human perception of flavour is usually closely related to the nature and amount of odour and taste components available within the sensory system (Overbosch *et al.*, 1991). Thus, it is important to consider the role of fat in the generation of flavour (taste, smell and trigeminal components) in processed meats and the actual effect of fat reduction on sensory profiles as the presence of fat has the unique ability to modify this flavour perception (Chevance and Farmer, 1999a; Mela and Marshall, 1992). Mottram and Edwards (1984) demonstrated that removal of the triglyceride fraction (subcutaneous or intramuscular fat) from a beef system could be achieved successfully without adversely altering the 'meaty' character of the system's odour. However, removal of both triglyceride and phospholipid fractions altered the meat odour which became 'roasted' or 'toasted' in terms of olfactory perception. This result suggests that physical removal of visible fat (the main source of triglycerides) from meat is possible since phospholipids are usually associated with the lean fraction of meat. However, the ratio of phospholipid : triglycerides as well as the interactions between these fractions cannot be ignored. This ratio of phospholipids : triglycerides will clearly influence the concentration of Maillard products and other volatiles produced during further meat processing and influence the net flavours produced during final consumption. Quantifying the actual flavour contribution from fat is difficult to elucidate and numerous studies employing model food systems have suggested that flavour release from a food is further dictated by the fat solubility of selected flavour volatiles and their rate of retention within the fat fraction (De Roos and Wolswinkel, 1993; Landly *et al.*, 1996).

The majority of aroma compounds within foods are fat soluble and partition coefficients suggest that they will be associated with the lipid phase at equilibrium; thus, fats act as a carrier or reservoir for these flavours (Chevance and Farmer, 1999a; Hatchwell, 1994). Moreover, the matrix of the food (dependent on the amount and type of fat in the system) greatly affects flavour release rates and profiles (De Roos 1997; Park *et al.*, 1990). Naturally, when fat is removed or reduced within a meat system, the perception of flavour is greatly altered (Chevance and Farmer 1999a,b) especially on replacement of the meat lipid fraction with fat substitutes (Chevance *et al.*, 2000). Several studies have reported on the ability of humans to detect fat in real and modified fluid dairy systems (Mela, 1988). However, the flavour becomes more difficult to elucidate for solid foods and a direct monotonically increasing relationship between percentage fat and perceived fattiness is not always evident (Yackinous and Guinard, 2000).

Information on flavour release systems in meat products (especially low-fat meats) is somewhat limited (Chevance and Farmer, 1999a,b). However, when the fat component is physically adjusted within a meat product it may: (i) lead to differences in the generation of compounds for which fat is a precursor; (ii) alter the types of interactions that occur in volatile aromatic compounds; and/or (iii) change the behaviour of some adjuncts (i.e. spices, seasonings, flavours, etc.) present within the meat system (De Roos, 1997; Ingham *et al.*, 1996; Park *et al.*, 1989).

Many researchers have reported super-critical carbon dioxide (SC-CO_2) extraction as a potential method for analytical extraction of cholesterol, lipids and fat-soluble volatiles from beef and other meats (Chao *et al.*, 1991; King *et al.*, 1989, 1993, 1996; Lin *et al.*, 1999). It has been suggested that this method may be more effective with precooked meat products owing to their reduced moisture content when compared with fresh meat products (King *et al.*, 1993). Determination of the fat and other volatile fractions within meat and other foods is an area that is set to evolve in the future and will hopefully lead to a greater understanding of the role of these lipid fractions in both flavour development and overall product quality (Berg *et al.*, 1997; Rozzi and Singh, 2002).

Studies have suggested that when preparing a low-fat meat product with increased levels of added water, the levels of added spices and other flavourings must be adjusted accordingly in order to maintain flavour consistency with traditional full-fat systems (Claus, 1991; Wirth, 1988). This suggests that the lipid fraction present in full-fat systems actually affects (absorbs/masks) some of the spice flavour and intensity in traditional full fat meat products and thus alters flavour release from the product (Ingham *et al.*, 1996). Reduction of salt (by 25%) is also recommended in order to successfully manufacture processed products with a minimum of 10% fat (Claus, 1991; Wirth, 1988).

The application of heat during meat cookery further influences the behaviour of fats, which melt at various temperatures (based on individual melting points), and this in turn influences the composition, texture, appearance, flavour profile (rates of oxidation) and overall eating quality of cooked meat products. The application of heat during processing also leads to the development of specific Maillard formation products which can further influence overall meat flavour

(Chevance and Farmer, 1999a). Cambero *et al.* (1992) reported a significant correlation between cooking temperature of beef broth and the concentration of certain flavour compounds namely: free amino acids (FAAs), carnosine and inosine 5′-monophosphate (IMP) responsible for the enhancement of the broth's beefy flavour. As results correlated with organoleptic scores, it was concluded that a wide mixture of FAAs, peptides of low molecular weight (< 6300 Da) and IMP played an important role in the flavour intensity of beef broth. This result further suggests that flavour development in low, reduced and full-fat meat systems is based on a complex series of chemical interactions involving more than one active compound.

14.5 Warmed-over flavour

Precooked, ready-to-eat meat products are usually stored frozen or at refrigeration temperatures prior to being purchased, reheated and consumed, giving rise to warmed-over flavour (WOF) development (Thongwong *et al.*, 1999). Moreover, the quality of heat-processed meat dishes is usually limited by this lipid oxidation (Kanner, 1994).

Thus, WOF has long been accepted as the term to describe the rancid or stale flavour detected in cooked meats within 48 h of refrigeration at 4 °C. This deterioration is in contrast to rancidity in raw meats, fatty tissues, lard and/or rendered fat which becomes evident after prolonged freezer storage (Gray *et al.*, 1996; Pearson and Gray, 1983). While the mechanism of WOF development is not fully understood, research suggests that it is associated with iron and autoxidation of polyunsaturated fatty acids and phospholipids (Gray and Pearson, 1987; Pearson *et al.*, 1977). Methods applied in the reduction of WOF may include prevention of its development using suitable antioxidants to prevent its onset (Gray *et al.*, 1996; McCarthy *et al.*, 2000a,b), or physical removal of both flavour and volatile compounds using methods such as supercritical fluid extraction (SC-CO_2) (Rizvi *et al.*, 1986; Rozzi and Singh, 2002; Thongwong *et al.*, 1999).

SC-CO_2 extraction of WOF volatiles from cooked, freeze-dried beef have yielded hexanal, heptanal, octanal, nonanal and 2,3-octanedione, in the volatile profile using dynamic headspace extraction and gas chromatography-mass spectrometry before and after CO_2 extraction. Isolation and identification of flavour compounds from fat fractions in meats have also been achieved using SC-CO_2 extraction in beef (Taylor *et al.*, 1997), pork (Lin *et al.*, 1999) as well as poultry (Taylor and Larick, 1995).

14.6 Meat proteins

In order to develop ingredients and ingredient blends suitable for the manufacture of low-fat meat products, meat processors must not only consider the formulations used and the technologies available, but must also evaluate the functionality and quality of the raw meat materials being utilised. A clear understanding of the key physico-chemical factors that influence the quality characteristics of meat products will facilitate the development of high-quality low-fat products. In view of the important role that meat proteins play in the characteristics of processed meat products, it is perhaps no surprise that protein functionality (i.e. water, fat and meat-binding ability) of raw meat materials is a potential avenue through which the properties of new low-fat products may be optimised (Colmenero, 1996).

Protein functionality may be defined as those physical and chemical properties that affect the behaviour of proteins in food systems during processing, storage, preparation and consumption with these properties being largely dependent on the type of food product being produced (Kinsella, 1981). In terms of meat systems, water binding, solubility, viscosity, emulsification and gelation are perhaps the factors of most importance. Functional properties are regarded as 'intermediate' properties in the sense that they are dictated by physiochemical properties of proteins, but they play a critical role in producing desirable product characteristics as shown: physiochemical properties → functionality → product quality (Xiong, 1996).

Processed meat manufacture usually entails the pre-selection of meat cuts (based on general quality, collagen and fat content) from animals, birds or seafoods and blending this raw material with a range of adjuncts including water, seasonings, extenders/binders (proteins, polysaccharides), sugars and flavourings, with these ingredients being manipulated using a range of processing technologies. Reduction of fat levels in meat product preparation clearly poses a number of technological challenges. As already outlined, adjusting the level of fat in processed meats can significantly alter product characteristics such as flavour, juiciness, mouthfeel, texture, cooking properties and storage stability (Cavestany *et al.*, 1994; Claus, 1991; Sofos and Allen, 1977).

An alternative classification or ranking of meat based on protein functionality has been proposed (Saffle and Galbreath, 1964), with functionality of various meat cuts based on the ultimate yield of salt (sodium chloride) solubilised protein. Meat bind constants were subsequently derived from these initial protein solubility determinations *via* quantitative assessment of the emulsifying capacity of meat extracts (Carpenter and Saffle, 1964). The initial bind values were later revised and defined as '*constant emulsification values*' (CEV) (Saffle, 1968). Further developments on the prediction of bind constants for meats resulted in the preparation of regression models based on moisture and protein levels of meat samples (Parks *et al.*, 1985). Meat research during the 1970s and 1980s led to a greater understanding of protein chemistry and its influence on the functionality of meat proteins (Acton and Dick, 1984; Acton and Saffle, 1972; Acton *et al.*, 1983; Gordon and Barbut, 1992a). The importance of protein and water binding, as well as fat binding in comminuted processed meats, has led to a re-evaluation of bind values. These subsequent revisions, together with development of alternative methodologies for the evaluation of meat functionality, have resulted in further modifications to the bind constant values (Labudde and Lanier, 1995).

In general, heat-induced gelation, water-holding capacity, fat-binding and emulsification are the principal functional properties required in meat products (Morrissey *et al.*, 1987). Meat batters formed during the production of comminuted meat products such as frankfurters, Bologna, some sausages and meat loaves may be described as multi-phase systems consisting of solubilised muscle proteins, muscle fibres, fat cells, fat droplets, water, salt and other ingredients (Gordon and Barbut, 1992a). Preparation of Bologna containing 13% and 11% protein has shown that more stable emulsions are obtained at higher protein concentrations and this is attributed to the encapsulation of fat globules by extracted protein molecules during processing (Claus *et al.* 1989; Lin and Mei, 2000). Two theories have been proposed to explain fat stabilisation within meat batters. The *emulsification theory* attributes fat stabilisation to the formation of an interfacial protein film around the fat globules. The *physical entrapment theory* proposes that fat particles in meat batters are physically entrapped within a highly viscous protein solution prior to heating and then within a gel protein matrix after thermal processing (Gordon and Barbut, 1992a; Morrissey *et al.*, 1987). The relative contribution of each process to meat batter stabilisation depends on the environmental conditions, the physical state and properties of the lean phases, processing conditions and the characteristics of the product being manufactured (Gordon and Barbut, 1992a). In addition, it is generally recognised that the formation of a protein gel matrix by myofibrillar proteins during thermal processing is largely responsible for the water entrapment within these products (Morrissey *et al.*, 1987).

As the content of fat decreases and the percentage of added water increases in low-fat meat batters, water-holding capacity replaces fat binding as a critical issue determining product quality and stability (Claus, 1991). During the preparation of meat batters, comminution of muscle in the presence of added salt and water physically disrupts the muscle tissue. This results in fibre swelling and solubilisation of salt-soluble muscle proteins, which increases the viscosity and water-holding capacity of the mix (Gordon and Barbut, 1992a; Morrissey *et al.*, 1987). During thermal processing, myofibrillar proteins in the continuous phase undergo conformational changes and participate in protein–protein interactions leading to the formation of a three-dimensional gel network which physically entraps water and fat particles within the mix (Gordon and Barbut, 1992a; Morrissey *et al.*, 1987).

Protein gels are usually defined as three-dimensional matrices or networks in which polymer–polymer and polymer–solvent interactions occur in an ordered manner resulting in the immobilisation of a large amount of water by a small amount of protein (Schmidt, 1981). Several theories have been proposed to explain the mechanism of protein gelation. Ferry (1948) proposed a two-step mechanism that involves initial denaturation of protein molecules, followed by formation of a three-dimensional network. The microstructure and properties of the gel matrix depend on the relative rates of denaturation and aggregation.

When the rate of protein aggregation is slow relative to the rate of unfolding, the denatured protein molecules are allowed to orient themselves and form an ordered fine gel network. In contrast, when aggregation occurs very rapidly, coarser, less ordered gel structures or coagula are formed (Ferry, 1948; Hermansson, 1978).

It is generally agreed that myosin is the major salt-soluble protein involved in thermal gelation in meat systems (Asghar *et al.*, 1985; Morrissey *et al.*, 1987). Thus, knowledge of the mechanism of myosin gelation, the molecular forces involved in this process and the effect of environmental conditions on the properties of myosin gels may ultimately facilitate manipulation of formulations and processing conditions to yield low-fat meat products with optimum textural and water-holding properties. Many studies have been carried out using model systems to determine the effects of environmental factors on the heat-induced gelation of myosin and to determine the major molecular transformations involved in the process.

The properties of microstructure of the muscle protein gel network formed during thermal processing dictates the textural and water-holding properties of low-fat comminuted meat systems (Claus, 1991). A critical balance between protein–protein interactions and protein–water interactions is necessary to give the desired textural and water-holding properties. If protein–protein interactions are too strong then the product may have a tight aggregated structure with poor water-holding properties and a very firm texture. In contrast, if protein–water interactions are dominant the product may lack structural integrity and have a very soft texture.

The importance of obtaining the optimum gel structure in meat batter systems is clearly illustrated by Gordon and Barbut (1990, 1992a). The authors demonstrated that meat batters prepared using 1.58% $CaCl_2$ instead of 2.5% NaCl underwent extensive protein–protein interactions during thermal processing, resulting in a very aggregated and discontinuous gel matrix which exhibited very high cooking losses. In a further study, Gordon and Barbut (1992b) investigated the ability of various chemical reagents to modify the textural, fat and water-holding properties of meat batters. Hydrogen peroxide (H_2O_2) oxidises free sulphydryl groups and β-mercaptoethanol (β-ME) reduces exposed disulphide bonds in proteins. It was found that meat batters containing β-ME or H_2O_2 exhibited similar fat and water losses as control batters. The authors concluded that disulphide bond formation within the gel matrix does not affect the fat or water-holding capacity of meat batters. However, H_2O_2 increased the hardness and cohesiveness of the cooked batter gels while β-ME decreased hardness and springiness compared with the control. These results indicate that disulphide bond formation is important in the development of an acceptable texture in meat batters.

Ethylene diamine tetraacetic acid (EDTA) containing batters exhibited high water losses during cooking due to extensive protein aggregation. Large well-interconnected channels throughout the matrix appeared to facilitate water loss from the EDTA-containing batters. Urea disrupts hydrogen and electrostatic bonds while increasing the availability of hydrophobic groups for bonding. Cooked urea-containing batters had similar hardness and springiness values as the controls and were very cohesive, exhibiting excellent fat and water-holding properties. The protein matrix of the urea-treated batters had a very fine highly interconnected appearance that accounts for their excellent water and fat-binding properties and high cohesiveness values. These results indicate that hydrophobic interactions, in addition to hydrogen bonding and electrostatic interactions, play an important role in the water holding and textural properties of meat batters.

In low-fat high-added water comminuted meat products, one's aim is to optimise the water-holding capacity of the system in order to minimise both cooking and purge losses; however, these resultant products usually tend to have a soft texture. Statistical models have been developed that enable processors to predict the effects of using different combinations of fat and added water on a given product trait (Claus *et al.*, 1989). However, these models are of limited value since optimising one trait, such as product firmness, may occur at the expense of other sensory and storage characteristics. Furthermore, predictive accuracy of these models is influenced by such factors as collagen content of meat, smoke-house conditions and product type (Claus, 1991). Overall there is a need to develop new integrated models that take into consideration all of the commercially important characteristics of low-fat comminuted products.

14.7 Technologies utilised in fat reduction of processed meats

14.7.1 Visual grading

Traditional methods employed in the selection of raw meat materials for the manufacture of processed meats and in particular low-fat products have based raw material grading on visual lean values and/or compositional analysis (Hale, 1994). Clearly product quality specifications are important criteria in ensuring an efficient vendor rating, as well as a consistent high-quality raw meat material. The tighter the quality specifications employed, the more efficient the processing operation and ultimate productivity levels achieved.

This selection process is slowly evolving and will possibly become more elaborate, based on the inclusion of factors such as indirect (breeding for leanness) and direct (transgenic animals) genetic manipulation of animals (Solomon *et al.*, 2000), dietary history as well as other animal husbandry-related issues (i.e. organic production, etc.).

The grading scheme presented in Table 14.4 illustrates the typical meat selection (visual) standards employed commercially. These score sheets indicate that as grade or class ranking increases, the quality of the meat decreases, with quality deterioration in this instance being defined as an increase in both fat and connective/collagen tissue concentrations within the meat.

The type/quality of meat product being processed, as well as the ultimate fat level desired, play an important role in the selection of the meat classes or grades selected. If an acceptable low-fat meat product is to be produced, good

Table 14.4 Grading/classification system used for both beef and pork meat in the manufacture of processed meat products

	Water (%)	Fat (%)	Connective tissue (%)	Lean (%)	Total protein (%)
Beef Class					
1	75	4	1.5	19.5	21
2	72	8	3.0	17.0	20
3	69	12	3.4	15.6	19
4	64	18	4.5	13.5	18
5	50	35	3.8	11.2	15
Pork Class					
1	75	5	1.0	19.0	20
2	73	8	1.5	17.5	19
3	70	11	2.9	16.1	19
4	53	33	2.1	11.9	14
5	32	60	1.2	6.8	8
6	40	50	3.0	7.0	10
7	17	78	2.5	2.5	5
8	8	90	0.3	1.7	2
9	25	70	2.5	2.5	5
10	40	50	7.0	3.0	10
11	20	75	3.2	1.8	5
12	55	30	9.7	5.3	15

quality lean meat is obviously not only desirable, but also a basic requirement. As low levels of fat are required in formulating low-fat meat products (<10% fat), meat grades 1 and 2 are usually required, based on data presented in Table 14.4. The advent of machine image technology provides a rapid, alternative means for measuring meat quality consistently based on reflectance characteristics (Gerrard *et al.*, 1996; McDonald and Chen 1991, 1992). Perhaps the advent of this technology will lead to the establishment of effective on-line techniques to quantitatively determine the fat content of meat cuts and their suitability for low-fat meat processing. While trimming and/or selection of visually lean meats for further processing facilitates the reduction of fat content in final products (Ahmed *et al.*, 1990, 1991), it is not always cost effective owing to the price of the lean meat and/or the level of trimming and preparation required, which in turn elevates the price of the recovered lean meat.

14.7.2 Use of extenders/binders

A second option in fat reduction (or dilution) within low-fat meat products is made possible through the use of suitable extenders or binders (proteins, polysaccharides, etc.) that possess a reduced calorific value (Claus *et al.*, 1989; Keeton, 1996). While water is an effective low-calorie adjunct, its usage rate in low-fat meat manufacture is limited owing to the negative textural and quality issues that arise when used in excess. Moreover, the regulatory aspects of added water levels in final meat products further controls its rate of addition in low fat meat formulations. The number of functional (i.e. fat, water and meat binding) adjuncts currently available for use in low-fat meat processing are exhaustive, however they may be generally categorised as follows:

- **Protein:**
  – *Meat-based* (gelatine, collagen, blood fractions, surimi).
  – *Non-meat-based* (soya, pea, wheat, dairy fractions).
- **Polysaccharides:**
  – *Hydrocolloids* (*iota*, *kappa* and *lambda* carrageenans, alginates, agars, etc.).
  – *Galactomannans* (guar gum, locust bean gum, Tara gum, gum Arabic, etc.).
  – *Starches* (potato, tapioca, waxy maize, wheat, pea, oat, etc.).
  – *Complex starches* (oat fibre, wheat fibre, pea fibre, inulin, Konjac flour, etc.).
  – *Other sources* (maltodextrin, high and low methoxy pectin, cherries, solubilised cellulose, carboxyl methyl cellulose, microcrystalline cellulose, etc.).
- **Fermentation products**: xanthan gum, gellan gum.
- **Enzymes**: Transglutaminase.

Application of functional ingredients to low-fat meat systems may take several forms including dry addition, pre-hydrated, pre-emulsified, or incorporation as a preformed gel (pseudo-fat). Use of ingredient blends in order to mimic the textural and other quality characteristics of fat in low-fat meat products reveals the complexity of such multicomponent meat gel systems and the effects of altering the fat : protein : water balance in such low-fat systems. Regardless of the mode of addition or blend employed, the principal function of added binders/extenders in low fat (high added water) meat processing is that of product extension while maintaining the characteristic textural properties of traditional full fat products (Bullock *et al.*, 1995; Ockerman and Chao, 1996). Table 14.5 highlights some of the more recent studies that have been carried out using functional ingredients in the preparation of low-fat meat products.

The preparation of fortified, low-fat 'healthy' products is a market with considerable growth potential (Sloan, 2002). Goldberg (1994) further identified 12 categories of ingredient (of animal and plant origin) that have beneficial effects on human health including (i) dietary fibre, (ii) oligosaccharides, (iii) sugars/alcohols, (iv) amino acids, peptides, proteins, (v) glucosides, (vi) alcohols, (vii) isoprenenoids and vitamins, (viii) cholines, (ix) lactic acid bacteria, (x) minerals, (xi) polyunsaturated fatty acids and (xii) others (i.e. phytochemicals, antioxidants, etc.). The inclusion of such ingredients in order to further enhance the nutritional qualities of traditional and low-fat meats is an area that holds numerous opportunities for improving the image of processed meat products.

Table 14.5 Selected functional ingredients successfully utilised in the manufacture of low-fat meat products

Ingredient	Ingredient addition rate (%)	Product type	% fat level	Functional properties	Reference
Concentrated blood plasma (CBP)	1.5, 2.5, 3.5	Beef patty	10	Blood fractions substituted for lean meat. CBP gave soy-type flavours with RCP giving bloody and metallic off-flavours compared with control. Changes in colour, cook losses and oxidative stability of test patties over control. Blood fractions may be used in processed foods where the colour and flavour might be masked by other components.	Guzman *et al.* (1995)
Beef collagen	10–20	Frankfurter	10–20	The addition of 20% connective tissue improved processing yields and decreased cohesiveness of 10% fat/30% water added frankfurters.	Eilert *et al.* (1996)
Semi refined pork connective tissue	10–30	Bologna	7–10	Heating (70 °C × 30 min) pork connective tissue (PCT) increased water binding and textural properties of PCT gels. The range of textures produced makes it a very functional texture modifying aid for use in low-fat meats.	Osburn and Mandigo (1997)
Soya protein	4	Frankfurter	11	Of 8 binders evaluated, modified waxy maize starch, isolated soy protein, and isolated muscle protein had sensory and textural properties most similar to the high-fat (21) control. Product containing isolated soy protein had a higher purge loss.	Yang *et al.* (2001)

	3	Frankfurter	12–20	Soya protein increased hardness and off-flavour, as well as decreasing juiciness, saltiness, and flavour intensity of test frankfurters. Recommended that soy protein should be added to meat product at less than 3.0% to minimise this effect.	Matulis *et al.* (1995)
Pea protein	2	Frankfurter	15	Pea protein had a weakening effect on the texture of test products containing pre-emulsified fat compared with full fat control (18%).	Su *et al.* (2000)
Pea inner fibre	1.6	Beef patty	10,14,18	Pea fibre improved tenderness and cooking yields with little patty volume reduction	Anderson and Berry (2001)
Caseinate	2	Frankfurter	16	Utilisation of preformed fat emulsions containing soy protein isolate or sodium caseinate as stabilisers sustained the desired texture lost due to salt reduction and/or high water addition when compared with controls (18% fat).	Su *et al.* (2000)
Dairy proteins	1, 3, 5	Smoked sausage	15	Addition of caseinate increased firmness, whiteness, elasticity and rancidity. Addition of whey proteins increased graininess, stickiness, colour, fatness, juiciness and smokiness, textural analysis correlated with sensory scores.	Baardseth *et al.* (1992)
Whey protein	0–4	Pork sausage	<3	Addition of whey protein/carrageenan gels to sausages improved product texture and organoleptic scores when assessed against full fat (20%) controls.	Lyons *et al.* (1999)

Table 14.5 Continued

Ingredient	Ingredient addition rate (%)	Product type	% fat level	Functional properties	Reference
Konjac flour/starch	1	Bologna	1.4	Konjac blend in combination with 2% SPI identified as having textural characteristics similar to regular Bologna (30% fat) based on sensory flavour test and Instron TPA results.	Chin *et al.* (2000)
Carrageenan	0.4	Meat batter	11	Improved emulsion stability and water holding capacity on addition of soya isolate (1.4%) over low-fat (11%) control.	Lin and Mei (2000)
Iota carrageenan	0.4	Frankfurter	12–20	Carrageenan increased test product hardness at salt levels <1.7% and decreased juiciness at fat levels >15%. Flavour intensity increased as carrageenan and fat level increased using 1.3% salt. Addition of 1.65% salt increased off-flavour intensity. Off flavour decreased as fat content increased and carrageenan concentration decreased.	Matulis *et al.* (1995)
Alginate	0.15	Beef patty	5–10	Low-fat beef patties containing a combination of alginate (0.15%) and carrageenan (0.5%) were similar to control (20% fat) for the properties of yield and texture.	Lin and Keeton (1998)
Alginate	0.8	Meat batter	11	Increased emulsion stability and water holding at higher cooking temperatures due to a more heat-stable alginate gel. Possible protective effect of gums and soy protein (1.4%) on meat proteins is proposed.	Lin and Mei (2000)

Dehydrated potato extract	0–2%	Beef patties	0–2	Similar yields and sensory properties to full-fat (11%) products, an effective anti-oxidant and water-binding ingredient.	Katsanidis *et al.* (2001)
Waxy starch hull-less barley	4	Pork Bologna	1	4% Addition of hull-less waxy barley flour or meal gave the best purge control; 4% normal starch barley, wheat flour and potato starch were intermediate; 0.25% *kappa*-carrageenan or 1% soy protein concentrate had little effect on water holding or texture. Formulations with wheat flour and waxy barley meal scored firmest, while Bologna with potato starch required the most force to compress. Wheat flour improved product texture but decreased spice flavour.	Shand (2000)
Oat bran	0–3	Frankfurter	11–15	Two oat fibres (bleached, and high water adsorption) were assessed. Results indicated that addition of both types of oat fibre produced greater yields, and lighter, less red colour. Purge was reduced with oat fibre at 3%. Product hardness increased for Bologna with both fibre types. The extent of product change, however, was different for the 2 oat fibre varieties.	Steenblock *et al.* (2001)
Solubilised cellulose	0–2%	Beef patties	0–2%	More moist product with increased yields compared to the full fat (11%) product, enhanced storage stability of patties when used in combination with 1.5% potato extract	Katsanidis *et al.* (2001)

14.7.3 Meat-based proteins

Recovery of functional meat protein from meat by-products, including porcine rind, connective tissue, blood protein, surimi and isolated meat protein (IMP) has been studied in recent years. Collagen prepared from the corium layer of beef hide has been successfully incorporated into meat systems as a water-binding agent (Eilbert *et al.*, 1993; Kenney *et al.*, 1986) and a number of commercial collagen protein sources are currently available (e.g. Collapro®). Use of gelatinised pork rind has also been shown to improve the texture and juiciness of low-fat comminuted meat products (Osburn and Mandigo, 1997). The fractionation and concentration of blood plasma proteins has been successfully achieved using membrane and gel filtration techniques. Functional blood plasma (e.g. Vepran®) and other fractions (e.g. Harimex® thrombin/fibrinogen clotting systems) are currently available and possess excellent meat binding properties (Dill and Landmann, 1988; Guzman *et al.*, 1995).

One of the most exciting developments in recent years is the production of myofibrillar protein concentrates usually referred to as surimi (Yang *et al.*, 2001). Surimi in the presence of added water and salts undergoes protein–protein interactions on heating to form the continuous matrix or surimi hydrogel (Lee, 1987; Lee *et al.*, 1992). This protein source is used as an intermediate product for the manufacture of a variety of fabricated seafood products and has also been successfully utilised as a meat and water-binding adjunct in the manufacture of processed meat products (Carballo *et al.*, 1992; Chen and Trout, 1991; Venugopal and Shahidi, 1995). Fish surimi may be added as a functional ingredient to processed meat products up to a maximum level of 5% addition; higher addition levels can result in an undesirable fishy aroma in final products.

Edible meat by-products have also been suggested as potential sources of functional meat protein where innovative or alternative technologies are developed for offal treatment (Brekke and Eisels, 1981). However, the impact of increasing negative consumer perception towards animal by-products has resulted in a decreased interest in their use as functional ingredients in processed meat formulation.

14.7.4 Non-meat proteins

Non-meat proteins employed in low-fat meat processing are usually sourced as isolates (>80% protein) and concentrates (30–80% protein) and are incorporated into meats at optimum residual powder levels of 2–3% and 4–6%, respectively. Addition of non-meat proteins in low-fat meat formulations is believed to partially compensate for the potential loss of some water-binding properties due to higher water addition rates and reduced salt levels in such products. Perhaps the most widely reported non-meat protein employed in meat processing is that of soya protein (Dexter *et al.*, 1993; Sofos and Allen, 1977; Yang *et al.*, 2001). However, use of soya isolate in emulsion type products in excess of 3% has been reported to increase hardness and off-flavour, and decrease juiciness, saltiness and flavour intensity (Matulis *et al.*, 1995b). Other non-meat protein sources that have been assessed in low-fat meat processing include: pea, wheat, dairy (whey proteins, caseinates, total milk protein, etc.) and oat flours as highlighted in Table 14.5. Incorporation of non-meat proteins in low-fat meat processing usually results in elevated protein levels together with improvements in product yield, product stability (water fat and meat binding), formulation costs and product textural properties (organoleptic issues) as well as a reduction in calorific values and improvement in nutritional status (Troy *et al.*, 1999).

14.7.5 Polysaccharides

Polysaccharides have been utilised in the manufacture of low-fat meats because of their ability to bind water and act as gelling agents in emulsified meat systems (Bloukas *et al.*, 1997; Mittal and Barbut, 1994; Wallingford and Labuza, 1983). Carrageenans have been utilised in a range of meat products such as ground beef, roasted turkey breast, fresh pork sausage and Bologna (Bater *et al.*, 1992; Brewer *et al.*, 1992; Egbert *et al.*, 1991; Trius *et al.*, 1994a). Ledward (1994) suggested that the interactions that occur between the carboxylate groups of anionic polysaccharides (such as alginate and carrageenan) and 'buried' basic groups of proteins exposed following heat denaturation are of significant importance. These interactions can produce more stable complexes than those formed with the native protein molecules. Konjac flour (E425) has also been used successfully in the manufacture of low-fat fresh pork sausages (Osburn and Keeton, 1994), Bologna (Chin *et al.*, 1998) and meatballs (Hsu and Chung, 2000). Numerous starches have also been employed in processed meat manufacture to improve water binding, reduce purge loss and stabilise meat batters (Berry and Wergin, 1993; Carballo *et al.*, 1995; Claus and Hunt, 1991; Khalil, 2000; Lyons *et al.*, 1999; Skrede, 1989). Gums have also been employed in low-fat meat manufacture on their own and in combination with carrageenans and have the ability to modify the mouthfeel and texture of meat products as well as enhance the performance of carrageenans when blended (Foegeding and Ramsey, 1986; Huffman *et al.*, 1991; Mittal and Barbut, 1994).

The use of oat fibre has also been reported to enhance moisture retention in meat products and serve as a natural source of dietary fibre (Hughes *et al.*, 1997). Oat products have achieved a very positive consumer image because of the modest but inverse dose–response relationship between dietary oat fibre and serum cholesterol concentrations (Shinnick *et al.*, 1990). However, oat fibre may also lead to increased product hardness that may be deemed a positive or negative for consumer acceptability depending on the type of product application considered (Steenblock *et al.*, 2001)

14.8 Processing technologies

On a commercial scale, it is easier for processors to employ a dry addition of non-meat ingredients. However, in order to extend the functionality of binders/

extenders, especially non-meat proteins in comminuted meat products, pre-emulsified fat (PEF) prepared with non-meat proteins as a stabiliser have been employed for several years, especially in Europe (Tyutyundzhiev *et al.*, 1979). When PEF is used, more salt-soluble meat proteins are spared for fat and water binding because part of the fat and water is stabilised completely by the non-meat proteins. Thus, utilisation of PEF with proteins (i.e. sodium caseinate, non-fat dry milk, and gelatin) and starch (corn, maize, wheat or pea) as stabilisers in reduced-fat and low-salt frankfurters can extend the water-holding capacity of myofibrillar proteins as well as improving textural properties and yields of final products (Bishop *et al.*, 1993; Lin and Zayas, 1987; Su *et al.*, 2000; Zayas, 1985). Moreover the substitution of saturated fatty acids with more desirable unsaturated fatty acids (Liu *et al.*, 1991a,b) allows for further manipulation of this technique.

The method of ingredient addition during processing as well as the mechanical methods employed in the physical manipulation of lean meat (e.g. chopping/grinding methods) will clearly have a significant influence on the overall quality and consistency of final products produced. Factors such as extraction time, speed of agitation, and ultimate size of meat particles will all influence the rate of salt-soluble protein extractability because of their relevance to membrane disruption and penetration of salt ions into the meat tissue (Keeton, 1994; Lin and Keeton, 1994; Wild *et al.*, 1991). Moreover, the temperature profiles of meat during processing will determine the functional quality of the extracted protein (Ripoche *et al.*, 2001; Sutton *et al.*, 1995).

14.9 Antioxidants

Lipid oxidation of raw meats may be effectively reduced or inhibited by dietary supplementation of vitamin E (Morrissey *et al.*, 1998) or minimising structural damage in raw meat materials (Cross *et al.*, 1987). In terms of processing, the antioxidant effect of spices (i.e. essential oils and extracts), smoke (phenols and related substances), nitrite, ascorbate and other natural compounds cannot be ignored in the manufacture of low- and full-fat meat products as they significantly influence the flavour profiles of processed products (Chevance and Farmer, 1999a). Other additives such as nitrites and phosphates (Igene *et al.*, 1985; Liu *et al.*, 1992), phytic acid (Graf and Panter, 1991; Empson *et al.*, 1991), citric acid or EDTA have been reported to reduce lipid oxidation in meat products. Synthetic antioxidants such as butylated hydroxyanisole (BHA), butylated hydroxytoluene (BHT), tertiary-butylated hydroxyquinone (TBHQ) and propyl gallate have also been reported to be effective antioxidants in meat preparations (Ladikos and Lougovois, 1990; Lai *et al.*, 1991). However, these synthetic additives are less readily accepted or desirable because of safety concerns and negative consumer perception (Addis and Hassel, 1992). Dietary supplementation of animals with vitamin E has also been reported as an effective means of reducing lipid oxidation in final meats (Morrissey *et al.*,

1998). Thus, the level of research on the selection and isolation of natural anti-oxidative ingredients and fractions for use in meat processing have increased (Gray and Crackel, 1992; Guntensperger *et al.*, 1998; Ho *et al.*, 1995; Löliger, 1991; Löliger and Wille, 1993; McCarthy *et al.*, 2001a,b) and is expected to grow for the foreseeable future.

The selection of suitable antioxidants for a given system depends on the compatibility and the effectiveness of the antioxidant, regulatory issues, solubility, dispersibility and the stability of the antioxidant during processing (Giese, 1996). While oxidatively induced off-flavours and discoloration have been extensively studied and the mechanisms are well understood, causes for alterations in physical characteristics of muscle foods due to exposure to oxidising environments have not been clearly identified (Xiong and Decker, 1995; Xiong *et al.*, 1993). Therefore, our current understanding on the role of protein oxidation in meat processing and meat quality is still quite limited (Xiong, 1996). Wan *et al.* (1993) showed a marked improvement in functional properties (e.g. gel-forming ability) of myofibrillar proteins when lipid oxidation was completely inhibited. Although there are similarities between lipid oxidation and protein oxidation (as both involve hydrogen abstraction), protein oxidation clearly differs from lipid oxidation since the most susceptible sites in proteins are usually not the residues containing double bonds (Xiong, 1996).

Controlled oxidative processes can be potentially beneficial in processing of some food products. Studies by Liu and Xiong (1996a,b) and Srinivasan and Xiong (1996) showed that mild oxidative modification of myofibrillar proteins could also facilitate protein gelation. However, most science literature has shown that under oxidative conditions, muscle proteins exhibit deteriorations in functional properties including solubility, gel-forming ability, water-binding capacity and viscosity (Decker *et al.*, 1993; Jarenback and Liljemark, 1975; Kelleher *et al.*, 1994; Smith, 1987; Xiong and Decker 1995). This deterioration in protein functionality and ultimate product quality further highlights the need for care in the selection of effective antioxidant ingredients suitable for the type of product and process being employed, as well as the storage/display conditions being employed.

14.10 Packaging and storage

In processed products, effective packaging and sterilisation techniques greatly enhance storage stability. Exclusion of oxygen, in combination with protection against light and use of lower storage temperatures, are highly effective in controlling lipid oxidation (Gray *et al.*, 1996; Güntensperger and Escher, 1994). Issues relating to the packaging and storage of low-fat meat products are similar to those of traditional full-fat products; however, it is perhaps worth noting that the elevated water content of such reduced fat products naturally affects product colour, purge loss and freeze/thaw stability (Ho *et al.*, 1995). Naturally, the type of laminates employed will influence the overall quality of the final product and its ultimate shelf-life.

Freezing and frozen storage can induce the formation of ice crystals that physically disrupt the meat system, reducing protein functionality. Berry (1993), for example, showed that rapid freezing of low-fat (6%) beef patties at −43 °C compared with −20 °C improved instrumental and sensory tenderness scores of low-fat products. Moreover, this effect is more pronounced as the water content of the low-fat systems and storage times increase (Colmenero, 1996). The application of vacuum packaging to high added water low-fat meat products can also influence product purge levels and stability, and is a factor that should be taken into consideration during processing. Finally, the microbiological status of high added water low-fat meat systems containing added carbohydrates (i.e. sugars, starches and other polysaccharides) should be carefully monitored and suitable preservatives added in order to ensure adequate shelf-life stability of these low-fat meat products.

14.11 Current regulations and labelling guidelines of low-fat products

The development of effective labelling guidelines at an international level is realised through Codex Alimentarius. For instance, in the case of fat levels in food products, it has developed such guidelines for the most commonly used nutrition claims such as 'low', 'rich', 'light', etc. (Table 14.6).

Changes in the regulation of low-fat meat products were introduced by the USDA in 1988. This amendment permitted the substitution of fat with added water (where added water = % moisture − 4 × % protein) provided their total does not exceed 40% and the fat content is no greater than 30% in cooked sausages (Chin *et al.*, 1998; Trius *et al.*, 1994; Yang *et al.*, 2001) as illustrated in Fig. 14.1. However, Claus *et al.* (1989) reported that such changes in product formulation did not necessarily result in a less tender product.

Council Directive 90/496/EEC provides a definition of 'nutrition claim' as follows:

> Any representation and any advertising message which states, suggests or implies that a foodstuff has particular nutrition properties due to the energy (calorific value) it: (1) provides, (2) provides at a reduced or increased rate or (3) does not provide and/or due to the (4) nutrients it contains, (5) contains in reduced or increased proportions or (6) does not contain. A reference to qualities or quantities of a nutrient does not constitute a nutrition claim in so far as it is required by legislation.

Although it is true that the majority of nutrition claims concern nutrients or substances that have a nutritional function, (i.e. protein, carbohydrates, fat, macro-nutrients), there is an increasing number of claims for other alternative substances, such as fibre, antioxidants and lactic bacteria, which do not have a nutritional effect

Table 14.6 Claims and conditions warranting the health-related claims for different nutrients (and other substances)

Claim	Conditions
Low energy	**Codex**: less than 40 kcal/100 g and less than 20 kcal/100 ml **Conditions in use in some EU Member States**: less than 50 kcal/100 g and less than 20 kcal/100 ml
Energy-free/without energy	**Codex**: less than 4 kcal/100 ml
Low fat	**Codex**: no more than 3 g/100 g and 1.5 g/100 ml **Conditions in use in some Member States**: No more than 3 g per 100 g for solids or per 100 ml for liquids.
Fat-free/without fat	**Codex**: no more than 0.15 g per 100 g or 100 ml
Low saturates or saturated fatty acids	**Codex**: no more than 1.5 g per 100 g for solids, 0.75 g/100 ml for liquids **Conditions in use in some Member States**: Level of saturates in the fat at most 25% and polyunsaturates level at least 60%, and the product contains at least 5 g of fat in a reasonable daily consumption level. No more than 1.5 g per 100 g for solids or per 100 ml for liquids and should not make up more than 10% of the total energy of the product.
Saturates or saturated fatty acids-free/without saturates or saturated fatty acids	**Codex**: no more than 0.1 g per 100 g or 100 ml
Low sodium or salt	**Codex**: for low sodium: no more than 0.12 g/100 g; for very low sodium: 0.04 g/100 g **EU**: under Community legislation, low sodium and very low sodium foodstuffs are covered by the Directive on Foods for Particular Nutritional Uses. **Conditions in use in some Member States**: for low sodium: no more than 0.04g sodium per 100 g or 100 ml
Sodium or salt-free/without sodium	**Codex**: no more than 0.005 g/100 g salt

but rather a physiological effect. Some argue therefore that the definition of nutrition claims should be amended to take this fact into account. While the review of current EU Directives on nutritional claims may continue, Table 14.7 outines the key information that is currently required on packaged food products.

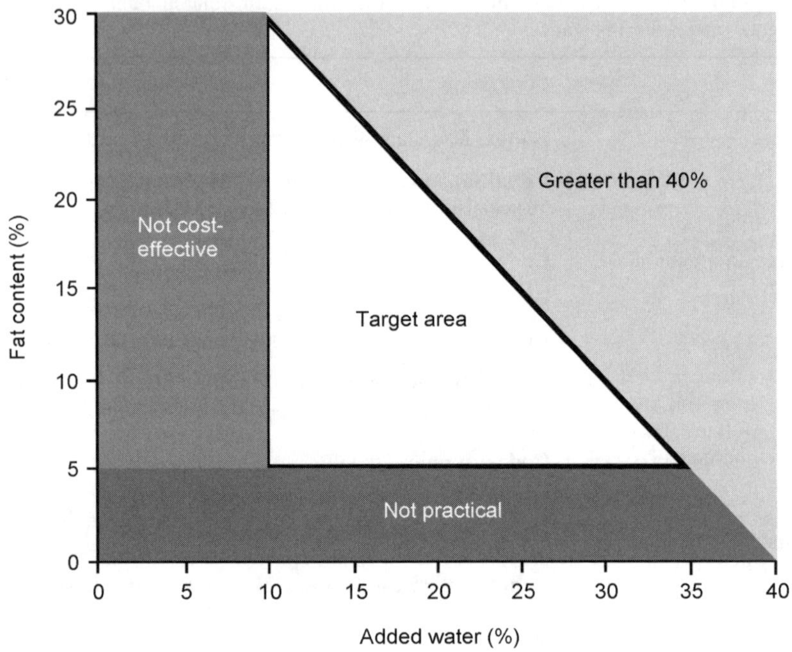

Fig. 14.1 Test area for selecting various combinations of fat and added water that complies with the 40% rule for comminuted meats (Claus, 1991).

EU Council Directive 2000/13/EC provides that the labelling, presentation and advertising of foodstuffs should not mislead the consumer as to the characteristics of the foodstuff, or by attributing to the product effects or properties it does not possess, or by suggesting that the foodstuff possesses special characteristics when in fact all similar products possess such characteristics. Moreover, Directive 2000/13/EC has been amended (Directive 2001/101/EC) to provide a more accurate definition for the term meat used in prepared meat products with other parts of animals suitable for human consumption, such as offal (heart, intestine, liver, etc.) or fat being labelled as such and not as 'meat'. Furthermore, there is provision for a certain part of the fat content, where it adheres to the muscles, to be treated as meat, subject to the maximum limits laid down in the definition.

14.12 Meat culinary issues

As highlighted throughout this chapter, the influence of heat is perhaps the single most important criterion in the successful preparation of a palatable meat product. Application of heat to meat products physically alters the properties of protein, water, fat and other adjuncts and further influences the types of

Table 14.7 Outline of the list of nutritional information for presentation on food products within the EU

	1
Energy	[*x*] kJ and [*x*] kcal
Protein	[*x*] g
Carbohydrate	[*x*] g
of which	
– sugars	[*x*] g
– polyols	[*x*] g
– starch	[*x*] g
Fat	[*x*] g
of which:	
– saturates	[*x*] g
– mono-unsaturates	[*x*] g
– polyunsaturates	[*x*] g
– cholesterol	[*x*] mg
Fibre	[*x*] g
Sodium	[*x*] g
[Vitamins][2]	[*x* units][3]
[Minerals][2]	[*x* units][3]

Notes:
1. [*x*] to be substituted by the appropriate amount.
2. The name(s) to be given as used in the Table of vitamins and minerals.
3. [*x* units] to be substituted by the amount using the units in the Table of vitamins and minerals, and, to give the %RDA.

Where it is required to give additional information relating to any substance which belongs to, or is a component of, one of the items listed, it shall appear as follows:

[item][1]	[*x*] g or mg
of which	
– [substance or component][2]	[*x*] g or mg

Notes:
1. [item] to be the relevant item from the above list.
2. [substance or component] to be the relevant name.

It should be noted that all nutritional values are
a) Calculated per 100 g or 100 ml
b) Listed per quantified serving or portion (if the number of portions in the pack is stated)
c) Calculated for the food as sold, except where detailed preparation instructions are given, they may be the amounts after such preparation (however this must be expressly indicated)
d) Determined as an average (factoring seasonal variation, patterns of consumption, etc.) based on: i) the manufacturer's analysis of the food, ii) a calculation from the actual mean values of the ingredients used in product preparation and/or iii) a calculation from generally established and accepted data.

In calculating energy values, the following conversion factors shall be used:

- 1 g carbohydrate (excluding polyols) = 17 kJ (4 kcal)
- 1 g polyols = 10 kJ (2.4 kcal)
- 1 g protein = 17 kJ (4 kcal)
- 1 g fat = 37 kJ (9 kcal)
- 1 g ethanol = 29 kJ (7 kcal)
- 1 g organic acid = 13 kJ (3 kcal)

chemical interactions that can occur between these ingredients. This series of physicochemical interactions in turn influences the wholesomeness (texture, flavour, juiciness, etc.), safety (microbiological status) and colour (Maillard browning, etc.) of the cooked meat product.

The interaction of lipids and Maillard reactants has been proposed as a possible contributor of meat aroma (and flavour). The pathways by which these interactions take place may include:

- the reaction of carbonyl compounds from lipids with amino groups of cysteine and ammonia produced by Strecker degradation;
- the reaction of amino groups in phosphatidylethanolamine with sugar-derived carbonyl compounds;
- the interaction of free radicals from oxidised lipids in the Maillard reaction;
- the reaction of hydroxy and carbonyl lipid oxidation products with free hydrogen sulphide (Farmer and Mottram, 1990).

While meat cookery is a time and temperature-dependent process (based on pasteurisation requirements), the rate of heating and temperatures employed will naturally have a significant impact on a product's final eating qualities. Berry (1998) reported that meat pH <5.7 was an important consideration in reducing pink colour in final cooked beef patties as is the thawing rate (Bigner-George and Berry, 2001). Addition of extenders/binders may further influence the cooking profiles of low-fat products (Anderson and Berry, 2001; Lin and Berry, 1996).

The type of cooking method (electric broiling, charboiling, roasting, grilling, frying, microwave, hybrid cooking systems, etc.), the target temperature and heating profile (i.e. delta cooking) to be achieved, as well as the desired degree of '*doneness*' are some of the more important factors to consider in thermal processing (Colmenero, 1996).

14.13 Conclusions

The consumer-driven demand for organoleptically acceptable, healthier processed meat products is a challenge to the processor and meat technologists alike. Future developments in genetics, animal breeding and feed programmes, together with a greater understanding of muscle growth and biochemistry, will lead to further improvements not only in meat quality and tenderness, but also in lean meat content of carcasses. Advances in analytical techniques, including the development of novel methodologies will allow for improvements in selection criteria in terms of meat grade, protein functionality and isolation/extraction of meat and fat flavour compounds. Greater understanding of protein chemistry and functionality and their interaction with other ingredients (fat, water, binders/extenders and seasonings/salts) can only lead to improvements in product quality and consistency. It has been shown that effective chemical and physical manipulation of meat will improve its functionality by way of enhanced fat, water and meat-binding properties.

While the addition of high levels of lean meat (and water) to low-fat products may cause undesirable changes in product quality characteristics, such as juiciness and texture, much work is still required to determine the conditions necessary for optimal protein performance within low-fat meat systems. Moreover, the price of low-fat meat products is usually a limiting factor in their manufacture and sale. Addition of nutraceutical type ingredients with health-promoting properties may be a possible marketing tool in order to enhance the sale of fortified, low-fat meat products. Research on the utilisation of novel processing techniques as well as optimisation of traditional processing methodologies for low-fat meat manufacture will be both an exciting and potentially rewarding area in terms of future low-fat meat product development. In conclusion, modification of traditional, as well as development of novel meat product manufacturing techniques and an understanding of the key functionality required in low-fat meat products will ensure a healthy future in low-fat meat manufacture.

14.14 References

ACTON, J.C., and DICK, R.L. (1984) Protein-protein interactions in processed meats. *Annual Reciprocal Meat Conference Proceedings*. **37**: 36–43.

ACTON, J.C., and SAFFLE, R.L. (1972) Emulsfying capacity of muscle protein: phase volumes at emulsion collapse. *Journal of Food Science* **37**: 904–906.

ACTON, J.C., ZEIGLER, C.R., and BURGE, D.L. (1983) Functionality of muscle constituents in the processing of comminuted meat products. *CRC Critical Reviews in Food Science and Nutrition* **18**: 99–121.

ADDIS, P.B., and HASSEL, C.A. (1992) Safety issues with antioxidants in foods. In: *Food Safety Assessment*. Eds Finley, J.W., Robinson, S.F., Armstring, D.J., Washington, DC: American Chemical Soc **484**: 346–376.

AHMED, P.O., MILLER, M.F., LYON, C.E., VAUGHTERS, H.M., and REAGAN, J.O. (1990) Physical and sensory characteristics of low-fat fresh pork sausage processed with various levels of added water. *Journal of Food Science* **55**: 625–628.

AHMED, P.O., MILLER, M.F., YOUNG, L.L., and REAGAN, J.O. (1991) Hot-fat trimming and electrical stimulation effects on beef quality. *Journal of Food Science* **56**: 1484–1488, 1499.

AHN, D.U., WOLFE, F.H., and SIM, J.S. (1995) Dietary alpha-linolenic acid and mixed tocopherols, and packaging influences on lipid stability in broiler chicken breast and leg muscle. *Journal of Food Science* **60**: 1013–1018.

ANDERSON, E.T., and BERRY, B.W. (2001) Sensory, shear, and cooking properties of lower-fat beef patties made with inner pea fiber. *Journal of Food Science* **65**: 805–810.

ANDERSON, P.T. (2000) Mechanisms by which metabolic modifiers alter growth rate and carcass composition of meat animals. *Reciprocal Meat. Conference Proceedings* **52**: 31–36.

ASGHAR, A., SAMEJIMA, K., and YASUI, T. (1985). Functionality of muscle proteins in gelation mechanisms of structured meat products. *CRC Critical Reviews in Food Science and Nutrition*, **22**, 27–106.

BAARDSETH, P., NAES, T., MIELNIK, J., SKREDE, G., HOLLAND, S., and EIDE, O. (1992) Dairy ingredients effects on sausage sensory properties studied by principle component analysis. *Journal of Food Science* **57**: 822–828.

BATER, B., DESCAMPS, O., and MAURER, A.J. (1992) Quality characteristics of hydrocolloid-added oven-roasted turkey breasts. *Journal of Food Science* **57**: 1068–1070.

BENDER, A.K. (1998) The effect of heat on protein-rich foods. In: *Food Quality and Nutrition*. ed. W.K Downey. Applied Science Publishers, 411–426.

BERG, H., MAGARD, M., JOHANSSON, G., and MATHIASSON, L. (1997) Development of a supercritical fluid extraction method for determination of lipid classes and total fat in meats and its comparison with conventional methods. *Journal of Chromatography A* **785**: 345–352.

BERRY, B.W. (1993) Fat level and freezing temperature affect sensory, shear, cooking and compositional properties of ground beef patties. *Journal of Food Science* **58**: 34–37, 42.

BERRY, B.W. (1997) Effects of formulation and cooking method on properties of low-fat beef patties. *Journal of Foodservice Systems*. **9**: 211–228.

BERRY, B.W. (1998) Cooked colour in high pH beef patties as influenced by fat content and cooking from the frozen or thawed state. *Journal of Food Science* **63:** 797–800.

BERRY, B.W., and WERGIN, W.P. (1993) Modified pre-gelatinized starch in low-fat ground beef patties. *Journal of Muscle Foods* **4**: 305–320.

BIGNER-GEORGE, M.E., and BERRY, B.W. (2001) Thawing prior to cooking affects sensory, shear force, and cooking properties of beef patties. *Journal of Food Science* **65**: 2–8.

BISHOP, D.J., OLSON, D.G., and KNIPE, C.L. (1993) Pre-emulsified corn oil pork fat or added water affect quality of reduced fat Bologna quality. *Journal of Food Science* **58**: 484–487.

BLOUKAS, J.G., PANERAS, E.D., and PAPADIMA, S. (1997) Effect of carrageenan on processing and quality characteristics of low-fat frankfurters. *Journal of Muscle Foods* **8**: 63–83.

BREKKE, C.J. and EISELS, T.A. (1981) The role of modified proteins in the processing of muscle foods. *Food Technology* **35** (5): 231–234.

BREWER, M.S., MCKEITH, F.K., and BRITT, K. (1992) Fat, soy and carrageenan effects on sensory and physical characteristics of ground beef patties. *Journal of Food Science* **57**: 1051–1052, 1055.

BROADHURST, C.L. and WINTHER, M. (2000) Evening primrose oil: Pharmacological and clinical applications. In: *Herbs, Botanicals and Teas as Functional Foods and Nutraceuticals*. eds Mazza G. and Oomah B.D., Technomic Pub. Co., Inc., Lancaster, PA, 265–291.

BULLOCK, K.L., HUFFMAN, D.L., EGBERT, W.R., BRADFORD, D.D., MIKEL, W.B., and JONES, W.R. (1995) Non-meat ingredients for low-fat ground beef patties. *Journal of Muscle Foods* **6**: 37–46.

CAMBERO, M.I., SEUSS, I., and HONIKEL, K.O. (1992) Flavour compounds of beef broth as affected by cooking temperature. *Journal of Food Science* **57**: 1285–1290, 1239.

CANADIAN PAEDIATRIC SOCIETY (CPS) (1994) *Nutrition Recommendations Update: Dietary Fat and Children*. Report of the Joint Working Group of the Canadian Paediatric Society (CPS) and Health Canada Reference No. N94-01.

CARBALLO, J., CAVESTANY, M., and COLMENERO, F.J. (1992) Rheological changes during thermal gelation of meat batters containing surimi from Alaska pollack (*Theragra chalcogramma*) or sardine (*Sardinia pilchardus*). *Journal of the Science of Food and Agriculture* **59**, 117–122.

CARBALLO, J., BARRETO, G., and JIMENEZ COLMENERO, F. (1995) Starch and egg white influence on properties of Bologna sausage as related to fat content. *Journal of Food Science* **60** 673–677.

CARPENTER, J.A., and SAFFLE, R.L. (1964) A simple method of estimating the emulsifying capacity of various sausage meats. *Journal of Food Science* **29**: 774–781.

CAVESTANY, M., JIMÉNEZ COLMENERO, F., SOLAS, M.T., and CARBALLO, J. (1994) Incorporation of sardine surimi to bologna sausage containing different fat levels. *Meat Science* **38:** 27–37.

CHAO, R.R., MULVANEY, S.J., BAILEY, M.E., and FERNANDO, L.N. (1991) Supercritical CO_2 conditions affecting extraction of lipid and cholesterol from ground beef. *Journal of Food Science* 56: 183–187.

CHEN, C.M., and TROUT, G.R. (1991) Sensory, instrumental texture profile and cooking properties of restructured beef steaks made with various binders. *Journal of Food Science* **56**: 1457–1460.

CHEVANCE, F.F.V., and FARMER, L.J. (1999a) Identification of major volatile odour compounds in Frankfurters. *Journal of Agricultural Food Chemistry* **47**: 5151–5160.

CHEVANCE, F.F.V., and FARMER, L.J. (1999b) Release of volatile odour compounds from full-fat and reduced fat Frankfurters. *Journal of Agricultural Food Chemistry* **47**: 5161–5168.

CHEVANCE, F.F.V., FARMER, L.J., DESMOND, E.M., NOVELLI, E., TROY, D.J., and CHIZZOLINI, R. (2000) Effect of some fat replacers on the release of volatile aroma compounds from low-fat meat products. *Journal of Agricultural Food Chemistry* **48**: 3476–3484.

CHIN, K.B., KEETON, J.T., LONGNECKER, M.T., and LAMKEY, J.W. (1998) Functional, textural and microstructural properties of low-fat bologna (model system) with a konjac blend. *Journal of Food Science* **63**: 801–807.

CHIN, K.B., KEETON, J.T., MILLER, R.K., LONGNECKER, M.T, and LAMKEY J.W. (2000) Evaluation of konjac blends and soy protein isolate as fat replacements in low-fat bologna. *Journal of Food Science* **65**: 756–763.

CLAUS, J.R. (1991) Fat reduction in comminuted meat systems. *Reciprocal Meat Conference Proceedings* **44**: 93–99.

CLAUS, J.R., and HUNT, M.C. (1991) Low-fat, high added-water bologna formulated with texture-modifying ingredients. *Journal of Food Science* **56**: 643–647, 652.

CLAUS, J.R., HUNT, M.C., and KASTNER, C.L. (1989) Effects of substituting added water for fat on the textural, sensory and processing characteristics of Bologna. *Journal of Muscle Foods* **1**: 1–21.

CLAUS, J.R., HUNT, M.C., KASTNER, C.L., and KROPF, D.H. (1990) Low-fat high added water bologna: effects of massaging, pre-blending and time of addition of water and fat on physical and sensory characteristics. *Journal of Food Science* **55**: 338–341, 345.

COLMENERO, F.J. (1996) Technologies for developing low-fat meat products. *Trends in Food Science and Technology* **7**: 41–48.

COLMENERO, F.J., CARBALLO, J., and COFRADES, S. (2001) Healthier meat products: their role as functional foods. *Meat Science* **59**: 5–13.

Council Directive 2000/13/EC of the European Parliament and of the Council relating to the labelling, presentation and advertising of foodstuffs, *OJ* L 109 p.29 of 6.5.2000.

Council Directive 90/496/EEC on nutrition labelling of foodstuffs, *OJ* L 276p. 40 of 6.10.1990.

CROSS, H.R., LEU, R., and MILLER, M.F. (1987) Scope of warmed-over flavour and its importance to the meat industry. In: *Warmed-over Flavour of Meat*. Academic Press, London, pp. 1–17.

DECKER, E. A., CRUM, A.D., SHANTHA, N.C., and MORRISSEY, P.A. (1993) Catalysis of lipid oxidation by iron from an insoluble fraction of deep diaphragm muscle. *Journal of Food Science*, **58**: 233–236, 238.

DE ROOS, K.B. (1997) How lipids influence food flavor. *Food Technology* **51**: 60–62.

DE ROOS, K.B., and WOLSWINKEL, K. (1993) Non-equilibrium partition model for predicting flavour release in the mouth. *Trends in Flavour Research: Proceedings of the 7th Weurman Flavour Research Symposium, Noordwijkerhout*. Elsevier Science Publishers, Amsterdam, 15–32.

DEXTER, D.R., SOFOS, J.N., and SCHMIDT, G.R. (1993) Quality characteristics of turkey bologna formulated with carrageenan, starch milk protein and soya protein. *Journal of Muscle Foods* **4**: 207–223.

DIKEMAN, M.E. (2000) Effects of metabolic modifiers used in animal production on meat quality. *Reciprocal Meat. Conference Proceedings* **52**: 36–62.

DILL, C.W., and LANDMANN, W.A. (1988) Food grade proteins from edible blood. In: *Edible Meat By-Products*. eds Pearson, A.M. and Dutson, T.R. Elsevier Applied Science, London, 127–145.

DINARDO, K., MULLICH, J., and MELVILLE, N.A. (2004) Obesity a popular issue in technical program review. *Food Technology* **58**: 50–65.

DIXON, L.B., CRONIN, F.J., and KREBS-SMITH, S.M. (2001). Let the pyramid guide your food choices: capturing the total diet concept. *Journal of Nutrition* **131**: 461–472.

DREWNOWSKI, A. (1990) Diet and health: a commentary on current dietary recommendations and their use in public health. *For a Better Nutrition in the 21st Century: Proceedings of the 27th Nestle Nutrition Workshop*, Lausanne.

DREWNOWSKI, A. (1997) Why do we like fat? *Journal of the American Dietetic-Association*, S58–S62.

DREWNOWSKI, A., and SCHWARTZ, M. (1990) Invisible fats: sensory assessment of sugar/fat mixtures. *Appetite* **14**: 203–217.

DUNFORD, N.T. (2001) Health benefits and processing of lipid-based nutritionals. *Food Technology* **55**: 38–44.

EGBERT, W.R., HUFFMAN, D.L., CHEN, C., and DYLEWSKI, D.P. (1991) Development of low-fat ground beef. *Food Technology* **45**: 64–73.

EILERT, S.J., BLACKMER, D.S., MANDIGO, R.W., and CALKINS, C.R. (1993) Meat batters with modified beef connective tissue. *Journal of Food Science* **58**, 691–696.

EILERT, S.J., MANDIGO, R.W., and SUMNER, S.S. (1996) Phosphate and modified beef connective tissue effects on reduced fat, high water-added frankfurters. *Journal of Food Science* **61**: 1006–1011, 1029.

EMPSON, K.L., LABUZA, T.P., and GRAF, E. (1991) Phytic acid as a food antioxidant. *Journal of Food Science* **56**: 560–563.

FARMER, L.J., and MOTTRAM, D.S. (1990) Interaction of lipid in the Maillard reaction between cysteine and ribose: the effect of a triglyceride and three phospholipids on the volatile products. *Journal of the Science of Food and Agriculture* **53**: 505–525.

FERRY, J.D. (1948) Protein gels. *Advances in Protein Chemistry* **4**: 1–78.

FOEGEDING, E.A., and RAMSEY, S.R. (1986) Effect of gums on low-fat meat batters. *Journal of Food Science* **51**: 33–36, 46.

GERRARD, D.E., GAO, X., and TAN, J. (1996) Beef marbling and colour score determination by image processing. *Journal of Food Science* **61**: 145–148.

GIESE, J. (1996). Antioxidants: tools for preventing lipid oxidation. *Food Technology* **50**: 73–81.

GOLDBERG, I. (1994) Introduction. In: *Functional Foods: Designer foods, Pharmafoods, Nutraceuticals*. ed. Goldberg, I. Chapman and Hall, Inc., New York, 3–19.

GORDON, A., and BARBUT, S. (1990). The microstructure of raw meat batters prepared with monovalent and divalent chloride salts. *Food Structure*, **9**: 279–295.

GORDON, A., and BARBUT, S. (1992a) Mechanisms of meat batter stabilisation: a review. *CRC Critical Reviews in Food Science and Nutrition*, **32**: 299–332.

GORDON, A., and BARBUT, S. (1992b) Effect of chemical modification on the stability, texture and microstructure of cooked meat batters microstructure. *Food Structure*, **11**, 133–146.

GRAF, E., and PANTER, S.S. (1991) Inhibition of warmed-over flavour development by polyvalent cations. *Journal of Food Science* **56**: 1055–1058, 1067.

GRAY, J.I., and CRACKEL, R.L. (1992) Oxidative flavour changes in meat: their origin and prevention. In: *The Chemistry of Muscle-Based Foods*. eds Johnston, D.E., Knight, M.K., and Ledward, D.E. The Royal Society of Chemistry, Cambridge, 145–168.

GRAY, J.I., and PEARSON, A.M. (1987) Rancidity and warmed-over flavor. In: *Re-structured Meat and Poultry Products, Advances in Meat Research*, Vol. 3, Ch. 6. eds A.M. Pearson and T.R. Dutson. Van Nostrand Reinhold, New York, 221–269.

GRAY, J.I., GOMMA, E.A., and BUCKLEY, D.J. (1996) Oxidative quality and shelf life of meats. *Meat Science* **43**: S111–S124.

GREGG, L.L., CLAUS, J.R., HACKNEY, C.R., and MARRIOT, N.G. (1993) Low-fat, high added water bologna from massaged, minced batter. *Journal of Food Science* 58: 259–264.

GüNTENSPERGER, B., and ESCHER, F.E. (1994) Oxidative changes of heat-sterilized meat in trays. *Journal of Food Science* **59**: 689–692.

GUNTENSPERGER, B., HAMMERLI-MEIER, D.E., and ESCHER, F.E. (1998) Rosemary extract and precooking effects on lipid oxidation in heat-sterilized meat *Journal of Food Science* **63:** 955–957.

GUZMAN, J.C., MCMILLAN, K.W., BIDNER, T.D., DUGAS-SIMS, S., and GODBER, J.S. (1995) Texture colour and sensory characteristics of ground beef patties containing bovine blood plasma. *Journal of Food Science* **60**: 657–660.

HA, J.K., and LINDSAY, R.C. (1991) Volatile alkylphenols and thiophenol in species-related characterizing flavours of red meats. *Journal of Food Science* **56**: 1197–1202.

HA, Y.L., GRIMM, N.K., and PARIZA, W.M. (1989) Newly recognized anticarcinogenic fatty acids: Identification and quantification in natural and processed cheeses. *Journal of Agriculture and Food Chemistry* **37**: 75–81.

HALE, D.S. (1994) Grading. In: *Muscle Foods*. eds D.M. Kinsman, Kotula, A.W and Breidenstein. Chapman and Hall, London, 186–223.

HANIN, I. (1979) Commercially available 'lecithin': Proposed guidelines for nomenclature and methodology. In: *Nutrition and Brain.* Eds Barbeau A., Growdon J.H., and Wurthman R.J., Vol.5, Raven Press, New York, 443–445.

HATCHWELL, L.C. (1994) Implications of fat on flavour. In: *Flavour-Food Interactions: Proceedings of a Symposium, Washington DC, August 1994*. ACS, Washington, DC, 14–23.

HERMANSSON, A.-M. (1978) Physico-chemical aspects of soy proteins structure formation. *Journal of Texture Studies*, **9**: 33–58.

HO, C.P., HUFFMAN, D.L., BRADFORD, D.D., EGBERT, W.R., MIKEL, W.B., and JONES, W.R. (1995) Storage stability of vacuum packaged frozen pork sausage containing soy protein concentrate, carrageenan or antioxidants. *Journal of Food Science* **60**: 257–261.

HSU, S.Y., and CHUNG, H.Y. (2000) Interactions of konjac, agar, curdlan gum, kappa-carrageenan and reheating treatment in emulsified meatballs. *Journal of Food Engineering* **44:** 199–204.

HU, F.B., RIMM, E., SMITH-WARNER, S.A., FESKANICH, D., STAMPFER, M.J., ASCHERIO, A., SAMPSON, L., and WILLETT, W.C. (1999) Reproducibility and validity of dietary patterns assessed with a food-frequency questionnaire. *American Journal of Clinical Nutrition* **69**: 243–249.

HU, F.B, RIMM, E.B, STAMPFER, M.J., ASCHERIO, A., SPIEGELMAN, D., and WILLETT, W.C. (2000) Prospective study of major dietary patterns and risk of coronary heart disease in men. *American Journal of Clinical Nutrition* **72**: 912–921.

HUFFMAN, D.L., EGBERT, R.W., CHEN, C.-M., and DYLEWSKI, D.P. (1991) Technology of low-fat ground beef. *Reciprocal Meat Conference Proceedings* **44:** 73–79.

HUGHES, E., COFRADES, S., and TROY, D.J. (1997) Effects of fat level, oat fibre and carrageenan on Frankfurters formulated with 5, 12 and 30% fat. *Meat Science* **45**: 273–281.

IGENE, J.O., YAMAUCHI, K., PEARSON, A.M., and GRAY, J.I. (1985) Mechanisms by which nitrite inhibits the development of warmed-over-flavour (WOF) in cured meat. *Food Chemistry* **18**: 1–18.

INGHAM, K.E., TAYLOR, A.J., CHEVANCE, F.F.V., and FARMER, L.J. (1996) Effect of fat content on volatile release from foods. In: *Flavour Science Recent Developments*. eds A.J. Taylor and Mottram, D.S. Proceedings of the Eighth Weurman Flavour Research Symposium. Royal Society of Chemistry Cambridge, 386–391.

JARENBACK, L., and LILJEMARK, A. (1975). Ultrastructural changes during frozen storage of cod III. Effects of linoleic acid and linoleic acid hydroperoxides on myofibrillar proteins. *Journal of Food Technology*, **10**: 437–452.

JOHNSTON, P.V. (1995) Flaxseed oil and cancer: a-Linolenic acid and carcinogenesis. In: *Flaxseed in Human Nutrition*. Eds Cunnane, S.C. and Thompson L.U., AOCS Press, Champaign, Ill. pp. 207–218.

KANNER, J. (1994) Oxidative processes in meat and meat products: quality implications. *Meat-Science* **36**: 169–189.

KATSANIDIS, E., MEYER, D.C., EPLEY, R.J., ADDIS P.B., and RUAN R. (2001) Solubilized cellulose and dehydrated potato extract in cooked, low-fat comminuted beef. *Journal of Food Science* **66**: 758–761.

KEETON, J.T. (1991) Fat substitutes and fat modification in processing. *Reciprocal Meat Conference Proceedings* **44**: 79–91.

KEETON, J.T. (1994) Low-fat meat products – technological problems with processing. *Meat Science* **36**: 261–276.

KEETON, J.T. (1996) Non-meat ingredients for low/non-fat processed meats. *Reciprocal Meat Conference*, **49**: 23–31.

KELLEHER, S.D., HULTIN, H.O., and WILHELM, K.A. (1994). Stability of mackerel surimi prepared under lipid-stabilizing processing conditions. *Journal of Food Science*, **59**: 269–271.

KENNEY, P.B., HENDRICKSON, R.O., CLAYPOOL, P.L., and RAO, B.R. (1986) Influence of temperature, time and solvent on the solubility of corium collagen and meat proteins. *Journal of Food Science* **51**: 227–280, 287.

KHALIL, A.H. (2000) Quality characteristics of low-fat beef patties formulated with modified corn starch and water. *Food Chemistry* **68**: 61–68.

KING, J.W., JOHNSON, J.H., and FRIEDRICH, J.P. (1989) Extraction of fat tissue from meat products with supercritical carbon dioxide. *Journal of Agricultural and Food Chemistry* **37**: 951–954.

KING, M., HAMILTON, B.L., MATTHEWS, M.A., RULE, D.C., and FIELD, R.A. (1993) Isolation and identification of volatiles and condensable material in raw beef with supercritical carbon dioxide extraction. *Journal of Agricultural and Food Chemistry* **41**: 1974–1981.

KING, J.W., ELLER, F.J., SNYDER, J.M., JOHNSON, J.H., MCKEITH, F.K., and STITES, C.R. (1996) Extraction of fat from ground beef for nutrient analysis using analytical supercritical fluid extraction. *Journal of Agricultural and Food Chemistry* **44**: 2700–2704.

KINSELLA, J.E. (1981) Relationship between structure and functional properties of food proteins. In: *Food Proteins* Ch. 3. Eds P.F. Fox and J.J. Condon. Applied Science Publisher, New York, 51–103.

KUSHI, L.H., LENART, E.B., and WILLETT W.C. (1995) Health implications of Mediterranean diets in light of contemporary knowledge. 2. Meat, wine, fats, and oils. *Am J Clin Nutr* **61**: 1416–1427.

LABUDDE, R.A., and LANIER, T.C. (1995) Protein functionality and development of bind values. *Annual Reciprocal Meat Conference Proceedings*, **48**: 59–68.

LADIKOS, D., and LOUGOVOIS, V. (1990) Lipid oxidation in muscle foods: a review. *Food Chemistry* **35**: 295–314.

LAI, S.M., GRAY, J.I., SMITH, D.M., BOOREN, A.M., CRACKEL, R.L., and BUCKLEY, D.J. (1991) Effects of oleoresin rosemary, tertiary butylhydroquinone and sodium tripolyphosphate on the development of oxidative rancidity in restructured chicken nuggets. *Journal of Food Science*; **56**: 616–620.

LANDLY, P., COURTHAUDON, J.L., DUBOIS, C., and VOILLEY, A. (1996) Effect of interface in model food emulsions on the volatility of aroma compounds. *Journal of Agricultural Food Chemistry* **44**: 526–530.

LAW, M. (2000). Dietary fat and adult diseases and the implications for childhood nutrition: an epidemiologic approach. *American Journal of Clinical Nutrition* **72**: 1291–1296.

LEDWARD, D.A. (1994) Protein-polysaccharide Interactions. In: *Protein Functionality in Food Systems*. Eds Hettiarachchy, N.S. and Ziegler, G.R., Marcel Dekker, New York, 225–259.

LEE, C.M. (1987) Surimi manufacturing and fabrication of surimi based products. *Food Technology* **40**: 115–124.

LEE, C.M., WU, M.C., and OKADA, M. (1992) Ingredient and formulation technology for surimi-based products. In: *Surimi Technology*. Eds Lanier, T.C. and Lee, C.M., Marcel Dekker, New York, 273–302.

LIN, C.S., and ZAYAS, J.F. (1987) Microstructural comparison of meat emulsions prepared with corn protein emulsified and unemulsified fat. *Journal of Food Science* **52**: 267–271.

LIN, K.W., and KEETON, J.T. (1994) Determination of optimum particle size for low-fat precooked ground beef patties. *Journal of Muscle Foods* **5**: 63–76.

LIN, K.W., and MEI, M.Y. (2000) Influences of gums, soy protein isolate, and heating temperatures on reduced-fat meat batters in a model system. *Journal of Food Science* **65**: 48–52.

LIN, T.Y., WANG, Y.J., LAI, P.Y., LEE, F.J., and CHENG, J.T.S. (1999) Cholesterol content of fried-shredded pork extracted by supercritical carbon dioxide. *Food Chem* **67**: 89–92.

LIU, G., and XIONG, Y.L. (1996a). Contribution of lipid and protein oxidation to rheological differences between chicken white and red muscle myofibrillar proteins. *Journal of Agricultural and Food Chemistry* **44**: 779–784.

LIU, G., and XIONG, Y.L. (1996b). Storage stability of antioxidant-washed myofibrils from chicken white and red muscle. *Journal of Food Science*, **61**: 890–894.

LIU, H.F., BOOREN, A.M., GRAY, J.I., and CRACKEL, R.L. (1992) Antioxidant efficacy of oleoresin rosemary and sodium tripolyphosphate in restructured pork steaks. *Journal of Food Science* **57**: 803–806.

LIU, M.N., and BERRY, B.W. (1996) Variability in colour, cooking times, and internal temperature of beef patties under controlled cooking conditions. *Journal of Food Protection* **59**: 969–975.

LIU, M.N., HUFFMAN, D.L., EGBERT, W.R., McCASKEY, T.A., and LIU, C.W. (1991a) Soy protein and oil effects on chemical, physical and microbial stability of lean ground beef patties. Journal of Food Science; **56**: 906–912.

LIU, M.N., HUFFMAN, D.L., and EGBERT, W.R. (1991b) Replacement of beef fat with partially hydrogenated plant oil in lean ground beef patties. *Journal of Food Science* **56**: 861–862.

LÖLIGER, J. (1991) Natural antioxidants. *Lipid Technology* **3**: 58–61.

LÖLIGER, J., and WILLE, H.J. (1993) Natural antioxidants. *Oils and Fats International* **9**: 18, 20–22.

LYONS, P.H., KERRY, J.F., MORRISSEY, P.A., and BUCKLEY, D.J. (1999) The influence of added whey protein/carrageenan gels and tapioca starch on the textural properties of low fat pork sausages. *Meat Science* **51:** 43–52.

MANN, J., SKEAFF, M., TRUSWELL, S., HU, F.B., SACKS, F., WILLETT, W.C., HOOPER, L., SUMMERBELL, C.D., THOMPSON, R.L., CAPPS, N.E., SMITH, G.D., RIEMERSMA, R.A., and EBRAHIM, S. (2001) Dietary fats and prevention of cardiovascular disease. *British Medical Journal* **323**: 1000.

MARSHALL, R.J. (1990) Combined instrumental and sensory measurement of the role of fat in food texture. *Food Quality and Preference* **2**: 117–124.

MARSHALL, T., KENNEDY, E., and OFFUTT, S. (2000). Exploring a fiscal food policy: the case of diet and ischaemic heart disease. Commentary: Alternative nutrition outcomes using a fiscal food policy. *British Medical Journal* **320**: 301–305.

MARURI, J.L., and LARICK, D.K. (1992) Volatile concentration and flavour of beef as influenced by diet. *Journal of Food Science* **57**: 1275–1281.

MATULIS, R.J., McKEITH, F.K., SUTHERLAND, J.W., and BREWER, M.S. (1995a) Sensory characteristics of frankfurters as affected by fat, salt, and pH. *Journal of Food Science* **60**: 28–47.

MATULIS, R.J., McKEITH, F.K., SUTHERLAND, J.W., and BREWER, M.S. (1995b) Sensory characteristics of frankfurters as affected by salt, fat, soy protein, and carrageenan. *Journal of Food Science* **60**: 48–54.

McCANCE, R.A., and WIDDOWSON, E.M. (1991) Meat and meat products. In: *The Composition of Foods*, 5th edition. RSC, Letchworth, 123–187.

McCARTHY, T.L., KERRY, J.P., KERRY, J.F., LYNCH, P.B., and BUCKLEY, D.J. (2001a) Assessment of the antioxidant potential of natural food and plant extracts in fresh and previously frozen pork patties. *Meat Science* **57**: 177–184.

McCARTHY, T.L., KERRY, J.P., KERRY, J.F., LYNCH, P.B., and BUCKLEY, D.J. (2001b) Evaluation of the antioxidant potential of natural food/plant extracts as compared with synthetic antioxidants and vitamin E in raw and cooked pork patties. *Meat Science* **57**: 45–52.

McDONALD, T., and CHEN, Y.R. (1991) Visual characterization of marbling in beef ribeyes and its relationship to taste parameters. *Transactions of the ASAE* **34**(6): 2499–2504.

McDONALD, T., and CHEN, Y.R. (1992) A geometric model of marbling in beef longissimus dorsi. *Transactions of the ASAE* **35**: 1057–1062.

McDONALD, B.E., and FITZPATRICK, K. (1998) Designer vegetable oils. In: *Functional Foods, Biochemical and Processing Aspects*, ed. Mazza G., Technomic Pub. Co. Inc., Lancaster, PA. pp. 265–291.

McMILLIN, K.W., BIDNER, T.D., FELCHLE, S.E., DUGAS, S.M., and KOH, K.C. (1991) Flavour and oxidative stability of ground beef patties as affected by source and storage. *Journal of Food Science* **56**: 899–902.

MELA, D.J. (1988) Sensory assessment of fat content in fluid dairy products. *Appetite* **10**: 37–44.

MELA, D.J., and MARSHALL, R.J. (1992) Sensory properties and perceptions of fats. In: *Dietary Fats: Determinants of Preference, Selection and Consumption*. Elsevier Applied Science Publishers, London, 43–57.

MELTON, S.L. (1990). Effects of feeds on flavour of red meat: a review. *Journal of Animal Science* **68**: 4421–4435.

MITTAL, G.S., and BARBUT, S. (1994) Effects of carrageenans and xanthan gum on the texture and acceptability of low fat frankfurters. *Journal of Food Processing Preservation* **18**(3): 201–216.

MOLONEY, A. (1999) The quality of meat from beef cattle: Is it influenced by diet? *R&H Hall Technical Bulletin* Issue no. 4.

MORRISSEY, P.A., MULVIHILL, D.M., and O'NEILL, E. (1987). Functional properties of muscle proteins. In: *Developments in Food Proteins – 5*. ed. B.J.F. Hudson. Elsevier Applied Science Publishing, London, 195–257.

MORRISSEY, P.A., SHEEHY, P.J., GALVIN, K., KERRY, J.P., and BUCKLEY, D.J. (1998) Lipid stability in meat and meat products. *Meat Science* **49**: S73–S86.

MOTTRAM, D.S., and EDWARDS, R.A. (1984) The role of triglycerides and phospholipids in the aroma of cooked beef. *Journal of the Science of Food and Agriculture* **34**: 517–522.

NAKAMURA, Y., TONOGAI, Y., TSUMARA, Y., SHIBATA, T., and UCHIYAMA, M. (1997) Effect of dietary squalene on the fecal steroid excretions and the lipid levels of serum and the liver in the rat. *Nutr. Res.* **17**: 243–257.

NATIONAL TASKFORCE ON OBESITY (2005) *The Policy Challenges Obesity*. The Report of the National Taskforce On Obesity, Ireland, 1–132.

NICOLASI, R.J., ROGER, E.J., AUSMAN, L.M., and ORTHOEFER, F.T. (1992) Rice bran oil and its health benefits. In: *Rice Science and Technology*. eds Marshall W.E. and Wadsworth J.I., Marcel Dekker, New York, 421–437.

OCKERMAN, H.W., and CHAO, W.H. (1996) Fat replacer in meat: a review. *Meat Focus International* **5**: 453–455.

OOMAH, B.D., and MAZZA, G. (1999) Health benefits of phytochemicals from selected Canadian crops. *Trends Food Sci. Technol.* **10**: 193–198.

OSBURN, W.N., and KEETON, J.T. (1994) Konjac flour gel as fat substitute in low-fat *prerigor* fresh pork sausage. *Journal of Food Science* **59**: 484–489.

OSBURN, W.N., and MANDIGO, R.W. (1997) Pork skin connective tissue gel utilisation in reduced-fat bologna. *Journal of Food Science* **62**, 1176–11829.

OVERBOSCH, P., AFTEROF, W.G.M., and HARING, P.G.M. (1991) Flavour release in the mouth. *Food Review International* **7**: 137–184.

PANERAS, E.D., BLOUKAS, J.G., and PAPADIMA, S.N. (1996) Effect of meat source and fat level on processing and quality characteristics of frankfurters. *Lebensmittel-Wissenschaft und Technologie* **29**: 507–514.

PANIANGVAIT, P., KING, A.J., JONES, A.D., and GERMAN, B.G. (1995) Cholesterol oxides in foods of animal origin. *Journal of Food Science* **60**: 1159–1174.

PARK, J., RHEE, K.S., KEETON, J.T., and RHEE, K.C. (1989) Properties of low-fat frankfurters containing monounsaturated and omega-3 polyunsaturated oils. *Journal of Food Science* **54**: 500–504.

PARK, J., RHEE, K.S., and ZIPRIN, Y.A. (1990) Low-fat frankfurters with elevated levels of water and oleic acid. *Journal of Food Science* **55**: 871–872, 874.

PARKS, L.L., CARPENTER, J.A., RAO, V.N.M., and REGAN, J.O. (1985) Prediction of bind value constants of sausage ingredients from protein or moisture content. *Journal of Food Science* **50**, 1564–1567.

PEARSON, A.M., and GRAY, J.I. (1983) Mechanism responsible for warmed-over flavor in cooked meat. In: *The Maillard Reaction in Foods and Nutrition*. eds G.R. Waller and M.S. Feather, Symp. Ser. 215. Am. Chem. Soc., Washington, DC, 287–300.

PEARSON, A.M., LOVE, J.D., and SHORLAND, F.B. (1977) Warmed-over flavor in meat, poultry and fish. *Advances in Food Research* **23**: 1–74.

REISER, R., and SHORLAND, F.B. (1990) Meat fats and fatty acids. In: *Meat and Health: advances in meat research*, Vol. 6. eds A.M. Pearson and T.R. Dutson, Elsevier Science, New York, 21–62.

RIPOCHE, A., LE GUERN, L., MARTIN, J.L., TAYLOR, R.G., and VENDEUVRE J.L. (2001) Sausage structure analysis. *Journal of Food Science* 66: 670–674.

RIZVI, S.H., DANIELS, J.A., BENADO, A.L., and ZOLLWEG, J.A. (1986) Supercritical fluid extraction: operating principles and food applications. *Food Technology* **40**: 57–64.

ROMANS, J.R., COSTELLO, W.J., CARLSON, C.W., GREASER, M.L., and JONES, K.W. (1994) *The Meat We Eat*. Interstate Publisher Inc., Danville, IL.

ROZZI, N.L., and SINGH, R.K. (2002) Supercritical fluids and the food industry Dept. of Food Science and Technology. *Comprehensive Reviews in Food Science and Food Safety* **1**: 33–44.

RUST, R., and OLSEN, D. (1988) Making good 'lite' sausage. *Meat and Poultry* **34**: 10.

SAFFLE, R.L. (1968) Meat emulsions. *Advances in Food Research* **16**, 105–160.

SAFFLE, R.L., and GALBREATH, J.W. (1964) Quantitative determination of salt-soluble meat protein in various types of meat. *Food Technology* **18**: 1943–1944.

SAWYER, R. (1975) 'The composition of meat: analytical aspects'. In: *Meat*. eds D.J.A Cole and R.A Lawrie, Butterworths, London, 287–301.

SCHAEFER, E.J. (2002) Lipoproteins, nutrition, and heart disease. *American Journal of Clinical Nutrition* **75**: 191–212.

SCHMIDT, R.H. (1981) Gelation and coagulation. In: *Protein Functionality in Foods*. ed. J.P. Cherry, ACS Symposium Series No. 147, American Chemical Society, Washington, DC, 131–147.

SEIDELL, J.C. (1999) The burden of obesity and its sequelae. *Disease Management & Health Outcomes* **5**: 13–21.

SHAND, P.J. (2000) Textural, water holding, and sensory properties of low-fat pork bologna with normal or waxy starch hullless barley. *Journal of Food Science* **65**: 101–109.

SHAND, P.J., and SCHMIDT, G.R. (1990) New technology for low-fat meat products. *Reciprocal Meat Conference Proceedings* **43**: 37–52.

SHEARD, P.R., WOOD, J.D., NUTE, G.R., and BALL, R.C. (1998) Effects of grilling to 80 °C on the chemical composition of pork lion chops and some observations on the UK National Food Survey estimate of fat consumption. *Meat Science* **49**: 193–204.

SHINNICK, F.L., INK, S.L., and MARLETT, J.A. (1990) Dose response to a dietary oat bran fraction in cholesterol-fed rats. *Journal of Nutrition* **120:** 561–568.

SIMOPOULOS, A.P. (1999) Essential fatty acids in health and chronic disease. *American Journal of Clinical Nutrition* **70**: 560S–569S.

SKREDE G. (1989) Comparison of various types of starch when used in meat sausages. *Meat Science* **25**: 21–36.

SLATTERY, M.L., BOUCHER, K.M., CAAN, B.J., POTTER, J.D., and MA, K.N. (1998) Eating patterns and risk of colon cancer. *American Journal of Epidemiology* **148**: 4–16.

SLOAN, E.A. (2002) The top 10 functional food trends: the next generation. *Food Technology* **56**: 32–57.

SMITH, D.M. (1987) Functional and biochemical changes in deboned turkey due to frozen storage and lipid oxidation. *Journal of Food Science* **52**: 22–27.

SOFOS, J.N., and ALLEN, C.E. (1977) Effects of lean meat source and the levels of fat and soya protein on the properties of wiener-type products. *Journal of Food Science* **42**: 875–878.

SOLOMON, M.B., EASTRIDGE, J.S., PURSEL, V.G., BEE, G., and MITCHELL, A.D. (2000) Implications of biotechnology: meat quality and value. *Annual Reciprocal Meat Conference Proceedings* **53**: 94–102.

SRINIVASAN, S., and XIONG, Y.L. (1996) Gelation of beef heart surimi as affected by antioxidants. *Journal of Food Science* **61**: 707–711.

STEENBLOCK, R.L., SEBRANEK, J.G., OLSON, D.G., and LOVE, J.A. (2001) The effects of oat fiber on the properties of light bologna and fat-free frankfurters. *Journal of Food Science* **66**: 1409–1415.

STORER C.E., SOUTAR, G.N., and HAWKINS, M.H. (1998) Meat consumption patterns of meat consumption: some Australian evidence. *Australian Agribusiness Review* **6**: 1442–6951.

SU, Y.K., BOWERS, J.A., and ZAYAS J.F. (2000) Physical characteristics and microstructure of reduced-fat frankfurters as affected by salt and emulsified fats stabilized with non-meat proteins. *Journal of Food Science* **65**: 124–128.

SUTTON, D.S., HAND, L.W., and NEWKIRK, K.A. (1995) Reduced fat, high moisture beef frankfurters as affected by chopping temperature. *Journal of Food Science* **60**: 580–582, 586.

TAYLOR, D.L., and LARICK, D.K. (1995) Volatile content and sensory attributes of supercritical carbon dioxide extracts of cooked chicken fat. *Journal of Food Science* **60**: 1197–1200, 1204.

TAYLOR, S.L., ELLER, F.J., and KING, J.W. (1997) A comparison of oil and fat content in oilseeds and ground beef- using supercritical fluid extraction and related analytical techniques. *Food Research International* **30**: 365–370.

TEPPER, B.J., and KUANG, T. (1996) Perception of fat in a milk model system using multidimensional scaling. *Journal of Sensory Studies* **11**: 175–190.

THONGWONG, A., FERNANDO, L.N., GRÜN, I.U., and CLARKE, A.D. (1999) Reduction of warmed-over flavour volatiles from freeze-dried lean beef by supercritical CO_2 extraction. *Journal of Food Science* **64**: 387–389.

TRABER, M.G., and PACKER, L. (1995) Vitamin E: beyond antioxidant function. *American Journal of Clinical Nutrition* **62**: 1501S–9S.

TRIUS, A., SEBRANEK, J.G., RUST, R.E., and CARR, J.M. (1994a) Low-fat bologna and beaker sausage: effects of carrageenans and chloride salts. *Journal of Food Science* **59**: 941–945.

TRIUS, A. SEBRANEK, J.G., RUST, R.E., and CARR, J.M. (1994b) Carrageenans in beaker sausage as affected by pH and sodium tripolyphosphate. *Journal of Food Science* **59**: 946–951.

TROUTT, E.S., HUNT, M.C., JOHNSON, D.E., CLAUS, J.R., KASTENER, C.L., KROPF, D.H., and STRODA, S. (1992) Chemical, physical, and sensory characterisation of ground beef containing 5 to 30 per cent fat. *Journal of Food Science* **57**: 25–29.

TROY, D.J., DESMOND, E.M., and BUCKLEY, D.J. (1999). Eating quality of low-fat beef-burgers containing fat-replacing functional blends. *Journal of Science, Food and Agriculture* **79**: 507–516.

TYUTYUNDZHIEV, N., VELINOV, P., and TZANEVA, Z. (1979) Technological and histochemical methods for the determination of protein-fat emulsions stability in meat products. *Proc. European Meeting of Meat Research Worker* **25**: 511–516.

UK HEALTH COMMITTEE (2004) *Obesity Third Report of Session 2003–04*, Volume I (HC 23-1), 1–148.

VASS, A. (2002) Obesity causes 30 000 deaths a year, report says. *British Medical Journal* **324**: 192.

VENUGOPAL, V., and SHAHIDI, F. (1995) Value-added products from underutilised fish species. *CRC Critical Reviews in Food Science and Nutrition* **35**, 431–453.

WALLINGFORD, L., and LABUZA, T.P. (1983) Evaluation of the water binding properties of food hydrocolloids by physical/chemical methods, and in a low-fat meat emulsion. *Journal of Food Science* **48**: 1–5.

WAN, I., XIONG, Y.L., and DECKER, E.A. (1993) Inhibition of oxidation during washing improves the functionality of bovine cardiac myofibrillar protein. *Journal of Agricultural and Food Chemistry* **41**: 2267–2271.

WHINCUP, P.H., GILG, J.A., PAPACOSTA, O., SEYMOUR, C., MILLER, G.J., ALBERTI, K., and COOK, D.G. (2002) Early evidence of ethnic differences in cardiovascular risk: cross sectional comparison of British South Asian and white children. *British Medical Journal* **324**: 635.

WHO (1998) *Life in the 21st Century: A Vision for All.* World Health Report. WHO, Geneva.

WHO/FAO (1977) Dietary fats and oils in human nutrition. Report of an expert consultation. World Health Org., Food and Agric. Org., Rome.

WILD, J.L., SEBRANEK, J.G., and OLSON, D.G. (1991) Grinding time and pressure developed in beef and pork: effects of temperature and fat. *Journal of Food Science* **56**: 1171–1175.

WILLETT, W.C., SACKS, F., TRICHOPOULOU, A., DRESCHER, G., FERRO-LUZZI, A., HELSING, E., and TRICHOPOULOS D. (1995) Mediterranean diet pyramid: a cultural model for healthy eating. *American Journal of Clinical Nutrition* **61**: 1402–1406.

WILLIAMS, A.A. (1994) Flavour quality – understanding the relationship between sensory responses and chemical stimuli. What are we trying to do? The data, approaches and problems. *Food Quality and Preference* **5**: 3–16.

WILLIAMS, C. (1992) Consumer considerations. In: *Reduced Fat Food: Dietary Fats: Determinants of Preference, Selection and Consumption*. Elsevier Applied Science Publishers, London, 179–192.

WILLIS, W.M., and MARANGONI, A.G. (1999) Biotechnological strategies for the modification of food lipids. *Biotech. Gen. Eng. Rev.* **16**: 141–175.

WIRTH, F. (1988) Technologies for the manufacture of fat-reduced meat products. *Fleischwirtschaft* **68**: 160–165, 201.

XIONG, Y.L. (1996) Impacts on oxidation on muscle protein functionality. *Annual Reciprocal Meat Conference Proceedings* **49**: 79–86.

XIONG, Y. L., and DECKER, E. A. (1995). Alterations of muscle protein functionality by oxidative and antioxidative processes. *Journal of Muscle Foods* **6**: 139–160.

XIONG, Y.L., DECKER, E.A., ROBE, G.H., and MOODY, W.G. (1993). Gelation of crude myofibrillar protein isolated from beef under antioxidative conditions. *Journal of Food Science* 58: 1241–1244.

YACKINOUS, C., and GUINARD, J.X. (2000) Flavour manipulation can enhance the impression of fat in some foods. *Journal of Food Science* **65**: 1270–1283.

YANG, A., KEETON, J.T., BEILKEN, S.L., and TROUT G.R. (2001) Evaluation of some binders and fat substitutes in low-fat frankfurters. *Journal of Food Science* 66: 1039–1047.

ZABOLOTSKY, D.A., CHEN, L.F., PATTERSON, J.A., FORREST, J.C., LIN, H.M., and GRANT, A.L. (1995) Supercritical carbon dioxide extraction of androstenone and skatole from pork fat. *Journal of Food Science* **60**: 1006–1008.

ZAYAS, J.F. (1985) Structural and water binding properties of meat emulsions prepared with emulsified and unemulsified fat. *Journal of Food Science* **50**: 689–692.

ZUBILLAGA, M.P., and MAERKER, G. (1991) Quantification of three cholesterol oxidation products in raw meat and chicken. *Journal of Food Science* **56**: 1194–1196, 1202.

15

The use of fat replacers for weight loss and control

J. M. Jones, College of St. Catherine, Minnesota, USA and S. S. Jonnalagadda, Novartis Medical Nutrition, Minnesota, USA

15.1 Introduction

Obesity rates for both children and adults have increased dramatically in the US, the UK and Western Europe (WHO, 1998; Centers for Disease Control and Prevention, 2002; Nielsen *et al.*, 2002). The obesity epidemic is fueled by readily available, inexpensive food, especially energy-dense, high-fat foods and increased portion size, coupled which both lead to the over-consumption of calories (Swinburn and Egger, 2002; Rolls *et al.*, 2002; Nielsen and Popkin, 2003; Young and Nestle, 2003; Smiciklas-Wright *et al.*, 2003; Roe and Rolls, 2004). Since increases in the energy density of foods have also been shown to increase energy intake (Kral *et al.*, 2004; Devitt and Mattes, 2004; De Castro, 2004), it is reasonable to assume that ingestion of foods that lower energy density by any means, including the use of fat replacers, would result in lower overall food energy intake. Thus manipulation of the energy density of the diet can lower energy consumption by 20–25% and can lead to modest changes in body weight (Bell and Rolls, 2001; Kral *et al.*, 2002). These data indicate that a reduction in the proportion of fat in the diet by 10% can result in a corresponding reduction of 238 kcal/day of total energy intake and can produce a weight loss of ~3.2 kg. Therefore, lowering the fat content of foods, by using fat replacers, has potential for lowering the energy density of foods, which can be helpful in the struggle to maintain a healthy weight (Astrup *et al.*, 2000).

15.2 Fat replacers and their uses

Fat replacers are called by many synonyms with various nuances in their usage. The various names are distinguished in Box 15.1. Fat replacers in food must do two things if they are to help consumers with weight loss. First, they must replicate all or some of the functional properties of fat and, in so doing, impart the sensory properties attributed to fat such as a rich, creamy mouth feel and a tender texture. No one fat replacer is likely to provide all the functions of fat such as flavor, texture, lubrication, keeping quality, volume or heat transfer. Second, they must lower the fat and calorie content of the food. They do this either by enabling the holding of air and water or by being less well absorbed. Fat replacers are most frequently used to replace fat in products with a high fat content and are used in a variety of food products, including frozen desserts, processed meats, cheese, sour cream, salad dressings, snack chips and baked goods. At the height of the interest in low-fat foods, more than 1000 fat-modified foods were introduced, with fat modified snacks being the fastest growing category of products in supermarkets at the time (Schwenk and Guthrie, 1997; Calorie Control Council, 2004).

Box 15.1 Fat replacer terms

Fat replacers can provide some or all of the functions of fat
- Usually yield fewer calories than fat
- They may or may not provide the same nutrients as the fat they replace

Fat substitutes resemble conventional fats and oils and provide all food functions of fat
- Replace fat on a gram-for-gram basis
- Stable at cooking and frying temperatures, usually
- Yield less than 9 kcal/g
- In some cases they are not absorbed at all, so they yield no calories

Fat analogs provide food with many of the characteristics of fat
- Lower digestibility than common dietary fat
- Alter nutritional value

Fat extenders optimize the functionality of fat
- Allow a decrease in the usual amount of fat in the product

Fat mimetics mimic one or more of the sensory and physical functions of fat in the food
- Either carbohydrate, protein, or fat components alone or in combination
- Provide from 0 to 9 kcal/g
- Provide lubricity, mouthfeel and other characteristics of fat by holding water
- Unsuitable for fat functions such as frying, owing to additional water
- May be used for baking and at retort temperatures
- May be subject to excessive browning at high heat

15.3 Categories of fat replacers

There are three broad categories of fat replacers on the market. Since fat replacers may contain calories, food manufacturers using these products should ensure that the final product is not only reduced in fat, but also reduced in calories. In the end the food with fat replacers will be of little value for weight reduction if it fails to cause a significant reduction in calories.

15.3.1 Carbohydrate-based fat replacers

Carbohydrate-based fat replacers use carbohydrate polymers and dietary fibers, such as cellulose, dextrins, maltodextrins, polydextrose, gums, fiber, and modified starch, to replace fat. Carbohydrate-based fat replacers can provide up to 4 kcal/gm if the carbohydrate is fully digestible. Often the calories are lower than this since the fat replacers either are dietary fibers, which are not digested or only fermented to some degree or are digestible carbohydrates mixed with water so they provide 0–2 kcal/g. In some cases fibers, such as cellulose, are ground into microparticles that can form gels for use as fat substitutes, e.g. Oatrim® and Z-trim®. Carbohydrate-based fat replacers are used in a variety of foods including dairy-type products, frozen desserts, sauces, salad dressings, processed meats, baked goods, spreads, chewing gums, and sweets, but cannot replace fats in frying.

15.3.2 Protein-based fat replacers

Protein-based fat replacers are made from many different types of protein, but soy, egg, milk, or whey proteins are common. Microparticulation of protein into tiny, spherical particles that provide a creamy mouthfeel similar to fats helps protein to function as a fat replacer. Blending protein with carbohydrates is another way to create fat replacers. Several studies have shown that combinations of ingredients in fat replacer formulations create synergy that helps lower fat and helps retain desirable product texture (Conforti and Archilla, 2001; Conforti *et al.*, 2001; Ordonez *et al.*, 2001; Ruthig *et al.*, 2001; El-Nager *et al.*, 2002). Fat replacers from protein and protein blends do provide 4 kcal/g, but they may provide only 1–4 kcal/g either because they hold water or are used in lesser amounts than fat. For example, 1 g of Simplesse® can replace 3 g of fat in cream.

Protein-based fat replacers have been used in fat-free ice cream, low-fat cheese, low-fat baked goods, and reduced-fat versions of butter, sour cream, cheese, yogurt, salad dressing, margarine, mayonnaise, baked goods, coffee creamers, soups, and sauces. Often, a combination of these fat replacers can have tremendous potential in the development of fat-modified foods with greater acceptability while lowering the total energy and fat intake.

15.3.3 Fat-based fat replacers

Fat-based fat replacers include common fats that have had chemical alterations of fatty acids so that they deliver less than 9 calories per gram. Some fat-based fat replacers pass through the body partially or totally unabsorbed. Thus they provide less than 9 kcal/g or no calories at all. For example, Olestra (Olean®) is a sucrose polyester consisting of a mixture of hexa, hepta and octa esters of sucrose, esterified with long chain fatty acids. It has the organoleptic and thermal properties of fat, but cannot be hydrolyzed by gastric or pancreatic lipase. The unhydrolyzed molecule is too large to be absorbed in the gastrointestinal tract and, therefore, cannot be metabolized for energy with a net effect of yielding no calories. Other fat-based fat replacers, Salatrim (short and long chain triglyceride molecule) and Caprenin, a substitute for cocoa butter in candy bars, are only partially digested and absorbed, and provide 5 kcal/g. Some fat replacers, such as Enova™ oil, are structured diglycerides and are metabolized differently from triglycerides so that some of the energy is lost as heat rather than stored as adipose.

Emulsifiers can be another type of fat-based substances that can be used as a fat replacer. They may be used with water to replace all or part of the shortening content in cake mixes, cookies, icings, vegetable, and dairy products. They provide the same number of calories as fat, but since less is used in the formulation, the resultant product has less total fat and energy. Mono- and diglycerides are currently used in foods as fat replacers and other substances such as dialkyl dihexadecylmalonate, esterified propoxylated glycerol, and trialkoxytriartallate are in various stages of development.

15.4 Fat replacers and weight loss

Fat replacers can potentially impact overall diet quality and help with weight loss and maintenance. For example, salad dressings and spreads made with fat replacers can help enhance appeal of other nutritious foods such as vegetables and fruit. Thus, fat replacers may help increase the intake of satiety-producing low-calorie, high-fibre, nutrient-dense foods while adding few calories. In meat and other food items, fat replacers such as prunes, raisins, cherry paste, or wild rice replace some of the fat and increase the antioxidant value of foods while lowering calories.

15.4.1 Impact of protein-based fat replacers

Since these are from milk powder, whey, soy or legumes, they not only have potential to lower calories, but also can increase the protein in the diet or offer some nutritional advantages of the individual protein. Some preliminary data indicate that protein may have an impact on satiety and food consumption in the short term (Anderson and Moore, 2004; Layman and Baum, 2004). Furthermore, protein-based fat replacers have the potential to increase the protein in the diet and a high protein to carbohydrate ratio has been associated in studies with greater weight loss than diets with a lower ratio (Layman, 2004). Dairy-based proteins may add calcium, which has been shown in some studies to be related to weight loss (Zemel, 2004). Thus protein-based fat replacers might offer two benefits to the calorie-conscious eater.

15.4.2 Impact of fiber-based fat replacers

These may offer calorie savings while increasing fiber in the diet (Inglett, 2002). Some types of fiber have been shown to regulate food intake, to aid in both preventing weight gain and helping with weight maintenance (Toeller *et al.*, 2001; Howath *et al.*, 2001; Archer *et al.*, 2004; Laitinen *et al.*, 2004). One study with male diabetics shows the utility of a fiber-based fat replacer in dealing with obesity and complications associated with it. In this study those who chose diets rich in fiber-based fat replacers along with sugar replacers and other lifestyle changes reduced body weight and body mass index more than those eating the standard treatment plan. In addition there were greater decreases in HbA1C* and increases in HDL cholesterol (Reyna *et al.*, 2003). In like manner, inclusion of foods made with fat replacers such as Mimex or Oatrim® (a powdered soluble oat fiber containing beta-glucans) has been observed to not only lower blood lipids, and systolic blood pressure, and to improve glucose tolerance and antioxidant status, but also lower body weight (Inglett, 2002; Lairon *et al.*, 2003). Liu *et al.* (2003) noted that those in the Harvard Nurses' Health Study cohort who had the highest fiber intakes were least likely to gain weight.

15.4.3 Impact of fat-based fat replacers

Fat-based fat replacers have also been associated with caloric dilution (Glueck *et al.*, 1982), decreased caloric intake, and changes in appetite (Burley *et al.*, 1994). In a study with lean and overweight subjects eating foods prepared with fat emulsion of palm oil and oat oil (Olibra®) as a fat replacer, there was decreased total energy intake for up to 36 hours post-consumption. Use of Olibra® as a fat substitute in yogurt significantly reduced the energy and macronutrient intakes relative to use of milk fat (Burns *et al.*, 2000, 2001, 2002).

15.4.4 Impact of fat replacers

Use of fat replacers in foods such as mayonnaise, hotdogs, and chips has been shown to decrease the energy and fat in products by as much as 50%. In a study where subjects were offered either full-fat or fat-free Olestra containing chips, total fat intake was reduced from 32–43% on regular chips to 27–30% with

* Hemoglobin A1c is the best measure of glucose because it will be high only if glucose has been elevated for a sustained period of time.

Olestra chips (Miller *et al.*, 1998). In one study the use of fat-free chips did not have a positive impact on diets if consumers were regarded as moderate or high Olestra consumers. This subset increased total energy intake by 209 kcal/day and carbohydrate intake by 37 g/day, compared to a reduction of 87 kcal/day and 14 g/day, respectively, among those not moderate or heavy consumers ($P = 0.01$) (Satia-Bouta *et al.*, 2003). While the changes in percentage energy from carbohydrate and total fat were not significant in this study, the small changes in the energy intake over time may lead to increases in body weight, emphasizing the importance of reduced fat products to also be low in energy and not be consumed in excessive quantities.

Some studies showed greater weight loss with the use of fat replacers, Bray *et al.* (2002) and Lovejoy *et al.* (2000) observed weight loss of 6.3 kg over 6 months with fat-substituted diets, wherein Olestra substituted a portion of the full-fat diet, while decreasing digestible fat to 25% but retaining palatability comparable to diet with 33% of energy from fat. Significant reductions were also observed in body fat (−5.9 kg), total cholesterol (−10 mg/dl), and LDL-cholesterol (−12 mg/dl) compared with the regular (33% energy from fat) group. Likewise, Westrate *et al.* (1998) noted that providing free access to reduced fat products resulted in a reduction in energy intake and percentage energy from fat, while it was associated with an increase in percentage energy from carbohydrate, especially among individuals classified as high fat consumers. Body weight remained stable in reduced-fat group while it increased significantly by about 1 kg in full-fat group. In addition, cardiovascular disease risk factors such as blood lipids, and hemostatic factors were lower in the reduced-fat group compared to the full-fat group.

Kennedy and colleagues (Kennedy *et al.*, 1999, 2001) showed that the selection of low-fat grain mixtures, cakes, cookies and pies not only lowered fat and saturated fat, it resulted in a less energy-dense diet. The individuals consuming lower-fat foods were more likely to meet nutrient requirements than those consuming higher-fat foods even though they were eating 400–500 kcal less (Kennedy *et al.*, 2001).

Thus one strategy for combating the obesity epidemic may involve the switch from consumption of full-fat products to lower-calorie, reduced fat alternatives. Lyle *et al.* (1992) estimated that a 30% reduction in fat calories and a total calorie reduction of 800 kcal can be achieved per week if fat-free products from food categories such as cheese, sour cream, frozen desserts, commercial sweets, and baked goods, were substituted for their regular versions. The Olestra Post-Market Surveillance Study (Patterson *et al.*, 2000) showed that an intake of 2 g/day of Olestra replaced 18 kcal of fat/day (6570 kcal/year), equivalent to a 0.85 kg decrease in body weight.

Existing evidence suggests that reduced fat diets and foods are an important strategy, which can help lower energy density of foods and limit total fat and energy intake in fighting the obesity epidemic (Sigman-Grant *et al.*, 2003). Fat replacers, thus can play a useful role in maintaining the palatability of reduced fat foods without sacrificing the hedonic qualities of the food or putting the

Box 15.2 Safety of fat replacers

Consumer safety concerns over ingredients added to compensate for fat removal highlight the need to educate the general population about fat replacers and their proper use. Safety of most fat replacers is not an issue as the majority of fat replacers are widely used as food additives and have GRAS (Generally Recognized as Safe) status.

Fat replacers that are approved food additives have raised safety health concerns. Polydextrose can have a laxative effect, while Olestra may cause leaky and fatty stools and loss of fat-soluble vitamins. Olestra was approved in 1996 for use in savory snacks such as potato chips, crackers, and tortilla chips. Manufacturers were required to add vitamins A, D, E, and K to Olestra-containing foods to compensate for Olestra's effects on these vitamins, and to place a label informing consumers that Olestra may cause abdominal cramping, loose stools, inhibit absorption of fat soluble vitamins and other nutrients. Subsequent, scientific review has led the Food and Drug Administration (FDA) to conclude that the warning is no longer warranted (US Food and Drug Administration, 2003). There is limited evidence at the present time to suggest any long-term adverse consequences associated with the consumption of these or any other reduced-fat foods developed using the approved fat replacers.

population at a safety risk (Box 15.2) (Swanson *et al.*, 2002). Therefore, on a population level, replacing only 1–2 g of fat/day, by using fat replacers and fat-modified foods, can prevent excess weight gain and associated chronic diseases and help in promoting health (WHO, 1998; Eldridge *et al.*, 2002). On the other hand, foods prepared with fat replacers that neither lower calories nor encourage the consumption of foods that are central to the dietary recommendations may do little to improve the quality of the diet or to help with obesity. Excessive consumption of brownies, cookies, snack cakes and crisps (chips) and other such foods made with fat replacers may do little to help in the battle against obesity. This may be especially problematic if the consumer erroneously believes that fat-free means calorie-free and takes this as a license to consume unlimited amounts.

15.5 Conclusion

Fat replacers have facilitated the development of reduced fat and fat-free foods that have the taste and texture of high-fat foods with less fat and fewer calories. The food industry provided a variety of low-fat products and a segment of the public responded by consuming these products. The actual use of reduced-fat foods by the general population is influenced by dietary advice and recommendations, individual health concerns, sensory characteristics of products, usefulness in the dietary pattern, and willingness to accept the fat substitute. A US survey done in 2000 revealed that the top three reasons for using reduced-fat products were to stay in better overall health, to eat or drink healthier foods and beverages, and to reduce intake of fat and calories (Calorie Control Council, 2004). Thus when fat replacers enable the provision of palatable, lower-calorie foods, they can be one strategy in the battle to lose or maintain desirable weight. On the other hand, fat replacers that neither lower calories nor enable consumption of foods that are useful in weight reduction and maintenance plans may be of little use. In like manner, the over-consumption of foods containing fat replacers by consumers who are either misled by irresponsible manufacturers or misconstrue package claims and equate fat-free or reduced fat with a license to ingest unlimited amounts obviates any potential benefits of fat replacers in the diet. No food or fat replacer supplants the need for practicing moderation and good nutrition.

15.6 References

ANDERSON G H, MOORE S E (2004), 'Dietary proteins in the regulation of food intake and body weight in humans', *J Nutr*, **134**, 974S–979S.

ARCHER B J, JOHNSON S K, DEVEREUX H M, BAXTER A L (2004), 'Effect of fat replacement by inulin or lupin-kernel fibre on sausage patty acceptability, post-meal perceptions of satiety and food intake in men', *Br J Nutr*, **91**, 591–599.

ASTRUP A, GRUNWALD G K, MELANSON E L, SARIS W H, HILL J O (2000), 'The role of low-fat diets in body weight control: a meta-analysis of *ad libitum* dietary intervention studies', *Intl J Obes Relat Metab Disord*, 24, 1545–1552.

BELL E A, ROLLS B J (2001), 'Energy density of foods affects energy intake across multiple levels of fat content in lean and obese women', *Am J Clin Nutr*, 73, 1010–1018.

BRAY G A, LOVEJOY J C, MOST-WINDHAUSER M, SMITH S R, VOLAUFOVA J, DENKINS Y, DEJONGE L, ROOD J, LEFEVRE M, ELDRIDGE A L, PETERS J C (2002), 'A nine-month randomized clinical trial comparing a fat-substituted and fat-reduced diet in healthy obese men: the Ole Study', *Am J Clin Nutr*, 76, 928–934.

BURNS A A, LIVINGSTONE M B E, WELCH R W, DUNNE A ROBSON P J, LINDMARK L, REID C A, MULLANEY U, ROWLAND I R (2000), 'Short-term effects of yoghurt containing a novel fat emulsion on energy and macronutrient intakes in non-obese subjects', *Int J Obes Relat Metab Disord*, 24, 1419–1425.

BURNS A A, LIVINGSTONE M B E, WELCH RW, DUNNE A, REID A, ROWLAND I R (2001), 'The effects of yoghurt containing a novel fat emulsion on energy and macronutrient intake in lean, overweight and obese subjects', *Intl J Obes Relat Metab Disord*, 25, 1487–1496.

BURNS A A, LIVINGSTONE M B E, WELCH R W, DUNNE A, ROWLAND I R (2002), 'Dose–response effects of a novel fat emulsion (Olibra^{TM}) on energy and macronutrient intakes up to 36 h post-consumption', *Eur J Clin Nutr*, 56, 368–377.

BURLEY V J, COTTON J R, WESTSTRATE J A, BLUNDELL J E (1994), 'Effect on appetite of replacing natural fat with sucrose polyester in meals or snacks across one whole day'. In: Ditschuneit H, Gries FA, Hauner H, Schusdziarra V, Wechsler JG (eds) *Obesity in Europe*, Libbey, London, 227–233.

CALORIE CONTROL COUNCIL (2004), 'Fat replacers: Food ingredients for healthy eating', available at: http://www.caloriecontrol.org/fatreprint.html. Accessed 5/6/2004.

Caprenin http://www.chiroweb.com/archives/15/13/07.html.

Centers for Disease Control and Prevention: Monitoring the Nation's Health (2002), 'Dietary intake of macronutrients, micronutrients, and other dietary constituents: United States, 1988–94', *Vital and Health Statistic*, 11, 9–85.

CONFORTI F D, ARCHILLA L (2001), 'Evaluation of a maltodextrin gel as a partial replacement for fat in a high-ratio white-layer cake', *Intl J Consumer Sci*, 25, 238–245.

CONFORTI F D, NEE P, ARCHILLA L (2001), 'The synergistic effects of maltodextrin and high-fructose corn sweetener 90 in a fat-reduced muffin', *Intl J Consumer Sci*, **25**, 3–8.

DE CASTRO J M (2004), 'Dietary energy density is associated with increased intake in free-living humans', *J Nutr*, **134**, 335–341.

DEVITT A A, MATTES R D (2004), 'Effects of food unit size and energy density on intake in humans', *Appetite*, **42**, 213–220.

ELDRIDGE A L, COOPER D A, PETERS J C (2002), 'A role for olestra in body weight management', *Obesity Rev*, **3**, 17–25.

EL-NAGER G, CLOWES G, TUDORICA CM, KURI V, BRENNAN C S (2002), 'Rheological quality and stability of yog-ice cream with added inulin', *Intl J Dairy Tech*, **55**, 89–93.

Enova™ http://lowfatcooking.about.com/od/healthandfitness/p/enovaoil.htm

GLUECK C J, HASTINGS M M, ALLEN C, HOGG E, BAEHLER L, GARTSIDE PS, PHILLIPS D, JONES M, HOLLENACH E J, BRAIN B, ANASTASIA J V (1982), 'Sucrose polyester and covert caloric dilution', *Am J Clin Nutr*, **35**, 1352–1359.

HOWARTH N C, SALTZMAN E, ROBERTS S B (2001), 'Dietary fiber and weight regulation', *Nutr Rev*, **59**, 129–139.

INGLETT G (2002), 'Development of Beta-Glucan Compositions and Their Health Benefits', Annual Meeting Of The Institute Of Food Technologists June 19, 2002. Available at: http://www.ars.usda.gov/research/publications/publications.htm Accessed 6/14/2004.

KENNEDY E T, BOWMAN S A, POWELL R (1999), 'Dietary-fat intake in the US population', *J Am Coll Nutr*, **18**, 207–212.

KENNEDY E, BOWMAN S A, POWELL R (2001), 'Assessment of the effect of fat-modified foods on diet quality in adults, 19–50 years, using data from the Continuing Survey of Food Intake by Individuals', *J Am Diet Assoc*, **101**, 455–460.

KRAL T V, ROE L S, ROLLS B J (2002), 'Does nutrition information about the energy density of meals affect food intake in normal-weight women?', *Appetite*, **39**, 137–145.

KRAL T V, ROE L S, ROLLS B J (2004), 'Combined effects of energy density and portion size on energy intake in women', *Am J Clin Nutr*, **79**, 962–968.

LAIRON D, BERTRAIS S, VINCENT S, ARNAULT N, GALAN P, BOUTRON M C, HERCBERG S (2003), 'French Supplementation en Vitamines et Mineraux AntioXydants (SU.VI.MAX) Adult Cohort', 'Dietary fibre intake and clinical indices in the French Supplementation en Vitamines et Mineraux AntioXydants (SU.VI.MAX) adult cohort', *Proc Nutr Soc*, **6**, 11–15.

LAITINEN J, PIETILAINEN K, WADSWORTH M, SOVIO U, JARVELIN M R (2004), 'Predictors of abdominal obesity among 31-y-old men and women born in Northern Finland in 1966', *Eur J Clin Nutr*, **58**, 180–190.

LAYMAN, D K (2004), 'Dietary protein and weight'. IFT 2004. Annual meeting Las Vegas.

LAYMAN D K, BAUM J I (2004), 'Dietary protein impact on glycemic control during weight loss', *J Nutr*, **34**, 968S–973S.

LIU S, WILLETT W C, MANSON J E, HU F B, ROSNER B, COLDITZ G (2003), 'Relation between changes in intakes of dietary fiber and grain products and changes in weight and development of obesity among middle-aged women', *Am J Clin Nutr*, **78**, 920–927.

LOVEJOY J C, LEFEVRE M, BRAY GA, MOST-WINDHAUSER M, DENKINS Y M, ROOD J C, ELDRIDGE A, PETERS J (2000), *Beneficial Effects of a Low-fat Diet on Health Risk Factors is Mediated by Weight-loss in Middle Age Men*, North American Association for the Study of Obesity (NAASO), Long Beach, CA.

LYLE B J, MCMAHON K E, KREUTLER P A (1992), 'Assessing the potential dietary impact of replacing dietary fat with other macronutrients', *J Nutr*, **122**, 211–216.

MILLER D L, CASTELLANOS V H, SHIDE D J, PETERS J C, ROLLS B J (1998), 'Effect of fat-free potato chips with and without nutrition labels on fat and energy intakes', *Am J Clin Nutr*, **68**, 2, 282–290.

NIELSEN S J, POPKIN B M (2003), 'Patterns and trends in food portion sizes, 1977–1998', *JAMA*, **289**, 450–453.

NIELSEN S J, SIEGA-RIZ A M, POPKIN B M (2002), 'Trends in energy intake in U.S. between 1977 and 1996: similar shifts seen across age groups', *Obes Res*, **10**, 370–378.

Oatrim® http://www.ars.usda.gov/is/AR/archive/dec98/nutrim1298.pdf. Accessed 02/05.

Olestra http://www.olean.com. Accessed 02/05.

Olibra® http://www.lipid.se/olibra/main.html. Accessed 02/05.

ORDONEZ M, ROVIRA J, JAIME I (2001), 'The relationship between the composition and texture of conventional and low-fat frankfurters', *Intl J Fd Sci Tech*, **36**, 749–758.

PATTERSON R E, KRISTAL A R, PETERS J C, NEUHOUSER M L, ROCK C L, CHESKIN L J, NEUMARK-SZTAINER D, THORNQUIST M D (2000), 'Changes in diet, weight, and serum lipid levels associated with olestra consumption', *Arch Intern Med*, **160**, 2600–2604.

REYNA N Y, CANO C, BERMUDEZ V J, MEDINA M T, SOUKI A J, AMBARD M, NUNEZ M, FERRER M A, INGLETT G E (2003), 'Sweeteners and beta-glucans improve metabolic and anthropometrics variables in well controlled type 2 diabetic patients', *Am J Ther*, **10**, 438–443.

ROE L S, ROLLS B J (2004), 'Combined effects of energy density and portion size on energy intake in women', *Am J Clin Nutr*, **79**, 962–968.

ROLLS B J, MORRIS E L, ROE L S (2002), 'Portion size of food affects energy intake in normal-weight and overweight men and women', *Am J Clin Nutr*, **76**, 1207–1213.

RUTHIG D J, SIDER D, MECKLING-GILL K A (2001), 'Health benefits of dietary fat reduction by a novel fat replacer: Mimix', *Intl J Fd Sci Nutr*, **52**, 61–69.

SALATRIM (Benefat) http://www.danisco.com/emulsifiers/productrange/benefat.asp

SATIA-BOUTA J, KRISTAL A R, PATTERSON R E, NEUHOUSER M L, PETERS J C, ROCK C L, NEUMARK-SZTAINER D, CHESKIN L J, THORNQUIST M D (2003), 'Is olestra consumption associated with changes in dietary intake, serum lipids, and body weight?', *Nutrition*, **19**, 754–779.

SCHWENK N E, GUTHRIE J F (1997), 'Trends in marketing and usage of fat-modified foods: implications for dietary status and nutrition promotion', *Fam Eco Nutr Rev*, **10**, 16–32.

SIGMAN-GRANT M, WARLAND R, HSIEH G (2003), 'Selected lower-fat foods positively impact nutrient quality in diets of free-living Americans', *J Am Diet Assoc*, **103**, 570–576.

Simplesse® . http://www.cpkelco.com/simplesse/. Accessed 02/05.

SMICIKLAS-WRIGHT H, MITCHELL D C, MICKLE S J, GOLDMAN J D (2003), 'Cook A. Foods commonly eaten in the United States, 1989–1991 and 1994–1996: Are portion sizes changing?', *J Am Diet Assoc*, 103, 41–47.

SWANSON R B, PERRY J M, CARDEN L A (2002), 'Acceptability of reduced-fat brownies by school-aged children', *J Am Diet Assoc*, **102**, 856–859.

SWINBURN B, EGGER G (2002), 'Preventive strategies against weight gain and obesity', *Obesity Rev*, **3**, 289–301.

TOELLER M, BUYKEN A E, HEITKAMP G, CATHELINEAU G, FERRISS B, MICHEL G; EURODIAB IDDM COMPLICATIONS STUDY GROUP (2001), 'Nutrient intakes as predictors of body weight in European people with type 1 diabetes', *Int J Obes Relat Metab Disord*, **25**, 1815–1822.

US FOOD AND DRUG ADMINISTRATION (2003), 'Food additives permitted for direct addition to food for human consumption', **68**(150).

WESTSTRATE J A, VAN HET HOF K H, VAN DEN BERG H, VELTHUIS-TE-WIERIK E J M, DE GRAAF C, ZIMMERMANNS N J H, WESTERTERP K R, WESTERTERP-PLANTENGA M S, VERBOEKET-VAN DE VENNE W P H G (1998), 'A comparison of the effect of free access to reduced fat products or their full fat equivalents on food intake, body weight, blood lipids and fat-soluble antioxidants levels and haemostasis variables', *Eur J Clin Nutr*, **52**, 389–395.

WHO WORLD HEALTH ORGANIZATION CONSULTATION ON OBESITY (1998), *Obesity: Preventing and Managing the Global Epidemic*, World Health Organization: Geneva.

YOUNG L R, NESTLE M (2003), 'Expanding portion sizes in the US marketplace: implications for nutrition counseling', *J Am Diet Assoc*, **103**, 231–234.

ZEMEL, M (July 2004), 'Calcium and weight', IFT Annual Meeting, Las Vegas.

Z-trim® http://www.ars.usda.gov/is/pr/1996/z-trim896.htm Accessed 02/05.

16

Testing novel fat replacers for weight control

C. M. Logan, J. M. W. Wallace, P. J. Robson and M. B. E. Livingstone, University of Ulster, UK

16.1 Introduction

Food intake is largely controlled by human appetite (Blundell & Tremblay, 1995). Although appetite is influenced by a profusion of factors, the satiating power of food plays a major role in controlling the biological drive to eat. The term satiating power refers to the ability of food to suppress further food intake via physiological and biochemical mechanisms, collectively known as the satiety cascade (Blundell & Tremblay, 1995). It is now accepted that macronutrients exert independent effects on satiety, and although subject to debate, protein is regarded as the most satiating macronutrient and fat as the least satiating macronutrient (Cotton *et al.*, 1994; Blundell & MacDiarmid, 1997; Poppitt *et al.*, 1998). Moreover, studies demonstrate that dietary fat is positively associated with energy intake (Stubbs *et al.*, 1995a,b), and body weight (Blundell *et al.*, 1996; Bray & Popkin, 1998). The hedonic properties of dietary fat coupled with its high energy density, may partially explain the passive over-consumption associated with dietary fat intake (Blundell & MacDiarmid, 1997).

The effect of dietary fat on satiety and food intake may vary, however, depending on physiological and chemical properties of the constituent fatty acids (French, 1999; French, 2004). In particular, chain length and the degree of saturation of fatty acids have received considerable attention in trying to unravel the relationship between fat and satiety. Studies suggest that medium chain triglycerides are more satiating than long chain triglycerides, and therefore may be capable of limiting the consumption of excess energy associated with high-fat diets (Rolls *et al.*, 1988; Stubbs & Harbron, 1996). It has been suggested that this effect is exerted via post-absorptive activities (Van Wymelbeke *et al.*, 1998). Greater body weight and fat losses have been associated with the consumption of diacylglycerol oil compared to triacylglycerol oil, which may be due to differences in energy expenditure (Maki *et al.*, 2002). Studies also indicate that polyunsaturated fatty acids (PUFAs) elicit more potent satiating properties compared with monounsaturated fatty acids and saturated fatty acids (French *et al.*, 1998; Lawton *et al.*, 2000). Post-ingestive activities, namely hormonal responses and rate of gastric emptying, are the proposed mechanisms of action for the more potent satiating effects of PUFAs (Lawton *et al.*, 2000). In addition, emulsification properties, route of administration and gastrointestinal region have also been identified as important factors in determining the satiating potential of dietary fat (Welch *et al.*, 1985, 1988; Armand *et al.*, 1992) (see Chapter 7).

As the worldwide prevalence of obesity, and related morbidities and mortalities, continues to escalate, effective weight management strategies are urgently required. Ultimately, the development of a functional food that could attenuate the achievement of positive energy balance would be ideal (Dye & Blundell, 2002). Both the reduction of the fat content of food in order to reduce its energy content, and the incorporation of manipulated fatty acids into foods to strengthen satiating signals, have been considered (Dye & Blundell, 2002).

Olibra™, a relatively novel fat emulsion, is an example of a food ingredient that aims to reduce food intake by promoting and maintaining satiety. To our knowledge it is one of the first functional food products that attempt to control food intake by modulating satiety. Firstly, it is worth noting that prior to human intervention trials, the ability of Olibra™ fat emulsion to reduce short-term food intake was demonstrated in animal studies (unpublished data). This fat emulsion has been formulated from palm oil and oat oil fractions in the proportions 95:5, dispersed in water to give a total fat content of 42% (w/w). In human intervention studies to date, the emulsion has been incorporated into yoghurt, in which it partially replaces the milk fat normally found in such yoghurt. The percentage fatty acid composition of Olibra™ compared with milk fat is as follows: palmitic (16:0), 42.1 *vs* 26.8; stearic (18:0), 4.3 *vs* 11.5; other saturates, 2.1 *vs* 25.8; oleic (18:1), 40.1 *vs* 28.7; linoleic (18:2), 10.4 *vs* 1.4; and other unsaturates, 1.0 *vs* 5.8. Studies have demonstrated the ability of the emulsion incorporated into yoghurt to induce a short-term reduction in food intake (Burns *et al.*, 2000, 2001, 2002). However, the efficacy of the emulsion to bring about medium- to long-term reductions in food intake is currently under investigation.

16.2 Short-term studies

In the three initial short-term studies, the Olibra™ fat emulsion was incorporated into a 200 g portion of yoghurt, and its effects on food intake and appetite were evaluated in randomised, double-blind, placebo-controlled, within-subject crossover studies. The test yoghurt used in the first two studies was composed of 5 g Olibra™ fat and 1 g milk fat, corresponding to 12.5 g Olibra™ emulsion respectively, while the control yoghurt contained milk fat only. Both yoghurts were matched for energy and macronutrient content (800 kJ, 6.8 g protein, 6.0 g fat, 28.8 g carbohydrate per 200 g portion). In preparation for all studies, subjects fasted from 20.00 h the evening prior to the study. The first two trials ($n = 29$, $n = 30$) followed a similar protocol, thus data underwent separate and combined analysis and is referred to as one study. In this study, a sample of non-obese subjects consumed a defined breakfast providing 25% of estimated daily energy expenditure, fasted until lunch when they then received the yoghurt, and food intake was then covertly assessed 4 h post-consumption at an *ad libitum* meal. Subjects recorded food intake for the remainder of the day using weighed dietary records. A subsequent study investigated the effect of the emulsion on food intake in groups of non-overweight ($n = 20$), overweight ($n = 20$) and obese ($n = 20$) subjects. In addition, food intake was evaluated at 8 h post-consumption of the yoghurts in order to determine if the effect was sustained for this length of time. In this study, the yoghurt was consumed at breakfast, and food intake was covertly assessed 4 h post-consumption at an *ad libitum* lunch and again 4 h later at an *ad libitum* dinner. Subjects fasted between the consumption of the test yoghurt and the test lunch, and between test meals. Weighed food diaries were completed for the remainder of the study day and the post-study day.

The studies described above focused on the effect brought about by 12.5 g of the Olibra™ emulsion, and as results suggested a possible dose effect relative to body weight, this phenomenon was subsequently evaluated in non-overweight subjects ($n = 50$). In this study, subjects received for breakfast, in random order, a 200 g portion of yoghurt containing 15 g of fat with 0 g (control), 2, 4 or 6 g of the Olibra™ fat, corresponding to 0, 5, 10 and 15 g of Olibra™ emulsion respectively. Subjects fasted until 4 h post-consumption when food intake was assessed at an *ad libitum* meal by pre- and post-covert weighing. Food intake was again monitored using self-reported weighed food diaries for the remainder of the study day and the post-study day. In all studies appetite was assessed using visual analogue scales (VAS) at appropriate time-points throughout the study day.

16.2.1 Effects of Olibra™ emulsion on food intake and appetite

Overall, the first human study revealed a significant decrease of 14% in energy intake, in addition, intakes of fat, protein and carbohydrate and total weight of food eaten were significantly reduced 4 h post-consumption of the test yoghurt relative to control conditions (Burns *et al.*, 2000). These results were confirmed in the later study, and moreover, the reduction in food intake was sustained up to 8 h post-consumption (Burns *et al.*, 2001). Self-reported energy intakes also remained significantly lower for the remainder of the study day following consumption of the test yoghurt (40% in study one, 17% in study two) (Burns *et*

Table 16.1 Energy and macronutrient intakes following consumption of test yoghurt containing 12.5 g of Olibra™ emulsion relative to control conditions*

	Energy (MJ)	Fat (g)	Protein (g)	CHO (g)
Burns *et al.* (2000) (*n* = 59)				
4 h post-consumption				
Test	6.67	70.5	64.1	181.7
Control	7.75	86.9	72.9	202.2
% difference	−13.9	−18.9	−12.1	−10.1
Self-reported intakes for remainder of study day				
Test	0.6	4.4	2.1	19.3
Control	1.0	6.8	3.4	32.8
% difference	−40.0	−35.3	−38.2	−41.1
Burns *et al.* (2001) (*n* = 60)				
4 h post-consumption				
Test	4.26	54.1	36.7	101.9
Control	5.60	74.8	46.6	128.7
% difference	−23.9	−27.7	−21.2	−20.8
8 h post-consumption				
Test	4.23	45.3	37.7	119.5
Control	5.81	66.6	52.1	154.8
% difference	−27.2	−32.0	−27.6	−22.8
Self-reported intakes for remainder of study day				
Test	0.49	2.8	1.4	11.4
Control	0.96	6.9	4.3	24.8
% difference	−17.0	−59.4	−67.4	−54.0
Self-reported intakes for 24 h post-study day				
Test	6.35	58.1	60.5	202.6
Control	7.70	69.1	78.2	226.1
% difference	−17.5	−15.9	−22.6	−10.4

CHO (carbohydrate).
*All intakes under test conditions are significantly different from control conditions ($P < 0.05$)

al., 2000, 2001), and remained lower during the subsequent 24 h (18%) (Burns *et al.*, 2001). Reductions in food intake observed following the consumption of 12.5 g of the emulsion are summarised in Table 16.1. VAS scales revealed reduced hunger ratings, desire to eat and preoccupation with thoughts of food and an enhanced feeling of fullness after the test yoghurt throughout the study day (Burns *et al.*, 2001).

16.2.2 Response by BMI groups

The response to the Olibra™ emulsion appeared to differ between subjects when categorised according to their BMI (20–24.9 kg/m^2 – non-overweight, 25–29.9 kg/m^2 – overweight, >30 kg/m^2 – obese), these differences are presented in Table 16.2. Energy and macronutrient intakes and weight of food consumed were significantly reduced at 4 h post-consumption of the test yoghurt in the

Table 16.2 Percentage energy and macronutrient reductions following the consumption of test yoghurts containing various doses of Olibra™ emulsion relative to control conditions in subjects categorised according to their BMI

	4 h post-consumption				8 h post-consumption				Remainder of test evening				24 h subsequent to test day			
	Energy	Fat	Protein	CHO	Energy	Fat	Protein	CHO	Energy	Fat	Protein	CHO	Energy	Fat	Protein	CHO
Non-obese																
Dose 12.5 g[1]	−13.9	−18.9	−12.1	−10.1	Intake not assessed at this time				−40.0	−35.3	−38.2	−41.1	Intake not assessed at this time			
Non-overweight																
Dose 12.5 g[2]	−30.2	−33.9	−30.6	−26.9	−30.0	−31.7	−35.6	−23.9	−64.3	−66.9	−65.4	−63.7	−15.1	−16.8	−21.6	−9.5*
Dose 5 g[3]	−21.4	−23.6	−15.4	−17.8	Intake not assessed at this time				−52.6	−63.6	−42.0	−48.3	−27.6	−39.4	−20.7	−21.0
Dose 10 g[3]	−24.5	−23.8	−25.5	−24.1	Intake not assessed at this time				−59.4	−67.2	−56.9	−56.2	−27.0	−36.5	−19.9	−24.6
Dose 15 g[3]	−29.4	−30.7	−31.0	−26.5	Intake not assessed at this time				−68.3	−76.0	−57.5	−61.3	−35.0	−45.3	−23.5	−22.4
Overweight																
Dose 12.5 g[2]	−27.6	−31.9	−22.9	−24.0	−32.1	−40.6	−31.7	−23.6	0*	−37.0*	−55.0*	−17.8*	−12.2*	−17.7*	−18.9	−2.6*
Obese																
Dose 12.5 g[2]	−13.1*	−16.8*	−9.2*	−10.3*	−21.6	−24.2	−15.9	−21.1	−69.7*	−65.1*	−81.1*	−73.0*	−25.8	−12.4*	−28.1	−19.5

CHO (carbohydrate).
Non-obese (BMI < 30 kg/m^2), non-overweight (BMI 20–24.9 kg/m^2), overweight (BMI 25–29.9 kg/m^2), obese (BMI ≥ 30 kg/m^2).
Intakes differed from control conditions with the exception of intakes indicated with an asterisk (*).
[1] Burns *et al.* (2000).
[2] Burns *et al.* (2001).
[3] Burns *et al.* (2002).

non-overweight and the overweight groups, but not in the obese group (Burns *et al.*, 2001). In fact, this study revealed a stronger response 4 h post-consumption in the non-overweight subjects compared to the non-obese sample of subjects in the initial studies (30% *vs* 14%). Although the obese group also reduced their food intakes, reductions were not significantly lower relative to the control conditions. However, by 8 h post-consumption of the test yoghurt, all BMI groups demonstrated significantly reduced energy and macronutrient intakes and weight of food eaten (Burns *et al.*, 2001). Lower self-reported energy and macronutrient intakes reported during the evening following the consumption of the test yoghurt reached significance in the non-overweight group only. However, during the 24 h following the study day, energy intakes were significantly suppressed in the non-overweight and the obese subjects. The overweight group also demonstrated a lower energy intake during this time period, but this was not significantly different from control conditions (Burns *et al.*, 2001). Overall, it appears the non-overweight group was more responsive to the emulsion compared to the overweight and obese groups (Burns *et al.*, 2001).

16.2.3 Dose–response effects of Olibra™

The latter results suggest that the magnitude of response to Olibra™ may be lower in heavier subjects, perhaps because they ingest a lower dose relative to body weight. Hence the final short-term study investigated the dose–response effects of the emulsion on food intake in non-overweight subjects (Burns *et al.*, 2002). Results reveal significant reductions in energy intake of 21, 25 and 30% following consumption of test yoghurts containing 5, 10 and 15 g of the emulsion respectively. Corresponding macronutrient intakes and weight of food eaten were also significantly lower (Burns *et al.*, 2002). However, there was no consistent trend between dose levels (Burns *et al.*, 2002). Self-reported energy and corresponding macronutrient intakes remained significantly lower during the evening and the following 24 h after the test yoghurts at all dose levels relative to control conditions, but again intakes did not differ between doses (Burns *et al.*, 2002). Interestingly, there were no differences in appetite ratings between varying doses relative to the control treatment (Burns *et al.*, 2002). Difference in energy and macronutrient intakes following consumption of various doses of the Olibra™ emulsion relative to control conditions are presented in Table 16.2.

16.2.4 Gender differences in response to Olibra™

The response to the emulsion differs considerably between men and women (Table 16.3). In the first study, although females generally decreased intakes more than males, the treatment effect was independent of either sex or body size (Burns *et al.*, 2000). However, in a later study, the treatment effect was gender-dependent, in that males, relative to female subjects, consumed more food at a test meal following consumption of both the test and control treatments (Burns *et al.*, 2001). This could imply that the optimal dose of Olibra™ fat emulsion

Table 16.3 Percentage difference in energy intakes among male and female subjects 4 h post-consumption of varying doses of Olibra™ emulsion relative to control conditions

Dose	Female: % difference	Male: % difference
12.5 g[1]	−18	−11
5 g[2]	−25	−16
10 g[2]	−34	−11
15 g[2]	−34	−23

[1] Burns *et al.* (2000).
[2] Burns *et al.* (2002).

may vary between males and females. Alternatively, males may be simply more responsive to the 'plate-cleaning phenomenon'.

The inconsistent response to varying doses of the emulsion among males and females are difficult to interpret. Overall, both males and females significantly lowered energy intakes 4 h post-consumption of a yoghurt containing doses as low as 5 g of Olibra™ emulsion, with a greater response observed in females than males (25% *vs* 16%). The response to the emulsion increased among the female group up to the 10 g dose (34%), thereafter, there was no further increase associated with the 15 g dose. The male group, on the other hand, showed a lower response to the 10 g dose level (11%), but the response increased following the 15 g dose (23%) (Burns *et al.*, 2002). Self-reported intakes did not differ between men and women for the remainder of the evening, or during the following 24 h after the test yoghurts, at any of the dose levels (Burns *et al.*, 2002).

While comparing results from various studies, similar reductions in energy intakes were observed in male subjects at 4 h post-consumption of 12.5 g and 10 g of the emulsion (11%) (Burns *et al.*, 2000, 2002). Results are not as consistent for females, with an 18% reduction in energy intake 4 h post-consumption of 12.5 g of the emulsion compared to a 34% reduction following consumption of 10 g of the emulsion (Burns *et al.*, 2000, 2002). Differences between subject groups and unaccounted differences within subject groups are likely to explain some of these differences. In any case, however, females tend to demonstrate a stronger response to the Olibra™ fat emulsion compared with males.

16.2.5 Inter-individual variability in responses

Individual responses to the Olibra™ fat emulsion show substantial variation. While some subjects are extremely responsive to the emulsion, resulting in energy reductions as high as 67% 4 h post-consumption, others remain unresponsive to the satiating properties of the emulsion. Both initial and more recent medium-term studies demonstrate the presence of non-responders, but evidence of lack of responsiveness is particularly evident in the more recent trials. When data from initial studies testing the 12.5 g dose of Olibra™ emulsion are combined, 27% of subjects ($n = 32$) did not respond to the emulsion. In the most recent trial to date, 54% of subjects ($n = 15$) failed to reduce their food intake. Analysis preformed on all available data assessing the 12.5 g dose of Olibra™ emulsion revealed a similar number of responders among males (33%) and females (31%) (Figs 16.1a,b). Additionally, non-responders were evident in all BMI groups (Figs 16.2a–c), with similar proportions of non-responders in the

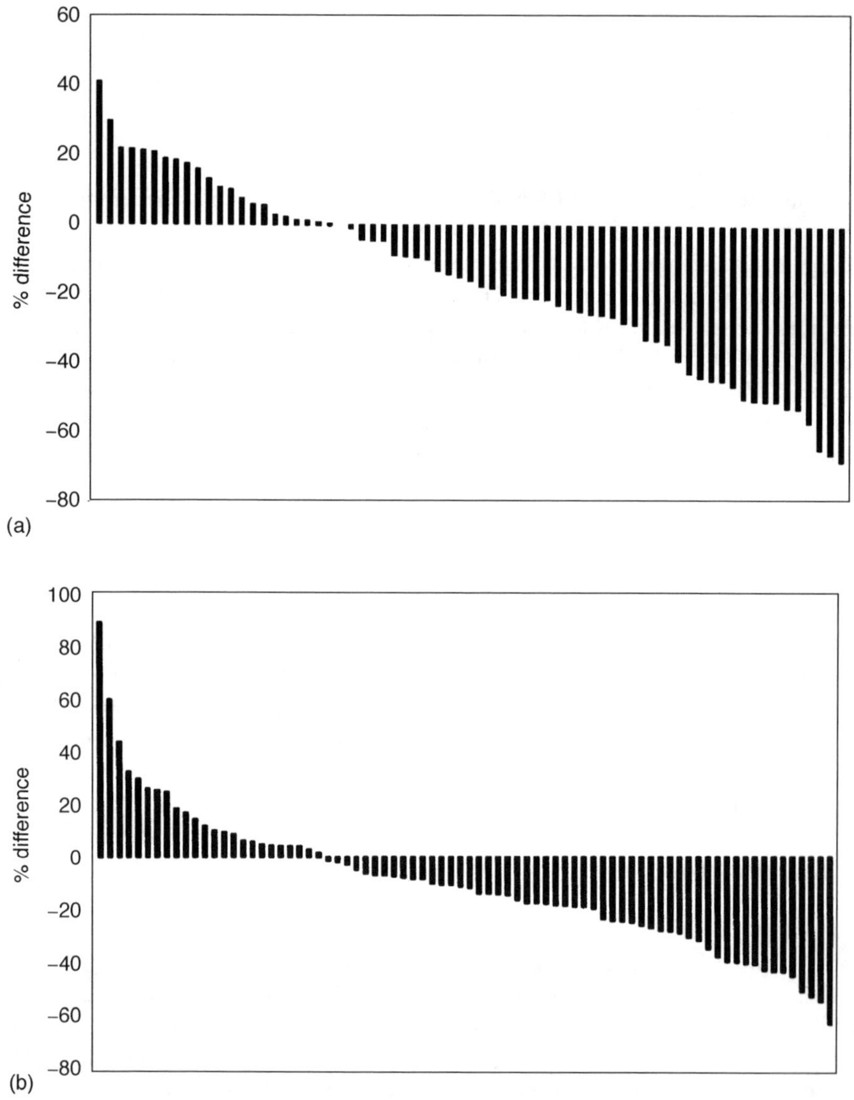

Fig. 16.1 (a) Percentage difference in energy intake in males 4 h post-consumption of test yoghurt relative to control conditions ($n = 69$), (b) percentage difference in energy intake in females 4 h post-consumption of test yoghurt relative to control conditions ($n = 78$).

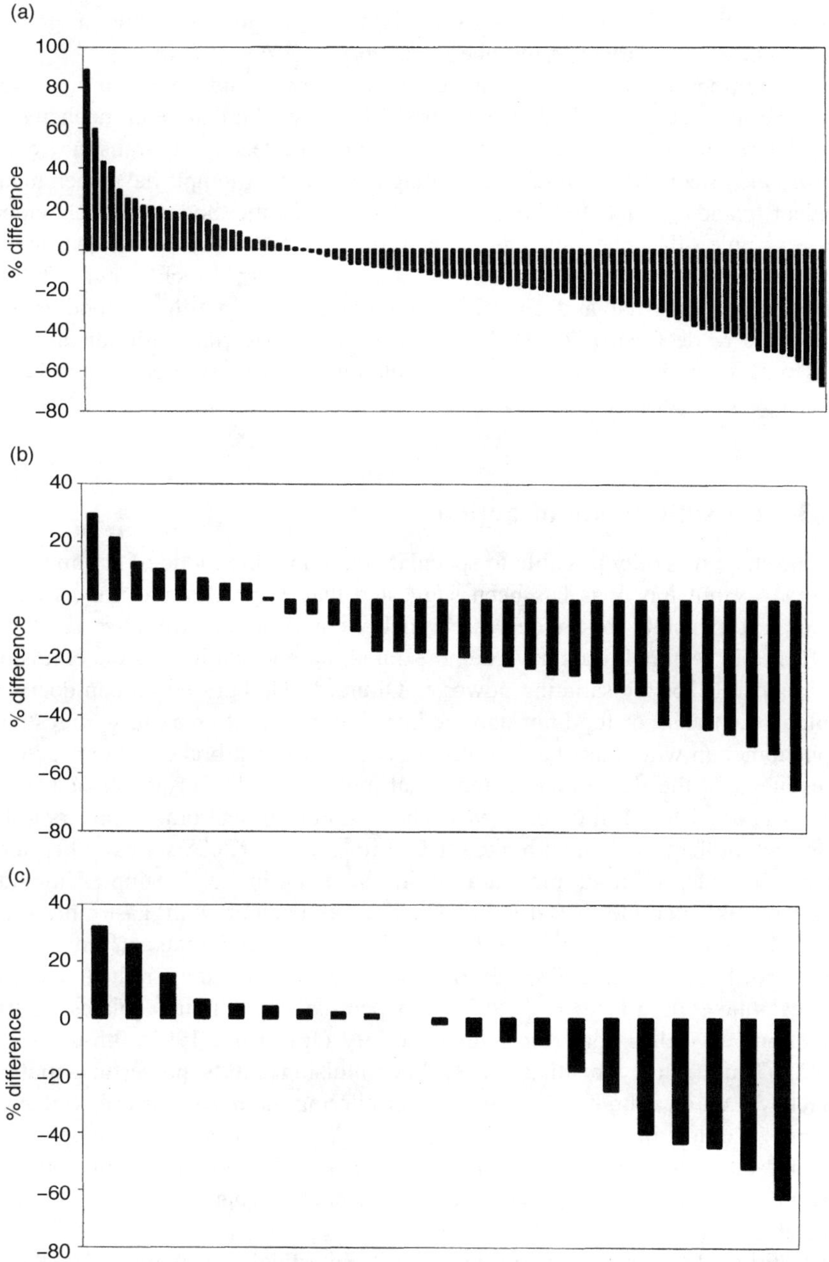

Fig. 16.2 (a) Percentage difference in energy intake in non-overweight subjects 4 h post-consumption of test yoghurt relative to control conditions ($n = 93$), (b) percentage difference in energy intake in overweight subjects 4 h post-consumption of test yoghurt relative to control conditions ($n = 33$), (c) percentage difference in energy intake in obese subjects 4 h post-consumption of test yoghurt relative to control conditions ($n = 21$).

non-overweight (30%) and the overweight (27%) groups, while a greater prevalence was observed in the obese category (48%).

In addition to difference in appetite preferences and variation in dose–responses expressed on a body weight basis, it is assumed that other mechanisms may determine the effectiveness of this fat emulsion. Personality traits may exert a profound effect on food intake and eating behaviour. Attempts have been made to identify and establish links between such characteristics and eating behaviour. For example, the phenomenon of restrained eating may be of particular relevance in such studies (Green & Blundell, 1996; Lluch *et al.*, 2000). Additionally, external and environmental factors play a role in food intake (Stroebele & de Castro, 2004). It is probable that in certain individuals these cues may over-ride normal appetite regulation. This is an area that is being investigated at present.

16.3 Possible mode of action

At this stage it is only possible to speculate on a possible mode of action of the Olibra™ emulsion. It is has been suggested that a specific and non-aversive effect is responsible for the decreased energy consumption (Burns *et al.*, 2000, 2001, 2002). Animal trials have demonstrated that the stability of the emulsion is responsible for the satiating power of Olibra™. Undigested fat can delay or prolong the transit of food through the intestine in order to maximise digestion, a phenomenon which has been referred to as the jejunal brake in the proximal intestines and the ileal brake in the distal intestines (MacFarlane *et al.*, 1983; Spiller *et al.*, 1984; Lin *et al.*, 1996). The fat-induced ileal brake appears to be more potent than the jejunal brake (H. C. Lin *et al.*, 1997). A series of peptides have been identified to play a role in the ileal brake. Examples include glucagon-like peptide 1 (GLP-1), which is associated with gastrointestinal motility regulation, increased satiety and reduced food intake (Flint *et al.*, 1998; Naslund *et al.*, 1998, 1999), enterostatin which may reduce fat and energy intake (L. Lin *et al.*, 1997), and peptide YY which regulates gastric secretions as well as gastrointestinal motility (Jin *et al.*, 1993; Pironi *et al.*, 1993). Thus, it may be that the Olibra emulsion exerts powerful satiating effects via the ileal brake by prolonging or altering the release or effect of such factors. The ileal brake and release of peptide YY appear to be dose-dependent (Pironi *et al.*, 1993), supporting the hypothesis that the Olibra™ emulsion may operate, at least partially, via the ileal brake mechanism and associated mediators.

Additionally, factors that influence gastrointestinal transit may also throw some light on the inter-subject differences in response to the emulsion. For example, age may influence gastric motility and release of related gastro-intestinal hormones (Madsen, 1992; MacIntosh *et al.*, 1999). BMI may also influence gastrointestinal transit (Madsen, 1992). Additionally, shorter colonic transit was observed in men compared with women (Meier *et al.*, 1995), and if this is the case, the prolonged presence of the emulsion in the gut may contribute to the greater response to the emulsion observed in females (Burns *et al.*, 2000, 2002). Furthermore, the influence of the menstrual cycle on colonic transit in women may partially explain the inconsistency of results among females (Meier *et al.*, 1995; Jung *et al.*, 2003).

16.4 Implications for product development and future trends

The exact role and efficacy of the Olibra™ fat emulsion in body weight management remain to be fully elucidated. To date, studies reveal no evidence of compensation for energy reduction associated with the Olibra™ emulsion. However, this is merely an assumption drawn from short-term studies. Longer-term studies are required to establish whether the effects of the Olibra™ emulsion on food intake and satiety persist in those who reduce food intake in response to the emulsion and, in turn, if these effects induce desirable outcomes on body weight management. Energy compensation or habituation to the emulsion leading to lack of responsiveness are the two possible outcomes that may result from longer-term consumption of the emulsion.

More recent investigations suggest that the effects of Olibra™ emulsion were not evident in the medium term (up to 3 weeks) (unpublished data). However a range of factors associated with the latter study may have influenced results. Firstly, the study was set in a sociable environment, seating between 10–12 subjects per test meal. Such factors are known to influence eating behaviour (de Castro & de Castro, 1989; Webber *et al.*, 2004). Secondly, self-reported food intake records may have confounded the results (Livingstone *et al.*, 1990). Although it could be argued that this may be the case in the previous studies, mis-reporting appears to be a problem that has intensified since it was first identified as a problem in studies assessing food intake (Heitmann *et al.*, 2000). Thirdly, eating behaviour is likely to be influenced by a free lunch in which a wide range of foods served in extra large portion sizes are presented (Rolls, 1985; Rolls *et al.*, 2002; Sorensen *et al.*, 2003). This may have assumed greater relevance of late, given that many people have become preoccupied, even obsessed, with food, eating and body image. It could be postulated that a combination of these factors could account for the fact that a proportion of subjects remained unresponsive to the satiating effects of Olibra™. Consequently, to reveal the true potential of functional foods aiming to control food intake, it is important to identify the characteristics of subjects who do not eat according to physiologically driven appetite cues.

Another limitation of these crossover studies is a carry-over effect of the treatment from one study day to another. This carry-over effect is a combination of three different effects: (1) systematic differences between the two groups of subjects, (2) differences in 'carry-over' between the two treatments, and (3) treatment × period interaction, all of which cannot be distinguished from one another in a two × two crossover design. Additionally, a period effect may also confound data. Although, a double-blind, crossover study is regarded as the most powerful study design, this methodology is not without shortfalls.

None of the short-term studies revealed any adverse effects or discomfort associated with the consumption of the test yoghurt. Both test and control yoghurts were rated similarly in regards to pleasantness of taste (Burns *et al.*, 2000, 2001, 2002). Additionally, consumption of the emulsion over a 3-week period did not elicit any undesirable effects on blood profile (unpublished data).

The studies to date show that the effects of the Olibra™ emulsion are evident by 4 h post-consumption, at least in non-obese subjects. However, given that the protocol requires subjects to fast between yoghurt consumption and the test meal, it is unclear whether appetite suppression would be evident earlier and whether other food intake during this period would influence the satiating capacities of the emulsion. At present, attempts are being made to develop a product that induces instant satiety to improve the action of the existing emulsion. Further research is required to establish the possible interaction between various foods or specific nutrients and the Olibra™ emulsion. Identification of other potential food vehicles for the emulsion is another area for future development, primarily the incorporation of a powdered version of the emulsion into solid foods.

16.5 Other fat replacements used in the control of body weight

Increased consumer awareness and concerns regarding the fat content of food has resulted in the manufacture of fat-modified foods. Identification of fat replacement strategies is a developing industry, as exemplified by the fact that over 100 fat substitutes have been formulated since they were initially developed over a decade ago (Lawton, 1998). Fat replacers, also referred to as fat substitutes or fat mimetics, are ingredients that replicate some of the properties of dietary fat, but yield less energy. They can be classified according to their macronutrient base. The majority of replacers are carbohydrate-based and examples of trade names include Litesse, Maltrin and Slendid (Warshaw *et al.*, 1996). Examples of protein-based fat replacers are Simplesse, Dairy-lo and Veri-lo and fat-based replacers include Caprenin, Olean and Salatrim (Warshaw *et al.*, 1996). Olestra, a fat-based substitute prepared from sucrose polyesters is among the most widely studied, and is sold under the brand name Olean. Olestra mimics the physical properties of triacylglycerol, but cannot be digested or absorbed and hence does not contribute to metabolisable energy, proving an ideal zero-calorie replacement of dietary fat (Dye & Blundell, 2002). Trials have demonstrated a dose–response reduction in energy and fat intake during a single test meal containing Olestra, resulting in a reduction in daily fat intake, but Olestra did not influence total daily energy intake (Rolls *et al.*, 1992). Studies ranging in duration from 2 weeks to 9 months, reveal a partial compensation for the reduction in energy intake, nevertheless, weight loss and reduction in body fat was achieved (Bray *et al.*, 2002; Roy *et al.*, 2002).

16.6 Summary and conclusions

Overall, the initial studies investigating the potential of Olibra™ fat emulsion to extend satiety and limit food intake reveal promising results, at least in the short term. The reduced food intake following consumption of yoghurt containing this emulsion indicates that it has potential as a functional food to assist in the control of obesity. Furthermore, compensation for reduction in energy intakes was not evident within the 24 h period subsequent to the test days. A dose–response paradigm, indicating an increase in the effects of the Olibra™ fat emulsion with increasing dose levels, was evident within a mixed-sex sample. In fact, the lowest emulsion dose investigated (5 g) produced significant effects, suggesting that even lower doses may be effective (Burns *et al.*, 2002). Interestingly, varying responses to this fat emulsion were not only observed between body sizes but also between sexes.

At this stage it is important not to over-interpret these results for a number of reasons. Firstly, the studies demonstrating a reduction in energy have been short-term studies, in which food intakes were accurately assessed up to 8 h post-consumption, and relying on self-reported intakes thereafter. Effects of prolonged use of this emulsion in regards to compensation for energy reduction or habituation must be established. Secondly, if lower food intake is sustained in the medium term, it is probable that this is not an effective therapy for the general population. People whose eating behaviour is in accordance with physiological appetite cues are likely to reap the benefits of the emulsion and, as with most weight loss strategies, it is likely to be a slow process even in these individuals. However, as characteristics of responders and non-responders are yet to be confirmed, it is probable that non-responders have a greater need for assistance in controlling food intake. Finally, and most importantly, it is unclear whether the reduction in food intake will be reflected in body weight reduction and subsequently in modification of risk factors for diseases associated with obesity.

The burgeoning rates of obesity clearly indicate that there is a huge market for functional foods with the ability to regulate body weight. The opportunity and need for collaboration between academia and industry for the development of such functional foods have been highlighted (Dye & Blundell, 2002; Hill & Peters, 2002). Indeed, the success of these novel products will inevitably be revolutionary in regards to the treatment of obesity among individuals who respond to such treatments, however, it would be naïve to assume that this strategy alone would be able to control obesity. Other important factors associated with body weight, such as appropriate food choices and physical activity, should not be ignored. Therefore, the ultimate affirmation of the Olibra™ emulsion is likely to be as an adjunct to other lifestyle changes in the treatment and management of obesity.

16.7 Sources of further information

For more information visit www.lipid.se

16.8 References

ARMAND M, BOREL P, YTHIER P, DUTOT G, MELIN C, SENFT M, LAFONT H & LAIRON D (1992) Effects of droplet size, triacylglycerol composition, and calcium on the hydrolysis of complex emulsions by pancreatic lipase: an in vitro study. *Journal of Nutritional Biochemistry* **3**, 333–341.

BLUNDELL JE & MACDIARMID JI (1997) Fat as a risk factor for overconsumption: satiation, satiety, and patterns of eating. *Journal of the American Dietetic Association* **97**, Suppl., S63–S69.

BLUNDELL JE & TREMBLAY A (1995) Appetite control and energy (fuel) balance. *Nutrition Research Reviews* **8**, 225–242.

BLUNDELL JE, LAWTON CL, COTTON JR & MACDIARMID JI (1996) Control of human appetite: implications for the intake of dietary fat. *Annual Review of Nutrition* **16**, 285–319.

BRAY GA & POPKIN BM (1998) Dietary fat intake does affect obesity! *American Journal of Clinical Nutrition* **68**, 1157–1173.

BRAY GA, LOVEJOY JC, MOST-WINDHAUSER M, SMITH SR, VOLAUFOVA J, DENKINS Y, DE JONGE L, ROOD J, LEFEVRE M, ELDRIDGE AL & PETERS JC (2002) A 9-mo randomized clinical trial comparing fat-substituted and fat-reduced diets in healthy obese men: the Ole Study. *American Journal of Clinical Nutrition* **76**, 928–934.

BURNS AA, LIVINGSTONE MBE, WELCH RW, DUNNE A, ROBSON PJ, LINDMARK L, REID CA, MULLANEY U & ROWLAND IR (2000) Short-term effects of yoghurt containing a novel fat emulsion on energy and macronutrient intakes in non-obese subjects. *International Journal of Obesity* **24**, 1419–1425.

BURNS AA, LIVINGSTONE MBE, WELCH RW, DUNNE A, REID CA & ROWLAND IR (2001) The effects of yoghurt containing a novel fat emulsion on energy and macronutrient intakes in non-overweight, overweight and obese subjects. *International Journal of Obesity* **25**, 1487–1496.

BURNS AA, LIVINGSTONE MBE, WELCH RW, DUNNE A & ROWLAND IR (2002) Dose-response effects of a novel fat emulsion (Olibra™) on energy and macronutrient intakes up to 36 h post-consumption. *European Journal of Clinical Nutrition* **56**, 368–377.

COTTON JR, BURLEY VJ, WESTSTRATE JA & BLUNDELL JE (1994) Dietary fat and appetite: similarities and differences in the satiating effect of meals supplemented with either fat or carbohydrate. *Journal of Human Nutrition and Dietetics* **7**, 11–24.

DE CASTRO JM & DE CASTRO ES (1989) Spontaneous meal patterns of humans: influence of the presence of other people. *American Journal of Clinical Nutrition* **50**, 237–247.

DYE L & BLUNDELL J (2002) Functional foods: psychological and behavioural functions. *British Journal of Nutrition* **88**, Suppl. 2, S187–S211.

FLINT A, RABEN A, ASTRUP A & HOLST JJ (1998) Glucagon-like peptide 1 promotes satiety and suppresses energy intake in humans. *Journal of Clinical Investigation* **101**, 515–520.

FRENCH S (2004) Effects of dietary fat and carbohydrate on appetite vary depending upon site and structure. *British Journal of Nutrition* **92**, Suppl. 1, S23–S26.

FRENCH S, MUTUMA S, FRANCIS J, READ N & MEIJER G (1998) The effect of fatty acid composition on intestinal satiety in man. *International Journal of Obesity* **22**, Suppl. 3, S82.

FRENCH SJ (1999) The effects of specific nutrients on the regulation of feeding behaviour in human subjects. *Proceedings of the Nutrition Society* **58**, 533–540.

GREEN SM & BLUNDELL JE (1996) Effect of fat- and sucrose-containing foods on the size of eating episodes and energy intake in lean dietary restrained and unrestrained females: potential for causing overconsumption. *European Journal of Clinical Nutrition* **50**, 625–635.

HEITMANN BL, LISSNER L & OSLER M (2000) Do we eat less fat, or just report so? *International Journal of Obesity* **24**, 435–442.

HILL JO & PETERS JC (2002) Biomarkers and functional foods for obesity and diabetes. *British Journal of Nutrition* **88**, Suppl. 2, S213–S218.

JIN H, CAI L, LEE K, CHANG T, LI P, WAGNER D & CHEY WY (1993) A physiological role of peptide YY on exocrine pancreatic secretion in rats. *Gastroenterology* **105**, 208–215.

JUNG HK, KIM DY & MOON IH (2003) Effects of gender and menstrual cycle on colonic transit time in healthy subjects. *Korean Journal of Internal Medicine* **18**, 181–186.

LAWTON CL (1998) Regulation of energy and fat intakes and body weight: the role of fat substitutes. *British Journal of Nutrition* **80**, 3–4.

LAWTON CL, DELARGY HJ, BROCKMAN J, SMITH FC & BLUNDELL JE (2000) The degree of saturation of fatty acids influences post-ingestive satiety. *British Journal of Nutrition* **83**, 473–482.

LIN HC, ZHAO X & WANG L (1996) Jejunal brake. Inhibition of intestinal transit by fat in the proximal small intestine. *Digestive Diseases and Sciences* **41**, 326–329.

LIN HC, ZHAO X & WANG L (1997) Intestinal transit is more potently inhibited by fat in the distal (ileal brake) than in the proximal (jejunal brake) gut. *Digestive Diseases and Sciences* **42**, 19–25.

LIN L, CHEN J & YORK DA (1997) Chronic ICV enterostatin preferentially reduced fat intake and lowered body weight. *Peptides* **18**, 657–661.

LIVINGSTONE MBE, PRENTICE AM, STRAIN JJ, COWARD WA, BLACK AE, BARKER ME, MCKENNA PG & WHITEHEAD RG (1990) Accuracy of weighed dietary records in studies of diet and health. *British Medical Journal* **300**, 708–712.

LLUCH A, KING NA & BLUNDELL JE (2000) No energy compensation at the meal following exercise in dietary restrained and unrestrained women. *British Journal of Nutrition* **84**, 219–225.

MACFARLANE A, KINSMAN R, READ NW & BLOOM SR (1983) The ileal brake: ileal fat slows small bowel transit and gastric emptying in man. *Gut* **24**, A471–A472.

MACINTOSH CG, ANDREWS JM, JONES KL, WISHART JM, MORRIS HA, JANSEN JBMJ, MORLEY JE, HOROWITZ M & CHAPMAN IM (1999) Effects of age on concentrations of plasma cholecystokinin, glucagon-like peptide 1, and peptide YY and their relation to appetite and pyloric motility. *American Journal of Clinical Nutrition* **69**, 999–1006.

MADSEN JL (1992) Effects of gender, age, and body mass index on gastrointestinal transit times. *Digestive Diseases and Sciences* **37**, 1548–1553.

MAKI KC, DAVIDSON MH, TSUSHIMA R, MATSUO N, TOKIMITSU I, UMPOROWICZ DM, DICKLIN MR, FOSTER GS, INGRAM KA, ANDERSON BD, FROST SD & BELL M (2002) Consumption of diacylglycerol oil as part of a reduced-energy diet enhances loss of body weight and fat in comparison with consumption of a triacylglycerol control oil. *American Journal of Clinical Nutrition* **76**, 1230–1236.

MEIER R, BEGLINGER C, DEDERDING JP, MEYER-WYSS B, FUMAGALLI M, ROWEDDER A, TURBERG Y & BRIGNOLI R (1995) Influence of age, gender, hormonal status and smoking habits on colonic transit time. *Neurogastroenterology and Motility* **7**, 235–238.

NASLUND E, GUTNIAK M, SKOGAR S, ROSSNER S & HELLSTROM PM (1998) Glucagon-like peptide 1 increases the period of postprandial satiety and slows gastric emptying in obese men. *American Journal of Clinical Nutrition* **68**, 525–530.

NASLUND E, BARKELING B, KING N, GUTNIAK M, BLUNDELL JE, HOLST JJ, ROSSNER S & HELLSTROM PM (1999) Energy intake and appetite are suppressed by glucagon-like peptide-1 (GLP-1) in obese men. *International Journal of Obesity* **23**, 304–311.

PIRONI L, STANGHELLINI V, MIGLIOLI M, CORINALDESI R, DE GIORGIO R, RUGGERI E, TOSETTI C, POGGIOLI G, MORSELLI LABATE AM, MONETTI N, GOZZETTI G, BARBARA L & GO VLW (1993) Fat-induced ileal brake in humans: a dose-dependent phenomenon correlated to the plasma levels of peptide YY. *Gastroenterology* **105**, 733–739.

POPPITT SD, McCORMACK D & BUFFENSTEIN R (1998) Short-term effects of macronutrient preloads on appetite and energy intake in lean women. *Physiology and Behaviour* **64**, 279–285.

ROLLS BJ (1985) Experimental analyses of the effects of variety in a meal on human feeding. *American Journal of Clinical Nutrition* **42**, 932–939.

ROLLS BJ, GNIZAK N, SUMMERFELT A & LASTER LJ (1988) Food intake in dieters and nondieters after a liquid meal containing medium-chain triglycerides. *American Journal of Clinical Nutrition* **48**, 66–71.

ROLLS BJ, PIRRAGLIA PA, JONES MB & PETERS JC (1992) Effects of olestra, a noncaloric fat substitute, on daily energy and fat intakes in lean men. *American Journal of Clinical Nutrition* **56**, 84–92.

ROLLS BJ, MORRIS EL & ROE LS (2002) Portion size of food affects energy intake in normal-weight and overweight men and women. *American Journal of Clinical Nutrition* **76**, 1207–1213.

ROY HJ, MOST MM, SPARTI A, LOVEJOY JC, VOLAUFOVA J, PETERS JC & BRAY GA (2002) Effect on body weight of replacing dietary fat with olestra for two or ten weeks in healthy men and women. *Journal of the American College of Nutrition* **21**, 259–267.

SORENSEN LB, MOLLER P, FLINT A, MARTENS M & RABEN A (2003) Effect of sensory perception of foods on appetite and food intake: a review of studies on humans. *International Journal of Obesity* **27**, 1152–1166.

SPILLER RC, TROTMAN IF, HIGGINS BE, GHATEI MA, GRIMBLE GK, LEE YC, BLOOM SR, MISIEWICZ JJ & SILK DBA (1984) The ileal brake – inhibition of jejunal motility after ileal fat perfusion in man. *Gut* **25**, 365–374.

STROEBELE N & DE CASTRO JM (2004) Effect of ambience on food intake and food choice. *Nutrition* **20**, 821–838.

STUBBS RJ & HARBRON CG (1996) Covert manipulation of the ratio of medium- to long-chain triglycerides in isoenergetically dense diets: effect on food intake in *ad libitum* feeding men. *International Journal of Obesity* **20**, 435–444.

STUBBS RJ, HARBRON CG, MURGATROYD PR & PRENTICE AM (1995a) Covert manipulation of dietary fat and energy density: effect on substrate flux and food intake in men eating ad libitum. *American Journal of Clinical Nutrition* **62**, 316–329.

STUBBS RJ, RITZ P, COWARD WA & PRENTICE AM (1995b) Covert manipulation of the ratio of dietary fat to carbohydrate and energy density: effect on food intake and energy balance in free-living men eating *ad libitum*. *American Journal of Clinical Nutrition* **62**, 330–337.

VAN WYMELBEKE V, HIMAYA A, LOUIS-SYLVESTRE J & FANTINO M (1998) Influence of medium-chain and long-chain triacylglycerols on the control of food intake in men. *American Journal of Clinical Nutrition* **68**, 226–234.

WARSHAW H, FRANZ M, POWERS MA & WHEELER M (1996) Fat replacers: their use in foods and role in diabetes medical nutrition therapy. *Diabetes Care* **19**, 1294–1301.

WEBBER AJ, KING SC & MEISELMAN HL (2004) Effects of social interaction, physical environment and food choice freedom on consumption in a meal-testing environment. *Appetite* **42**, 115–118.

WELCH I, SAUNDERS K & READ NW (1985) Effect of ileal and intravenous infusions of fat emulsions on feeding and satiety in human volunteers. *Gastroenterology* **89**, 1293–1297.

WELCH I, SEPPLE CP & READ NW (1988) Comparisons of the effects on satiety and eating behaviour of infusion of lipid into the different regions of the small intestine. *Gut* **29**, 306–311.

Part III

Using polyunsaturated and other modified fatty acids in food products

17

Developing products with modified fats

E. Flöter and A. Bot, Unilever Research and Development Vlaardingen, The Netherlands

17.1 Introduction

A food company can only have a sustainable business provided consumers buy its products repeatedly. No matter how exquisite the technology behind the manufacturing, no matter how subtle the microstructure of the product, it is the consumer who decides whether a newly developed product is a success or a failure. Surprisingly, most textbooks on food products digress extensively on the manufacturing and the microstructure of products, spend possibly a few paragraphs on their perception, but almost ignore the factors that will be the most apparent to the consumer at the moment of purchase or use. This chapter intends to avoid that pitfall by inverting the traditional order from molecular to macroscopic scale in which this type of text is usually written. Instead, this chapter discusses spread products in the reverse order of the supply chain, starting from the supermarket perspective. The elaboration of the technical issues that a food manufacturer faces to make consumers buy its product is concluded with a specific focus on issues that crop up when aiming for improvement of the fat composition of products.

17.1.1 In the supermarket

The shelves of the supermarket contain a wide range of spreads and shallow frying products. Apart from marketing-related external design aspects, it will be apparent that these products come mainly in three different packaging formats: wrappers, tubs and bottles. A look at the history of margarine and the development of packaging material illustrates from where these formats emerge. It was in the 1860s that French Emperor Louis Napoleon III offered a prize to anyone who could make a satisfactory substitute for butter. He was interested in an affordable new food suitable for use by the armed forces and the lower classes. The French chemist Hippolyte Mège-Mouriés invented such a substance and called it oleomargarine. Its short form 'margarine' evolved to become the generic term for such products. The product of Mège-Mouriés was based on edible tallow, which, when combined with butyrin and water, made a cheap, more-or-less palatable butter substitute.

Historically, paper wrappers were the cheapest packaging materials available for branded products, with foils as a more expensive alternative. As modern plastics did not exist, the products were designed to be physically stable in such packaging. This required the product to be quite firm. Since margarine was originally introduced as a cheap alternative to butter, which is quite firm too, this was not considered to be a problem, although it did affect the spreadability of the product in a negative way. In the second half of the twentieth century, however, the introduction of the refrigerator in the kitchen and the invention of alternative versatile packaging materials such as polyethylene (PET) and polypropylene (PP) introduced many possibilities for new products. More or less simultaneously new views on the role of specific fatty acids in nutrition and health received attention. In particular the roles of saturated, unsaturated and polyunsaturated fatty acids were clearly formulated (e.g. Keys *et al.*, 1965). To generate the desired specific health benefits, an increase in the level of unsaturated fatty acids in products was necessary. This change in product formulation towards preferred usage of liquid oils instead of fats made the wrapper or stick format less suitable. Initially special products rich in polyunsaturated fatty acids relating to blood cholesterol control were sold in tins. Eventually plastic tubs were introduced that could support the product, especially during stacking of products in warehouses and on supermarket shelves. The advantage of plastic tubs is that their barrier properties against external influences can be tuned much easier to the specific needs of a certain product.

The introduction of softer products also allowed separation into the two main product use categories that are available today: a spreading product and a shallow frying product. Although these functionalities were historically provided via multipurpose wrapper products the search for healthier alternatives led to the introduction of a new product format, liquid margarine for cooking packed in a bottle, whereas the spreading product is best provided in tub format. By tailoring the products to a specific consumer use, the manufacturer increases the likelihood that its products will be purchased by the consumer.

17.1.2 In your fridge

When comparing butter and margarine, it is not only the origin of their raw materials that differs (animal source for butter, vegetable for most current margarines), but the shelf-life of these products also differs significantly. Butter, even when stored in the refrigerator, tends to develop a rancid note rather quickly. Margarine or spreads, in contrast, can typically be stored for periods of months, usually around three. This longer shelf-life improves consumer convenience because the purchased product does not have to be consumed quickly. As spreading products are exposed to changing environments, at least migrating between the kitchen table and the refrigerator, the product should also be able to withstand a certain amount of temperature cycling. Keepability of products involves a number of aspects: safety of the product, avoidance of spoilage of the product, and textural and taste stability of the product.

17.1.3 During application

On the table

The true test of margarine or a spread product is when it is spread on a slice of bread. The product appearance, the ease of scraping or scooping it out of the tub and the actual ease of spreading can be directly linked to the product properties. The ease of spreading on bread or toast depends on the yield stress of the margarine, which in a first approximation is proportional to the square of the solid fat content (SFC) of the fat composition used.

The SFC depends on temperature. Consequently the fat composition has to be chosen carefully in relation to the envisaged product application and temperature exposure during the product life. As mentioned before the SFC at refrigeration temperature for spreading margarine is typically lower than for butter. This explains the difference in direct ease of spreading. At higher temperatures (ambient, depending on the country of use, can vary between 20 and 35 ºC) the amount of solid fat must be sufficient to guarantee the integrity of the product. Products suited for baking need to satisfy other criteria. They have to contribute some structure to the dough during the preparation process. Therefore these products are typically characterised by increased firmness. This necessitates (in particular for puff-pastry baking) specific profiles of the solid fat content as a function of temperature (de Bruijne and Bot, 1999; Bot *et al.*, 2003). The melting point of triacylglycerols, the primary molecular species present in fats and oils, is directly linked to their three fatty acid residues attached to the glycerol backbone. Triacylglycerols containing unsaturated fatty acids tend to have a lower melting point than those based on saturated fatty acids (Garti and Sato, 1988). Therefore the SFC of a healthy fat blend is lower, and consequently the product is softer.

Apart from instabilities caused by the melting behaviour of the fat composition, there are other instabilities caused by droplet coalescence resulting from shear, especially during spreading of so-called low-fat spreads. The shear forces applied during spreading of low-fat spreads lead to coalescence of the water droplets in the product and subsequent exudation of water from the product structure. This product defect is prevented by structuring of the water phase in order to give it a yield stress, e.g. by gelatin, and thus prevent coalescence of the droplets.

In the mouth

Apart from the product properties at the temperature of application, also the melting behaviour will be of importance. A spread that is firm in the tub, should not be firm in the mouth. This property can also be tuned by choosing a proper melting profile for the fat blend that is used in a product. The melting profile is determined by the choice of raw materials used in the fat blend. Ideally, the SFC of the fat composition would be unaffected by temperature in the range below the application temperature (to avoid sensitivity to temperature cycling), and melt relatively steeply in the interval between application temperature and mouth temperature (Bot *et al.*, 2003). Practical limitations, including the composition of available raw materials, mean that this ideal situation is not really achievable and some kind of compromise has to be designed. However, it remains essential that the fat crystals melt or dissolve in the mouth as a consequence of temperature and mastication, resulting in the disintegration of the spread product. If this is not the case the product will result in a waxy mouthfeel, insufficient flavour release, and a dry sensation due to the absence of oil lubrication.

In the frying pan

The temperature in the frying pan is much higher than in the mouth and, independent of the type of fat composition used in the spread's formulation, product melting and product disintegration are achieved relatively quickly. However, in order to achieve the application temperatures of 150 °C and above, it is necessary to evaporate the water released from the product. For obvious reasons, this takes longer the lower the fat, and higher the water content of the product. This causes the typical sizzle accompanied by slight foam formation (Mellema and Benjamins, 2004). Products specifically designed for shallow frying applications contain combinations of lecithin and salt in order to reduce the spitting of hot fat, the so-called spattering.

17.2 Product characteristics

17.2.1 Texture and texture stability

Consumers expect margarine to be quite stable over shelf-life, unlike products such as bread which have a completely different texture when eaten fresh or after a few days. Margarine should not change during storage, or as a result of mild temperature cycling as experienced during transport or consumer use. Spreadability is the most apparent physical property that could change and is intimately related to the firmness of the product. As already mentioned, the fat crystal network predominantly determines the firmness of margarine.

Fat-continuous spread products such as margarine (80% fat level) and halvarines (40% fat level) are best characterised as suspension–emulsion systems. A dispersed water phase is embedded into a fat crystal network. This network forms a sponge-like structure that is filled with oil. This is illustrated in

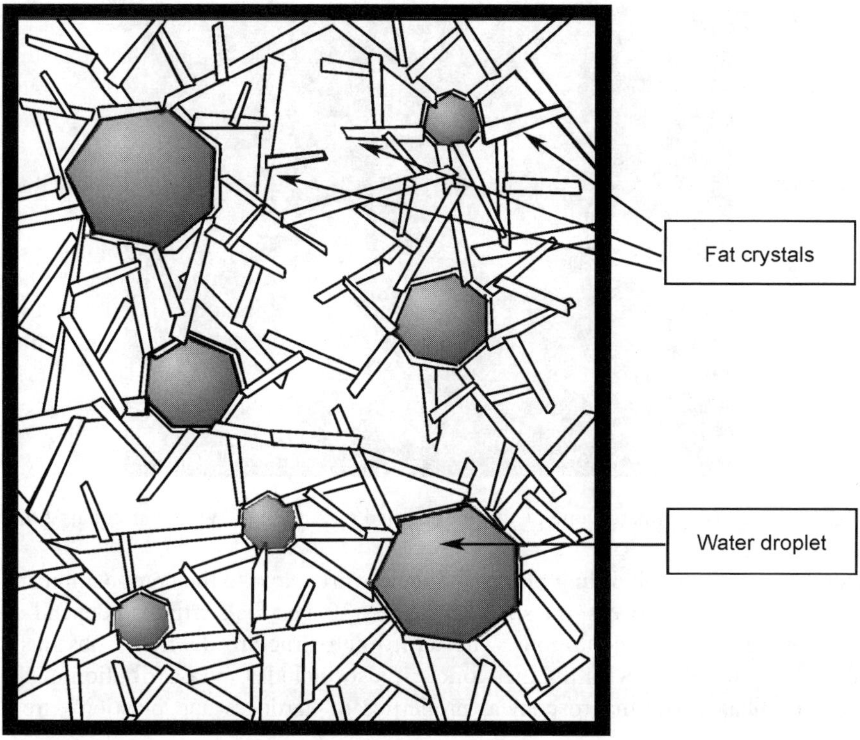

Fig. 17.1 Schematic representation of spread culture. Water droplets (dark grey circles) are covered by fat crystals (white sticks); fat crystals form a sponge-like structure that binds the liquid oil (light grey background).

Fig 17.1 and 17.2. From the schematic representation it can be appreciated that the task of the solid fat material is twofold: to stabilise the water droplet surface and to build the sponge-like structure that is able to bind the oil through adhesive forces. The electron micrograph illustrates that for the depicted 60% fat spread the individual droplets are located very close to each other.

The contribution of the solid fat to the perceived macroscopic product structure can be described in a hierarchical fashion. This is illustrated in Fig. 17.3. The molecular composition of the mixture of fats and oils determines the structuring potential. Different compounds have melting points at different temperatures, and the composition of the mixture translates these into the solidification behaviour of the final fat blend. However, fats have the ability to crystallise in at least three different molecular arrangements in the crystalline structure. This ability is called polymorphism. The different structures have different physical properties and thus different solidification behaviour. Which form appears and how stable it is depends on the composition of the mixture and the actual crystallisation process (Sato, 1999, 2001). Besides the organisation of the molecules in the crystal, the size and shape of the crystals are important, as

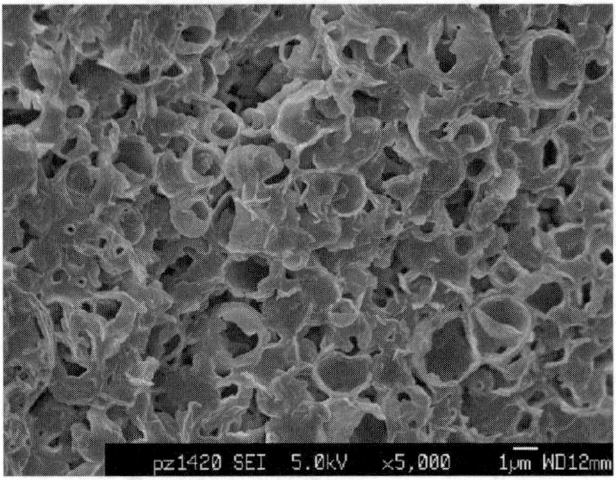

Fig. 17.2 Electron microscope picture of de-oiled 60% spread. White bar equals 1 μm.

they form the actual building blocks of the network. Next to the composition and the crystallisation process, the size and shape of the crystals will also depend on the storage time and conditions. The term microstructure describes obviously more than the pure crystalline network – it also includes the distribution of the aqueous phase. The macroscopical properties of hardness and plasticity are a

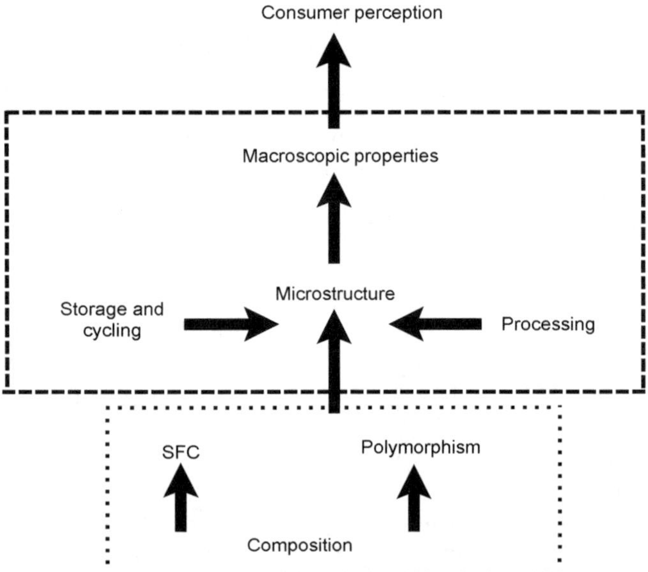

Fig. 17.3 Hierarchical influences on fat-based structural aspects perceived by the consumer. Boxes indicate main influences.

direct derivative of the microstructure and are important determinants of the consumer perception.

A few possible sources of instability in the product are related to the desired product structural attributes, described above. Significant supercooling of the fat blend in the spread after processing may lead to uncontrolled crystallisation of the hardstock in the tub. This leads to an increase in firmness over time, which is undesirable because product properties should be retained over the stated shelf-life of the product. Furthermore, it could lead to the formation of large crystals in the product, which may be detectable by the consumer, when crystals of 20 μm or more in size are formed. Other defects are re-crystallisation defects, such as the formation of the more stable β-crystal polymorphs from the typical β' modification encountered in margarine ('sandiness'). Alternatively, large crystals in the β polymorph and in triple fatty acid chain length stacking can occur in fat blends rich in symmetric disaturated and monounsaturated triacylglycerols such as POP, POS and SOS (de Bruijne and Bot, 1999; Watanabe *et al.*, 1992). Here P stands for palmitic acid, S for stearic acid and O for oleic acid. This phenomenon is referred to as 'tropical graininess'.

Other changes in the product texture may occur as a result of temperature cycling during storage. Repeated dissolution and precipitation of crystalline fat will lead to a coarsening of the fat crystals, and an increase of 'primary' bonds between fat crystallites at the expense of 'secondary' bonds. Secondary bonds are associated with van der Waals interactions between crystals and give rise to plastic rheology of the spread, whereas primary bonds refer to sintered crystals which give rise to brittle structures (Bot *et al.*, 2003).

17.2.2 Appearance

The appearance of margarine is one of the attributes by which a consumer will determine the quality of the product. In general, a homogeneous product is preferred, and deviations are considered to be defects. A well-known example is oil exudation from the continuous phase in the emulsion, especially if the fat crystal network is too coarse or too sparse. The first indicates a possible processing problem, the second is a general sensitivity that occurs in products using relatively soft fat blends. As is explained by the Darcy law (Darcy, 1856), both large pores and many pores will promote oil exudation (de Bruijne and Bot, 1999). Traditionally, oil exudation is a defect that may occur with wrapped products that are stacked during storage in the warehouse. Modern softer margarine, however, is potentially even more sensitive to this phenomenon because the fat crystal network is so much more delicate in these products. Another well-known defect is the development of more intense yellow coloured spots in the product as a result of local drying.

17.2.3 Safety and properties of the emulsion

It goes without saying that products should not constitute a health risk to the consumer, whether the product is consumed directly or after storage. This is largely under the control of the manufacturer, by attention to strict specification on ingredients, and via a hazard analysis and critical control points analysis (HACCP) of the manufacturing processes. Furthermore, the barrier properties of the packaging and the hygiene of the filling operation are important to ensure that no product is left on the exterior of the packaging. However, safety is also in the hands of the consumer, i.e. the extent to which the instructions on the package regarding storage and usage are complied with by the consumer.

The best way to avoid any product safety issues, however, is to make sure that the product cannot become a safety issue in the first place. For the products under consideration in this chapter, outgrowth of micro-organisms is the main danger. The alarming aspect of microbiological growth is that given enough nutrients and the potential for growth, a minor contamination of the product can potentially make a product unsafe over time. Since food products tend to contain sufficient nutrients for microbiological growth, starvation is not an option and other means of prevention of microbiological growth should be introduced in order to ensure safety of the product. There are two ways to do this. Microbiological growth occurs in an aqueous environment, and the conditions in the aqueous phase can be made unpleasant for any micro-organisms, e.g. by including preservatives such as sorbate, dropping the pH or by having high salt levels, or combinations of these. Another route is compartmentalisation of the aqueous phase. Margarine-related products mainly depend on the latter strategy to achieve their microbial stability: by dispersing the aqueous phase in small droplets in a continuous oil phase, any potential contamination cannot grow to become a danger to the consumer. There are two important requirements. The water droplets need to be small enough, typically below 7 μm (Verrips and Zaalberg, 1980; Verrips *et al.*, 1980), and the droplets need to remain that small during storage. Small, (kinetically) stable droplets can be found in so-called emulsions, systems of intimately mixed phases that are immiscible on a molecular length scale. Margarine would classify as a water-in-oil or w/o emulsion. Droplet size depends on the power input during the emulsification process and droplet size reduces with increasing power input:

$$D_{\min} \sim \epsilon^{-2/5} \gamma^{3/5} \rho^{-1.5} \qquad 17.1$$

where ϵ is the energy density, γ the interfacial tension and ρ the density of the continuous phase and assuming turbulent break-up for which the final droplet is similar to the size of the energy-bearing eddies (Walstra, 2005). Typical values encountered in practice are $10^4 < \epsilon/(\mathrm{W/m^3}) < 10^{12}$ and $1 < \gamma/(\mathrm{mN/m}) < 40$. Tools to change the droplet size in practice are the emulsification device to change ϵ and the addition of emulsifiers to change γ.

In a factory-scale environment, a range of emulsification devices can be found: shear mixers, colloid mills, pin stirrers, high-pressure homogenisers. For each application, equipment is selected that gives just about the right droplet size, as preparing smaller droplets than actually required increases the energy cost, and thus results in a competitive disadvantage in the marketplace. For margarine production, usually a combination of scraped surface heat exchangers

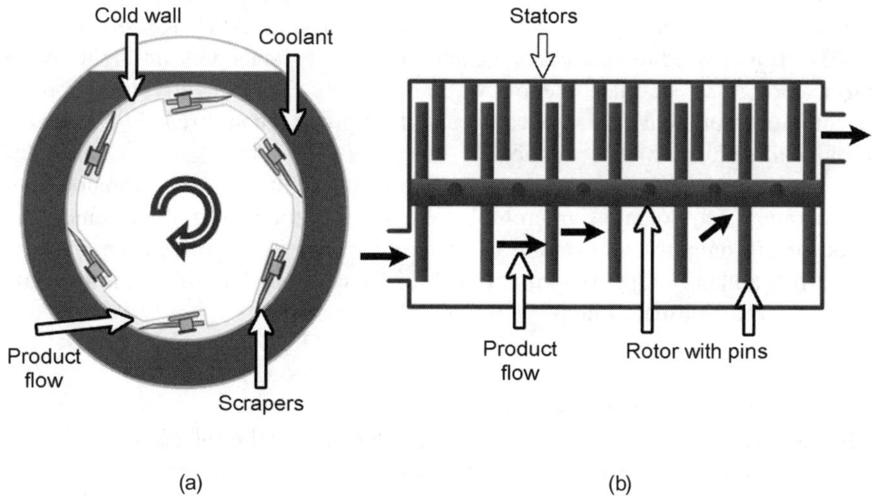

Fig. 17.4 Schematic representation of main votator units. (a) Cross-sectional cut of scraped surface heat exchanger (also A-unit). (b) Axial cut of pin-stirrer or kneading unit (C-unit).

and pin stirrers is selected which is incorporated in a so-called votator (see Fig. 17.4). This enables the production of 3–7 μm water droplets for a regular margarine composition. For low-fat products the droplet sizes are often in excess of this range and consequently other measures of preservation have to be taken.

The formation of small droplets is facilitated by the presence of small molecular weight emulsifiers, such as mono- and diacylglycerols, food acid esters of monoacylglycerols, sorbitan esters, polysorbate, polyglycerol polyricinoleate (PGPR) and lecithin, which all decrease the w/o interfacial tension γ. A typical γ_{ow} for a water–triacylglycerol interface is 30 mN/m, but this drops to values in the range of 3 mN/m in the presence of small molecular weight emulsifiers. By choosing the emulsifier mix one can manipulate the stability of the emulsion. Primarily this is the stability of the emulsion, but secondly emulsifiers with a tendency to form oil-in-water emulsions promote the disintegration process once the emulsion-stabilising solid fat starts melting in the mouth. A typical example for the latter is whey protein.

The stability of the emulsion is further helped by the formation of fat crystals during margarine processing (fat crystals are quite efficient in emulsions, and it is possible to make a margarine without having to use emulsifiers in the recipe). Fat crystals help to stabilise w/o emulsions by so-called Pickering stabilisation (Pickering, 1907). Fat crystals adsorb at the oil water interface. Any emulsifier promotes the formation of an emulsion in which the emulsifier is located predominantly in the continuous phase, as described by the Bancroft rule (Bancroft, 1913), and this results in the case of fat crystals in the formation of a w/o emulsion. Temperature cycling may have a negative effect on emulsion stability and thus on droplet size (Hodge and Rousseau, 2003; Rousseau *et al.*, 2003). At increased temperatures the amount of fat crystals present might not be large enough to stabilise the oil–water interface. Consequently the droplets become unstable and coalescence occurs. This process could reduce the microbiological stability of the product.

Note that the occurrence of condensation on top of the product during cooling or storage is a potential microbiological threat, because it undermines the concept of compartmentalisation of the water phase in the margarine. Process (cold-fill) and packaging (gap in the seal for the covering leaf of the tub to allow water vapour to escape) helps to tackle this problem.

17.2.4 Taste release and stability

The taste and flavour compounds in the product should be released during use. For spreads, this is released during cold use, but for cooking products it could involve release of flavour components at high temperatures as well. Flavour release of components that are dissolved in the oil phase depends mainly on the volatility of the flavour. Very volatile flavours will release easily during use, but could also disappear relatively easily from the flavour cocktail during the shelf-life of the product (which could be reduced by choosing optimal barrier properties of the packaging). The release of such flavours depends mainly on the heating of the product, e.g. in the mouth or in a frying pan. Components that are dissolved in the water phase, such as salt and acids, usually require coalescence or disintegration of the water droplets before they can be perceived. For this type of flavour the heating profile may play a role (in relation to coalescence), but the mixing will be very important as well to allow the water phase of the product to coalesce with the saliva in the mouth (Bot and Pelan, 2000). The typical taste experience for a given product can easily be enhanced through the presence of salt.

Margarine should have a pleasant taste and flavour in application, preferably in the buttery direction, and should deliver this experience over the full shelf-life of the product. Taste and flavour involve a number of separate issues. The taste components interact with taste buds on the tongue and tend to react to relatively stable compounds such as sodium chloride. The flavour components are detected by receptors in the nasal cavity. Therefore, flavours in spreads should have a certain degree of volatility at mouth temperature, whereas flavours in cooking products may be released specifically at high temperatures. The volatility of a flavour could be a complicating factor over the shelf-life of a product, because the escape of part of the components in the flavour cocktail could modify the sensory experience. Apart from this 'physical' change in composition of the flavour cocktail, chemical changes can also occur. Small molecular changes in either the flavour cocktail or even in the chemical composition of the lipid phase, especially through oxidation, may lead to the development of a specific off-taste in the product.

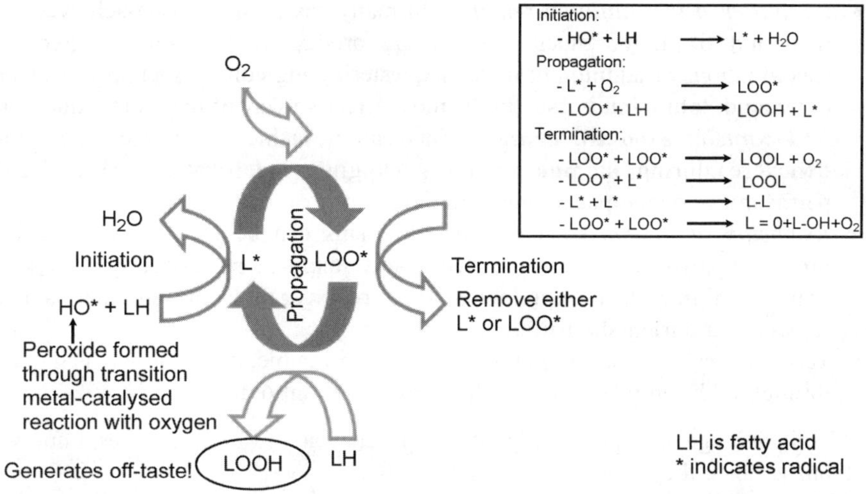

Fig. 17.5 Schematic representation of the pathways of the oxidation process.

Lipid oxidation is a complex three-stage process involving initiation, propagation and termination reactions. Initiation reactions involve light, heat or metal-ion catalysed break-down of peroxides: light can excite oxygen in a reactive singlet state from which it can react immediately with unsaturated fatty acid chain residues, heat and light can induce cleavage of peroxides or fatty acids leading to fatty acid radicals, and metal ions can catalyse a reaction ('autoxidation') in which peroxides are formed also leading to fatty acid radicals. Propagation steps involve the formation of lipohydroperoxides, and are catalysed by the fatty acid radicals. Termination involves reactions between two radicals, and results in the formation of dimers, polymers, ketones and alcohols. The primary products from these reactions do not contribute to the off-flavour of the oil. However, homocyclic and heterocyclic cleavage of unstable radicals or from lipohydroperoxides results in the formation of volatiles such as alkanes, aldehydes and ketones (see e.g. Allen and Hamilton, 1994; Chan, 1987). This is also depicted in Fig. 17.5. The off-taste of oxidised vegetable oils is most often described as rancid or cardboard-like, although a wide pallet of flavours can develop. Triacylglycerols containing polyunsaturated fatty acids (PUFAs) are most sensitive to oxidation, those containing monounsaturated fatty acids (MUFAs) less, and those containing saturated fatty acids (SAFAs) the least. The relative sensitivities of stearic (C18:0), oleic (C18:1), linoleic (C18:2) and linolenic acid (C18:3) to autoxidation have been reported to be ~10^{-4}–10^{-2}, ~1, ~20, ~50, respectively. Thus, unfortunately, healthy fat blends tend to be most sensitive to the formation of off-taste.

Knowledge on the reaction mechanism helps to counteract oxidation in products:

- *Inhibition of the initiation reaction.* In many cases, this can be achieved by reduction of active metal ions in the product, e.g. through ingredient specifications or addition of metal-sequestering ingredients such as EDTA or citric acid. Inhibition is usually the most effective way of reducing oxidation.
- *Reduction of exposure to light.* This can be achieved by reducing light exposure during storage or by packaging specifications (low light permeability of the packaging material).
- *Exclusion of oxygen from the product.* This can be controlled partly by process, partly by packaging with low oxygen permeability. Oxygen scavengers may help if a low amount of oxygen is present that is not replenished during shelf-life.
- *Termination of propagation reaction.* In principle, this can be achieved through addition of so-called 'chain-breaking' antioxidants.

Overall, storage and processing of the product at low temperatures improve stability, since they reduce the oxidation rate.

For margarine, many of these measures are taken. Oil specifications are usually relatively tight, and citric acid or EDTA is often added to low-fat spreads. Since products are stored most of the time in the dark, reduction of light exposure is not frequently exploited. Under typical conditions, the oxygen already present in the product is sufficient to cause oxidation. Other sources of oxygen, such as oxygen from the headspace or from permeation through the packaging material, do not contribute dramatically, as can be demonstrated by simple back-of-the-envelope calculations. The typical solubility of O_2 in oil at ambient temperature and normal partial oxygen pressure is ~30 mg/l oil (the solubility in water is three to five times smaller). Thus, a 500 g tub with 80% fat spread contains ~12 mg or ~10 ml O_2, which equals to the amount of oxygen in 50 ml headspace. The oxygen solubility at fridge temperature is roughly twice that at ambient temperature. The gas permeability of the packaging material (roughly 10^{-17}–10^{-16} $m^3\,m\,m^{-2}\,s^{-1}\,Pa^{-1}$) is typically low enough to prevent seeping in of comparable quantities of oxygen during closed shelf-life, although the fact that margarine packaging tends not to be sealed completely introduces other routes for the oxygen to come in. The use of chain-breaking antioxidants is not common.

An unresolved issue is still whether the microstructure of the emulsion can be used to confine oxidation: dispersion of the oxidising lipid in individual small droplets may increase the number of initiation reactions required to develop a noticeable off-taste. However, in fat-continuous products such as margarine, this is not a viable route.

17.3 Development of nutritionally improved products

In the previous sections the product attributes perceivable by the consumer and the respective underlying processing principles were discussed. In the following the effect of changed product formulations with respect to these attributes is addressed. In terms of optimising the product formulation there are four major directions:

- Reduction of the fat level.
- Minimisation of the content of saturated fats and elimination of *trans* fatty acids.
- Increase of polyunsaturated fatty acids, in particular n-3, EPA and DHA.
- Fortification with other health-relevant ingredients.

17.3.1 Fat reduction

Fat reduction for spread products is equal to an increased level of water in the product. As previously discussed, the water droplets are embedded into the fat crystal network, which stabilises the oil–water interface. With the increased size of this interface, assuming constant droplet sizes, more crystals are needed for its stabilisation. However, combinations of fat levels above 40% and commonly used fat compositions contain enough excess fat crystals for the interface stabilisation. It also deserves mention that for reduced fat products the distance between the individual droplets is dramatically decreased. Taking these two facts into account it is easily understood that low-fat products tend to be more sensitive to temperature challenging. Both droplet coalescence and oil exudation may occur. A common way to improve the stability of the low-fat products is the introduction of structure to the aqueous phase. This can be achieved through a choice from the long list of water-gelling agents. However, the effect of the gelling agent with respect to the disintegration of the product in the mouth has to be considered as well. Additionally, lower fat levels and the incorporation of water phase structuring interfere with the typical manufacturing process. Historically the aqueous phase is dispersed in the warm fat phase prior to the start of the first processing step, cooling. At fat levels below 50%, however, the starting system tends to be water-continuous and the emulsion has to be inverted within the process sequence of cooling and kneading in order to fabricate a fat-continuous product.

17.3.2 Minimising saturated and *trans* fatty acids

The presence of saturated and/or *trans* fatty acids in fat-based products is purely functional. They are the key building blocks to the product structure. As their limited nutritional value is discussed in other chapters of this book, this is not elaborated on here. However, it should be clear that the ultimate ambition is to fabricate products that are solely based on liquid oils. These products should still have the macroscopical properties that are appealing to the consumer. In line with the general consensus of the nutritional quality of saturated fatty acids (Keys *et al.*, 1965) and *trans* fatty acids (Hayakawa *et al.*, 2000), the first priority is currently to eliminate the trans fatty acids from product formulations. Chapter 21 of this book focuses on *trans* fatty acids. *Trans* fatty acids containing fats, as a product from partial hydrogenation, are highly versatile structuring agents. They crystallise quickly, form small crystals, and are fairly resistant to recrystallisation. Typically their elimination is achieved through substitution by carefully chosen structuring fats rich in SAFAs.

There are two sources of saturated fatty acids in the final fat composition, the highly saturated fats that supply structure to the products (hardstock fats) and the liquid oils that contain between 6.8% (canola oil) and 22% (cottonseed oil) SAFAs. Liquid oils account typically for the major fraction of the fat composition, and consequently the use of low SAFA oils is a very effective way to reduce SAFA level in a product. However, the choice of the liquid oil is often constrained by a number of other factors such as the contents of other fatty acids (especially PUFA), local consumer preference and, last but not least, price and availability. The other means to reduce the SAFA contents of the product formulation is a change of the structuring fat, the so-called hardstock. Optimal hardstock fats have a very low solubility, thus most of the added SAFA material is eventually in the solid state. This is best realised by using triacylglycerols containing only SAFAs. However, using only high-melting fully saturated triacylglycerols has an adverse effect on the melting properties of products in the mouth. In optimising this delicate balance, oil modification techniques, such as full hydrogenation, wet and dry fractionation, chemical interesterification, and enzymatic rearrangement in combination with the choice of the right starting material, are all widely used to fabricate superior hardstocks (Bockisch, 1993). As is easily appreciated, the use of these techniques is limited by the additional cost generated and a consumer preference for more natural products. Applying state-of-the-art hardstocks at levels above 10%, levels of saturated fatty acids in the range of 18–25% of the fat composition can currently be achieved.

17.3.3 Increase of nutritionally beneficial fatty acids

The discussion of the implications of increased nutritional value of the fat composition will be limited to increased levels of n-3 fatty polyunsaturated fatty acids (n-3 PUFA) (Wijendran and Hayes, 2004). The first step in formulating products with increased levels of PUFAs is the choice of the oil source. Similar to the approach used in the initial parts of this chapter, consideration of the incorporation of n-3 PUFA into margarine requires a 'reverse engineering' approach. Since a food manufacturer typically wants to claim the delivery of beneficial ingredient through the product, fulfilment of the constraints that allow statements such as 'rich in . . .' or 'a good source of . . .' and so forth on the pack is the starting point for the product design. At the same time the fat levels of the products tend to decrease so that simple mass balance considerations show how much of which raw material needs to be incorporated in the fat composition in order to allow for a claim. At high-fat levels canola oil might be a good source for the delivery of n-3 PUFA in the form of linolenic acid. In contrast to this is the concentration of linolenic acid in canola oil insufficient to deliver n-3 PUFA according to the requirements at reduced fat levels.

For this type of product, sources such as linseed oil need to be considered. However, these oils and also the resulting fat compositions have increased concentrations of highly unsaturated fatty acids so that they are very prone to oxidation. With reference to Section 17.2.4 it is obvious that the susceptibility to oxidation of eicosapentaenoic acid and docosahexaenoic acid (with five and six double bonds respectively) derived mainly from marine origin is much higher than for n-3 linolenic acid (with just three double bonds). To ensure best quality products with an enhanced nutritional profile it is thus necessary to take maximum precautions with respect to the presence of pro-oxidants. This does imply that the oil rich in the highly sensitive fatty acids must be treated with maximum care and that the product is specified for lowest levels of metals and other pro-oxidants.

17.3.4 Fortified products

The enhancement of the nutritional profile of fat-based products does not stop at improved compositions of the fat phase. Products with all kinds of fortification, ranging from sterols via probiotics to minerals such as calcium can be found in the marketplace. Depending on the type of fortification one can expect a change in the consumer-perceivable attributes of the product. Sterols or sterolesters added for reducing blood cholesterol levels (Katan *et al.*, 2003) might change the viscosity of the lipid phase of the product, with possible implications on the manufacturing process and the oral perception. Other ingredients, such as probiotics dissolving in the aqueous phase, do not impact directly on the product performance. However, if they contain pro-oxidants, their effect on sensitive fat compositions can be dramatic. On addition of nutritionally relevant ingredients in solid form, two aspects have to be taken into account: (i) the increased wear of manufacturing equipment due to abrasion and (ii) the possible oral detection of solid particles if their size is above a threshold level of 20 μm if they do not disintegrate quickly in the mouth.

17.4 Summary

Designing products with nutritionally enhanced characteristics is a challenge. Successful products need to deliver a credible health benefit and be good products with respect to their perceivable properties. The benchmark for the perceivable properties that can be assessed by the consumer directly on usage are the generic products. Alternative attempts to provide the consumer with visible cues in healthy products have not yet been successful. The key challenge for the food scientist is thus to significantly change the products in their composition but to at least maintain their primary quality attributes. In practice this means maintaining the product structure and delivering oral melting and taste sensation with a reduced fat phase that contains fewer saturated fatty acids. Additionally it can be expected that almost all nutrition-enhancing ingredients will increase the sensitivity of the product to chemical changes. These have, for obvious reasons, to be kept at a minimum. To achieve this, one either improves the raw material quality and manufacturing practices or takes chemical measures and introduces additional sequestering ingredients to inhibit oxidation.

17.5 References

J.C. ALLEN and R.J. HAMILTON, editors (1994), *Rancidity in Foods*, 3rd edition, Blackie Academic & Professional, Glasgow, UK.

W.D. BANCROFT (1913), Theory of emulsification, *Journal of Physical Chemistry*, **17**, 501–519.

D.W. DE BRUIJNE and A. BOT (1999), Fabricated fat-based foods, in *Food Texture: Measurement and Perception*, editor A.J. Rosenthal, Aspen, Gaithersburg, MD, USA, chapter 7, 185–227.

M. BOCKISCH (1993), *Nahrungsfette und Öle*, Handbuch der Lebensmitteltechnologie, Ulmer Verlag, Stuttgart, Germany.

A. BOT and E.G. PELAN (2000), Food emulsions inside and outside the mouth, *Food Ingredients and Analysis International*, **22**(6), 53–58.

A. BOT, E. FLÖTER, J.G. LAMMERS and E.G. PELAN (2003), Controlling the texture of spreads, in: *Texture in Foods, volume 1: Semi-solid Foods*, editor B.M. McKenna, Woodhead Publishing, Cambridge, UK, Chapter 14, 350–372.

H.W.-S. CHAN (1987), *Autoxidation of Unsaturated Lipids*, Academic Press, London, 1–16.

H. DARCY (1856), *Les Fontaines Publiques de la Ville de Dijon*, Dalmont, Paris.

N. GARTI and K. SATO (1988), *Crystallization and Polymorphism of Fats and Fatty Acids*, Marcel Dekker, New York.

K. HAYAKAWA, Y.Y. LINKO and P. LINKO (2000), The role of *trans* fatty acids in human nutrition, *Journal of Lipid Science and Techology*, **102**, 419–425.

S.M. HODGE and D. ROUSSEAU (2003), Flocculation and coalescence in water-in-oil emulsions stabilized by paraffin wax crystals, *Food Research International*, **36**, 695–702.

M.B. KATAN, S.M. GRUNDY, P. JONES, M. LAW, T. MIETTINEN, R. PAOLETTI *et al.* (2003), Efficacy and safety of plant stanols and sterols in the management of blood cholesterol concentrations, *Mayo Clinic Proceedings*, **78**, 965–978.

A. KEYS, J.T. ANDERSON and F. GRANDE (1965), Serum cholesterol response to changes in the diet, IV. Particular saturated fatty acids in the diet, *Metabolism*, **14**, 776–787.

M. MELLEMA and J. BENJAMINS (2004), Importance of the Marangoni effect in the forming of hot oil with phospholipids, *Colloids and Surfaces A: Physicochemical and Engineering Aspects*, **237**, 113–118.

S.U. PICKERING (1907), Emulsions, *Journal of the Chemical Society*, **91**, 2001–2021.

D. ROUSSEAU, L. ZILNIK, R. KHAN and S.M. HODGE (2003), Dispersed phase destabilisation in table spreads, *Journal of the American Oil Chemists' Society*, **80**, 957–961.

K. SATO (1999), Solidification and phase transformation behaviour of food fats a review, *Fett/Lipid*, **101**, 467–474.

K. SATO (2001), Crystallization behaviour of fats and lipids – a review, *Chemical Engineering Science*, **56**, 2255–2265.

C.T. VERRIPS and J. ZAALBERG (1980), The intrinsic stability of water-in-oil emulsions. 1. Theory, *European Journal of Applied Microbiology and Biotechnology*, **10**, 187–196.

C.T. VERRIPS, D. SMID and A. KERKHOF (1980), The intrinsic stability of water-in-oil emulsions. 2. Experimental, *European Journal of Applied Microbiology and Biotechnology*, **10**, 73–85.

P. WALSTRA (2005), Emulsions, in: *Fundamentals of Interface and Colloid Science, volume V: Soft Colloids*, editor J. Lyklema, Elsevier, Amsterdam, Chapter 8 (equation 8.2.12).

A. WATANABE, I. TASHIMA, N. MATSUZAKI, J. KURASHIGE and K. SATO (1992), On the formation of granular crystals in fat blends containing palm oil, *Journal of the American Oil Chemists' Society*, **69**, 1077–1080.

V. WIJENDRAN and K.C. HAYES (2004), Dietary n-6 and n-3 fatty acid balance and cardiovascular health, *Annual Review of Nutrition*, **24**, 597–615.

18

Using polyunsaturated fatty acids (PUFAs) as functional ingredients

C. Jacobsen and M. Bruni Let, Danish Institute for Fisheries Research, Denmark

18.1 Introduction

During the past 30 years there has been an increasing interest in polyunsaturated fatty acids (PUFAs) for food, nutritional and pharmaceutical applications. This is due to the increasing evidence that PUFAs have a wide range of nutritional benefits in the human body. There are two distinct families of PUFA, namely the n-3 and the n-6 families, and these families cannot be interconverted. The terms 'n-3' and 'n-6' refer to the position of the first double bond in the carbon chain as counted from the methyl terminus. The health benefits of n-3 long chain PUFA have received particular attention during the past decade, and from a nutritional point of view the three most important n-3 PUFAs are α-linolenic acid (LNA, C18:3 n-3), eicosapentaenoic acid (EPA, C20:5 n-3) and docosahexaenoic acid (DHA, C22:6 n-3). The molecular structures of EPA and DHA are shown in Fig. 18.1. The potential health effects of EPA and DHA include reduction of cardiovascular disease risk,[1–3] anti-inflammatory effects including reduction of symptoms of rheumatoid arthritis[4,5] and Crohns disease,[6] and reduction of the risk of certain cancer forms. DHA is particularly important in the development of brain and nervous tissue in the infant.[7]

Particularly, the evidence for the preventive effect of EPA and DHA on cardiovascular disease is strong. This is also demonstrated by the fact that the US Food and Drug Administration (FDA) in September 2004 announced the availability of a qualified health claim for reduced risk of coronary heart disease (CHD) on conventional foods that contain EPA and DHA n-3 fatty acids. This means that the following claim can be used on food products containing EPA and DHA in the US: S*upportive but not conclusive research shows that*

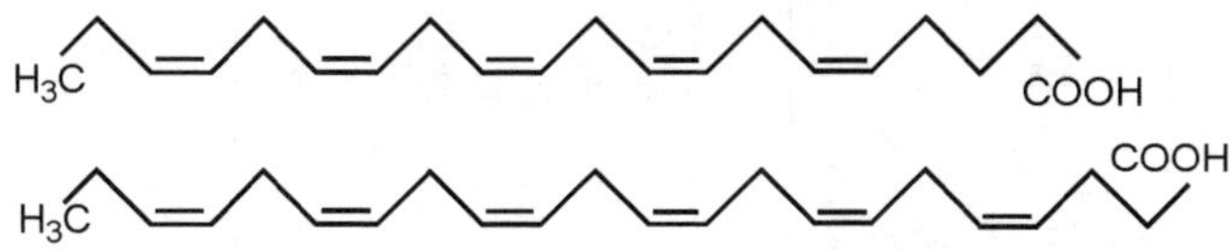

Fig. 18.1 Molecular structure of EPA and DHA n-3 fatty acids.

consumption of EPA and DHA omega-3 fatty acids may reduce the risk of coronary heart disease. One serving of [name of food] provides [x] grams of EPA and DHA omega-3 fatty acids.[8] The Joint Health Claims Initiative (JHCI) in the UK has also approved the following claim: *eating 3 g weekly (or 0.45 g daily) of long chain omega-3 polyunsaturated fatty acids as part of a healthy life style helps maintain heart health.*[9]

18.1.1 Sources for n-3 PUFA from plants and fish

Plant materials such as flaxseed, canola and soybean oil contain relatively high levels of n-3 PUFA in the form of LNA. However, n-3 and n-6 PUFA with 18 carbon atoms (LNA and linoleic acid) are competing for the same enzyme systems for conversion of the C18 fatty acids into PUFA with longer chain length (EPA from LNA and C20:4 n-6 from linoleic acid). Therefore, only a minor part of LNA is converted to EPA and DHA. This is particularly a problem if the intake ratio between n-3/n-6 PUFAs is low. This chapter will therefore mainly focus on EPA and DHA, and in the remainder of this chapter the term n-3 PUFA refers to EPA plus DHA and not LNA. The main source of EPA and DHA are seafood products, especially fatty fish. The n-3 PUFA are extracted from fish in connection with the production of fish meal.

The fish that are processed to produce crude fish oil (and fish meal) can usually be categorised as follows: (1) offal and waste from the edible fisheries, e.g. cutting from filleting industry, (2) fish of a quality that is not high enough to make the fish suitable for human consumption, or (3) fish types that are not considered acceptable or aesthetically pleasing for human consumption. The latter are caught especially for reduction to fish meal and fish oil. The most important fish species that are caught commercially and processed into fish oil are shown in Table 18.1. The fatty acid composition of the fish oil depends on the fatty acid composition of the feed and therefore substantial variation is observed within each species. Approximate data for the most important fatty acids are also shown in Table 18.1.

The total annual world production of fish oil during the past 10 years has been approximately 1.25 million tonnes.[11] The main producers are Japan, Scandinavia, Chile, Peru, USA and Russia. Most of the fish oil (56%) is going into salmonid production in Norway, Chile, Canada and in various European countries. With the current growth in aquaculture this figure may increase to 80–100% before 2010.[11] There may even be a risk that the demand for fish oil for use in aquaculture may exceed the production. However, approximately 25–30

Table 18.1 Sources of fish oil and their fatty acid compositions (from Allen[10])

	Fish species									
	Capelin	Herring	Norway pout	Mackerel	Sand eel	Menhaden	Sardine/ pilchard	Horse mackerel	Anchovy	Sprat
Main sources	Barents Sea, N. Atlantic	N. Atlantic, N. Sea, Norwegian Sea, Pacific Ocean	N. Sea, N. Atlantic, Barents Sea	N. Atlantic, Pacific Ocean, N. Sea	N. Sea	USA East Coast, Gulf of Mexico	Off S. Africa, Chile, Peru, Japan, Atlantic coasts of Canada and USA	S. Africa, Pacific Coast of South America	Off S. & W. Africa, Chile, Peru, and Mexico (Pacific Coast)	N. Sea
Fatty acids										
14:0	7	7	6	8	7	9	8	8	9	–
16:0	10	16	13	14	15	20	18	18	19	16
16:1	10	6	5	7	8	12	10	8	9	7
18:1	14	13	14	13	9	11	13	11	13	16
20:1	17	13	11	12	15	1	4	5	5	10
22:1	14	20	12	15	16	0.2	3	8	2	14
20:5	8	5	8	7	9	14	18	13	17	6
22:6	6	6	13	8	9	8	9	10	9	9
Total (principles)	86	86	82	84	88	75	83	81	83	78

million tonnes of fish are discarded annually. Efforts are being made to increase fish oil production by decreasing the amount of waste and increasing the amount of recycling of fish waste to fish meal and fish oil production. In addition, efforts are being made to reduce the amount of fish oil used per kg farmed fish produced, e.g. by substituting part of the fish oil with rapeseed oil. However, to obtain a satisfactory omega-3 level in farmed fish at the time of slaughtering it may be possible to substitute fish oil with rapeseed oil only at the beginning of the feeding period. Nevertheless, despite the expected growth in aquaculture, fish oil will still be available for human consumption in the years to come.

Certain fishing areas are heavily polluted with compounds such as PCBs (polychlorinated biphenyls), dioxins, lead and arsenic. PCB and dioxin are lipid soluble and therefore they will be extracted together with the fish oil during the fish oil manufacturing process. In July 2002, a new regulation was imposed in the EU where the limit for dioxin in fish oil was set at 6 ng WHO-PCDD/F-TEQ/kg. A similar regulation will be imposed for PCBs in the near future. Owing to the strict rules, new technologies have been developed to remove dioxin from fish oil. The most common method is to remove the dioxin by activated carbon, but new deodorisation techniques are also under development. Such new technologies will be required to remove PCBs as they cannot be removed effectively by activated carbon.

18.1.2 Microbial sources of n-3 PUFA

Micro-organisms capable of producing n-3 PUFA with a chain length above C20 include lower fungi, bacteria and marine microalgae (see Chapter 19).[12–16] The most promising micro-organisms for the production of n-3 PUFA seems to be the marine micro-algae as they are able to accumulate high amounts of n-3 PUFA. The advantage of algae oil compared with fish oil is thus that the oil contains higher levels of, in particular, DHA than fish oil, e.g. up to 52%.[17] Micro-algae are cultivated either in photo-autotrophic or in heterotrophic production systems. The disadvantage of the former is that they require the presence of light, which means that the production is dependent on the weather if carried out in open ponds. If the production is carried out in closed photo-bioreactors, the scale-up of the production is limited by the ability to effectively introduce light.[18] The production of EPA by photo-autotrophic growth has been intensively studied.[17] The yield of EPA by this production method is low, and the production is not commercially feasible. EPA content and productivity rates of some of the most promising microalgae are summarised in Medina *et al.*[19] In recent years, production of DHA by heterotrophic marine micro-organisms has received increased commercial attention and today DHA produced this way is used in several infant formula products.

Currently, Martek Biosciences uses *Schizochytrium* sp. for the production of DHA, which has been used for DHA-enriched egg and as feed for aquaculture.[17] Recently, the European Commission has approved the use of DHA-rich oil from

Schizochytrium sp. produced by Martek Biosciences in products such as dairy products, spreads, dressings, breakfast cereals and food supplements.[17] Martek Biosciences has also patented a process for the production of DHA-rich oil (25–60%) using *Crypthecodiniuim cohnii* and this DHA oil is currently used in several infant formula products.

18.2 Current problems in producing n-3 PUFA and using fish oils in food products

The main problem in relation to the use of n-3 PUFA in both pharmaceutical and food applications is their susceptibility to lipid oxidation. The chemistry behind lipid oxidation is therefore briefly summarised.

18.2.1 Lipid oxidation and antioxidation chemistry

The basic substrates for lipid oxidation reactions are unsaturated fatty acids with one or more double bonds. The susceptibility to lipid oxidation increases with the number of double bonds in the fatty acid. For example, the oxidisability of DHA is five times greater than that of linoleic acid.[20] There are three different types of oxidation; autoxidation, photo-oxidation and enzymatic oxidation. Autoxidation is a spontaneous free radical reaction with oxygen and consists of three main stages: initiation, propagation and termination. Photo-oxidation happens only in the presence of light and when the food system contains photosensitisers. Enzymatic oxidation is due to the presence of certain enzymes such as lipoxygenase in plant and animal systems.

The autoxidation reaction is initiated by initiators (e.g. metal ions, heat, protein radicals), which causes unsaturated fatty acids (LHs) to form carbon-centred alkyl radicals (L•) (Fig. 18.2). In the presence of oxygen these radicals propagate by a free radical chain mechanism to form peroxyl radicals (LOO•) and later hydroperoxides (LOOH). The hydroperoxides are the primary oxidation products of autoxidation. The free radical chain reaction propagates until two free radicals combine and form a non-radical product to terminate the chain.[20,21] The hydroperoxides can be decomposed by heat or in the presence of traces of transition metals and thereby alkoxyl and peroxyl radical intermediates (LO• and LOO•) are formed. These radicals propagate the free radical chain reaction.[20] Moreover, these radicals may be further decomposed to form a variety of non-volatile and volatile secondary oxidation products (in Fig. 18.2 aldehydes are mentioned as an example on volatile oxidation compounds).[20] The latter are termed 'volatiles' and include a wide range of carbonyl compounds (aldehydes, ketones and alcohols), hydrocarbons and furans that are responsible for flavour deterioration.[22–25] In contrast to the volatiles, hydroperoxides are essentially tasteless and odourless.

Photo-oxidation leads to oxidation of unsaturated fatty acids owing to exposure to light in the presence of photosensitisers. The latter will be activated by

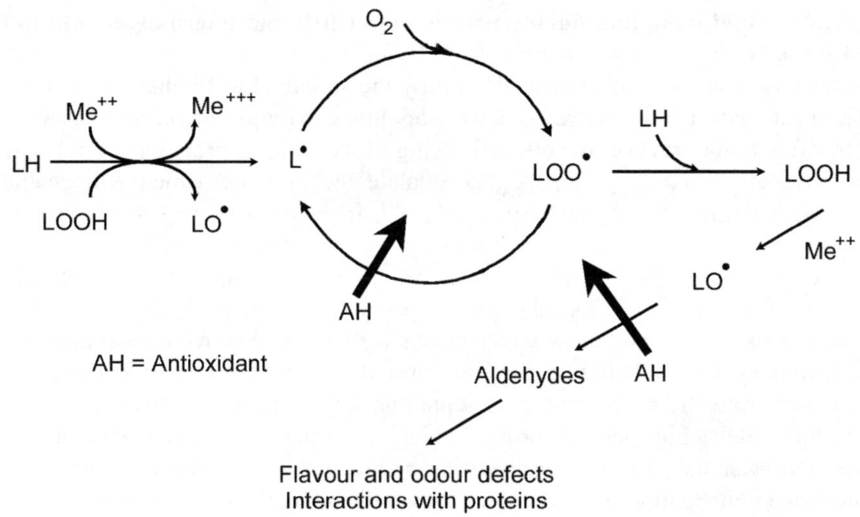

Fig. 18.2 Initiation and propagation of lipid oxidation and prevention of oxidation by free radical chain breaking antioxidants.

absorbing visible or near-UV light. Type I sensitisers then react with the substrate, generating substrate radicals, which can react with oxygen. Type II sensitisers react directly with triplet oxygen, transforming it into the short-lived, but highly reactive, high-energy form of singlet oxygen $^1O_2$, which reacts directly with the double bond of unsaturated fatty acids to form hydroperoxides (LOOH).[26] This is not a free-radical process and will lead to the formation of other lipid hydroperoxides and in turn also to other volatiles than those formed from free radical oxidation. In food systems, chlorophyll, riboflavin or haemeproteins, serve as photosensitisers.[24–27] The hydroperoxides are decomposed by the same reactions as described under autoxidation.

Lipid oxidation may to a certain extent be prevented by the addition of antioxidants, which are usually classified as either primary or secondary antioxidants. Primary antioxidants (AH) are also referred to as free radical scavengers because they act as chain-breaking antioxidants by donating electron/hydrogen to free radicals such as the lipid, peroxyl or the alkoxyl radical (Fig. 18.2). Thereby, they terminate the free radical chain reaction. Primary antioxidants include hindered phenols such as the synthetic antioxidants BHA (butylhydroxyanisole), BHT (butylhydroxytoluene), propyl gallate, naturally occurring compounds such as tocopherol and plant polyphenols such as carnosic acid. The secondary antioxidants act by a number of different mechanisms such as metal chelation, oxygen scavenging and replenishing hydrogen to primary antioxidants. Therefore, the secondary antioxidants often exert synergistic effects together with primary antioxidants.

18.2.2 Lipid oxidation during processing of fish and micro-algae into n-3 PUFA oils

Generally, fish are processed to fish oil by the so-called wet reduction method. The principal operations are cooking, pressing, separation of oil and water by centrifugation to recover the oil, and drying of the residual protein material. The purpose of the cooking step is to coagulate the proteins, which will enable mechanical separation of the liquids and solids in the pressing step. Moreover, fat cells are ruptured during the cooking step, whereby the oil is released into the liquid phase. During the pressing operation, two intermediate products are produced, namely the press cake and the press water. The press cake is dried to produce fish meal. The press water passes a screen to remove coarse particles followed by removal of fine particles in a decanter. Subsequently, the oil is removed from the press water in a separator. Impurities are removed from the resulting oil in a polisher. The protein and lipid fractions may also be separated in the step after the heating step by using a three-phase decanter centrifuge. As mentioned in Section 18.2.1, high temperatures, light, metal ions and haem proteins will catalyse lipid oxidation. Thus, the traditional oil extraction method will unavoidably lead to some oxidation of the fish oil. Lipid oxidation will be less severe if fresh raw materials of good quality are used. Thus, efforts should be made on board the fishing vessel to reduce transportation time and temperature, avoid exposure to light and reduce the squashing of the fish and thereby decrease the risk of bleeding, which will otherwise expose the lipids to haem proteins.

It is possible to reduce the fish processing temperature by extracting the lipids by an enzymatic hydrolysis process. In this process, proteins are hydrolysed by enzymes, whereby lipids can be released into the liquid phase at a much lower temperature (e.g. 60 °C) with a satisfying yield (Jacobsen *et al.*, unpublished findings). It may therefore be possible to produce fish oil of a better quality by an enzymatic extraction method.

Recently, several studies on the production of fish oil from by-products including the oxidative stability of these oils have been reported in the literature.[28–36] The effect of the processing conditions on the oxidative stability of herring oil when using a three-phase decanter to extract the oil from fresh unsalted herring by-products was reported by Aidos *et al.*[28] Surprisingly, it was observed that the decanter temperature did not influence the oxidative stability of the fish oil. In contrast, the oxidative stability was influenced by an interaction effect of the speed of the mono-pump and the speed of the decanter. The best oil stability was obtained when the oils were processed with the highest mono pump speed. Aidos *et al.*[29] compared the stability of herring oil produced from three different herring by-products: only heads, mixed and headless by-products. Oils from the heads had the highest oxidation level, despite the fact that it contained less PUFA than the other two by-products. It was suggested that a lower α-tocopherol content in the oils from the heads compared with the other oils and liberation of endogenous enzymes from the skin was responsible for the increased oxidation in the heads. In another study, the oxidative stability and flavour deterioration of herring oil produced from freshly produced or frozen unsalted herring by-products or salted *maatjes* by-products was compared.[30] As expected, oil produced from fresh unsalted by-product had a higher stability and a better sensory quality than oils produced from the other by-products. This supports the finding that the quality of the fish is of great importance to the quality of the resulting oil. Moreover, the increased oxidation in the oil produced from salted *maatjes*, which had a higher content of iron than the other by-products, indicates that both the presence of transition metals in the fish and the presence of salt will promote oxidation in the resulting oil.

The extraction of n-3 PUFA from micro-algae is a complicated process that involves the use of organic solvents. To the authors' knowledge data on the effect of the processing conditions on the oxidative stability of the oils have not been published.

18.2.3 Lipid oxidation and refining of fish oil

The general objective of processing crude fish oil is to remove impurities that cause the original product to have an unattractive colour or taste or that cause harmful metabolic effects.[37] At the same time, the processing should retain desirable nutritional components such as the n-3 PUFA and antioxidants such as tocopherol. Before refining, the crude oil is often stored in large bulk storage tanks. Insoluble impurities are precipitated during storage and can be drained off together with moisture and thereby reduce the increase in free fatty acids, which may otherwise promote oxidation. To further minimise oxidation during storage, Young[38] recommended that intake pipelines should be extended to the bottom of the tank and that contact with iron, copper and copper alloys should be eliminated. The procedure for refining unhydrogenated and unfractionated fish oil often involves the following steps (the reader may refer to Bimbo[39] for a more thorough review of the refining process).

- Degumming by treatment with phosphoric acid or other acids to remove phospholipids, proteinaceous compounds, trace metals and others. A high content of phospholipids will lead to emulsion formation in the subsequent refining steps and therefore make separation of oil and water difficult. Fish oils are low in phospholipids and therefore degumming is not necessary. However, the oil quality (i.e. oxidative stability) is often improved by the degumming step owing to the removal of trace metals.[39]
- Neutralisation by addition of an alkali solution such as caustic soda to remove free fatty acids, pigments, phospholipids, oil insolubles, water solubles and trace metals. The neutralisation process involves heating and is followed by one or more washing steps with water. The reduction in the content of free fatty acids will improve the sensory properties and oxidative stability of the oil. The free fatty acid content of refined fish oils should be as low as possible, preferably not higher than 0.1–0.2%.
- Bleaching is performed to improve the colour, flavour and oxidative stability of the oil and to remove impurities. Activated clay (bleaching earth) is used for the bleaching process. Bleaching involves the adsorption of coloured

compounds, peroxides and some volatile oxidation compounds as well as other impurities to the bleaching clay. Bleaching can either be carried out at atmospheric pressure or under vacuum. The latter may be performed in a batch or continuous process. The best oxidative stability is obtained by the use of continuous vacuum bleaching.[39]

- The last step in the refining process is the deodorisation step, which removes undesirable ingredients from the oil and compounds formed during the preceding steps in the refining process. The deodorisation process is basically a steam distillation process, which will remove compounds that are more volatile than the triglycerides. The deodorisation of fish oil is often carried out at a temperature around 190 °C. Owing to the high temperature peroxides are decomposed into secondary volatile oxidation products which are then distilled off. Deodorisation may be carried out in a batch, semicontinuous, continuous or thin film deodoriser. The difference between the first three processes and the thin film deodoriser is that the latter employs a thin film concept to strip volatiles from the oil at high transfer rates, whereas deodorisation in the first three processes takes place in one or more consecutive vessels/tanks. The deodorisation time and temperature in the thin film process are lower than in the other processes, and therefore the thin film deodorisation is a more gentle process than the traditional deodorisation method. This leads to a lower loss of tocopherol and a lower formation of undesirable components such as *trans* fatty acids and polyaromatic hydrocarbons.

18.3 Improving the sensory quality and shelf-life of n-3 PUFA-enriched foods

The very high susceptibility of n-3 PUFA oils towards oxidative deterioration invariably means that special precautions have to be taken in order to achieve stable and sensory acceptable PUFA-enriched products. When n-3 PUFA are added as an ingredient in a food product, the product is usually processed further in order to achieve the desired physical stability, functional and sensory properties. Such processing will imply further oxidative stress on the n-3 PUFA oils. Choice of processing conditions, packaging material and storage conditions are important extrinsic factors, which need to be addressed. Secondly, the intrinsic or physico-chemical properties of the individual food product can affect oxidative stability in both antioxidative and pro-oxidative directions. In the following section, different actions and approaches to achieve and maintain a good quality and oxidative stability of n-3 PUFA-enriched foods will be discussed.

18.3.1 Quality of the n-3 PUFA oil

Obviously, the quality, i.e. oxidative status, of the n-3 PUFA oil has a significant influence on the oxidative stability of foods enriched with this oil. The oxidative status of oils has traditionally been measured by the peroxide value (PV) and the anisidine value (AV). PV is a measure of the level of the primary oxidation products (lipid hydroperoxides) in the product, while the anisidine value is an unspecific measure of saturated and unsaturated carbonyl compounds. Several fish oil-producing companies guarantee that their fish oil has a PV lower than 1.0 meq/kg and an AV lower than 5. Recent studies performed with fish oil-enriched milk corroborated the importance of using a fish oil of high quality for incorporation into foods.[40,41] Thus, it was reported that milk emulsions based on cod liver oil with a slightly elevated PV of 1.5 meq/kg oxidised significantly faster than a tuna oil with a low PV of 0.1 meq/kg despite the fact that the tuna oil was more unsaturated than the cod liver oil.[40] It was hypothesised that trace metals present in the milk in combination with the slightly elevated level of lipid hydroperoxides were responsible for the rapid oxidative flavour deterioration of the milk based on cod liver oil owing to the ability of trace metals to decompose lipid hydroperoxides. A subsequent study supported these findings and also showed that a sensory panel was able to distinguish milk emulsions produced with fish oil with a PV of 0.1 meq/kg as being less fishy and rancid than when a fish oil with a PV of 0.5 meq/kg was used.[41]

18.3.2 Emulsion formulation

Emulsifiers

Many n-3 PUFA-enriched foods exist in the form of some kind of emulsion (e.g. salad dressing, spreads, milk, ice cream). These food systems require the addition of an emulsifier. Primarily, emulsifiers provide physical stability to the emulsions. However, emulsifiers are able to interact with other components/ingredients of the food product, and the choice of emulsifier can therefore be of significant importance for both physical and oxidative stability of the food product. Basically, emulsifiers are surface active molecules with amphiphilic properties, which can interact with the oil–water interface and reduce surface tension. Emulsifiers for food use are thus either macromolecules, such as proteins unfolding at the interface, or smaller surfactant molecules, such as phospholipids, free fatty acids, monoacylglycerols and synthetic surfactants.

Emulsifiers are able to influence lipid oxidation in different ways. In emulsions stabilised by proteins, pH will generally be either below or above the *pI* of the protein in order to avoid coalescence of droplets. This results in an either positive or negative surface charge of these droplets. Similarly, the use of some surfactants such as charged phospholipids may lead to a charged oil droplet. The surface charge of emulsion droplets is important for lipid oxidation catalysed by the presence of trace metal ions, such as Fe^{2+}. With a negative surface charge emulsion droplets will attract the potentially highly pro-oxidative trace metals, and bring them into closer proximity of the n-3 PUFA oil, thereby enhancing lipid oxidation. If instead an emulsifier, which creates a positive charge of the droplets, is chosen, trace metals are repelled and oxidation is likely to be reduced.[42,43] Another aspect is the fact that the solubility of trace metals generally increases at decreasing pH,[27] which potentially can promote oxidation.

As practically all food products contain some amount of trace metals, the choice of an appropriate emulsifier for PUFA-enriched foods should thus consider the pH of the given food.

An example of the effect of pH on oxidation was the finding that in fish oil-enriched mayonnaise lipid oxidation increased as pH decreased from 6.0 to 3.8.[44] The following hypothesis was suggested to explain this phenomenon: the egg yolk used as an emulsifier in mayonnaise contains large amounts of iron, which is bound to the protein phosvitin. At the natural pH of egg yolk (pH 6.0), the iron forms cation bridges between phosvitin and other components in egg yolk, namely low-density lipoproteins (LDL) and lipovitellin. These components are located at the oil–water interface in mayonnaise. When pH is decreased to 4.0, which is the pH in mayonnaise, the cation bridges between the before-mentioned egg yolk components are broken and iron becomes dissociated from LDL and lipovitellin. Thereby, iron becomes more active as a catalyst of oxidation.[44,45] In contrast, lipid oxidation in salmon oil-in-water model emulsions (5% oil) was greater and more rapid at pH 7.0 than at pH 3.0.[46] These contradicting results demonstrate that in complex multiphase systems, pH may affect lipid oxidation differently through various mechanisms, and it is often necessary to pacify trace metals by adding metal-chelating compounds.

Surfactants can also influence the location of the metal ions and lipid hydroperoxides by forming micelles. This is because under normal conditions, surfactants are present in excess in emulsions, and surfactants not associated with the emulsion droplets may form micelles in the continuous phase. Lipid hydroperoxides and/or metal ions could become associated with or solubilised in the micelles. When present in the micelles, these components cannot react with lipid components in the oil phase and this may in turn reduce lipid oxidation.[47,48]

Apart from influencing droplet surface charge, the emulsifier may otherwise affect the oxidative stability of the emulsions.[49–51] Protein emulsifiers may affect oxidative stability through the amino acid composition as some amino acids possess antioxidative properties.[52] For example, the sulphhydryl group of cysteine has been reported to have antioxidant activity owing to its ability to scavenge free radicals.[52] Other amino acids such as tyrosine, phenylalanine, tryptophan, proline, methionine, lysine and histidine have also been reported to have antioxidative effects.[51] In model emulsions it has also been suggested that the actual thickness of the interface layer of the droplets is important.[50,51] A thicker or more dense interface could provide enhanced protection of the emulsified oil by decreasing accessibility of water-soluble pro-oxidants. Finally, the food matrix components may also influence the release of secondary volatile oxidation products thereby affecting the release of fishy or rancid off-flavour developed during oxidation.[53,54] Thus, it may be possible to 'mask' the rancidity by choosing the right emulsifier.

Antioxidants and metal chelators

The most thoroughly investigated area regarding oxidative stabilisation of lipid systems concerns the addition of antioxidants and antioxidant systems, natural as well as synthetic antioxidants. However, compared with the number of studies performed in oil-in-water model emulsion, relatively few studies on the antioxidant mechanism in real food emulsions have been reported. In complex food systems, several factors influence the efficacy of the different types of antioxidants, and it is clearly an important issue to address during the manufacture of stable n-3 PUFA-enriched foods. The use of antioxidants in microencapsulated n-3 PUFA oil is dealt with as a special case in Section 18.3.3 concerning microencapsulation of n-3 PUFA oils.

The localisation or partitioning of antioxidants into the different phases of a food system seems to be of major importance. This is probably because the antioxidants need to be located close to where oxidation occurs. Therefore, when choosing an antioxidant for a particular food system both the mode of action (chain breaking, O_2 scavenging or metal chelating) and the solubility/partitioning properties of the antioxidant should be considered. Several studies have shown that in model oil-in-water emulsions, non-polar antioxidants were more efficient than polar antioxidants.[55–57] It was suggested that the non-polar antioxidants were located in the oil droplets, where oxidation would propagate, whereas polar antioxidants would be solubilised in the water phase far from where the initiation and propagation of lipid oxidation take place. Furthermore, in fish oil-enriched mayonnaise, antioxidants such as Trolox, tocopherol, propyl gallate, gallic acid, ferulic acid, caffeic acid and catechin have been shown to interact with the interfacial layer of the emulsion.[58] As several authors have proposed that oxidation in emulsions is initiated at the interfacial layer, such interactions with antioxidants could also affect the activity and efficiency of the antioxidants. The antioxidative effect of propyl gallate, gallic acid, tocopherol, ascorbic acid or a mixture of ascorbic acid (8.6% w/w), lecithin (86.2% w/w) and tocopherol (5.2% w/w) (the so-called A/L/T system) in fish oil-enriched mayonnaise has been determined by sensory profiling, measurements of lipid hydroperoxides and volatiles and in some cases also by measurements of free radical formation.[44,45,59–62] Weak pro-oxidative effects of propyl gallate and gallic acid were observed.[59,62] Tocopherol was inactive as an antioxidant and it even seemed to have pro-oxidative effects at higher concentrations (>140 mg/kg).[60,61] Ascorbic acid (40–800 mg/kg) and the A/L/T system (200 mg/kg total concentration) were strong pro-oxidants (Table 18.2).[44,45,60] The pro-oxidative effect of these antioxidant systems was suggested to be due to the ability of ascorbic acid to promote the release of iron from the egg yolk located at the oil–water interface. The released iron would then be able to decompose pre-existing lipid hydroperoxides located near the oil–water interface or in the aqueous phase. The findings that tocopherol, gallic acid and propyl gallate were ineffective as antioxidants could either be due to their interaction with the emulsifier, or to the fact that these antioxidants are free radical scavengers that cannot prevent metal-catalysed oxidation happening at the oil–water interface.[59,61,62]

In contrast to these results, it was reported that γ-tocopherol (330 mg/kg), but not α-tocopherol was able to reduce lipid oxidation in fish oil-enriched milk.[63]

Table 18.2 Sensory scores in freshly produced mayonnaise with different addition levels of ascorbic acid illustrating the pro-oxidative effect of ascorbic acid (from Jacobsen *et al.*[45])

Amount of ascorbic acid added ppm (mM)	Fishy/train oil aroma	Rancid aroma	Fishy/train oil flavour	Rancid flavour	Metallic flavour
0 (0)[1]	$0.4 \pm 0.8^{a,2}$	0.5 ± 1.2^{a}	0.2 ± 0.6^{a}	0.3 ± 0.6^{a}	0.3 ± 0.8^{a}
40 (0.23)	1.1 ± 1.2^{ab}	1.5 ± 1.8^{a}	2.7 ± 2.2^{b}	1.7 ± 2.0^{abcd}	0.4 ± 0.7^{a}
80 (0.45)	1.9 ± 1.6^{ab}	1.4 ± 1.9^{a}	2.6 ± 1.4^{b}	1.2 ± 1.9^{abc}	0.8 ± 1.3^{a}
200 (1.14)	1.8 ± 1.4^{ab}	1.4 ± 2.2^{a}	3.2 ± 1.7^{b}	2.5 ± 2.2^{bcd}	0.8 ± 1.3^{a}
400 (2.27)	2.5 ± 2.2^{b}	1.7 ± 1.7^{a}	4.2 ± 2.4^{b}	3.0 ± 2.1^{d}	1.0 ± 1.5^{a}
800 (4.45)	1.6 ± 2.2^{ab}	2.0 ± 1.9^{a}	3.5 ± 2.4^{b}	2.3 ± 1.7^{bcd}	1.2 ± 1.5^{a}

[1]Values in parentheses show the concentration of ascorbic acid in mM.
[2]Values in the same column followed by the same letter are not significantly different ($P < 0.05$).

When both α- and γ- tocopherol were present, a slight pro-oxidative effect on oxidation was observed (Fig. 18.3). Likewise, EDTA at a concentration of 5 mg/kg did not have any effect. However, ascorbyl palmitate (300 mg/kg) was able to inhibit lipid oxidation in this food system (Fig. 18.3). It was suggested that ascorbyl palmitate exerted its antioxidative effect either via its ability to regenerate tocopherol, via its ability to act as a free radical scavenger, or via its metal-chelating properties. Ascorbyl palmitate is an amphiphilic molecule and can therefore be expected to be located at the oil–water interface where oxidation takes place. This location may have a positive influence on the antioxidative effect of ascorbyl palmitate.

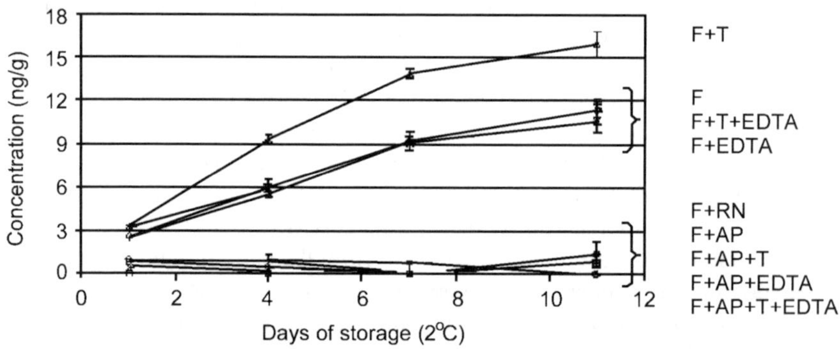

Fig. 18.3 Effect of 260 ppm α-tocopherol + 360 ppm γ-tocopherol (T), 5 ppm EDTA, or 300 ppm ascorbyl palmitate (AP) and combinations thereof on formation of *E,E*-2,4-heptadienal in milk drink with 1.0% milk fat and 0.5% fish oil. The fish oil milk emulsions were compared with milk with 0.5% fish oil and 0.5% rapeseed oil (F+RN). Ascorbyl palmitate was as efficient in reducing lipid oxidation as the addition of rapeseed oil. Addition of tocopherol or EDTA to the milk with ascorbyl palmitate did not reduce oxidation further (from Let *et al.*[63]).

Table 18.3 Sensory scores during storage at 20 °C for fishy off-flavour in fish oil enriched mayonnaise with and without 75 ppm EDTA. Sensory scale from 0 to 9 (from Jacobsen *et al.*[62])

	0 weeks	1 week	2 weeks	3 weeks	4 weeks
Mayonnaise without antioxidant	0.2 ± 0.4	2.1 ± 1.5	2.4 ± 1.6	2.8 ± 1.3	3.4 ± 1.8
Mayonnaise with 75 ppm EDTA	0.2 ± 0.3	0.2 ± 0.4	0.1 ± 0.3	0.3 ± 0.5	0.2 ± 0.3

In contrast to the poor effect of free radical scavengers in fish oil-enriched mayonnaise, the metal chelator EDTA efficiently inhibited lipid oxidation in mayonnaise enriched with fish oil (Table 18.3) or with structured lipid based on sunflower oil.[62,64,65] In fish oil-enriched milk, low levels of EDTA (5 mg/kg) were also able to reduce lipid oxidation significantly, although not completely, when fish oil with a peroxide value (PV) of 1.5 meq/kg was used.[40] However, when fish oil with a PV of 0.1 meq/kg was used, the emulsions were oxidatively stable and no effect of EDTA was observed. These data indicated that trace metal-catalysed lipid oxidation is very important in many food emulsions enriched with n-3 PUFA. Therefore, addition of metal-chelating compounds to such foods may be an efficient way of preventing oxidation.

In model emulsions of fish or algae oil in water, it has been shown that EDTA was pro-oxidant in molar ratios of EDTA to iron of 1:1 or lower, but otherwise effectively inhibited oxidation at molar ratios of 2:1 and 4:1.[66] In contrast, in fish oil-enriched mayonnaise a significant antioxidant effect of EDTA was found at an EDTA : iron ratio of 1:2.[65] It thus seems that the ratio between the actual concentration of trace metals and the metal chelating compound is of importance for inhibition of lipid oxidation, but also that this ratio is influenced by the particular composition of the food system.

Apart from addition of natural and synthetic purified antioxidants, another approach to obtain stable products enriched with n-3 PUFA is to mix these sensitive n-3 PUFA oils with more stable fats and oils. Claims have been made that vegetable oils, such as rapeseed oil, corn oil, sunflower oil and soybean oil, as well as animal fat, are able to stabilise fish oil against oxidation.[67–69] Subsequent studies have shown that products, such as milk (Table 18.4) and spreads, containing these stabilised oils were significantly more resistant against oxidation during storage, than products containing only fish oil.[70,71] It was suggested that vegetable oil and fish oil should be co-refined in order to obtain optimum stability, and that the protective effect of the vegetable oils were mainly based on the natural content of antioxidants present in these vegetable oils.[67,68] However, it was also claimed that the protection of unsaturated oils was based on a dilution of the unsaturated fatty acids with saturated fatty acids. Dilution of vegetable oils containing natural antioxidants with animal fats, such as beef tallow, containing no or relatively low amounts of natural antioxidants was claimed to enhance the oxidative stability.[69]

Table 18.4 Sensory scores during storage at 2 °C in milk drink enriched with fish oil (0.5%) or a mixture of fish oil and rapeseed oil (0.25% of each) illustrating the protective effect of rapeseed oil (from Let *et al.*[70])

	Fish odour			Fish taste		
	Day 1[1]	Day 4	Day 8	Day 1	Day 4	Day 8
Rapeseed	$0.4^{a} \pm 0.7$	$0.0^{a} \pm 0.1$	$0.2^{a} \pm 0.4$	$0.2^{a} \pm 0.5$	$0.1^{a} \pm 0.3$	$0.2^{a} \pm 0.3$
FR1+A	$0.3^{a} \pm 0.5$	$0.1^{a} \pm 0.3$	$0.3^{a} \pm 0.5$	$0.6^{ab} \pm 0.8$	$0.5^{a} \pm 0.7$	$0.3^{a} \pm 0.5$
FR2+A	$0.1^{a} \pm 0.3$	$0.3^{a} \pm 0.5$	$0.2^{a} \pm 0.3$	$0.2^{a} \pm 0.2$	$0.4^{a} \pm 0.5$	$0.5^{a} \pm 0.5$
FR3	$0.7^{a} \pm 0.9$	$0.2^{a} \pm 0.4$	$0.3^{a} \pm 0.5$	$1.0^{bc} \pm 0.7$	$0.5^{a} \pm 0.6$	$0.5^{a} \pm 0.7$
F1	$0.4^{a} \pm 0.4$	$1.3^{b} \pm 1.1$	$1.9^{b} \pm 1.7$	$1.0^{bc} \pm 0.8$	$2.3^{b} \pm 1.4$	$2.4^{b} \pm 1.5$
F2	$0.4^{a} \pm 0.4$	$1.5^{b} \pm 1.4$	$1.4^{b} \pm 1.1$	$1.3^{c} \pm 1.0$	$2.1^{b} \pm 1.2$	$2.4^{b} \pm 1.4$

[1]Average of all 12 assessors' determinations. The six emulsions were compared at each day (columnwise) in Tukey's test using 0.05 level of significance, and emulsions followed by same letter are not significantly different. *FR* 0.25% fish oil and 0.25% rapeseed oil. *F* 0.5% fish oil. *1* and *2* refer to different deodorisation procedures of the same cod liver oil. *3* refers to tuna oil. *A* refers to antioxidants added to the oil.

Finally, some carbohydrates have shown antioxidative activity in high concentrations due to their ability to scavenge free radicals.[72] Furthermore, sucrose has an increasing effect on the viscosity of the emulsion and this may decrease the diffusion coefficient of oxygen,[73] metals, other reaction products and reactants, which may in turn slow down oxidation rates. Fructose has been suggested as an efficient antioxidant in different meat formulations[74] and in emulsions such as salad dressings[75] both enriched with fish oil.

18.3.3 Process means for optimising quality and stability of n-3 PUFA-enriched food

Process and storage conditions

Production of PUFA-enriched foods includes basic operations such as homogenisation and mixing with other ingredients. Generally, the most important issues to address during production and storage of n-3 PUFA-enriched foods are control of oxygen access, control of temperature, and reduction of light.

Oxygen is necessary for propagation of lipid oxidation. It is therefore important to avoid contact between the n-3 PUFA oils and headspace oxygen, dissolved oxygen and trapped air bubbles both during processing as well as storage. Several studies have shown that a reduction in the access of oxygen retards lipid oxidation.[76] Reduction of oxygen can be achieved by processing under vacuum or in a nitrogen atmosphere. This would additionally reduce the amount of dissolved or trapped oxygen in the final product, which also is able to promote oxidation. In the final product exclusion of headspace oxygen can be reduced by packaging in an air-tight container impermeable to oxygen, and preferably under modified atmosphere.

The mechanisms of lipid oxidation change with temperature, especially above 60 °C. Additionally, lipid hydroperoxides from different fatty acids decompose into secondary volatile oxidation products at different temperatures.[27] Therefore, it is difficult to predict the effect of temperature on lipid oxidation during processing and storage of complex food systems, such as n-3 PUFA-enriched foods. However, as temperature affects oxidation rates in an exponential manner, limited temperature increases and otherwise strict control of temperature is required to achieve stable n-3 PUFA-enriched foods.

Apart from lipid autoxidation, n-3 PUFA-enriched foods may undergo photo-oxidation. Photo-oxidation requires light, oxygen and the presence of a photosensitising compound in the food as previously described. Therefore the access of light to n-3 PUFA-enriched foods should be restricted in order to enhance storage stability.

Finally, the physical structure of the oil-in-water emulsions obtained during processing of the n-3 PUFA-enriched foods may be of importance to lipid oxidation. To obtain a physically stable emulsion, the oil droplet size is reduced during emulsification, which results in the formation of a large interfacial area, increasing the contact between the oil and water phase. Initiation of lipid oxidation is suggested to occur at the interface,[27] as the oil droplets becomes exposed to the water soluble pro-oxidants and dissolved oxygen via diffusion through the interfacial membrane. However, the potential presence of antioxidants, unsaturated phospholipids, and other amphiphilic compounds at the interface as well as the physical packaging of the interfacial membrane are also able to affect oxidation,[27] and thus the impact of droplet size on oxidation is complex and depends on the composition of the particular food product. In fish oil-enriched mayonnaises with small droplet sizes, lipid oxidation was faster in the initial part of the storage period than in mayonnaise with larger droplets, whereas no effect of droplet size on oxidative flavour deterioration was observed in the later part of the storage period.[77] The following mechanism to explain these findings was suggested: in the initial oxidation phase, a small droplet size, i.e. a large interfacial area, would increase the contact area between iron located in the aqueous phase and lipid hydroperoxides located at the interface and this would increase oxidation. In the later stage, oxidation proceeds inside the oil droplet and therefore the droplet size is less important.

Pre-emulsification

One strategy to produce n-3 PUFA-enriched foods is to prepare a pre-emulsion of the n-3 PUFA oil, which is then to be added to the finished or semi-finished food product. This approach has long been known for example regarding fortification with fat-soluble vitamins and fish oil[78] and has been attempted in products such as different milk drinks and tofu.[79,80] A recent study by Park *et al.* has reported a procedure for the production of n-3 PUFA enriched surimi, using an algae oil stabilised by tocopherols, ascorbyl palmitate and rosemary extract, which was emulsified in water by whey protein isolate (WPI).[81] This emulsion was subsequently mixed with the semi-finished fish product and mixed into the final surimi product. Djordjevic *et al.* determined the optimum conditions for producing WPI-stabilised oil-in-water emulsions with a high content of n-3

PUFA and a low viscosity that could be used for incorporation of n-3 PUFA in foods.[82] Subsequently, they evaluated the oxidative stability of oil-in-water emulsions (25% oil) stabilised either by casein or WPI.[83] They found that PV was significantly higher in the WPI-stabilised emulsions compared with the casein-stabilised emulsions, but that there was no significant difference in the formation of headspace propanal. Moreover, they observed that it was difficult to dissolve casein at low pH, which makes it impractical to use this protein from a technological standpoint.[82] Another problem when using casein was that the viscosity increased steeply at high oil concentrations. Because of these findings they suggested that WPI-stabilised oil-in-water emulsions (pH 3) could be used to produce oxidatively and physically stable n-3 PUFA delivery systems.

The idea behind the pre-emulsification strategy is first of all to reduce the extent of processing of the oil, e.g. to reduce the amount of stresses such as heat, oxygen, and access of light, which are otherwise necessary for the production of the particular food product. Additionally, the contact between the n-3 PUFA oil and the potential pro-oxidant compounds of the food product during processing is reduced by adding the oil in an already stabilised pre-emulsion as the final step of processing. Finally, by using pre-emulsification it is possible to design a stable emulsion by choosing an optimum combination of emulsifier(s), anti-oxidants and, e.g., stabilisers. However, when designing such pre-emulsions, it seems necessary to take into account the composition and physical properties of the final product, to which the pre-emulsion is added. Complete avoidance of exposure of the n-3 PUFA oil and thus contact with remaining product ingredients in the final product is dependent on the physical stability of the pre-emulsion over time. If the pre-emulsion interacts with other product components, or if diffusion occurs across the emulsion droplet interface, the n-3 PUFA oil might in time get into contact with the remaining ingredients of the product.

Microencapsulation

Another approach to reduce contact between the oxidatively susceptible n-3 PUFA oils and atmospheric oxygen as well as the other ingredients of the food product is to use microencapsulated oils. This microencapsulation approach is used in a large variety of products, mainly in dry formulations and products such as milk and infant formula powders. Microencapsulation of fats and oils basically consists of an emulsion stabilised by modified starch or hydrocolloids and/or proteins, which is either spray or freeze dried to produce a powder. A non-emulsifying water-soluble material such as sugar or hydrolysed starch is used as filler.[84] Similar to fluid emulsions the oxidative stability of micro-encapsulated PUFA oils depends on processing conditions and the choice of emulsifier and antioxidant addition.[84,85] The individual processing steps have been shown to stress the oil, resulting in increasing PV.[86,87] Additionally, the oxidative stability of microencapsulated n-3 PUFA oil depends on molecular diffusion through the protective wall matrix and maintenance of the structural integrity that keeps emulsified lipids within each powder particle.

Kagami *et al.*[85] investigated the effect of different emulsifiers and fillers, and found that encapsulates stabilised by sodium caseinate in combination with highly branched cyclic dextrin produced from waxy corn starch were more stable than encapsulates made with sodium caseinate and maltodextrin, or combinations of whey protein and highly branched cyclic dextrin.

Another study by Keogh *et al.*[84] regarding emulsifiers showed that a low level of off-flavour and a shelf-life of 31 weeks at 4 °C can be obtained using only dairy ingredients as encapsulate material of a fish oil powder. The results also showed that the shelf-life increased when the free non-encapsulated fat and vacuole volume of the powder decreased. They did not find any effect of the surface fat. A study by Velasco *et al.*[88] on the oxidative stability of fish oil powder stabilised by ascorbic acid, lecithin and tocopherol stored in open Petri dishes found that oxidation was slower in the free oil fraction compared with the encapsulated fraction.

Several studies have investigated the effects of different antioxidants in encapsulates. Hogan *et al.* investigated the antioxidative effects of tocopherol and its hydrophilic analogue Trolox C in fish oil encapsulates prepared from herring oil, emulsified and stabilised by sodium caseinate and maltodextrin, respectively.[89] They observed that all antioxidants had reduced oxidation in the powders after 14 days of storage at 4 °C. Similarly, Baik *et al.*[87] showed that α-tocopherol inhibited oxidation significantly in microencapsulated menhaden oil, while ascorbyl palmitate was much less efficient. However, it should be noticed that PV was high in both studies ranging from 10 meq/kg in the freshly produced powders to 60 meq/kg after 1 to 4 weeks of storage. It is possible that the effects of the antioxidants would be less pronounced in powders with lower initial PV.

Heinzelmann *et al.*[86] showed that optimum shelf-life of an encapsulated fish oil was achieved by a combination of ascorbic acid, lecithin and tocopherol (A/L/T system). In the study by Velasco oxidation of a fish oil powder was slightly delayed by the A/L/T system compared with a non-stabilised powder. The oxidative stability seemed more dependent on the storage conditions, which was either light or dark with or without air.[88] Oxidation was stopped in the microencapsulated fish oil stabilised by ascorbic acid, lecithin and tocopherol which was stored under vacuum.

Finally, other storage conditions such as relative humidity have been shown to influence oxidation of microencapsulated fat and surface fat differently during storage.[90] However, this study was performed on encapsulated milk fat. Oxidation of encapsulated fat was maximum at a water activity (a_w) of 0.52, and decreased with decreasing a_w, minimum oxidation of surface fat was observed at an a_w of 0.52. In the study by Baik *et al.*, the relative humidity had only very slight effect on the oxidative stability of fish oil encapsulate effectively stabilised by α-tocopherol, as determined by thiobarbituric acid reactive species (TBARS).[87]

18.3.4 Recommendations

On the basis of the above summary of how lipid oxidation can be reduced during production of fish oil and in products enriched with n-3 PUFA the following strategies to avoid lipid oxidation are suggested:

- Reduce transportation time, exposure to heat and light and minimise bleeding of fish to be used for fish oil production.
- Do not use too high a temperature during refining and deodorisation of the fish oil and reduce exposure to light and oxygen to a minimum.
- Exclude oxygen from the food system, for example by packaging under vacuum.
- Store the enriched products at chilled temperatures.
- Ensure that ingredients have a low content of hydroperoxides, transition metals and other pro-oxidants. It seems to be especially important that n-3 PUFA oils have a low PV. Therefore, these oils should be stored at low temperatures (<0 °C), in the dark, with reduced oxygen and the fish oils should be used as fast as possible after deodorisation as hydroperoxides will form even at temperatures below 0 °C.
- Beware that the choice of emulsifier may significantly affect lipid oxidation rates. Therefore, when applying n-3 oils in a new food product it may be necessary to reformulate the conventional recipe to include other emulsifier types.
- Use metal chelators such as EDTA, citric acid, proteins, polysaccharides and metal chelating plant polyphenols to prevent lipid hydroperoxide decomposition.
- Addition of free radical chain breaking antioxidants may further reduce lipid oxidation. Select antioxidants that will be located where they are required, i.e. normally near the oil–water interface where the decomposition of lipid hydroperoxides takes place.
- Optimise the processing conditions. In some food systems the particle/droplet size will affect the oxidation rates, in other foods they may not. Therefore, this issue should be taken into consideration. In addition, the emulsification process may disrupt natural membranes that may protect the fish oil from protein-bound metals. Emulsification processes should be optimised to minimise lipid oxidation.

18.5 Future trends

As mentioned in the introduction to this chapter the Food and Drug Administration allowed a qualified health claim on n-3 PUFA-enriched food products in September 2004 and later a similar health claim was also allowed in the UK. It may be expected that this will lead to a growing industrial interest in exploiting the health effects of these oils in the US and in the UK. A new regulation on health claims is also expected in the EU in 2006. Whether health claims on n-3 PUFA will also be allowed in the rest of the EU is not known at this time. Nevertheless, because of the increased public awareness about the beneficial effects of the n-3 PUFA it is expected that more new food products enriched with n-3 PUFA will enter the marketplace in the coming years.

The infant's requirements for DHA has received substantial attention recently. Therefore, a promising new area is food for the infant. For example, several infant formulas enriched with DHA are now on the market. It is likely that efforts will also be made to develop other types of baby foods enriched with n-3 PUFA in the years to come.

Ice cream producers are now also targeting health-conscious consumers. Recently, a number of new fat-reduced ice cream formulations as well as calcium-enriched ice creams have entered the market. Efforts are currently being made to develop ice cream enriched with n-3 LC PUFA.

Dairy products are the fastest growing product within the functional food area.[91] So far, functional dairy products have mostly been 'functional' due to the addition of probiotic bacteria and the consumers already perceive some dairy products as being healthy. Therefore, milk drinks and yoghurts may be a good vehicle for n-3 PUFA enrichment and we may see a number of new products in this category in the future.

This chapter has mainly dealt with EPA and DHA from marine sources. However, with the increased focus on the beneficial effects of n-3 PUFA in general products enriched with LNA will most likely also receive more attention from the industry. Efforts are also being made to develop plants with a high level of EPA and DHA by genetic engineering (see Chapter 20).

Traditionally, the industry has mainly used free radical chain-breaking synthetic antioxidants for the prevention of oxidation in foods. However, this strategy seems to be less efficient in preventing lipid oxidation in emulsified food systems enriched with n-3 PUFA. With our increased understanding of the important role of trace metals, emulsifiers and processing conditions in the lipid oxidation processes, more efforts will be dedicated to use this knowledge to develop alternative strategies to retard lipid oxidation in real foods with n-3 PUFA oils. One such strategy may be an increased use of both synthetic and natural metal chelators. Another strategy may be to design oxidatively stable oil-in-water emulsion delivery systems for each particular food system.

18.5 Sources of further information

The Omega-3 Information Network at:
PO Box 24, Tiverton,
Devon EX16 4QQ, UK
Tel: (44) 1884-257547, Fax: (44) 1884-242757
E-mail: rayrice@eclipse.co.uk

International Fishmeal & Fish Oil Organisation
2 College Yard, Lower Dagnall Street

St Albans, Hertfordshire AL3 4P4, UK
E-mail: secretariat@iffo.org.uk

Oils and Fats International
dmg world media (uk) ltd
Queensway House, 2 Queensway, Redhill
Surrey RH1 1QS, UK
Tel: +44 (0) 1737 855068, Fax: +44 (0) 1737 855470
Email: anitarevis@uk.dmgworldmedia.com

NutriVit: http://www.nutrivit.org/whatsnew/index.htm
The Fish Foundation: http://www.fish-foundation.org.uk/references.htm

Fish Oil. Technology, Nutrition and Marketing. Hamilton, R.J. and Rice, R.D. (eds) PJ Barnes & Asscociates, Bucks, UK, 1995.

18.6 References

1. HARRIS W S, 'Fish oils and plasma-lipid and lipoprotein metabolism in humans – a critical review', *J. Lipid Res*, 1989 **30** 785–807.
2. PRISCO D, FILIPINI M, PANICCIA R, GENSINI G F, SERNERI G G N, 'Effect of n-3 fatty-acid ethyl-ester supplementation on fatty-acid composition of the single platelet phospholipids and on platelet functions', *Metabolism*, 1995 **44** 562–569.
3. SHAHAR E, FOLSOM A R, WU K K, DENNIS B H, SHIMAKAWA T, CONLAN M G, DAVIS C E, WILLIAMS O D, 'Associatons of fish intake and dietary n-3 polyunsaturated fatty-acids with a hypocoagulable profile – the atherosclerosis risk in communities (Aric) study', *Arterioscler Thromb*, 1993 **13** 1205–1212.
4. KREMER J M, LAWRENCE D A, PETRILLOW G F, 'Effects of high-dose fish oil on rheumatoid arthritis after stopping nonsteroidal antiinflammatory drugs', *Arthritis Rheum*, 1995 **38** 1107–1114.
5. BROUGHTON K S, JOHNSON C S, PACE B K, LIEBMAN M, KLEPPINGER K M, 'Reduced asthma symptoms with n-3 fatty acid ingestion are related to 5-series leukotriene production', *Am J Clin Nutr*, 1997 **65** 1011–1017.
6. BELLUZZI A, BOSCHI S, BRIGNOLA C, MUNARINI A, CARIANI G, MIGLIO F, 'Polyunsaturated fatty acids and inflammatory bowel disease', *Am J Clin Nutr*, 2000 **71** 339–42.
7. UAUY-DAGACH R, 'Marine oils: the health benefits of *n-3* fatty acids', *Nutrition Reviews*, 1996 **54** 102–108.
8. http://www.fda.gov/bbs/topics/news/2004/NEW01115.html
9. http://jhci.org.uk/approv/omega.htm
10. ALLEN D A, 'Fish oil compositions' in Hamilton R J and Rice R D, *Fish oil. Technology, nutrition and marketing.* Wycombe, P J Barnes & Associates, 1995, 95–108.
11. www.iffo.org.uk/tech/alaska.htm
12. BAJPAI P, BAPAI P K, WARD O P, 'Production of docosahexaenoic acid by *Traustochytrium aureum*', *Appl Microbial Biotechnol*, 1991 **35** 706–710.
13. KENDRIKC A, RATLEDGE C, 'Lipids of selected molds grown for production of n-3 and

n-6 polyunsaturated fatty acids', *Lipids*, 1992 **27** 15–20.

14. GUNSTONE F D, HARWOOD J L, PADLEY F B, *The lipid handbook*, London, Chapman and Hall, 1994.
15. KYLE D J, 'Production and use of a single cell oil which is highly enriched in docosahexaenoic acid', *Lipid Technol*, 1996 **8** 107–110.
16. KYLE D J, 'Production and use of a single cell oil highly enriched in arachidonic acid', *Lipid Technol*, 1997 **9** 116–121.
17. SIJTSMA L, 'Marine micro-organisms as new sources of n-3 polyunsaturated fatty acids (PUFA)' in Arnoldi A *Functional foods, cardiovascular disease and diabetes*, Cambridge, Woodhead Publishing, 2004, 333–350.
18. PULZ O, 'Photobioreactors: production systems for phototrophic microorganisms', *Appl Microbial Biotechnol*, 2001 **57** 287–293.
19. MEDINA A R, GRIMA E M, GIMÉNEZ A G, GONZÁLEZ M J I, 'Downstream processing of algal polyunsaturated fatty acids', *Biotechnol Advances*, 1998 **16** 517–580.
20. FRANKEL E N, *Lipid Oxidation*, Dundee, The Oily Press, 1998.
21. GUTTERIDGE J M C, HALLIWELL B, 'The measurement and mechanism of lipid peroxidation in biological systems', *Trends Biochem Sci*, 1990 **15** 129–135.
22. GRAY J I, GOMAA, E A, BUCKLEY D J, 'Oxidative quality and shelf life of meats', *Meat Sci*, 1996 **43** 111–123.
23. KITTS D D, 'An evaluation of the multiple effects of the antioxidant vitamins', *Trends Food Sci Technol*, 1997 **8**, 198–203.
24. AHMAD J I, 'Free radicals and health: Is vitamin E the answer?', *Food Sci Technol Today*, 1996 **10** 147–152.
25. KANNER J, 'Oxidative processes in meat and meat products: quality implications', *Meat Sci*, 1994 **36** 169–189.
26. BELITZ, H-D, GROSCH W, *Food Chemistry*, 2nd edn, Berlin, Heidelberg, Germany, Springer-Verlag, 1999, 992 pp.
27. FRANKEL E N, 'Recent advances in lipid oxidation. Review', *J Sci Food Agric*, 1991 **54** 495–511.
28. AIDOS I, KREB N, BOONMAN M, LUTEN J B, BOOM R M, VAN DER PADT A, 'Influence of production process parameters on fish oil quality in a pilot plant', *J Food Science*, 2003 **68** 581–587.
29. AIDOS I, MASBERNAT-MARTINEZ S, LUTEN J B, BOOM R M, VAN DER PADT A, 'Composition and stability of herring oil recovered from sorted byproducts as compared to oil from mixed byproducts', *J Agric Food Chem*, 2002 **50** 2818–2824.
30. AIDOS I, SCHELVIS-SMIT R, VELDMAN M, LUTEN J B, VAN DER PADT A, BOOM R M, 'Chemical and sensory evaluation of crude oil extracted from herring byproducts from different processing operations', *J Agric Food Chem*, 2003 **51**, 1897–1903.
31. AIDOS I, VAN DER PADT A, BOOM R M, LUTEN J B, 'Upgrading of maatjes herring byproducts: Production of crude fish oil', *J Agric Food Chem*, 2001 **49** 3697–3704.
32. AIDOS I, JACOBSEN C, JENSEN B, LUTEN J B, VAN DER PADT A, BOOM R M, 'Volatile oxidation products formed in crude herring oil under accelerated oxidative conditions', *Eur J Lipid Sci Technol*, 2002 **104** 808–818.
33. AIDOS I, VAN DER PADT A, BOOM R M, LUTEN J B, 'Quality of crude fish oil extracted from herring byproducts of varying states of freshness', *J Food Sci*, 2003 **68** 458–465.
34. AIDOS I, LOURENCE S, VAN DER PADT A, LUTEN J B, BOOM R M, 'Stability of crude herring oil produced from fresh byproducts: influence of temperature during storage', *J Food Sci*, 2002 **67** 3314–3320.

35. AIDOS I, VAN DER PADT A, LUTEN J B, BOOM R M, 'Seasonal changes in crude and lipid composition of herring fillets, byproducts and respective produced oils', *J Agric Food Chem* 2002 **50** 4589–4599.
36. SKÅRA T, SIVERTSVIK M, BIRKELAND S, 'Production of salmon oil from filleting byproducts effects of storage conditions on lipid oxidation and content of omega-3 polyunsaturated fatty acids', *J Food Sci*, 2004 **69** 417–421.
37. CHANG S S, 'Processing of fish oils' in Stansby M E, *Fish oil. Technology, nutrition and marketing*, Westport, Conn, AVI Publishing Co., 1967, 206–221.
38. YOUNG F V K, 'The refining and hydrogenation of fish oil', *Fish Oil Bulletin*, Vol. 17, International Association of Fish Meal Manufacturers, 1985, 27 pp.
39. BIMBO A P, 'Processing of fish oils' in Stansby M E, *Fish oils in nutrition*, New York, Van Nostrand Reinhold, 1990, 181–225.
40. LET, M B, JACOBSEN C, MEYER A S, 'Oxidative flavour deterioration of fish oil enriched milk', *Eur J Lipid Sci Technol*, 2003 **9** 508–517.
41. LET M B, JACOBSEN C, MEYER A S, 'Sensory stability and oxidation of fish oil enriched milk is affected by milk storage temperatures and oil quality', *Internat Dairy J*, 2005 **15** 173–182.
42. MEI L, DECKER E A, McCLEMENTS D J, 'Evidence of iron association with emulsion droplets and its impact on lipid oxidation', *J Agric Food Chem*, 1998 **46** 5072–5077.
43. MEI L, McCLEMENTS D J, WU J, DECKER E A, 'Iron-catalyzed lipid oxidation in emulsion as affected by surfactant, pH and NaCl', *Food Chem*, 1998 **61** 307–312.
44. JACOBSEN C, TIMM M, MEYER A S, 'Oxidation in fish oil enriched mayonnaise: ascorbic acid and low pH increase oxidative deterioration', *J Agric Food Chem*, **2001** 49 3947–3956.
45. JACOBSEN C, ADLER-NISSEN J, MEYER A S, 'The effect of ascorbic acid on iron release from the emulsifier interface and on the oxidative flavor deterioration in fish oil enriched mayonnaise', *J Agric Food Chem*, 1999 **47** 4917–4926.
46. MANCUSO J R, McCLEMENTS D J, DECKER E A, 'The effects of surfactant type, pH, and chelators on the oxidation of salmon oil-in-water emulsions', *J Agric Food Chem*, 1999 **47** 4112–4116.
47. CHO Y J, McCLEMENTS D J, DECKER E A, 'Ability of surfactant micelles to alter the physical location and reactivity of iron in oil-in-water emulsion', *J Agric Food Chem*, 2002 **50** 5704–5710.
48. NUCHI C D, HERNANDEZ P, McCLEMENTS D J, DECKER E A, 'Ability of lipid hydroperoxides to partition into surfactant micelles and alter lipid oxidation rates in emulsions', *J Agric Food Chem*, 2002 **50** 5445–5449.
49. HU M, McCLEMENTS D J, DECKER E A, 'Impact of whey protein emulsifiers on the oxidative stability of salmon oil-in-water emulsions', *J Agric Food Chem*, 2003 **51** 1435–1439.
50. HU M, McCLEMENTS D J, DECKER E A, 'Lipid oxidation in corn oil-in-water emulsions stabilized by casein, whey protein isolate, and soy protein isolate', *J Agric Food Chem* 2003 **51** 1696–1700.
51. SILVESTRE M C P, CHAIYASIT W, BRANNAN R G, McCLEMENTS D J, DECKER E A, 'Ability of surfactant headgroup size to alter lipid and antioxidant oxidation in oil-in-water emulsions', *J Agric Food Chem*, 2000 **48** 2057–2061.
52. TONG L M, SASAKI S, McCLEMENTS D J, DECKER E A, 'Mechanisms of the antioxidant activity of a high molecular weight fraction of whey', *J Agric Food Chem*, 2000 **48** 1473–1478.
53. RUTH S M, KING C, GIANNOULI, P, 'Influence of lipid fraction, emulsifier fraction, and

mean particle diameter of oil-in-water emulsions on the release of 20 aroma compounds', *J Agric Food Chem*, 2002 **50** 2365–2371.

54. DRUAUX C, VOILLEY, A, 'Effect of food composition and microstructure on volatile flavour release', *Trends Food Sci Technol*, 1997 **8** 364–368.
55. PORTER W L, 'Paradoxical behavior of antioxidants in food and biological systems', *Toxicol Ind Health*, 1993 **9** 93–122.
56. FRANKEL E N, HUANG S-W, KANNER J, GERMAN, J B, 'Interfacial phenomena in the evaluation of antioxidants: Bulk oils vs emulsions', *J Agric Food Chem*, 1994 **42** 1054–1059.
57. HUANG S-W, HOPIA A, FRANKEL E N, GERMAN J B, 'Antioxidant activity of α-tocopherol and Trolox in different lipid substrates: Bulk oils vs oil-in-water emulsions', *J Agric Food Chem* 1996, **44** 444–452.
58. JACOBSEN C, SCHWARZ K, STOECKMANN H, MEYER A S, ADLER-NISSEN J, 'Partitioning of selected antioxidants in mayonnaise', *J Agric Food Chem*, 1999 **47** 3601–3610.
59. JACOBSEN C, HARTVIGSEN K, LUND P, MEYER A S, ADLER-NISSEN J, HOLSTBORG J, HØLMER G, 'Oxidation in fish oil enriched mayonnaise: 1. Assessment of propyl gallate as antioxidant by discriminant partial least squares regression analysis', *Z Lebensm Unters Forsch*, 1999 **210** 13–30.
60. JACOBSEN C, HARTVIGSEN K, LUND P, ADLER-NISSEN J, HØLMER G, MEYER A S, 'Oxidation in fish oil enriched mayonnaise: 2. Assessment of the efficacy of different tocopherol antioxidant systems by discriminant partial least squares regression analysis', *Eur Food Res Technol*, 2000 **210** 242–257.
61. JACOBSEN C, HARTVIGSEN K, LUND P, THOMSEN M K, SKIBSTED L H, HØLMER G, ADLER-NISSEN J, MEYER A S, 'Oxidation in fish oil enriched mayonnaise: 4. Effect of tocopherol concentration on oxidative deterioration', *Eur Food Res Technol*, 2001 **212** 308–318.
62. JACOBSEN C, HARTVIGSEN K, THOMSEN M K, HANSEN L F, LUND P, SKIBSTED L H, HØLMER G, ADLER-NISSEN J, MEYER A S, 'Lipid oxidation in fish oil enriched mayonnaise: Calcium disodium ethylenediaminetetraacetate, but not gallic acid, strongly inhibited oxidative deterioration', *J Agric Food Chem*, 2001 **49** 1009–1019.
63. LET M B, JACOBSEN C, PHAM K A, MEYER A S, 'Protection against oxidation of fish oil enriched milk emulsions through addition of rapeseed oil or antioxidants', *J Agric Food Chem*, 2005 **53** 5429–5437.
64. JACOBSEN C, XU X, NIELSEN N S, TIMM-HEINRICH M, 'Oxidative stability of mayonnaise containing structured lipids produced from sunflower oil and caprylic acid', *Eur J Lipid Sci Technol*, 2003 **105** 449–458.
65. NIELSEN N S, PETERSEN A, MEYER A S, TIMM-HEINRICH M, JACOBSEN C, 'The effects of lactoferrin, phytic acid and EDTA on oxidation in two food emulsions enriched with long chain polyunsaturated fatty acids' *J Agric Food Chem*, 2004 **52** 7090–7099.
66. FRANKEL E N, SATUE-GRACIA T, MEYER A S, GERMAN J B, 'Oxidative stability of fish and algae oils containing long- chain polyunsaturated fatty acids in bulk and in oil-in-water emulsions', *J Agric Food Chem*, 2002 **50** (7) 2094–2099.
67. PADLEY FB, FREEMAN I P, POLMAN R G, VAN LOOKEREN G J, 'Marine/vegetable oil blend and products made therefrom', Patent EP0304115, 1989.
68. POLMAN R G, LAMMERS J G, PIERCE J H, 'Edible fatty composition containing bleached fish oils', Patent GB 2 241 503 (A), 1991.
69. PERLMAN D, HAYES K C, 'Modified fat blends', Patent US 5382442, 1995.
70. LET M B, JACOBSEN C, FRANKEL E N, MEYER A S, 'Oxidative flavour deterioration of fish oil enriched milk: effects of oil type and ethylenediaminetetraacetate (EDTA)', *Eur*

J Lipid Sci Technol, 2003 **105** 518–528.
71. KOLANOWSKI W, SWIDERSKI F, LIS E, BERGER S, 'Enrichment of spreadable fats with polyunsaturated fatty acids omega-3 using fish oil', *Internat J Food Sci Nutr*, 2001 **52** 469–476.
72. COUPLAND J N, McCLEMENTS D J, 'Lipid oxidation in food emulsions', *Trends Food Sci Technol*, 1996 **7** 83–91.
73. SIMS R J, FIORITI J A, TRUMBETAS J, 'Effect of sugar and sugar alcohols on autoxidation of safflower oil in emulsions', *J Am Oil Chem Soc*, 1979 **56** 742–745.
74. SCHROEDER L R, MUFFETT D J, 'Processed meat products containing fish oils stabilized with fructose', Patent US 5116629, 1992.
75. SCHROEDER L R, MUFFETT D J, 'Food products containing fish oils stabilized with fructose', Patent US 4913921, 1990.
76. GENOT C, MEYNIER A, RIAUBLANC A, 'Lipid oxidation in emulsions', in Kamal-Eldin A, *Lipid oxidation pathways*, Champaign IL, AOCS Press, 2003, 190–244.
77. JACOBSEN C, HARTVIGSEN K, LUND P, THOMSEN M K, SKIBSTED L H, ADLER-NISSEN J, HØLMER G, MEYER A S, 'Oxidation in fish oil enriched mayonnaise: 3. Assessment of the influence of the emulsion structure on oxidation by discriminant partial least squares regression analysis', *Eur. Food Res Technol*, 2000 **211** 86–98.
78. ANONYMOUS, 'Improvements in or relating to the manufacture of concentrated sweetened milk products and substances derived therefrom', Patent GB458399, 1936.
79. XINHUA L, 'Enhanced milk containing polyunsaturated fatty acid', Patent CN1108891, 1995.
80. NADACHI Y, UCHIDA Y, HATANO K, KARISHU M, KOGA K, OGAWA K, 'Process for producing DHA-containing tofu or soybean milk drink, or dry powder thereof', Patent US5976606, 1999.
81. PARK Y, KELLEHER S D, McCLEMENTS J D, DECKER E A, 'Incorporation and stabilization of omega-3 fatty acids in surimi made from cod, *Gadus morhua'*, *J Agric Food Chem*, 2004 **52** 597–601.
82. DJORDJEVIC D, KIM H-J, McCLEMENTS D J, DECKER E A, 'Physical stability of whey protein-stabilized oil-in-water emulsions at pH 3: potential omega-3 fatty acid delivery systems (Part A)', *J Food Sci*, 2004 **69** 351–355.
83. DJORDJEVIC D, KIM H-J, McCLEMENTS D J, DECKER E A, 'Physical stability of whey protein-stabilized oil-in-water emulsions at pH 3: Potential omega-3 fatty acid delivery systems (Part B)', *J Food Sci*, 2004 **69** 356–361.
84. KEOGH M K, O'KENNEDY B T, KELLY J, AUTY M A, KELLY P M, FUREBY A, HAAHR A M, 'Stability to oxidation of spray-dried fish oil powder microencapsulated using milk ingredients', *J Food Sci*, 2001 **66** 217–224.
85. KAGAMI Y, SUGIMURY S, FUJISHIMA N, MATSUDA K, KOMETANI T, MATSUMURA Y, 'Oxidative stability, structure and physical characteristics of microcapsules formed by spray drying of fish oil with protein and dextrin wall materials', *J Food Sci*, 2003 **68** 2248–2255.
86. HEINZELMANN K, FRANKE K, JENSEN B, HAAHR A M, 'Protection of fish oil from oxidation by microencapsulation using freeze-drying techniques', *Eur J Lipid Sci Technol*, 2000 **102** 114–121.
87. BAIK M Y, SUHENDRO E L, NAWAR W W, McCLEMENTS D J, DECKER E A, CHINACHOTI P, 'Effects of antioxidants and humidity on the oxidative stability of microencapsulated fish oil', *J Am Oil Chem Soc* 2004 **81** 355–360.
88. VELASCO J, DOBARGANES M C, MÁRQUEZ-RUIZ G, 'Oxidation of free and encapsulated

oil fractions in dried microencapsulated fish oils', *Grasas y Aceites* 2000 **51** 439–446.

89. HOGAN S A, O'RIORDAN E D, O'SULLIVAN, 'Microencapsulation and oxidative stability of spray-dried fish oil emulsions', *J Microencapsulation* 2003 **20** 675–688.
90. HARDAS N, DANVIRIYAKUL S, FOLEY J L, NAWAR W W, CHINACHOTI P, 'Effect of the relative humidity on the oxidative stability and physical stability of encapsulated milk fat', *J Am Oil Chem Soc*, 2002 **79** 151–158.
91. BOLAND M, MACGIBBON A, HILL J, 'Designer milks for the new millennium', *Livest Prod Sci,* 2001 **72** 99–109.

19

New marine sources of polyunsaturated fatty acids (PUFAs)

T. A. B Sanders, King's College London, UK, and H. E. Theobald, British Nutrition Foundation, UK

19.1 Introduction: the need for new sources of PUFAs

Several recent dietary guidelines have advocated an increased consumption of long chain *n-3* polyunsaturated fatty acids (PUFAs) because of evidence that the consumption of these fatty acids is associated with a decreased risk of cardiovascular disease. There is also growing recognition that long chain PUFAs particularly arachidonic acid (20:4*n-6*; AA) and docosahexaenoic acid (22:6*n-3*; DHA) may be required in the diets of the neonate and that the maternal supply of DHA is largely dependent on the amount of DHA in her diet. The major long chain *n-3* PUFA in human diets are eicosapentaenoic acid (20:5n-3; EPA) and DHA; their major dietary source is seafood (Meyer *et al.* 2003). Only small amounts are found in lean red meat, organ meats such as liver and brain, and eggs, and only trace amounts are present in dairy products. Consequently, attempts to increase the dietary intake of these fatty acids imply an increased intake of fish. This chapter considers the major barriers to increasing intakes from fish and considers alternative sources of long chain PUFAs from single cell oils.

19.1.1 Sustainability

It is now widely recognised that fish stocks throughout the world are becoming seriously depleted. Fish stocks in the North West Atlantic have collapsed and a similar pattern has emerged in the North Sea. Globally, current rates of fish catch are not sustainable (Pauly *et al.* 2005). While fish farming, particularly of salmon and trout, which are rich in EPA and DHA, may seem a logical alternative it is currently heavily dependent upon a supply of oil-rich marine fish. It is estimated that it takes about 10 kg of fish to produce 1 kg of farmed salmon. Consequently, there is a need to develop plant-based alternative feeds for farmed fish. While needs of fish for protein can easily be provided from land-based plant sources such as soybeans, there remains a need to provide a source of EPA and DHA in the feed.

19.1.2 Dioxins, PCBs and other persistent contaminants

Fish is a fragile food resource and contamination of the marine food chain can result in the accumulation of a variety of persistent toxic chemicals. Most attention has been focused on dioxins and related compounds but recently (Hites *et al.* 2004) attention has been drawn to the accumulation in fish of chemicals used as fire retardants particularly polybrominated diphenyl ethers which have 'gender bending' effects. Fish oils usually contain significant amounts (1 ppm) of polychlorinated biphenyls (PCBs) and trace amounts of dioxins (Foran *et al.* 2005). These compounds accumulate in the marine food chain. Dioxins are toxic substances produced during many industrial processes involving chlorine such as waste incineration, chemical and pesticide manufacturing and pulp and paper bleaching. Acute toxicity is rare and results in damage to the immune system and chloroacne – as exemplified by an attempt to poison the presidential candidate (later president) in Ukraine in 2004.

The gradual accumulations of PCBs and dioxins have no immediate effect on health, even at the highest levels found in foods, but potential risks to health come from long-term exposure. The most potent dioxin 2,3,7,8-tetrachlorodibenzo-*p*-dioxin (TCCD) is a known human carcinogen and endocrine disruptor. TCCD is a ligand for the arylhydrocarbon (AhR) receptor and blocks the synthesis of oestrogen receptor ERα. The toxicity of other dioxins and chemicals like PCBs that act like dioxin are measured in relation to TCDD in units called tetrachlorodibenzo-*p*-dioxin equivalents (TEQ) by comparing their relative binding to the AhR receptor.

PCBs have been used since the early 1930s, mainly in electrical equipment as coolants, but their manufacture and general use stopped in the 1970s. Nevertheless, substantial amounts of PCBs have been released into the environment particularly in developing countries where there is a lack of effective regulation against pollution. PCBs dumped in the tropics evaporate into the atmosphere and condense in the polar regions, contaminating the marine food chain. Both dioxins and dioxin-like PCBs are persistent organic pollutants that degrade slowly and accumulate by moving up the food chain in fatty tissues. The highest concentrations of PCBs and dioxins are found in the liver, and high concentrations have been found in the blood, milk and tissues of marine mammals, and also in humans residing in polar regions. The adverse toxic effects of dioxins and dioxin-like PCBs are likely to be greatest on the developing foetus and may increase the risk of hormone-related cancers in adults such as breast cancer and prostate cancer. Adverse effects on the offspring of women who consumed pilot whale blubber during pregnancy have been reported in the Faroe Islands and in women who consume 'sport's' fish from the Great Lakes in North America. However, it is uncertain whether the adverse effects are attributable to the PCBs and dioxins or whether these compounds are global markers for other marine toxins such as heavy metals (mercury, cadmium).

Fish and animals, particularly animals that have been fed fish oil/fish meal, are the most significant dietary sources of dioxins and dioxin-like PCBs. Although there has been a decline in dioxin and PCB exposure, more stringent regulation has meant that many unpurified fish oils and samples of oily fish exceed the recommended safe levels. The tightening regulatory noose has forced many fish oil processors to introduce additional refining processes to reduce the concentrations of these contaminants to barely detectable levels. This has become of particular concern in the area of infant feeding where the Tolerable Daily Intake for dioxins and dioxin-like PCBs should be below 2 pg TEQ/kg body weight. This has been an important driver for increasing the demand for sources of DHA that are free from dioxins and PCBs for use in infant formula.

19.1.3 Vitamins A and D and cholesterol

Retinol and vitamin D are found in relatively high concentrations in fish liver oils. Indeed the levels in halibut liver and shark liver oil are regarded as toxic. Traditionally cod liver oil has played an important role in providing vitamins A and D as well as EPA and DHA in Northern Europe. However, there is a concern that high intakes of retinol increase the risk of bone fractures in older women (Lips 2003). It is uncertain whether this applies to cod liver oil which also contains vitamin D. High intakes of retinol in pregnancy are teratogenic and excessive intakes of retinol have been linked to an increased risk of birth defects such as cleft palate. Consequently, it is recommended that intakes of retinol greater than 3300 μg/day should be avoided by women during their reproductive years (Dolk *et al.* 1999). For this reason regulatory authorities are considering means of restricting the intake of retinol from supplements.

Both fish body and fish liver oils contain significant amounts of sterols (~600 mg/100 g) mainly as cholesterol. The intake of cholesterol from fish oil is generally not of significance. However, de Oliveira *et al.* (1996) have shown that the consumption of 300 g shrimp/day increased LDL cholesterol by 7% which is attributable to the dietary cholesterol. Owing to consumer awareness regarding cholesterol in food, which has arisen as a result of nutritional labelling, there is also a demand for sources of EPA and DHA that are free from cholesterol.

19.1.4 Needs of vegetarians and vegans

A significant proportion of the world's population does not consume meat or fish for a variety of reasons. It is, therefore, appropriate to consider how their needs for EPA and DHA could be met. Vegetarians, who do not eat meat or fish, and vegans, who also exclude eggs and dairy products from their diets, have very low or negligible intakes of EPA and DHA. On the other hand, vegetarians and vegans tend to have a relatively high intake of linoleic acid (18:2*n-6*, LA), which is largely derived from plant sources. EPA and DHA can also be synthesised in the body from α-linolenic acid (18:3*n*-3, ALA); however, this conversion is limited in humans, possibly more in men than in women (Sanders 1999; Davis & Kris-Etherton 2003). The conversion may be further suppressed by a high intake of LA since the elongation and desaturation of ALA and LA involve the same rate-limiting Δ-6 desaturase enzyme. Indeed, trials have shown that ALA supplementation increases plasma EPA and docosapentaenoic acid (22:5 *n*-3; DPA) but has little effect on DHA. As a result, vegetarians and vegans, who have a low dietary intake of DHA (and a correspondingly high intake of LA) have lower amounts of EPA and DHA in blood and adipose tissue compared with omnivores. If long chain *n-3* fatty acids are required in human diets, there is a need to develop sources that are acceptable to vegans and vegetarians.

19.2 Microbial sources of PUFA

Single cell oils (SCO) have been defined as the edible oils obtained from micro-organisms being similar in type and composition to those oils and fats from plants and animals (Ratledge 2005). Early research in the first part of the 20th century, mainly by German chemists, identified a number of micro-organisms capable of synthesising fat (>20% of their biomass as triacylglycerol). The oil accumulation of these oleaginous micro-organisms could be increased by starving the cells of a supply of nitrogen. The medium had to be formulated with a high carbon : nitrogen ratio (typically 30 to 50:1). One of the first attempts to produce fat from these sources was in Germany during World War II. Oil-rich biomass from *Geotrichum candidum* was grown on waste lactose or other agricultural waste and fed to horses and probably people. Work conducted in the 1960s on identifying possible sources of arachidonic acid (AA) focused on yeast and other related fungi. More recent work identifying sources of EPA and DHA has focused on algae.

19.2.1 Fungal sources

Gamma linolenic acid (18:3*n*-6; GLA) was shown to occur in a group of lower fungi known as Zygomycetes (Table 19.1). The first SCO produced from this family using *Mucor circinelloides* in large-scale fermentors (220 m^3) was by J & E Sturge (Selby, North Yorkshire, UK). The oil was sold under the trade name of Oil of Javanicus and also a GLA-Forte™. This oil contained 18% by weight GLA compared with evening primrose oil which typically contains 8–10%. The fungal oil, although superior to evening primrose oil in several

Table 19.1 Fat content and fatty acid composition of *Zygomycetes* fungi used for commercial synthesis of PUFA (from Ratledge 2005)

	Mucor circinelloides	*Mortierella alpina*
Oil content g/100 g	25	50
Fatty acid composition wt%		
16:0	22	8
18:0	6	11
18:1	40	14
18:2n*n*-6	11	7
18:3*n*-6	18	4
20:3*n*-6	–	4
20:4*n*-6	–	49

respects, had difficulty being sold to a suspicious public in the UK. Research in Japan identified another Zygomycetes fungus, *Mortierella alpina*, as having the capacity to synthesise arachidonic acid (AA). The commercial production of this oil was undertaken in the UK using the facilities and technology developed to make mycoprotein (Quorn™, Marlowe Foods Ltd, UK). The arachidonic acid SCO (ARASCO™) produced by this process typically contains 49% AA by weight and is used in the manufacture of infant formula.

Mortierella alpina, when grown at low temperature (<20 °C) and supplemented with ALA, can produce EPA instead of AA. However, the costs of producing EPA by this technique are considerably greater than that for AA as it requires a lengthy cultivation period.

19.2.2 Algal sources

The high proportions of EPA and DHA in oily fish result from the accumulation of lipids synthesised by marine algae. The major primary producer of these fatty acids appears to be marine microalgae, of which the Dinophyta (dinoflagellates) are second only to diatoms as primary producers in coastal waters. Dinoflagellate species of microalgae produce the most commonly known microalgal toxins (such as the potent neurotoxins tetradoxin and saxitoxins). Toxins from dinoflagellates cause paralytic shellfish poisoning and diaorrhetic shellfish poisoning and are probably responsible for 'ciguatera poisoning' in certain areas of the Caribbean and Pacific Ocean. Consequently, the selection of strains of dinoflagellates need to ensure that the algae do not produce toxins. Table 19.2 shows the fatty acid composition of oil derived from different dinoflagellates. Oil from *Crypthecodinium cohnii*, which contains virtually no EPA and cholesterol, was developed as a source of DHA for infant formula by Martek Inc. (Columbia, Maryland, USA) as DHASCO™. By strain selection and optimising production conditions it has been possible to produce a triacylglycerol with 40–45% DHA and virtually no EPA. The other major fatty acids in DHASCO™ are myristic acid (5–20%), palmitic acid (5–20%) and oleic acid (10–40%).

Table 19.2 Fatty acid composition (wt%) of some dinoflagellates (from Wynn *et al.* 2005)

	Gonyaulax digenesis	*Crypthecodinium cohnii*	*Cochlodinium heteroblatum*
16:0	22	20	33
16:1	2	1	4
18:0	2	1	1
18:1	8	14	6
18:3*n*-6	–	–	–
18:3*n*-3	–	2	–
18:4*n*-3	1	–	1
18:5*n*-3	8	–	8
20:4*n*-6		–	–
20:5*n*-3	11	–	8
22:5*n*-3	–	–	–
22:6*n*-3	28	30	25

Thraustochytrids are probably a more significant global source of DHA in the marine environment. Thraustochytrids are microalgae or microalgae-like micro-organisms and are not related to the toxin-forming dinoflagellates or blue-green algae. Thraustochytrids are found throughout the world in estuarine and marine habitats. Their nutritional mode is primarily saprotrophic (obtain food by absorbing dissolved organic matter) and as such are generally found associated with organic detritus, decomposing algal and plant material. The earliest research of thraustochytrids placed them in the fungus kingdom because of their heterotrophic nature and superficial resemblance to chytrids. Current analyses using molecular biology techniques have demonstrated that thraustochytrids are not fungi, and they are related to the heterokont algae. There is still controversy on whether thraustochytrids are Heterokonta that have lost their chloroplasts or, as some of the most recent analyses suggest, the thraustochytrids may be the earliest member of the Heterokonta representing the form prior to acquisition of chloroplasts. It was discovered that *Schizochytrium* spp. were able to synthesise large amounts of DHA. By altering the source and level of sodium salts it was found that *Schizochytrium* spp. could be cultured to produce DHA in high yield. The oil also contains significant amounts of the *n-6* homologue of DHA, docosapentaenoic acid (22:5*n-6*, DPA).

Metz *et al.* using modern molecular biological techniques have shown that DHA in *Schizochytrium* spp. and probably other thraustochytrids is derived via a novel metabolic pathway related to the polyketide synthase pathway that does not involve ALA as substrate (Metz *et al.* 2001). Biomass from *Schizochytrium* spp. was first approved as an animal feed ingredient in the USA and later oil from *Schizochytrium* sp. was produced for commercial food use (DHA Gold^{TM} or DHASCO-S^{TM}). Table 19.3 shows the typical composition of refined oil from *Schizochytrium* spp.

Table 19.3 Fatty acid composition of oil from *Schizochytrium* sp. (from Sandes *et al.* 2005)

Fatty acid	Wt %
14:0	7.5
16:0	20.4
16:1	0.4
18:0	0.5
18:1	0.6
18:2*n*-6	0.5
20:4*n*-6	0.7
20:4*n*-3	0.9
20:5*n*-3	1.8
22:5*n*-6	15.5
22:6*n*-3	38.0

19.3 Production methods

Single cell oils are generally prepared by batch fermentation reactions and lipids are extracted following disruption of the cells using a solvent such as hexane. The hexane/oil mix is separated from the oil-depleted biomass and passed to an evaporator to remove the solvent. The crude oil is then stored at low temperature under nitrogen (to prevent oxidation) prior to further processing. The crude oil is then subjected to processing similar to that used for vegetable oils: alkali refining, bleaching, winterisation and deodorisation. Vitamin E and permitted antioxidants are then added to the oil. Owing to the novel (microbial) origin of the SCO, they have been subject to thorough safety evaluation in Europe to meet the requirements of the Novel Foods Directive and the requirement of the Food and Drugs Administration in the USA.

19.3.1 Safety evaluation of single cells oils as novel foods

The European Union Novel Foods Directive which came into force in 1997 requires that all novel foods and processes undergo a thorough evaluation before they can be used for food production. ARASCO™, DHASCO™ and DHA Gold™ have all undergone such an evaluation in the European Union that involved full toxicological testing as well as detailed specification of the production process and a thorough risk analysis. In the United States, the legal situation is somewhat different and the concept of substantial equivalence is more widely used. For example, the Food and Drug Administration agreed that DHASCO™ was substantially equivalent to menhaden oil, which is granted Generally Recognised as Safe (GRAS) status. Although SCO are widely used as minor ingredients in infant formula, it is to be noted there have been relatively few well-controlled published studies in adults using higher intakes.

19.3.2 Human feeding studies

Several studies have used purified algal triacylglycerol to investigate the effects of DHA on blood lipids and cardiovascular risk factors. Some early studies suggested a reduction in TAG concentration and an increase in HDL cholesterol concentration in normolipidaemic omnivores, at doses between 1.62 and 6.0 g/day (Ågren *et al.* 1996; Conquer & Holub 1996; Davidson *et al.* 1997; Nelson *et al.* 1997). No adverse reactions were noted but the number of subjects in the studies were small and study duration was short. Davidson *et al.* (1997) noted a tendency for non-HDL cholesterol to be greater in subjects with hyperlipidaemia. More recently, Theobald *et al.* (2004) conducted a year-long study, using a crossover design to investigate the effect of a low dose of 1.5 g DHASCO™/day (providing 0.7 g DHA/day) versus a placebo, taken for a 3-month period, with a 4-month washout period between the two treatments. Effect on cardiovascular risk factors as well as blood counts, liver function tests, renal function and biochemical indices of inflammation was measured in 39 middle-aged men and women (Tables 19.4–19.6). DHASCO™ was found to raise LDL cholesterol by 7% but did not result in any toxicological changes in safety parameters, i.e. liver and renal function and blood counts. In another study, 68 vegan men were given 200 mg DHA/day or placebo for 3 months. The DHA supplement increased plasma concentrations of DHA by ~42% and the proportion of DHA in erythrocytes by 41% (Fig. 19.1). There were no significant changes in plasma lipoprotein concentrations; blood counts and liver function tests were unaffected by treatment (Sanders TAB and Lloyd-Wright Z, unpublished observations).

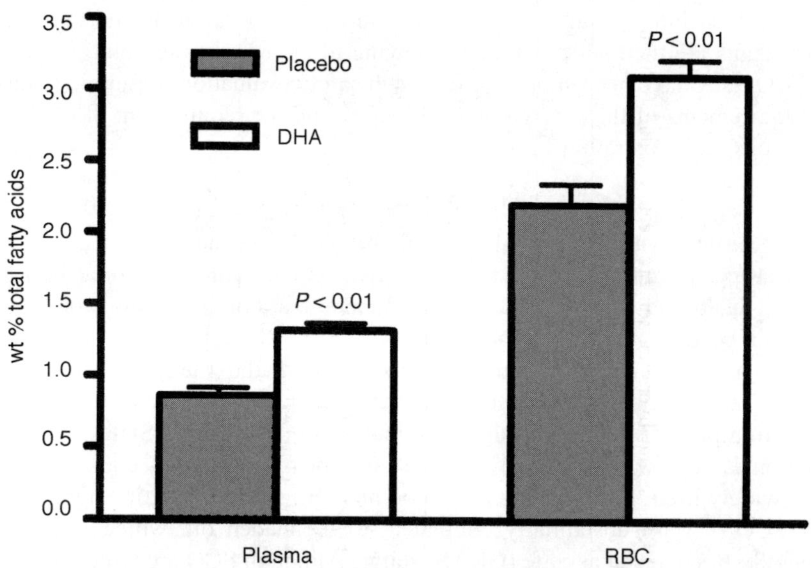

Fig. 19.1 Influence of 200 mg DHA/day for 3 months on the proportions (wt%) of DHA in plasma and erythrocyte lipids in vegans (mean values with SEM).

Table 19.4 Serum liver function pre-treatment and following 1.5 g of DHASCO™/day or placebo treatment in middle-aged healthy men and women

	DHA $n = 38$				Placebo $n = 38$			
	Pre-DHA		Post-DHA		Pre-placebo		Post-placebo	
	Mean	SEM	Mean	SEM	Mean	SEM	Mean	SEM
Total protein (g/l)	20.1	0.6	21.6	0.6	19.5	0.6	22.1	0.6
Albumin (g/l)	42.7	0.4	42.4	0.4	42.8	0.4	42.2	0.4
Bilirubin (μmol/l)	11.2	1.5	11.3	1.2	10.6	1.0	10.8	1.3
Alkaline phosphatase (U/l)	59.5	2.9	60.2	2.6	58.4	2.5	58.8	2.8
Aspartate transaminase (U/l)	19.1	0.9	19.6	1.1	19.4	1.1	19.4	0.7
Gamma glutamyl transferase (U/l)	20.1	1.4	21.6	1.6	19.5	1.4	22.1	2.5

No significant differences between treatments or periods.

Table 19.5 Full blood counts following pre-treatment and following 1.5 g of DHASCO^{TM}/day or placebo treatment in middle-aged healthy men and women

	DHA $n = 38$				Placebo $n = 38$			
	Pre-DHA		Post-DHA		Pre-placebo		Post-placebo	
	Mean	SEM	Mean	SEM	Mean	SEM	Mean	SEM
Haemoglobin (g/dl)	13.6	0.2	13.3	0.2	13.6	0.2	13.3	0.2
RBC (10^{12}/l)	4.5	0.1	4.4	0.1	4.5	0.1	4.4	0.1
PCV	0.4	0.0	0.4	0.0	0.4	0.0	0.4	0.0
MCV (fl)	91.1	0.5	91.3	0.5	90.8	0.6	91.2	0.6
MCH (pg)	30.2	0.2	30.2	0.2	30.2	0.2	30.2	0.2
MCHC (g/dl)	33.1	0.1	33.1	0.1	33.2	0.1	33.1	0.1
Platelets (10^9/l)	248	8.8	233	9.1	242	0.1	238	8.9
WBC (10^9/l)	5.8	0.3	5.2	0.3	5.6	0.3	5.5	0.2
Neutrophils (10^9/l)	3.2	0.1	3.07	0.2	3.2	0.2	3.18	0.2
Lymphocytes (10^9/l)	1.67	0.1	1.45	0.1	2.11	0.5	1.6	0.1
Monocytes (10^9/l)	0.48	0.0	0.49	0.0	0.51	0.0	0.51	0.0
Eosinophils (10^9/l)	0.2	0.0	0.21	0.0	0.18	0.0	0.19	0.0
Basophils (10^9/l)	0.04	0.0	0.03	0.0	0.03	0.0	0.03	0.0

No significant differences between treatments or periods.
RBC = red blood cell count.
PCV = packed cell volume.
MCV = mean corpuscular volume.
MCH = mean corpuscular haemoglobin.
MCHC = mean corpuscular haemoglobin concentration.
WBC = white blood cell count.

Table 19.6 Biochemical indices of inflammation renal function pre-treatment and following 1.5 g of DHASCO™/day or placebo treatment in middle-aged healthy men and women

	DHA $n = 38$				Placebo $n = 38$			
	Pre-DHA		Post-DHA		Pre-placebo		Post-placebo	
	Mean	SEM	Mean	SEM	Mean	SEM	Mean	SEM
IL-6 (μg/l)	2.32	0.39	2.7	0.54	2.4	0.52	2.4	0.29
vWF (iu/ml)	0.94	0.05	0.84	0.05	0.9	0.06	0.93	0.06
sCRP (mg/l)	1.62	0.35	2.63	0.55	1.8	0.33	1.69	0.34
ACR (mg/mmol)	0.94	0.24	0.83	0.27	0.71	0.16	0.87	0.22

ACR = microalbumin/creatinine ratio.
vWF = von Willebrand Factor antigen.
sCRP = high sensitivity C-reactive protein assay.
No significant differences between treatments.

Sanders *et al.* (2005) undertook a thorough safety evaluation of a 4 g/day dose of oil derived from *Schizochytrium* spp. taken for 4 weeks as part of the submission for Novel Foods Approval for DHA-Gold™. A placebo-controlled parallel design in 79 healthy men and women was used and the active treatment provided 1.5 g DHA, 0.6 g DPA, 0.04 g monounsaturated fatty acids and 1.2 g saturated fatty acids (mainly myristic and palmitic acid). The placebo provided 0.6 g polyunsaturated (mainly linoleic acid), 2.7 g monounsaturated (mainly

Table 19.7 Liver function test results in subjects allocated to placebo ($n = 39$) or 4 g oil from *Schizochytrium* sp. (DHA treatment $n = 40$)

		Mean	Median	SD	Min	Max	Outside lab normal range
Baseline total protein (g/l)	Placebo	70.1	70	2.6	66	78	0
	DHA	71.7	72.5	3.6	63	78	0
End of study total protein (g/l)	Placebo	69.3	69	3.9	61	78	0
	DHA	70.6	71	4.3	62	79	0
Baseline albumin (g/l)	Placebo	44.0	44	2.0	40	49	0
	DHA	44.4	44	2.0	40	48	0
End of study albumin (g/l)	Placebo	43.7	44	2.5	39	49	0
	DHA	43.5	43	2.6	37	49	0
Baseline globulin (g/l)	Placebo	26.1	26	2.7	21	32	0
	DHA	27.3	27.5	2.9	22	33	0
End of study globulin (g/l)	Placebo	25.5	25	3.0	21	32	0
	DHA	26.9	27	3.0	22	34	0
Baseline bilirubin (μmol/l)	Placebo	10.6	10	3.5	5	17	0
	DHA	12.6	10	7.8	5	46	3
End of study bilirubin (μmol/l)	Placebo	10.5	9	3.6	6	23	1
	DHA	11.8	10.5	5.5	6	35	3
Baseline alkaline phosphatase	Placebo	76.3	72	21.6	36	137	2
(Unit/l)	DHA	65.0	66	18.2	37	111	0
End of study alkaline phosphatase	Placebo	73.3	71	23.1	34	136	0
(Unit/l)	DHA	63.2	59.5	19.2	35	117	1
Baseline aspartate transaminase	Placebo	24.8	21	18.0	15	129	1
(Unit/l)	DHA	22.8	22	6.2	13	37	0
End of study aspartate	Placebo	21.2	19	5.1	14	38	0
transaminase (Unit/l)	DHA	23.3	22	6.0	15	42	0
Baseline gamma glutamyl	Placebo	15.8	12	11.1	2	49	0
transferase (Unit/l)	DHA	16.3	15	10.9	1	47	0
End of study gamma glutamyl	Placebo	16.2	13	11.3	6	70	1
transferase (Unit/l)	DHA	18.2	15.5	11.4	3	54	0

No significant differences between treatments.
Laboratory normal range for:
Total protein 60–80 g/l
Albumin (35–50)
Bilirubin <20 μmol/l
Alkaline phosphatase <130 units/l
Aspartate transaminase <50 units/l
Gamma glutamyl transferase <55 units/l

Table 19.8 Erythrocyte and platelet counts, haemoglobin and haematological indices in subjects allocated to placebo ($n = 39$) or *Schizochytrium* sp. (DHA treatment $n = 40$)

		Mean	Median	SD	Min	Max	No. above or below lab range Above	Below
Baseline RBC 10^{12}/l	Placebo	4.68	4.65	0.44	3.84	5.61	1	4
	DHA	4.54	4.57	0.47	3.84	5.60	0	6
End of study RBC 10^{12}/l	Placebo	4.62	4.51	0.48	3.87	5.69	1	1
	DHA	4.57	4.58	0.43	3.79	5.64	0	3
Baseline haemoglobin (g/dl)	Placebo	13.71	13.85	1.33	11.30	16.00	1	0
	DHA	13.49	13.75	1.23	11.30	15.30	0	0
End of study haemoglobin (g/dl)	Placebo	13.46	13.00	1.52	11.20	16.30	0	1
	DHA	13.49	13.60	1.13	11.40	15.80	0	1
Baseline PCV	Placebo	0.43	0.43	0.04	0.36	0.50	2	3
	DHA	0.42	0.43	0.04	0.35	0.51	0	6
End of study PCV	Placebo	0.42	0.40	0.04	0.36	0.51	0	6
	DHA	0.42	0.42	0.03	0.36	0.47	0	4
Baseline MCV (fl)	Placebo	91	90	4.6	80	103	7	0
	DHA	92	93	4.2	83	100	8	0
End of study MCV (fl)	Placebo	90	89.8	4.1	78.8	99.3	4	1
	DHA	91	91.6	4.0	80.9	97.9	5	0
Baseline MCH (pg)	Placebo	29.3	29.1	1.6	24.6	32.0	1	2
	DHA	29.8	30.0	1.3	25.9	31.8	0	1
End of study MCH (pg)	Placebo	29.2	29.3	1.6	24.6	32.3	2	2
	DHA	29.6	30.0	1.4	26.2	31.7	0	2
Baseline MCHC (g/dl)	Placebo	32.3	32.3	1.1	29.2	34.3	1	9
	DHA	32.3	32.3	0.8	30.0	33.9	0	3
End of study MCHC (g/dl)	Placebo	32.4	32.4	0.77	31.1	34.0	0	7
	DHA	32.4	32.4	0.76	31.0	34.3	0	5
Baseline platelet count (10^9/l)	Placebo	243	234	50	164	345	0	0
	DHA	256	245	49	154	409	0	0
End of study platelet count (10^9/l)	Placebo	238	244	50	161	349	0	0
	DHA	246	236	40	174	377	0	0

No significant differences between treatments.

Table 19.9 White blood cell counts in subjects allocated to placebo (n = 30) or oil from *Schizochytrium* sp. (DHA treatment n = 40)

		Mean	Median	SD	Min	Max	No. above or below lab range	
							Above	Below
Baseline WBC 10^9/l	Placebo	5.31	5.24	1.20	3.58	10.21	1	4
	DHA	5.49	5.15	1.42	3.52	10.41	0	6
End of study WBC 10^9/l	Placebo	5.15	4.99	1.36	3.49	8.60	0	8
	DHA	5.69	5.35	1.66	2.90	11.15	1	4
Baseline neutrophil count 10^9/l	Placebo	2.93	2.84	1.01	1.45	7.78	2	10
	DHA	2.92	2.59	1.05	1.58	6.56	0	17
End of study neutrophil count 10^9/l	Placebo	2.89	2.83	1.06	1.01	5.75	0	14
	DHA	2.88	2.55	1.35	0.77	8.58	1	18
Baseline lymphocyte count 10^9/l	Placebo	1.64	1.66	0.40	0.92	2.73	1	8
	DHA	1.80	1.74	0.45	0.94	3.01	0	5
End of study lymphocyte count 10^9/l	Placebo	1.58	1.52	0.42	0.84	2.97	0	8
	DHA	1.95	1.86	0.63	0.93	3.95	0	4
Baseline monocyte count 10^9/l	Placebo	0.53	0.54	0.17	0.24	1.00	0	0
	DHA	0.53	0.51	0.22	0.02	1.19	1	2
End of study monocyte count 10^9/l	Placebo	0.59	0.48	0.33	0.25	1.73	3	0
	DHA	0.60	0.50	0.31	0.21	1.74	4	0
Baseline eosinophil count 10^9/l	Placebo	0.18	0.12	0.15	0.03	0.60	5	0
	DHA	0.20	0.15	0.17	0.05	0.88	3	0
End of study eosinophil count 10^9/l	Placebo	0.16	0.12	0.12	0.00	0.50	3	1
	DHA	0.22	0.19	0.17	0.03	0.93	3	0
Baseline basophil count 10^9/l	Placebo	0.03	0.02	0.02	0.00	0.06	1	3
	DHA	0.03	0.03	0.02	0.00	0.11	1	1
End of study basophil count 10^9/l	Placebo	0.03	0.03	0.02	0.00	0.09	0	2
	DHA	0.04	0.03	0.02	0.01	0.09	0	0

No significant differences between treatments.

Table 19.10 Serum-sensitive C-reactive protein (CRP), creatinase kinase activity and plasma glucose concentrations in subjects allocated to placebo or oil from *Schizochytrium* sp. (DHA treatment $n = 40$)

		Mean	Median	SD	Min	Max	Valid n	Above or below normal range
Baseline CRP (mg/l)	Placebo	1.99	1.00	3.94	0.30	24.20	38	2
	DHA	2.41	0.90	4.42	0.20	26.50	40	5
End of study CRP (mg/l)	Placebo	2.06	0.90	3.21	0.20	17.10	39	4
	DHA	2.49	1.30	2.81	0.20	12.6	40	6
Baseline creatine kinase (units/l)	Placebo	113.4	91.0	94.7	30.0	608.0	39	4
	DHA	123.7	103.0	79.8	43.0	511.0	40	11
End of study creatine kinase (units/l)	Placebo	113.7	101.0	77.5	45.0	430.0	39	5
	DHA	123.2	109.5	72.8	46.0	374.0	40	7
Baseline plasma glucose (mmol/l)	Placebo	4.7	4.7	0.4	3.5	5.50	39	0
	DHA	4.7	4.7	0.5	3.6	5.60	40	0
End of study plasma glucose (mmol/l)	Placebo	4.7	4.6	0.3	3.8	5.40	39	0
	DHA	4.7	4.8	0.5	3.6	6.20	40	0

Laboratory normal ranges:
Sensitive C-reactive protein <5 mg/l
Creatine kinase <150 units/l
Plasma glucose >3 and <7 mmol/l
There were no significant differences between treatments.

Table 19.11 Reported side-effects of treatments following placebo oil from *Schizochytrium* sp. (DHA treatment $n = 40$)

	Placebo $n = 39$	DHA $n = 40$	Fischer's exact test
Did you experience any of the side-effects listed?	11	14	NS
Headache	1	5	NS
Stomach pain	0	4	NS
Nausea	0	1	NS
Bloating	3	5	NS
Flatulence	3	0	NS
Diarrhoea	0	1	NS
Constipation	2	1	NS
Itching	2	0	NS
Eruptions	0	1	NS
Fatigue	1	2	NS
Dizziness	2	1	NS
Heavy period[1]	1	0	NS

[1] $n = 30$ premenopausal menstruating women.
There were no significant differences (NS) between DHA and placebo.

oleic acid) and 0.5 g saturated fatty acids (mainly palmitic acid). Responses were assessed by measurements made at baseline and after 4 weeks of treatment. Full blood counts, liver function tests and indices of inflammation were measured in addition to cardiovascular risk factors and subjects were asked to record any side-effects. The DHA supplement led to a 10.4% increase in LDL cholesterol and a 9.0% increase in HDL cholesterol (both highly statistically significant) but there were no adverse toxicological changes in safety parameters (Tables 19.7–19.11).

19.4 Future trends

The potential of microbial systems to produce designer lipids has now been realised. At one stage it was believed that the production of lipids from microbial sources would not be economically competitive and there were concerns about contamination with microbial toxins. However, it has now been demonstrated that it is possible to produce oil of a higher quality and purity than from conventional sources. The success of speciality SCOs in the manufacture of ingredients for use in infant formula has been a beacon of economic success. A challenge will be to produce EPA in economical amounts from SCOs. The potential to genetically engineer micro-organisms to produce specific fatty acids is likely to lead to new designer lipids. Although there is widespread prejudice against the application of genetic engineering to food groups, it needs to be recognised that the use of genetic modification in a contained environment such as this is little different from that used to produce enzymes.

19.5 Sources of further information

COHEN Z, RATLEDGE C. *Single Cell Oils*. American Oil Chemist's Society, Champaign, Illinois, 2005.

SANDERS T, EMERY P. *The Molecular Basis of Human Nutrition*. Taylor & Francis, London, 2003.

19.6 References

AGREN JJ, HANNINEN O, JULKUNEN A *et al.* Fish diet, fish oil and docosahexaenoic acid rich oil lower fasting and postprandial plasma lipid levels. *Eur J Clin Nutr* 1996; **50**: 765–71.

CONQUER JA, HOLUB BJ. Supplementation with an algae source of docosahexaenoic acid increases (n-3) fatty acid status and alters selected risk factors for heart disease in vegetarian subjects. *J Nutr* 1996; **126**: 3032–9.

DAVIDSON MH, MAKI KC, KALKOWSKI J, SCHAEFER EJ, TORRI SA, DRENNAN KB. Effects of docosahexaenoic acid on serum lipoproteins in patients with combined hyperlipidemia: a randomized, double-blind, placebo-controlled trial. *J Am Coll Nutr* 1997; **16**: 236-43.

DAVIS B C, KRIS-ETHERTON P M. Achieving optimal essential fatty acid status in vegetarians: current knowledge and practical implications. *Am J Clin Nutr* 2003; **78** (suppl): 640S–6S.

DE OLIVEIRA E SILVA ER, SEIDMAN CE, TIAN JJ, HUDGINS LC, SACKS FM, BRESLOW JL. Effects of shrimp consumption on plasma lipoproteins. *Am J Clin Nutr* 1996; **64**: 712–17.

DOLK HM, NAU H, HUMMLER H, BARLOW SM. Dietary vitamin A and teratogenic risk: European Teratology Society discussion paper. *Eur J Obstet Gynecol Reprod Biol* 1999; **83**: 31–6.

FORAN JA, CARPENTER DO, HAMILTON MC, KNUTH BA, SCHWAGER SJ. Risk-based consumption advice for farmed Atlantic and wild Pacific salmon contaminated with dioxins and dioxin-like compounds. *Environ Health Perspect* 2005; **113**: 552–6.

HITES RA, FORAN JA, SCHWAGER SJ, KNUTH BA, HAMILTON MC, CARPENTER DO. Global assessment of polybrominated diphenyl ethers in farmed and wild salmon. *Environ Sci Technol* 2004; **38**: 4945–9.

LIPS P. Hypervitaminosis A and fractures. *N Engl J Med* 2003; **348**: 347–9.

METZ JG, ROESSLER P, FACCIOTTI D *et al.* Production of polyunsaturated fatty acids by polyketide synthases in both prokaryotes and eukaryotes. *Science* 2001; **293**: 290–93.

MEYER B J, MANN N J, LEWIS J L, MILLIGAN G C, SINCLAIR A J, HOWE P R. Dietary intakes and food sources of omega-6 and omega-3 polyunsaturated fatty acids. *Lipids* 2003; **38**: 391–8.

NELSON GJ, SCHMIDT PC, BARTOLINI GL, KELLEY DS, KYLE D. The effect of dietary docosahexaenoic acid on plasma lipoproteins and tissue fatty acid composition in humans. *Lipids* 1997; **32**: 1137–46.

PAULY D, WATSON R, ALDER J. Global trends in world fisheries: impacts on marine ecosystems and food security. *Philos Trans R Soc Lond B Biol Sci* 2005; **360**: 5–12.

RATLEDGE C. Single Cell Oils for the 21st Century. In *Single Cell Oils* eds, Cohen Z, Ratledge C. American Oil Chemist's Society, Champaign, Illinois, 2005.

SANDERS TAB. Essential fatty acid requirements of vegetarians in pregnancy, lactation, and infancy. *Am J Clin Nutr* 1999; **70** (Suppl): S555–S559.

SANDERS TAB, GLEASON K, GRIFFIN B, MILLER GJ. Influence of an algal triacylglycerol containing docosahexaenoic acid (22:6n-3) and docosapentaenoic acid (22:5n-6) on cardiovascular risk factors in healthy men and women. *Br J Nutr* 2005; in press.

THEOBALD HE, CHOWIENCZYK PJ, WHITTALL R, HUMPHRIES SE, SANDERS TA. LDL cholesterol-raising effect of low-dose docosahexaenoic acid in middle-aged men and women. *Am J Clin Nutr* 2004; **79**: 558–63.

WYNN G, *et al.* Searching for PUFA-rich microalgae. In *Single Cell Oils* eds, Cohen Z, Ratledge C. American Oil Chemist's Society, Champaign, Illinois, 2005.

20

Producing polyunsaturated fatty acids (PUFAs) from plant sources

J. A. Napier, Rothamsted Research, UK

20.1 Introduction

There is now considerable evidence as to the health-beneficial properties of a balanced diet that is enriched with the so-called fish oils (long chain polyunsaturated fatty acids, *n-3* LC-PUFAs) (von Schacky, 2003). Many aspects of these studies are discussed in the preceding chapters of this volume, so only a brief reiteration will be presented here. The earliest identification of fatty acids as playing an important role in human nutrition was provided by the pioneering studies of Burr and Burr, carried out in the 1920s (Burr and Burr, 1929; Burr, 1981). These identified two essential fatty acids (EFAs) which, if absent from mammalian diet, resulted in a number of deficiency symptoms, in particular altered skin properties. These two EFAs were identified as linoleic acid ($18{:}2\Delta^{9,12}$, *n-6*; abbreviated to LA) and α-linolenic acid ($18{:}3\Delta^{9,12,15}$, *n-3*; abbreviated to ALA), and mammals lack the endogenous capacity to synthesis both these fatty acids, explaining the essential requirement to derive them from dietary intake. Fortunately, most plants and plant seed oils are rich in the two EFAs, meaning that dietary deficiency is unusual under normal nutrition. The observation of Burr and Burr helped establish the importance of fatty acids in human nutrition, as well as highlighting the importance of dietary intake in organisms in which endogenous biosynthetic capacity is impaired or non-existent.

Interest in the human nutritional properties of the LC-PUFAs prevalent in fish oils was initially based on observations of communities that had naturally high consumption levels of fish (e.g. Inuit populations in Greenland). Epidemiological studies revealed that despite diets that were very rich in fat (through the consumption of large amount of fatty fish), the incidence of cardiovascular disease (CVD) was much lower than might have been predicted (Bang *et al.*,

1976). This led to the hypothesis that the health benefits of a fish-rich diet were derived from the concomitant consumption of high levels of *n-3* LC-PUFAs, fatty acids that accumulate in fish oils (but not in plants or meat) (Dyerberg and Bang, 1982). Subsequent epidemiological studies in other populations that have high levels of fish consumption, such as Japan, have confirmed the beneficial nature of fish oils, as have a number of controlled studies in which the consumption of fish, fish oils or *n-3* LC-PUFAs have been shown (on the whole) to be protective against CVD (reviewed by Calder, 2004). Perhaps of equal significance are the data provided by the GISSI Prevenzione Investigators (1999), in which the importance of *n-3* LC-PUFAs in preventing subsequent mortality in subjects who had previously experienced myocardial infarction (i.e. CVD). This intervention study is considered to provide clear evidence for the protective properties of *n-3* LC-PUFA fish oils (Calder, 2004, for an excellent discussion of this topic).

One key aspect to understanding the importance of *n-3* LC-PUFAs to human nutrition relates to the very inefficient biosynthetic capacity of mammals for these fatty acids. As noted above, LA and ALA are essential components due to an innate and total inability of mammals to endogenously synthesise these fatty acids (Wallis *et al.*, 2002). When they are obtained from dietary sources, among the several endogenous biochemical pathways that metabolise the EFAs is their conversion to LC-PUFAs. This is mediated by aerobic desaturation and fatty acyl chain elongation (this process will be described in detail in subsequent sections), resulting in the conversion of LA to arachidonic acid ($20{:}4\Delta^{5,8,11,14}$, *n-6*; abbreviated to ARA) and ALA to eicosapentaenoic acid ($20{:}5\Delta^{5,8,11,14,17}$, *n-3*; abbreviated to EPA) and docosahexaenoic acid ($22{:}6\Delta^{4,7,10,13,16,19}$, *n-3*; abbreviated to DHA). It should be noted that EPA and DHA are the two *n-3* LC-PUFAs, whereas ARA is an example of an *n-6* LC-PUFA, and current evidence indicates that only the *n-3* class of LC-PUFAs are protective against CVD (Calder, 2004). There are several important points relating to mammalian LC-PUFA biosynthesis: firstly, there is no conversion of substrates from *n-6* to *n-3* (thus, it is not possible to endogenously convert dietary LA to ALA, or ARA to EPA) (Sayanova and Napier, 2004). Secondly, the endogenous biosynthetic conversion of EFAs to ARA and EPA is remarkably inefficient, producing low levels of LC-PUFAs from dietary intake. Finally, the biosynthesis in mammals of the C_{22} *n-3* LC-PUFA DHA appears to involve both fatty acyl chain elongation and peroxisomal β-oxidative chain shortening, making its endogenous formation somewhat complicated (Leonard *et al.*, 2004). In view of all these observations, it is perhaps unsurprising that LC-PUFAs are now considered to be a vital component of human nutrition.

20.2 The role of long chain PUFAs (LC-PUFAs) in humans

PUFAs play key roles in cellular metabolism, including the regulation of membrane fluidity, electron and oxygen transport, as well as thermal adaptation.

However, from a medical point of view, perhaps the most important function of C_{20} PUFAs is that they are central to the biosynthesis of a class of compounds termed eicosanoids (i.e. metabolites of eicosa [C_{20}] PUFAs), serving as precursors for these regulating molecules. The eicosanoids consist of prostaglandins (PGs) and thromboxanes (TXs), which are collectively identified as protanoids, and the leukotrienes (LTs) (Funk, 2001). These compounds perform a number of essential physiological functions including regulation of immune system, blood clotting, neurotransmission and cholesterol metabolism (Funk, 2001). The importance of the eicosanoids in human biology is highlighted by the award of the Nobel Prize for Physiology and Medicine to Bergström, Samuelsson and Vane in 1982 'for their discoveries concerning prostaglandins and related biologically active substances'. Eicosanoids are formed when physical or chemical insults elicit the release of PUFAs from their phospholipid backbone (through the action of phospholipases) and subsequent oxygenation by local oxygenase enzymes. The type of eicosanoids produced (and hence the body's responses) are determined by a multiplicity of different factors including: cell-type stimulated, oxygenase enzymes present (cyclo-oxygenase, lipoxygenase) and the actual levels of substrate C_{20} PUFAs in the cell membrane.

Eicosanoids derived from *n-6* fatty acids have different metabolic properties from those derived from *n-3* fatty acids. In general, eicosanoids are classified into distinct series of chemicals: for example, series-1 and series-3 which are anti-inflammatory, whereas series-2 is pro-inflammatory. This designation is based on the oxygenating enzyme and substrate. For example, cyclo-oxygenase (COX) metabolises ARA to yield series-2 prostaglandins, whereas COX metabolism of EPA yields series-3 prostaglandins. Eicosanoids derived from the *n-6* ARA are generally pro-inflammatory, pro-aggregatory and immuno-active (Hwang, 2000). In contrast, eicosanoids derived from *n-3* EPA have little or no inflammatory activity and act to modulate platelet aggregation and immune-reactivity (Funk, 2001). Thus, there is considerable interest in the anti-inflammatory effects of *n-3* (e.g. EPA) derived eicosanoids and their potential as targets for intervention.

The primary synthesis of either *n-6* or *n-3* C_{20} PUFAs appears to be catalysed by the same biosynthetic enzymes that generally appear to have no particular preference for either substrate. Thus, the balance in dietary intake of *n-6* and *n-3* fatty acids will contribute to the types and amounts of eicosanoids in the body and so influence the strength of the inflammatory response. Consequential changes in the fatty acid composition of cell membranes can modify the inflammatory, immune and aggregatory responses of tissues, though this understates the complexity of cellular homeostasis. This concept provides the basis for the use of LC *n-3* PUFAs as therapeutic agents in the treatment of chronic inflammatory conditions such as rheumatoid arthritis, asthma, psoriasis and Crohn's disease (Simopoulos, 1991). Moreover, there is considerable interest in the possibility that LC *n-3* fatty acids may also be involved in the prevention of non-insulin dependent diabetes as it was shown that a diet low in these fatty acids may favour the development of insulin resistance (Browning,

2003). However, evidence for this is highly conflcting between animal and human studies. Additionally LC *n-3* PUFAs have been shown to be potent triglyceride-lowering agents, may promote increased oxidation of fatty acids in the liver and have beneficial effects on vascular reactivity (see Chapter 5). It is for these reasons that dietary intake of *n-3* PUFAs has been proposed to be protective from metabolic syndrome (Graham *et al.*, 2004; Nugent, 2004). Metabolic syndrome is a multi-component disorder characterised by reduced insulin sensitivity, alterations in circulatory lipids, especially triglycerides, hypertension and abdominal obesity, conveying an increased risk to cardio-vascular disease. In particular, obesity and insulin resistance (as indicators of metabolic syndrome) are now highly prevalent in both Western Europe and North America (Clarke, 2001). PUFA composition of cell membranes is, to a considerable extent, dependent on dietary intake and the typical Western/US diet is relatively deficient in *n-3* fatty acids compared with the diets of our ancestors. Today the ratio of *n-6* to *n-3* EFAs in such diets is about 25:1, and when compared with a likely ancestral dietary ratio of <2:1, indicative of a current relative deficiency in *n-3* fatty acids. The balance between the intake of *n-6* and *n-3* fatty acids may also be as important as the actual levels of individual dietary fatty acids, though further studies are required to clarify the former (Chapter 5) though this has been postulated to lead to the acquisition of symptoms analogous to metabolic syndrome (Clarke, 2001; Groop, 2000; Horrobin *et al.*, 2002).

There are two key *n-3* LC-PUFAs readily used by the body: EPA and DHA; DHA is synthesised directly from EPA as outlined below. These *n-3* PUFAs (particularly DHA) are highly concentrated in the brain and appear to be especially important for cognitive and behavioural function. DHA is also found in retinal cells and is likely to play a key role in the acquisition and maintenance of ocular vision in infants (Uauy *et al.*, 2001). In addition, these C_{20+} *n-3* PUFAs may be useful in the treatment or prevention of cardiovascular disease symptoms. Moreover, mild anti-inflammatory effects, possibly a result of increased PG-E1 and PG-E3 prostaglandins, may be helpful in the treatment of arthritis and other inflammatory diseases.

20.3 Dietary sources of essential fatty acids (EFAs) and LC-PUFAs

At present the only significant direct human dietary sources of *n-3* C_{20+} PUFAs are derived from marine fish oils, such as those extracted from salmon, cod liver and tuna. However, EPA and DHA occur widely in many unicellular protist species, especially those of marine origin (Metz *et al.*, 2001; Napier, 2002; Wallis *et al.*, 2002). Some fungi, mosses and bacteria also synthesise significant amounts of EPA and DHA. However, higher plants (the major dietary source of EFAs) do not generally contain LC-PUFAs, either in the seed storage triacyl-glycerols or in their membrane lipids (Sayanova and Napier, 2004). Some *Crucifera* species (especially the Brassica family) contain C_{20+} fatty acids, but these are usually in the form of monounsaturates such as erucic acid (22:1Δ^{13}, *n-9*), and not associated with any health benefit normally conferred by LC-PUFAs. In terms of the presence of fatty acids normally associated with the biosynthesis of LC-PUFAs, a few taxonomically unrelated plant species contain the C_{18} PUFAs γ-linolenic acid (18:3$\Delta^{6,9,12}$, *n-6*; abbreviated to GLA) and stereadonic acid (18:4$\Delta^{6,9,12,15}$, *n-3*; abbreviated to STA). These Δ^6-desaturated fatty acids are found (for example) in some members of the *Boraginacea*, and also in the *Primulaceae* (Sayanova *et al.*, 1999). Surprisingly, plants such as borage contain both GLA and STA in the seed lipids, but these fatty acids are almost completely absent from their vegetative tissue, whereas in *Primula* species the opposite is true. Considerable efforts have been expended in the search for a plant species that accumulates LC-PUFAs, and given the immense chemical diversity present in the Plant Kingdom, it is noteworthy that there is an almost total absence of these fatty acids from higher plants. Recently, a primitive Australian gymnosperm species, *Agathis robusta*, was demonstrated to contain low but significant amounts of ARA and EPA in its seed oils, leading the authors to speculate that this represented an intermediate between the modern angiosperms (which lack LC-PUFAs) and the Bryophytes (mosses) and liverworts, which are known to contain ARA and EPA (Wolff *et al.*, 1999).

Given the already discussed importance of LC-PUFAs in human health and nutrition, the lack of amenable sources in the form of vegetable oils can be considered as a major constraint. As mentioned above, the primary dietary source of LC-PUFAs such as EPA and DHA is via the consumption of fish, which contains these LC-PUFAs either in the liver or in the flesh, depending on the species. In fact fish, like other animals, are relatively inefficient at the synthesis of LC-PUFAs, and the abundance of these fatty acids in fish oils simply reflects the prevalence of these fatty acids in the aquatic environment; the accumulation of LC-PUFAs in fish is predominantly as a result of their dietary acquisition, rather than innate biosynthetic capacity (Tocher and Ghioni, 1999). The aquatic ecosystems contain many micro-organisms that actively synthesise and accumulate high amounts of *n-3* LC-PUFAs such as EPA and DHA, and these form the bottom of the PUFA food-web. The current pre-dominant source of LC-PUFAs is fish oils but, as noted by many commentators, the natural reserves of marine fish stocks are in perilous decline, towards a point of being unsustainable (reviewed in Opsahl-Ferstad *et al.*, 2003). This includes fish that are used for human consumption (such as cod and haddock), as well as the so-called 'trash' species such as sand eels, which are used exclusively in aquaculture. In that respect, attempts have been made to establish cultivation systems that will allow the growth of LC-PUFA accumulating marine micro-organisms. For example, the diatom *Phaeodactylum tricornutum* (which accumulates high amounts of EPA) and heterotrophic marine alga *Crypthecodinium cohnii* (which is rich in DHA) have been shown to be economically viable in controlled culture systems (De Swaaf *et al.*, 2003; Lebeau and Robert, 2003). Similarly, microbial fermentation systems have been used to generate ARA from the fungus *Mortierella alpina* (Zhu *et al.*, 2003)

In view of the importance of LC-PUFAs in human health and nutrition and the concomitant decline in marine fish stocks, there is an obvious need for a sustainable and environmentally benign source of these important fatty acids. As mentioned above, fermentation and culture systems may serve as sources of micro-organisms rich in LC-PUFAs. However, these systems can be expensive to maintain in continuous usage, and may have large environmental footprints. One additional alternative approach to the sustainable sourcing of LC-PUFAs is via the 'reverse-engineering' of the biosynthetic pathway into a suitable plant oilseed. Reverse-engineering can be considered a mechanism by which a process or device is replicated, without access to the original design plans. Thus, the steps required for the successful reconstitution of LC-PUFA biosynthesis in a transgenic plant are analogous to reverse-engineering (which is a term more often associated with replication of computer software or electronics), since the process requires firstly the identification of the endogenous genes required for synthesis, followed by their transfer to transgenic plants and finally their optimisation. In addition, an inherent understanding of the biosynthetic process is also required.

20.4 LC-PUFA biosynthetic pathways

The aerobic synthesis of LC-PUFAs is catalysed by two distinct biochemical reactions, which sequentially convert the EFAs LA and ALA into ARA, EPA and in some organisms, DHA. In the predominant (and, hence, 'conventional') LC-PUFA biosynthetic pathway, the first committed step is the Δ^6-desaturation of LA and ALA, to yield GLA and STA, respectively. This enzymatic reaction inserts a double bond at the Δ^6 (i.e. between C6 and C7 of the EFA substrate), leading to the classification of this process as 'front-end' desaturation (since the new double bond is inserted between the carboxyl 'front' of the fatty acid substrate and pre-existing double bonds such as that at the Δ^9 position) (Napier *et al.*, 1997). Front-end desaturation is the characteristic process by which aerobic LC-PUFA biosynthesis proceeds and understanding it is central to any attempts to reverse-engineer the pathway in transgenic plants (Napier *et al.*, 2003). Once GLA and STA have been generated, these two fatty acids are then subject to the second key process in LC-PUFA biosynthesis, fatty acyl elongation, in which they are chain-elongated by two carbons to yield the C_{20} fatty acids di-homo-γ-linolenic acid (20:3$\Delta^{8,11,14}$, *n-6*; abbreviated to DHGLA) and eicosatetraenoic acid (20:4$\Delta^{8,11,14,17}$, *n-3*; abbreviated to ETetA), respectively. A second round of front-end desaturation then occurs, in which a double bond is introduced between C5 and C6, by the Δ^5-desaturase. This yields the two primary C_{20} LC-PUFAs ARA and EPA, from the Δ^5-desaturation of DHGLA and ETetA, respectively. Thus, the conventional conversion of LA and ALA to ARA and EPA requires three enzymatic steps, namely Δ^6-desaturation, Δ^6-elongation (so-called as this process is specific for substrates containing a Δ^6 double bond) and Δ^5-desaturation. For recent reviews, see Huang *et al.*, 2004; Sayanova and Napier, 2004; Wallis *et al.*, 2002.

Early biochemical characterisations of LC-PUFA biosynthesis revealed that not all organisms used this conventional aerobic pathway for the synthesis of ARA and EPA. In particular, radiolabelling tracer studies observed the synthesis of ARA in the absence of Δ^6-desaturation in a range of diverse organisms. This led to identification of the so-called 'alternative' pathway, in which the elongation steps precedes desaturation (reviewed in Sayanova and Napier, 2004). In this alternative pathway, EFA substrates LA and ALA are chain-elongated to yield eicosadienoic acid (20:2$\Delta^{11,14}$, *n-6*; abbreviated to EDA) and eicosatrienoic acid (20:3$\Delta^{11,14,17}$, *n-3*; abbreviated to EtriA), respectively. These C_{20} fatty acids are then Δ^8-desaturated, to yield DHGLA and ETetA respectively, with these two products undergoing Δ^5-desaturation as for the conventional pathway, to yield ARA and EPA. Thus, C_{20} Δ^5 front-end desaturation is a common feature of both the conventional and alternative pathways for the synthesis of ARA and EPA.

Although ARA is considered to be the end-point in the synthesis of the *n-6* class of LC-PUFAs, further modification of the *n-3* EPA occurs in some organisms. In mammals, it is now clear that the conversion of EPA to DHA involves two additional cycles of C_2-elongation, yielding tetracosapentaenoic acid (24:5$\Delta^{9,12,15,18,21}$, *n-3*) which then undergoes Δ^6-desaturation to produce tetracosahexaenoic acid (24:6$\Delta^{6,9,12,15,18,21}$, *n-3*). This C_{24} PUFA is then subjected to limited peroxisomal β-oxidation, in which it is chain-shortened by two carbons to yield the final product DHA (Leonard *et al.*, 2004). There are number of unresolved issues regarding this route (known as the Sprecher pathway) for the synthesis of DHA, not least of all the mechanism by which substrates are transferred to the peroxisomes for limited β-oxidation (Sprecher and Chen, 1999). Recently, evidence has been presented that the same Δ^6-desaturase is responsible for the synthesis of C_{18} GLA and C_{24} THA (D'andrea *et al.*, 2002). However, it is clear that the mammalian biosynthetic route for DHA is somewhat complicated, which may also be reflected in the inefficient endogenous synthesis of this LC-PUFA.

Although the Sprecher pathway is now widely accepted as the predominant biosynthetic route in mammals, it appears that a more simple process is present in some aquatic micro-organisms that accumulate DHA. In this pathway, EPA undergoes one cycle of elongation to yield docosapentaenoic acid (22:5$\Delta^{7,10,13,16,19}$, *n-3*, abbreviated to DPA) which is then Δ^4-desaturated to produce DHA (Qiu, 2003). This pathway has been observed in both marine and freshwater micro-organisms. Interestingly, it has been found both in organisms that use the conventional EPA biosynthetic route, and also the alternative C_{20} Δ^8-desaturase system. The so called Δ^4-desaturase pathway for the synthesis of DHA is considerably simpler than the Sprecher pathway, with the former containing only two reactions (elongation, desaturation) compared with the latter's four (elongation, elongation, desaturation, β-oxidation). It is for this reason that most attempts to identify the genes encoding the DHA biosynthetic pathway have focused on the Δ^4-desaturase route (Meyer *et al.*, 2004).

20.5 Genes, technologies and resources

As discussed above, one of the primary steps in attempts to introduce the 'trait' for the synthesis of LC-PUFAs into plants by genetic engineering (Tucker, 2003) is to have a thorough understanding of the biochemical basis of the various biosynthetic pathways. Once these rationales have been characterised, the next step is the identification, by cloning and functional analysis, of the genes encoded in the LC-PUFA biosynthetic activities. Given the considerable importance of LC-PUFA biosynthesis, it is perhaps surprising that the genes that encode the desaturases and elongating activities have been identified only in the last decade (Sayanova and Napier, 2004). Although considerable effort was deployed in attempts to biochemically purify these enzyme activities, the majority of these were unsuccessful mainly due to the membrane-associated nature of these proteins. However, the advent of large-scale DNA sequencing projects (both genomic and cDNA expressed sequence tags, ESTs) in the early 1990s helped provide underpinning knowledge of fatty acid desaturase genes, in particular the soluble chloroplastic desaturase responsible for the synthesis of monounsaturated fatty acids such as oleic and palmitic acids. Perhaps more significantly, genetic approaches pioneered by Somerville and Browse (see the 1996 review by these authors) allowed for the isolation of *Arabidopsis* mutants defective in the synthesis of the EFAs LA and ALA. Subsequent mapping and cloning of the genes identified by this genetic approach gave the first insights into the molecular biology of membrane-bound desaturases, and revealed a number of highly conserved amino acid motifs which were shown to be essential for desaturase enzyme activity (reviewed in Shanklin and Cahoon, 1998).

Building on these observations, it was reasoned that related enzyme activities such as those required for LC-PUFA front-end desaturation might also be expected to contain these conserved motifs, facilitating the cloning of such genes from a suitable LC-PUFA accumulating organism. The efficacy of this approach was demonstrated by cloning of the Δ^6-desaturase, the first committed step of the conventional pathway for ARA and EPA synthesis. This was cloned by using a degenerate polymerase chain reaction (PCR) strategy to isolate candidate open reading frames (ORFs) from a higher plant species that accumulates GLA, common borage (*Borago officinalis*) (Sayanova *et al.*, 1997). One particular candidate gene, which was structurally distinct from the previously identified desaturases of *Arabidopsis*, was functionally characterised by expression in transgenic tobacco plants. Analysis of the fatty acids present in these transgenic tobacco lines revealed the presence of GLA and STA, resulting from the Δ^6-desaturation of LA and ALA, respectively (Sayanova *et al.*, 1997). These data provided the first identification of the Δ^6-desaturase ORF, as well as the formal demonstration that the same enzyme produced both *n-6* and *n-3* products.

Building on this, an orthologue (i.e. related sequence) of the plant gene was cloned from the nematode *Caenorhabditis elegans* and functionally characterised by heterologous expression in yeast as the first example of an animal Δ^6-desaturase (Napier *et al.*, 1998). Not only did this indicate the conserved nature of the Δ^6-desaturase between Kingdoms, but also pointed towards the feasibility of 'cloning by homology', i.e. a candidate gene can be reasonably identified from an appropriate genomic or EST database on the basis of similarity to predefined sequences. In the case of the Δ^6-desaturase, this was made easier by our observation that these enzymes contained an N-terminal domain not present in any of the *Arabidopsis* membrane-bound desaturases. This N-terminal extension showed homology to the electron donor cytochrome b_5, implying that the Δ^6-desaturase required physical proximity to an electron transport chain. The unexpected presence of the N-terminal cytochrome b_5 extension leads us to hypothesise that this domain may be related to the process of front-end desaturation, and therefore this motif could be diagnostic for microsomal desaturases involved in PUFA biosynthesis (Napier *et al.*, 1997, 2003). Subsequent work by our research group and others (notably the groups of Ernst Heinz in Hamburg, and Pradip Mukerji in Columbus, Ohio) has confirmed the presence of a cytochrome b_5 N-terminal domain in all current examples of PUFA desaturases (reviewed in Napier *et al.*, 2003; Sperling *et al.*, 2003). These include the Δ^6-desaturase, the paralogous Δ^5-desaturase, the related alternative pathway C_{20} Δ^8-desaturase and distantly related Δ^4-desaturase for DHA synthesis.

It is also clear from a number of studies that the cytochrome b_5 domain is absolutely required for enzyme activity, since site-directed mutagenesis of the conserved haem-binding motif completely ablated enzyme activity (Sayanova *et al.*, 1999). It is worth noting that the N-terminal cytochrome b_5 domain has been identified in several enzymes that are not involved in PUFA biosynthesis. One intriguing example is the sphingolipid Δ^8-desaturase, which introduces a Δ^8-desaturation into the long chain base of higher plant sphingolipids (Sperling *et al.*, 1998). This activity seems to be ubiquitous in higher plants, and the sphingolipid Δ^8-desaturase is closely related (~70% identical at the polypeptide level) to the few examples of plant Δ^6-desaturases that have been identified. It is tempting to speculate that the presence of a Δ^6-desaturase activity in higher plants is the result of divergence from the ubiquitous sphingolipid desaturase activity. If this is the case, then it seems likely that the presence of Δ^6-desaturated fatty acids in plants represents a (pseudo) convergent evolution, when compared with the presence of structurally related Δ^6-desaturases found in animals.

The breakthrough identification of the first front-end desaturase led to the identification and characterisation of ORFs for all PUFA desaturases. The presence of large-scale genomic resources provided searchable platforms for identification of candidate genes, and simple yeast heterologous expression systems provide a rapid method for functional characterisation. A number of these PUFA desaturases were also characterised by expression in transgenic plants, which confirmed their activity in these heterologous systems. For a full description of recent progress in the identification and characterisation of PUFA desaturases, see the reviews of Sayanova and Napier (2004) and Sperling *et al.* (2003).

The second key enzymatic reaction in the synthesis of LC-PUFAs is the microsomal elongation reaction, in which a C_{18} substrate PUFA (usually containing a front-end Δ^6-desaturation) is C_2-elongated to yield the C_{20} PUFA (Fig. 20.1). The various different routes for the aerobic biosynthesis are shown in Fig. 20.1. The precursor essential fatty acids linoleic and α-linolenic acid are the predominant fatty acids synthesised by plants. These then enter the mammalian food web and are subsequently metabolised to C_{20+} LC-PUFAs. The alternative Δ^8-desaturase/Δ^9-elongase pathway is shown, as are the two alternative routes for DHA synthesis. In the case of EPA/DHA synthesising microalgae, C_{20+} PUFAs are synthesised directly from saturated substrates (since such organisms contain both 'plant' and 'animal' components of the pathway). For simplicity, only the *n-6* section of the alternative pathway is shown. Note that the alternative pathway and the conventional pathway share the same final step (Δ^5-desaturation). The 'substrate dichotomy' present in LC-PUFA biosynthesis is indicated by glycerolipid-linked reactions marked with a solid arrow, and acyl-CoA reactions with open arrows.

Progress on the identification of the microsomal elongase has been slower, not least of all as this reaction encompasses four distinct and sequential enzymes, namely condensation (of malonyl-CoA and the PUFA acyl-CoA, β-keto-reduction, dehydration and enoyl-reduction. ORFs from *C. elegans* and *M. alpina* were identified by 'gain-of-function' (i.e. acquisition of the ability to elongate C_{18} PUFAs) experiments in yeast (Beaudoin *et al.*, 2000; Parker-Barnes *et al.*, 2000). The identified nematode and fungal ORFs showed homology to the yeast ELO genes, which are required for the synthesis of (saturated) LC-fatty acids found in sphingolipids. While the ELO-like genes are assumed to be condensing enzymes, this remains to be unequivocally demonstrated. One inferred observation from the identification of the ELO-like PUFA-elongating activity was that the expression of these single ORFs was still able to reconstitute a PUFA-specific elongase; there was no requirement for the co-expression of any of the other three components of the elongase. This may indicate that the initial condensing enzyme (in the form of the ELO-like ORFs) confers specificity on the elongase, with the other three reactions then acting in a non-specific manner. This is in agreement with data on the expression of the unrelated plant condensing enzyme Fae1p in yeast, which confers a 'gain-of-function' in the elongation of monounsaturated fatty acids (Millar *et al.*, 1998).

The identification of both PUFA desaturases and PUFA-specific elongating activities provides the genetic resources with which to undertake the reverse-engineering of LC-PUFA biosynthesis into a suitable transgenic plant. The generation of transgenic plants is now a well-established technology, usually enabled by *Agrobacterium*-mediated transformation systems. Many oilseed species (e.g. brassicas, linseed, tobacco) are amenable to this method, and a

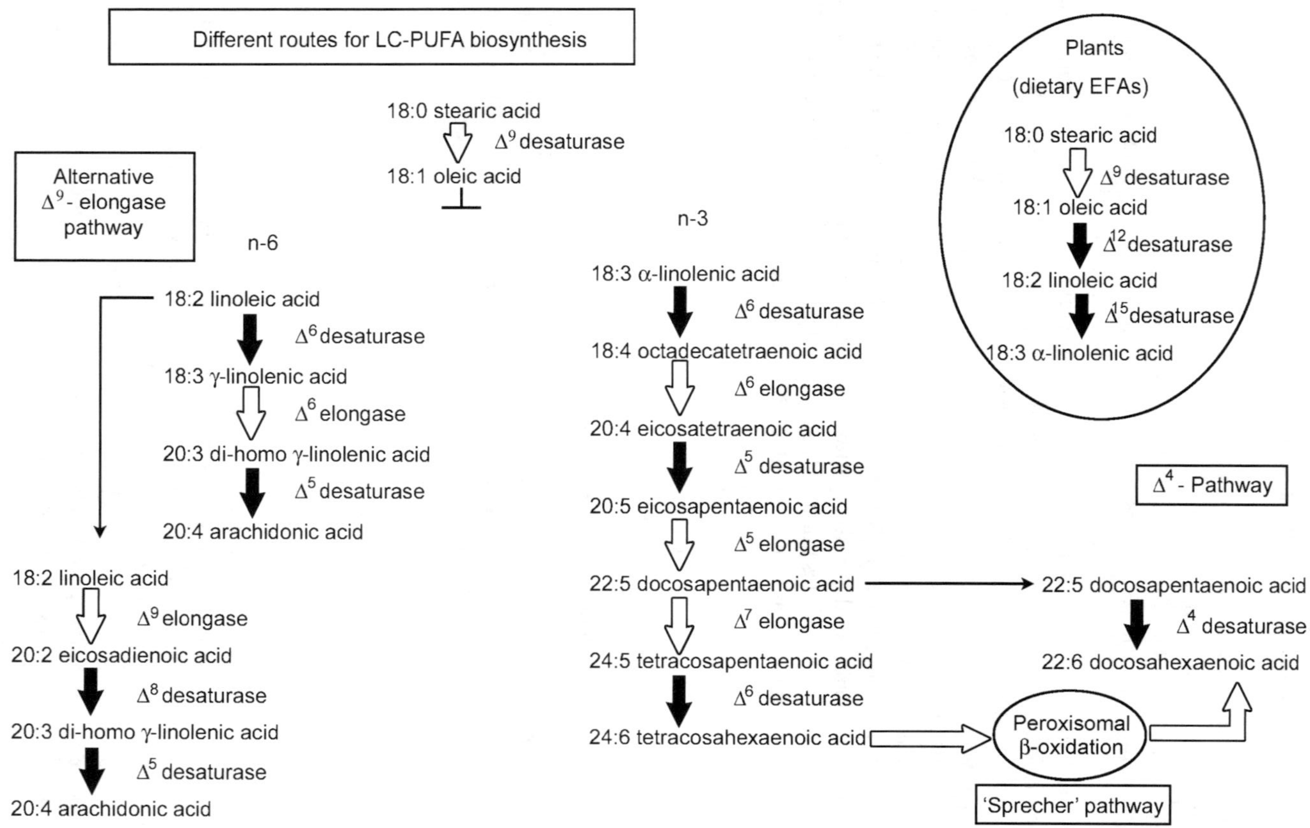

Fig. 20.1 Generalised pathway for the biosynthesis of LC-PUFAs.

range of different regulatory sequences (i.e. promoters) are available to direct the expression of the transgene in suitable manner (e.g. seed-specific). Having all these components in place has allowed significant progress in the heterologous reconstitution of LC-PUFA synthesis in transgenic plants, and the remaining sections of this chapter will focus on these research outputs.

20.6 The production of C_{20} LC-PUFAs in transgenic plants

Two significant attempts to synthesise LC-PUFAs in transgenic plants have recently been published, and these provide some key insights into feasibility of reverse-engineering this trait into oilseeds. The first study utilised a novel elongating activity present in the alternative pathway, a C_{18} Δ^9-elongating activity from the marine microalga *Isochrysis galbana*. Such a Δ^9-elongating activity utilises LA and ALA as substrates (in the form of CoAs), generating eicosadienoic acid (20:2$\Delta^{11,14}$, *n-6*; EDA) and eicostrienoic acid (20:3$\Delta^{11,14,17}$, *n-3*; ETriA) respectively. In that respect, it might be predicted that since the substrates for the Δ^9-elongating activity are already present in plants, this elongase might function more efficiently.

To fully reconstitute the alternative C_{20} PUFA biosynthetic pathway, transgenic *Arabidopsis* lines were generated by sequential transformation with the *Isochrysis* Δ^9-elongating activity, the *Euglena* C_{20} Δ^8-desaturase and the *M. alpina* Δ^5-desaturase. This resulted in the conversion of the C_{20} elongation products EDA and ETriA to 20:3 (*n-6*) and 20:4 (*n-3*) via Δ^8-desaturation, with concomitant Δ^5-desaturation of these products generating ARA and EPA, respectively (Qi *et al.*, 2004). These two LC-PUFAs accumulated in the leaf tissues of transgenic *Arabidopsis* plants to a combined level of ~10% total fatty acids, the majority being *n-6* ARA (Qi *et al.*, 2004). However, the resultant ratios of C_{20} *n-6*/*n-3* PUFAs did not reflect the levels of *n-6*/*n-3* substrates, which are predominantly ALA (*n-3*). In addition to accumulation of the desired products ARA and EPA, several other C_{20} PUFAs were also detected; these were identified as sciadonic acid (20:3$\Delta^{5,11,14}$) and juniperonic acid (20:4$\Delta^{5,11,14,17}$), two non-methylene-interupted PUFAs. which are likely to have been generated by the 'promiscuous' activity of the Δ^5-desaturase (Qi *et al.*, 2004). Whether this represents a perturbation of substrate-channelling (i.e. from CoA pool to glycerolipid) in the reconstituted alternative LC-PUFA biosynthetic pathway remains to be determined, though it is worth noting that the enzyme used in this study (the *M. alpina* Δ^5-desaturase) was also observed to synthesise unusual Δ^5-desaturated C_{18} fatty acids when expressed in transgenic canola. While sciadonic and juniperonic acids were not primary targets for the synthesis and accumulation in transgenic plants, both are found in a number of species of pine seeds, and as such have been widely consumed by humans without demonstrating any anti-nutritional effects.

A complementary study by Abbadi *et al.* (2004) on the expression of the conventional Δ^6-desaturase/elongase pathway has provided some further insights into the feasibility and constraints on LC-PUFA synthesis in transgenic oilseeds. Using genes encoding enzyme activities from a number of different PUFA-accumulating species, transgenic linseed and tobacco lines were generated expressing the Δ^6-desaturase, the Δ^6-elongase and the Δ^5-desaturase. These three activities were placed under the transcriptional regulation of a seed-specific promoter, and introduced into the transgenic plant as a single integration event. Analysis of the seeds of transgenic tobacco or linseed revealed very high levels (>20%) of Δ^6-desaturated fatty acids GLA and STA, yet only relatively low amounts (<2%) of ARA and EPA (Abbadi *et al.*, 2004). While these data clearly demonstrated the reconstitution of the conventional PUFA biosynthetic pathway in transgenic seeds, they also paralleled earlier observations in yeast on the inefficient synthesis of C_{20} PUFAs (Domergue *et al.*, 2003).

Further detailed biochemical analysis of the transgenic linseed expressing these activities revealed a number of interesting observations (Abbadi *et al.*, 2004). Firstly, although the Δ^6-desaturase and the Δ^6-elongase appeared to work at very different rates, the two transgenes were transcribed at similar levels. Secondly, although the Δ^6-desaturation products GLA and STA accumulate at high levels, these elongase substrates do not undergo elongation. This is likely to be due to their accumulation to high levels in the microsomal membranes, particularly at the *sn-2* position of phosphatidylcholine, rather than in the acyl-CoA pool (the substrate pool for microsomal elongases). Thus, there is inefficient exchange from phosphatidylcholine (the substrate for glycerolipid-linked Δ^6-desaturation of LA or ALA) into the acyl-CoA pool of the desaturation products GLA and STA. In addition, it was noted that there was an enrichment of *n-3* fatty acids (including the transgene-derived STA) in the triacylglycerols of the engineered linseed, indicating a channelling of this class of fatty acids. It seems very likely that this selective *n-3* channelling is mediated by an acyl-CoA-independent acyltransferases (such as phosphatidylcholine: diacylglycerol acyltransferase), also contributing to the reduced presence of Δ^6-desaturated fatty acids in the CoA pool for elongation.

Taking these observations together, it seems likely that a significant constraint on the synthesis of LC-PUFAs via the conventional Δ^6-desaturase/elongase route is the dichotomy of substrate requirements exhibited by the two key enzyme reactions: glycerolipid-linked desaturation versus acyl-CoA-dependent elongation. However, the levels of ARA and EPA accumulating in the seeds of the transgenic linseed lines is still significant, even allowing for the clearly sub-optimal exchange and channelling of acyl-substrates. Thus, these results should be taken as highly encouraging for the successful synthesis of LC-PUFAs via this pathway.

Collectively, the data from the studies of Qi *et al.* (2004) and Abbadi *et al.* (2004) provide a clear demonstration that the heterologous reconstitution of LC-PUFA biosynthesis by transgenic reverse-engineering is feasible. Perhaps more importantly, these studies provide pointers towards rationales for the optimisation of the heterologous process, and so will underpin future improvements in the synthesis of LC-PUFAs in plants.

20.7 Towards the production of docosahexaenoic acid (DHA)

The accumulation of C_{20} LC-PUFAs ARA and EPA in transgenic plants expressing either the conventional or alternative desaturase/elongase pathways is a major achievement, and while the levels are relatively modest (<4% EPA), these still represent levels that could provide nutritional enhancement to the human diet (Green, 2004). However, an additional target for the alternative sustainable production of 'fish oils' in transgenic oilseeds is the synthesis and accumulation of DHA. The simplest route for DHA synthesis is by the C_2 elongation of EPA, via the action of a Δ^5-elongase (to elongate EPA to 22:5 *n-3*) and subsequent desaturation with the C_{22} Δ^4-desaturase. Thus, two additional transgenes need to be introduced into transgenic plants which already accumulate EPA. The cytochrome b_5-fusion C_{22} Δ^4-desaturase has been identified and functionally characterised from several aquatic micro-organisms and more recently, the identification of the C_{20} Δ^5-elongase (which elongates EPA to 22:5) will facilitate the heterologous reconstitution of DHA synthesis (Meyer *et al.*, 2004). Initial proof-of-concept experiments have been carried out in yeast and revealed low but significant levels of DHA in strains that have been engineered to contain activities of the conventional LC-PUFA biosynthetic pathway (i.e. the C_{18} Δ^6-elongase, C_{20} Δ^5-desaturase, C_{20} Δ^5-elongase and the C_{22} Δ^4-desaturase) (Meyer *et al.*, 2004; Pereira *et al.*, 2004). A very high proportion of exogenously supplied STA was elongated to ETetA by the transgenic yeast, probably because of the high availability of the substrate as an acyl-CoA. Although EPA is efficiently elongated to DPA by the newly identified Δ^5-elongase, and DPA correctly Δ^4-desaturated to DHA, the resultant levels of DHA are low (~1% of total fatty acids); this appears to be due to the very poor conversion of ETetA to EPA by the microsomal Δ^5-desaturase (Meyer *et al.*, 2004). As discussed above, the microsomal desaturation reactions that underpin LC-PUFA biosynthesis predominantly utilise substrates at the *sn-2* position of PC, and the inefficiency of the Δ^5-desaturase may simply reflect the lack of glycerolipid-linked substrate (even though total levels of ETetA are high). In that respect, the data on the heterologous reconstitution of the C_{20}-to-C_{22} LC-PUFA biosynthetic pathway in yeast confirm the bottlenecks observed for the C_{18}-to-C_{20} pathway in both yeast and transgenic plants. In particular, the dichotomy of substrates required for elongation and desaturation indicates the need for additional factors (such as acyltransferases) to improve the efficiency of this process.

Attempts to accumulate DHA in transgenic plants are currently underway to determine additional constraints on heterologous LC-PUFA biosynthesis in these organisms. In that respect, it will be of considerable interest to assess the possibility of using the non-aerobic polyketide synthase-like system (Metz *et al.*, 2001) to synthesise DHA in transgenic plants, since this biosynthetic route does not apparently require acyl-exchange (at least during the processive synthesis of DHA).

20.8 Conclusions

The possibility of 'reverse-engineering' LC-PUFA biosynthesis into transgenic plants has now been successfully demonstrated for C_{20} LC-PUFAs ARA and EPA. These important breakthroughs have also provided new insights into the maintenance of lipid homeostasis in plants, and the key role of acyl-exchange enzymes in LC-PUFA reconstitution. This knowledge will underpin future attempts to engineer the synthesis of C_{22} LC-PUFAs such as DHA. Additionally, clear targets for the enhancement of this heterologous synthesis can also be identified, such as maximising the synthesis of *n-3* LC-PUFAs and concomitantly reducing the levels of *n-6* (Sayanova and Napier, 2004).

It is therefore not unreasonable to believe that LC-PUFA-synthesising transgenic plants are making rapid progress towards providing a sustainable alternative to our diminishing marine fish stocks. It should also be remembered that since aquaculture is also dependent on fish oils for the correct nutrition of farmed fish species, transgenic-derived plant oils enhanced by the presence of LC-PUFAs might also be able to sustainably replace this additional demand (Opsahl-Ferstad *et al.*, 2003). In that respect, the use of transgene-derived LC-PUFAs in aquaculture may provide an alternative point of entry for these products into the food chain, alleviating the need for direct consumption of so-called genetically modified (GM) food. This may prove important, given the continued antipathy of the European (but not North American) public to the general concept of GM foodstuffs. Whether this lack of enthusiasm will continue in the face of food products engineered to contain health-beneficial factors such as LC-PUFAs remains to be determined, though in the meantime, basic research efforts to better understand PUFA biosynthesis continue apace (Napier *et al.*, 2004).

20.9 Acknowledgements

Rothamsted Research receives grant-aided support from the Biotechnology and Biological Sciences Research Council (BBSRC) UK. The author acknowledges the support of BASF Plant Sciences, Germany.

20.10 References

ABBADI A, DOMERGUE F, BAUER J, NAPIER JA, WELTI R, ZAHRINGER U, CIRPUS P, HEINZ E (2004) 'Biosynthesis of very long-chain polyunsaturated fatty acids in transgenic oilseeds: constraints on their accumulation', *Plant Cell* **16**, 2734–48.

BANG HO, DYERBERG J, HJOORNE N (1976) 'The composition of food consumed by Greenland Eskimos', *Acta Med. Scand.* **200**, 69–73.

BEAUDOIN F, MICHAELSON LV, HEY SJ, LEWIS MJ, SHEWRY PR, SAYONOVA O, NAPIER J (2000) 'Heterologous reconstitution in yeast of the polyunsaturated fatty acid biosynthetic pathway', *Proc. Natl. Acad. Sci. USA* **97**, 6421–6.

BROWNING LM (2003) '*n-3* Polyunsaturated fatty acids, inflammation and obesity-related disease', *Proc. Nutr. Soc.* **62**, 447–53.

BURR GO (1981) 'The essential fatty acids fifty years ago', *Prog. Lipid Res.* **20**, xxvii–xxix.

BURR GO, BURR MM (1929) 'A new deficiency disease produced by the rigid exclusion of fat from the diet', *J. Biol. Chem.* **82**, 345–67.

CALDER PC (2004) '*n-3* Fatty acids and cardiovascular disease: evidence explained and mechanisms explored', *Clin. Sci.* **107**, 1–11.

CLARKE SD (2001) 'Polyunsaturated fatty acid regulation of gene transcription: a molecular mechanism to improve the metabolic syndrome', *J. Nutr.* **131**, 1129–32.

D'ANDREA S, GUILLOU H, JAN S, CATHELINE D, THIBAULT JN, BOURIEL M, RIOUX V, LEGRAND P (2002) 'The same rat Δ^6-desaturase not only acts on 18- but also on 24-carbon fatty acids in very-long-chain polyunsaturated fatty acid biosynthesis', *Biochem. J.* **364**, 49–55.

DE SWAAF ME, SIJTSMA L, PRONK JT (2003) 'High-cell-density fed-batch cultivation of the docosahexaenoic acid producing marine alga *Crypthecodinium cohnii*', *Biotechnol. Bioeng.* **81**, 666–72.

DOMERGUE F, ABBADI A, OTT C, ZANK TK, ZAHRINGER U, HEINZ E (2003) 'Acyl carriers used as substrates by the desaturases and elongases involved in very long-chain polyunsaturated fatty acids biosynthesis reconstituted in yeast', *J. Biol. Chem.* **278**, 35115–26.

DYERBERG J, BANG HO (1982) 'A hypothesis on the development of acute myocardial infarction in Greenlanders', *Scand. J. Clin. Lab. Invest. Suppl.* **161**, 7–13.

FUNK CD (2001) 'Prostaglandins and leukotrienes: advances in eicosanoid biology', *Science* **294**, 1871–5.

GISSI-PREVENZIONE INVESTIGATORS (1999) 'Dietary supplementation with *n-3* polyunsaturated fatty acids and vitamin E after myocardial infarction: results of the GISSI-Prevenzione trial', Gruppo Italiano per lo Studio della Sopravvivenza nell'Infarto miocardico. *Lancet* **354,** 447–55.

GRAHAM IA, CIRPUS P, REIN D, NAPIER JA (2004) 'The use of very long chain polyunsaturated fatty acids to ameliorate metabolic syndrome: transgenic plants as an alternative sustainable source to fish oils', *Nutr. Bull.* **29**, 228–33.

GREEN AG (2004) 'From alpha to omega-producing essential fatty acids in plants', *Nat. Biotechnol.* **22**, 680–82.

GROOP L (2000) 'Genetics of the metabolic syndrome', *Br. J. Nutr.* **83** Suppl 1: S39–48.

HORROBIN DF, JENKINS K, BENNETT CN, CHRISTIE WW (2002) 'Eicosapentaenoic acid and arachidonic acid: collaboration and not antagonism is the key to biological understanding', *Prostaglandins Leukot. Essent. Fatty Acids* **66**, 83–90.

HUANG YS, PEREIRA SL, LEONARD AE (2004) 'Enzymes for transgenic biosynthesis of long-chain polyunsaturated fatty acids', *Biochimie* **86**, 793–8.

HWANG D (2000) 'Fatty acids and immune responses – a new perspective in searching for clues to mechanism', *Annu. Rev. Nutr.* **20**, 431–56.

LEBEAU T, ROBERT JM (2003) 'Diatom cultivation and biotechnologically relevant products. Part II: current and putative products', *Appl. Microbiol. Biotechnol.* **60**, 624–32.

LEONARD AE, PEREIRA SL, SPRECHER H, HUANG YS (2004) 'Elongation of long-chain fatty acids', *Prog. Lipid Res.* **43**, 36–54.

METZ JG, ROESSLER P, FACCIOTTI D, LEVERING C, DITTRICH F, LASSNER M, VALENTINE R, LARDIZABAL K, DOMERGUE F, YAMADA A, YAZAWA K, KNAUF V, BROWSE J (2001)

'Production of polyunsaturated fatty acids by polyketide synthases in both prokaryotes and eukaryotes', *Science* **293**, 290–93.

MEYER A, KIRSCH H, DOMERGUE F, ABBADI A, SPERLING P, BAUER J, CIRPUS P, ZANK TK, MOREAU H, ROSCOE TJ, ZAHRINGER U, HEINZ E (2004) 'Novel fatty acid elongases and their use for the reconstitution of docosahexaenoic acid biosynthesis', *J. Lipid Res.* **45**, 1899–909.

MILLAR AA, WRISCHER M, KUNST L (1998) 'Accumulation of very-long-chain fatty acids in membrane glycerolipids is associated with dramatic alterations in plant morphology', *Plant Cell* **10,** 1889–902.

NAPIER JA (2002) 'Plumbing the depths of PUFA biosynthesis: a novel polyketide synthase-like pathway from marine organisms', *Trends Plant Sci.* **7**, 51–4.

NAPIER JA, SAYANOVA O, STOBART AK, SHEWRY PR (1997) 'A new class of cytochrome b_5 fusion proteins', *Biochem. J.* **328**, 717–18.

NAPIER JA, HEY SJ, LACEY DJ, SHEWRY PR (1998) 'Identification of a *Caenorhabditis elegans* Δ^6-fatty-acid-desaturase by heterologous expression in *Saccharomyces cerevisiae*', *Biochem. J.* **330**, 611–14.

NAPIER JA, MICHAELSON LV, SAYANOVA O (2003) 'The role of cytochrome b_5 fusion desaturases in the synthesis of polyunsaturated fatty acids', *Prostaglandins Leukot. Essent. Fatty Acids* **68**, 135–43.

NAPIER JA, BEAUDOIN F, MICHAELSON LV, SAYANOVA O (2004) 'The production of long chain polyunsaturated fatty acids in transgenic plants by reverse-engineering', *Biochimie* **86**, 785–92.

NUGENT AP (2004) 'The metabolic syndrome', *Nutr. Bull.* **29**, 36–43.

OPSAHL-FERSTAD H-G, RUDI H, RUYTER B, REFSTIE S (2003) 'Biotechnological approaches to modify rapeseed oil composition for applications in aquaculture', *Plant Sci.* **165**, 349–57.

PARKER-BARNES JM, DAS T, BOBIK E, LEONARD AE, THURMOND JM, CHAUNG LT, HUANG YS, MUKERJI P (2000) 'Identification and characterization of an enzyme involved in the elongation of *n-6* and *n-3* polyunsaturated fatty acids', *Proc. Natl. Acad. Sci. USA* **97**, 8284–9.

PEREIRA SL, LEONARD AE, HUANG YS, CHUANG LT, MUKERJI P (2004) 'Identification of two novel microalgal enzymes involved in the conversion of the omega3-fatty acid, eicosapentaenoic acid, into docosahexaenoic acid', *Biochem. J.* **384**, 357–66.

QI B, FRASER T, MUGFORD S, DOBSON G, SAYANOVA O, BUTLER J, NAPIER JA, STOBART AK, LAZARUS CM (2004) 'Production of very long-chain polyunsaturated omega-3 and omega-6 fatty acids in plants', *Nat. Biotechnol.* **22**, 739–45.

QIU X (2003) 'Biosynthesis of docosahexaenoic acid (DHA, 22:6-4, 7,10,13,16,19): two distinct pathways', *Prostaglandins Leukot. Essent. Fatty Acids* **68**, 181–6.

SAYANOVA O, NAPIER JA (2004) 'Eicosapentaenoic acid: biosynthetic routes and the potential for synthesis in transgenic plants', *Phytochemistry* **65**, 147–58.

SAYANOVA O, SMITH MA, LAPINSKAS P, STOBART AK, DOBSON G, CHRISTIE WW, SHEWRY PR, NAPIER JA (1997) 'Expression of a borage desaturase cDNA containing an N-terminal cytochrome b_5 domain results in the accumulation of high levels of Δ^6-desaturated fatty acids in transgenic tobacco', *Proc. Natl. Acad. Sci. USA* **94**, 4211–16.

SAYANOVA O, NAPIER JA, SHEWRY PR (1999) 'Δ^6-Unsaturated fatty acids in species and tissues of the Primulaceae', *Phytochemistry* **52**, 419–22.

SHANKLIN J, CAHOON EB (1998) 'Desaturation and related modifications of fatty acids', *Annu. Rev. Plant Physiol. Plant Mol. Biol.* **49**, 611–41.

SIMOPOULOS AP (1991) 'Omega-3 fatty acids in health and disease and in growth and development', *Am. J. Clin. Nutr.* **54**, 438–63.

SOMERVILLE C, BROWSE J (1996) 'Dissecting desaturation: plants prove advantageous', *Trends Cell Biol.* **6**, 148–53.

SPERLING P, ZAHRINGER U, HEINZ E (1998) 'A sphingolipid desaturase from higher plants. Identification of a new cytochrome b_5 fusion protein', *J. Biol. Chem.* **273**, 28590–6.

SPERLING P, TERNES P, ZANK TK, HEINZ E (2003) 'The evolution of desaturases', *Prostaglandins Leukot. Essent. Fatty Acids* **68**, 73–95.

SPRECHER H, CHEN Q (1999) 'Polyunsaturated fatty acid biosynthesis: a microsomal-peroxisomal process', *Prostaglandins Leukot. Essent. Fatty Acids* **60**, 317–21.

TOCHER DR, GHIONI C (1999) 'Fatty acid metabolism in marine fish: low activity of fatty acyl Δ^5 desaturation in gilthead sea bream (*Sparus aurata*) cells', *Lipids* **34**, 433–40.

TUCKER G (2003) 'Nutritional enhancement of plants', *Curr. Opin. Biotechnol.* **14**, 221–5.

UAUY R, HOFFMAN DR, PEIRANO P, BIRCH DG, BIRCH E (2001) 'Essential fatty acids in visual and brain development', *Lipids* **36**, 885–95.

VON SCHACKY C (2003) 'The role of omega-3 fatty acids in cardiovascular disease', *Curr. Atheroscler. Rep.* **5**, 139–45.

WALLIS JG, WATTS JL, BROWSE J (2002) 'Polyunsaturated fatty acid synthesis: what will they think of next?', *Trends Biochem. Sci.* **27**, 467–70.

WOLFF RL, CHRISTIE WW, PEDRONO F, MARPEAU AM (1999) 'Arachidonic, eicosapentaenoic, and biosynthetically related fatty acids in the seed lipids from a primitive gymnosperm, *Agathis robusta*', *Lipids* **34**, 1083–97.

ZHU M, YU LJ, WU YX (2003) 'An inexpensive medium for production of arachidonic acid by *Mortierella alpina*', *J. Ind. Microbiol. Biotechnol.* **30**, 75–9.

21

Virtually *trans* free oils and modified fats

G. van Duijn, E. E. Dumelin and E. A. Trautwein, Unilever Research and Development Vlaardingen, The Netherlands

21.1 Introduction

Trans fatty acids are geometrical isomers of monounsaturated and polyunsaturated fatty acids having non-conjugated (interrupted by at least one methylene group $-CH_2-CH_2-$) carbon–carbon double bonds in the *trans* configuration, in which the hydrogen atoms linked to the carbon atoms on both sides of the double bond have an opposite position with respect to the double bond. In the *cis* configuration, these hydrogen atoms are on the same side of the double bond (see Fig. 21.1).

Several studies, including epidemiological as well as animal and human intervention studies, have provided evidence for unfavourable health effects of dietary *trans* fatty acids. There is strong evidence from epidemiological studies indicating that high intakes of *trans* fatty acids are associated with an increased risk for cardiovascular heart disease (CHD) and they have an adverse effect on blood lipid concentrations (Lichtenstein, 2000). Evidence for adverse effects of high *trans* fatty acid intakes regarding other health aspects such as the risk of cancer, age-related macular degeneration or type 2 diabetes is insufficient and conflicting (Ip and Marshall, 1996; Zock 2001; Joint WHO/FAO expert consultation, 2003; Scientific Panel, 2004).

Digestion and absorption of dietary *trans* fatty acids occur similarly to other fatty acids. After absorption, *trans* fatty acids follow the same metabolic routes and selective accumulation in body tissues does not occur. Ultimately, *trans* fatty acids are oxidised to provide energy.

Trans fatty acids inhibit the de-saturation of linoleic and alpha-linoleic acid in *in vitro* studies, but data from human studies indicate that an inhibition of essential fatty acid metabolism by *trans* fatty acids consumed with habitual diets

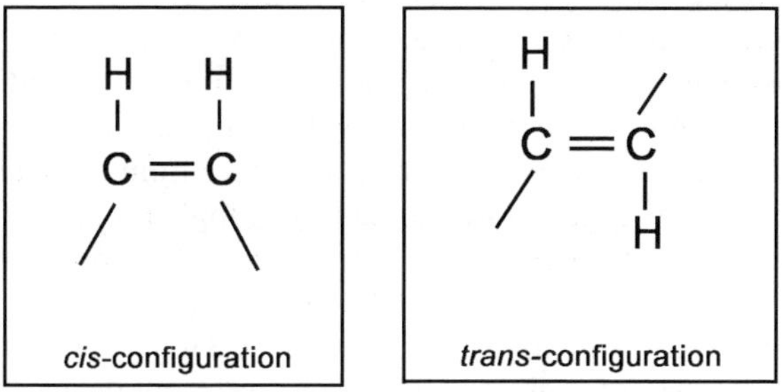

Fig. 21.1 Schematic presentation of the *cis* and *trans* configurations.

is unlikely and thus of no concern for human adults (Institute of Medicine, 2003). Nevertheless there are some reports on unfavourable effects of *trans* fatty acids on essential fatty acid metabolism and infant development. However, such an association has not been shown with certainty and more research is needed to resolve whether *trans* fatty acids have negative consequences early in life (Larque *et al.*, 2001).

There are three different sources of *trans* fatty acids in the diet:

- *Trans* fatty acids formed from partial hydrogenation of vegetable oils used to produce semi-solid or solid fats for the production of margarines, spreads shortenings, etc.
- *Trans* fatty acids from heat isomerisation formed during heat processing or frying of oils at high temperatures.
- *Trans* fatty acids formed from bio-hydrogenation, i.e. bacterial transformation of unsaturated fatty acids in the rumen of cattle and sheep.

The *trans* fatty acid content in partially hydrogenated oils fats can range up to 50% of total fatty acids, the majority of these *trans* fatty acids being elaidic acid. Ruminant fat, e.g. dairy foods, meat from cattle and from sheep, contains about 2–5% of *trans* fatty acids, mainly as vaccenic acid. The *trans* fatty acid profiles of ruminant fat and partially hydrogenated vegetable oils show considerable overlap, with many *trans* fatty acid isomers in common, though the isomers are present in different proportions.

21.1.1 Dietary *trans* fatty acids and risk of coronary heart disease

Several epidemiological studies have reported a positive relationship between the intake of *trans* fatty acids and the risk of CHD. Most of these studies have found that CHD risk was increased with higher intakes of *trans* fatty acids (Lichtenstein, 2000; Institute of Medicine, 2003). Hence, it was concluded that there is convincing evidence that *trans* fatty acid intake increases the risk of CHD (Joint WHO/FAO Expert Consultation, 2003).

There is some debate whether *trans* fatty acids from partially hydrogenated oils and ruminant fats differ or have similar effects regarding the increase in

CHD risk. So far, only a few studies have attempted to differentiate between intakes of these two *trans* fatty acid sources. A recent review of the available evidence concluded, based on data from epidemiological studies, that positive associations shown for *trans* fatty acids with CHD risk, up to an intake of 2.5 g/day, are similar for total *trans* fatty acids and those from ruminant fat or partially hydrogenated oils (Weggemans *et al.*, 2004). A higher intake of more than 3 g/d of total fatty acids and *trans* fatty acids from partially hydrogenated oils are also associated with increased risk of CHD. There is, however, insufficient data on ruminant *trans* fatty acid intake of more than 3 g/day to allow evaluation of impact on CHD risk, of high intakes of *trans* from ruminant sources. Thus, the scarce data available do not support different effects on CHD risk of *trans* fatty acids from ruminant fat and partially hydrogenated oils.

21.1.2 Intake of *trans* fatty acids and blood lipids

Dietary intervention studies with different human populations have shown that *trans* fatty acid intake increases plasma total and low-density lipoprotein (LDL) cholesterol, and decreases high-density lipoprotein (HDL) cholesterol and the ratio of total/HDL cholesterol as compared with *cis*-unsaturated fatty acids (Mensink *et al.*, 2003). Plasma triacylglycerol concentrations are also increased when *trans* fatty acids replace an isocaloric amount of a usual mix of other dietary fatty acids. These changes in plasma lipids are indicative of an adverse effect on the risk of CHD. Habitual diets contain many different *trans* fatty acid isomers which may not all have similar effects on blood lipids; however, there are only scarce data to draw conclusions on distinct effects of different *trans* fatty acids, e.g. from sources like ruminant fat or partially hydrogenated oils. Results from an animal study testing elaidic acid and vaccenic acid showed that both *trans* fatty acid isomers had similar effects on blood lipids (Meijer *et al.*, 2001). There are no human data that have directly compared the effects of specific ruminant *trans* fatty acids versus those from partially hydrogenated fats.

21.1.3 Overview of current dietary intakes of *trans* fatty acids

There are few data available on dietary intakes of *trans* fatty acids. Variation and changes in the *trans* fatty acid content of different foods, especially in processed foods, further complicate such estimates. The major contributors of total *trans* fatty acid intake are partially hydrogenated oils and ruminant fat. Prior to 1995, partially hydrogenated oils were the major source of *trans* fatty acids in Europe and North America. Subsequently, in Europe, manufacturers reduced the level of *trans* fatty acids in spreads. As a result, intakes of *trans* fatty acids from ruminant sources are now higher than intakes from partially hydrogenated oils in many European countries.

The most comprehensive study addressing *trans* fatty acid intakes in 14 European countries is the so-called TransFair study (Hulshof *et al.*, 1999). This study compared the intakes of fats and fatty acids between 14 European countries using recent data (post-1995) on food composition. The TransFair study also analysed *trans* fatty acid levels in common foods on the market in Europe in 1995/96 (Aro *et al.*, 1998a,b,c; van Erp-Baart *et al.*, 1998). The variation in *trans* fatty acid levels in fats and oils and products prepared with partially hydrogenated fats was substantial: products with almost no *trans* fatty acids could be found as well as frying fats with up to 50% and baked goods with up to 27% *trans* fatty acids. From the TransFair study, data are also available on the contribution of various foods, such as margarine, milk and meat, to *trans* fatty acid intake. These showed that the intake of *trans* fatty acids from ruminant sources was greater than that from partially hydrogenated fats in 9 out of the 14 countries studied. Major contributors to intakes from *trans* fatty acids from partial hydrogenation were bakery and fried foods.

Since the TransFair study was conducted, *trans* fatty acid levels in many foods and thus dietary intakes have continued to decrease (Precht *et al.*, 2000; Steinhart *et al.*, 2003; Harnack *et al.*, 2003). In Germany, for instance, *trans* fatty acids intake decreased from 4.1 g/day in 1992 to 2.3 g/day in 1997 for men and from 3.4 g/day in 1992 to 1.9 g/day in 1997 for women (Steinhart *et al.*, 2003). Therefore, total intakes of *trans* fatty acids are currently probably lower than those measured by the TransFair study and range from 0.5 to 2% of energy or 1 to 4 g/day. In the USA, the mean intake of *trans* fatty acids is about 2–3% of energy or 4–7 g/day (Lichtenstein 2000; Institute of Medicine, 2003)

21.1.4 Current dietary recommendations regarding *trans* fatty acids

There is no physiological requirement for *trans* fatty acids and therefore their intake should be as low as possible (Institute of Medicine, 2003). Recent dietary recommendations in most countries (e.g. Austria, Germany, Switzerland, UK, Netherlands) have set an upper limit for the intake of *trans* fatty acids most commonly of 1–2% of energy, which is equivalent to about 2–4 g/day. The World Health Organization recommends that the *trans* fatty acid intake of daily diets should be 1% of energy or less (Joint WHO/FAO Expert Consultation, 2003).

21.2 The formation of *trans* fatty acids during hydrogenation

21.2.1 Oils and fats for margarine production

Margarines (or fat continuous spreads) consist of an emulsion of dispersed small droplets of an aqueous phase in liquid oil stabilised by a structure of solid fat crystals (see Fig. 21.2). Both the aqueous and the oil/fat phases contain other minor dissolved components such as salt, flavours and emulsifiers. The solid fat crystals are important for three reasons:

- They supply the structure, hardness and texture to the product.
- They form a sponge-like structure that prevents the oil from leaking out of the product.

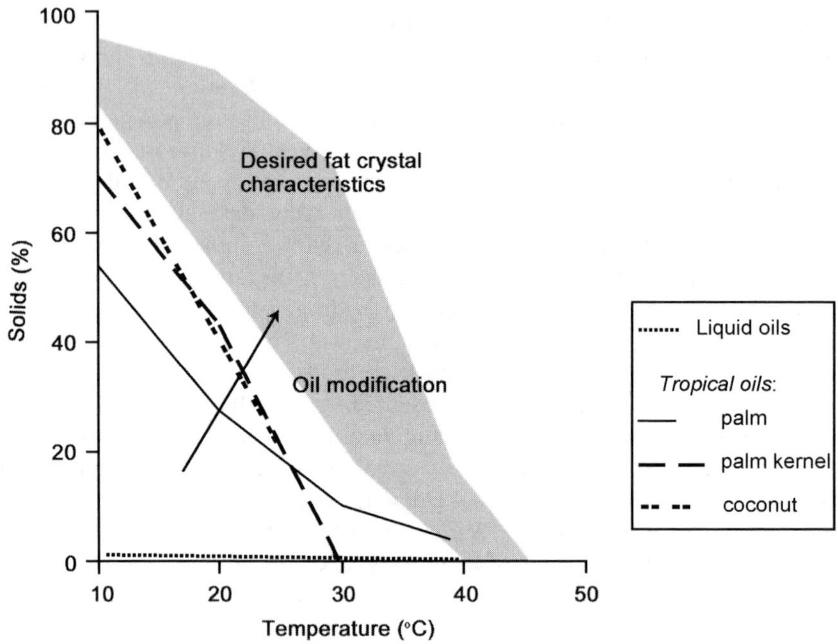

Fig. 21.2 The desired solid phase lines for margarine hardstocks (grey area) compared with the lines of naturally occurring oils and fats. Liquid oils are oils that are liquid at ambient temperature (20 °C), important liquid oils are soybean, rapeseed and sunflower oil. Tropical oils originate from tropical tree fruits, they are solid at 20 °C, important tropical oils are palm, palm kernel and coconut oil.

- They avoid coalescence of the dispersed aqueous phase droplets.

To what extent these functionalities are satisfied depends primarily on the amount of solid fat present, but also on the size, shape and mutual interaction of the crystals. These characteristics are mainly influenced by the solid fat content of the crystals (the solid fat content of fat blends is routinely measured using nuclear magnetic resonance (NMR) techniques, the solid fat content as a function of temperature is often referred to as N-line or solid phase line of the product).

The production of margarines with properties adapted to consumer needs requires the availability of solid fat crystals (often called hardstocks) with optimised solid phase lines. The solid phase line of an optimal hardstock has the following characteristics:

- It is not too high at 10 °C for a good spreading behaviour of a refrigerated product.
- It is not too low at 20 °C to contribute to a satisfying consistency and homogeneity at ambient temperature.
- It is low at 35 °C for a good oral melt and flavour release.

The area of solid phase lines fulfilling these criteria is indicated in Fig. 21.2.

Most of the oils and fats obtained from seeds (such as soybean, sunflower, rapeseed) are too low in solids in the temperature range 10–35 °C to give consistency to margarine. Tropical oils such as palm oil, palm kernel oil and coconut oil are higher in solids although their solid phase lines are still outside the optimal range indicated in Fig. 21.2. In theory, margarines could be produced using high levels of unmodified tropical oils as hardstock. However, this has an unfavourable effect on blood cholesterol since tropical oils are high in saturated fatty acids (coconut oil around 90%, palm kernel oil around 80%). Modification of the solid phase lines of naturally occurring oils and fats is required to produce optimal hardstocks.

21.2.2 *Trans* fatty acid formation

Hydrogenation of oils and fats has been applied on a large scale since the start of the twentieth century to produce hardstocks from a wide variety of feedstocks (mainly liquid oils and fish oil). Hydrogenation involves the addition of two hydrogen atoms across the unsaturated double bonds (C=C) in the fatty acid groups of the triacylglycerols. The more saturated fat resulting from this reaction has a higher melting point than the starting material. In the hydrogenation process, hydrogen gas is reacting with liquid oil at elevated temperatures and pressures in the presence of a solid catalyst. The catalyst consists normally of small nickel crystallites supported by an inorganic oxide, usually silica or alumina. Products with different solid phase lines can be obtained by stopping the hydrogen supply, and hence the reaction, when only a proportion of the double bonds has been saturated (partial hydrogenation). After stopping the reaction, the catalyst is removed by filtration and remaining traces of nickel are subsequently removed by post treatment to a level below 0.1 ppm.

As well as saturation, isomerisation of double bonds also takes place during the hydrogenation reaction. Two types of isomerisation reaction will occur:

- Geometric isomerisation (*cis* – *trans*).
- Positional isomerisation (shift of double bond along the fatty acid chain).

The mechanisms of hydrogenation and isomerisation are strongly connected. The addition of hydrogen to a double bond occurs in two steps. First a half-hydrogenated intermediate is formed in which the triacylglycerol molecule adsorbed to the catalyst surface by a single bond (part of the 'opened' double bond) can freely rotate. Addition of a second hydrogen atom to the other part of the 'opened' double bond results in hydrogenation, while re-donation of a hydrogen atom to the catalyst surface will yield either the original *cis* double bond or a positional or geometric (*trans*) isomer. Hence, the isomerisation reactions are promoted by a relative shortage of hydrogen at the catalyst surface. A low hydrogen pressure, and/or a low gas–liquid mass transfer, and/or a high temperature can cause this shortage. Also poisoning of the catalyst surface by sulphur will strongly promote isomerisation.

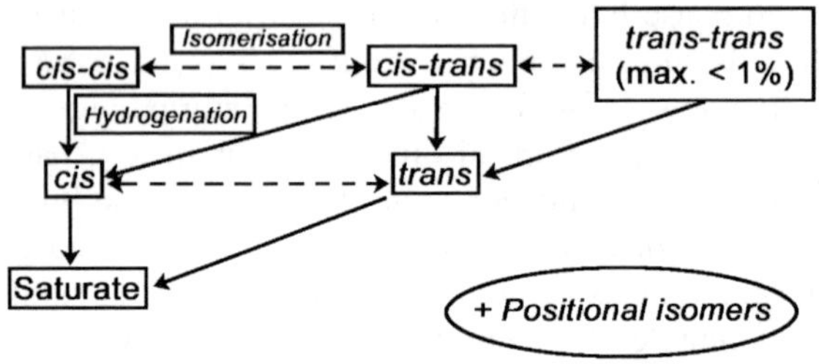

Fig. 21.3 A simplified reaction scheme for the hydrogenation and isomerisation of *cis-cis* diene.

A simplified reaction scheme for the hydrogenation/isomerisation of *cis–cis* diene is shown in Fig. 21.3; more complete reaction schemes are given in the literature (Rozendaal, 1976). *Trans*-containing dienes will be formed during the first phase of the reaction (*cis–trans* combinations and even a low level of *trans–trans* (< 1%)). In the course of the reaction, these dienes will be hydrogenated further to *trans* or *cis* monoenes. In partly hydrogenated hardstocks most of the *trans* will be in the form of *trans* monoenes, the level of *trans*-containing dienes will normally not exceed a few per cent.

The formation of *trans* fatty acids during the hydrogenation of soybean oil at two different temperatures using a fresh (non-poisoned) and a sulphur-poisoned catalyst is shown in Fig. 21.4. During the course of the reaction, the *trans* level rises until a maximum is reached. In thermodynamic equilibrium, 72% of the double bonds will be in the *trans* configuration and 28% in the *cis* configuration. The maximum obtainable *trans* level will be 72%; this will occur when all double bonds have passed the half-hydrogenated state under isomerisation-promoting conditions. In the example shown, this maximum *trans* level is almost reached at a degree of saturation of around 35%, during the hydrogenation at high temperature using the sulphur-poisoned catalyst. The maximum *trans* level at high temperature with the fresh catalyst is almost 40%; this level is reached at around 45% saturation. At low temperature (120 °C) with fresh catalyst a maximum of around 25% is reached at around 50% saturation. For commercial nickel on carrier catalysts, the reaction will not start at temperatures below 120 °C. After reaching the maximum, the *trans* level drops as both *cis* and *trans* unsaturated fatty acids are hydrogenated to saturated fatty acids. The *trans* level will be zero at full hydrogenation (all double bonds are saturated). The lowest curve in Fig. 21.4 represents the minimum *trans* level obtainable under industrial conditions with the currently available nickel-based catalysts.

Low *trans* levels can be obtained by hydrogenation with noble catalyst (platinum or palladium) sometimes in the presence of basic additives such as tetra ethyl ammonium hydroxide (TEAH) and NH_3. The obtained low *trans* products may be suited as high-stability frying oils while the potential benefits as margarine hardstocks are small because of the low solids formation and the

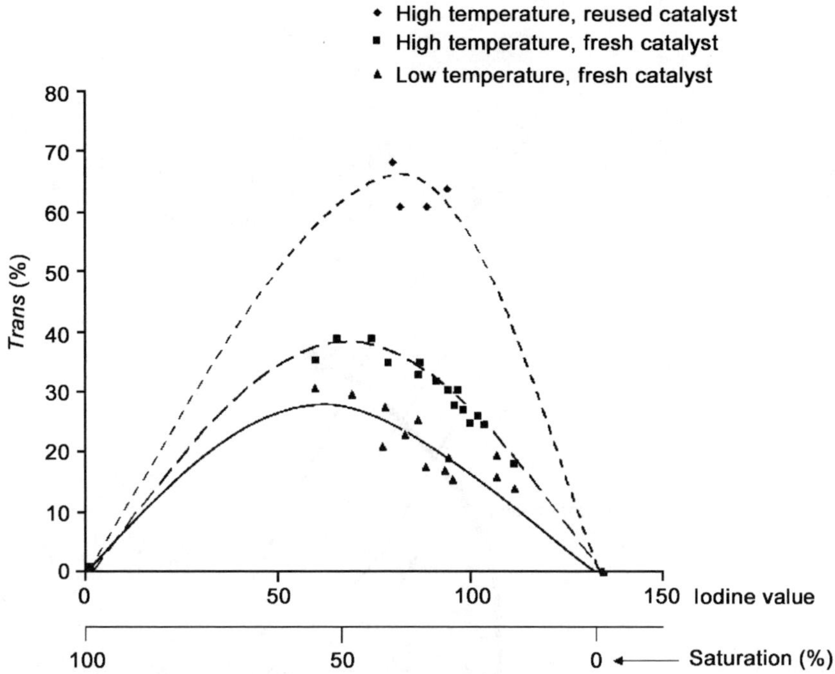

Fig. 21.4 The level of *trans* fatty acids as function of the iodine value and the degree of saturation. The graph shows lines for two different hydrogenation temperatures and for fresh and reused (sulphur-poisoned) catalyst.

very flat solid phase lines. The commercial case, of using noble catalyst for edible oil hydrogenation, has so far not been proved.

21.2.3 Partially hydrogenated products

During hydrogenation of liquid oil (e.g. soybean oil), the solid phase line will develop as shown in Fig. 21.5:

- Non-hydrogenated liquid oil has hardly any solids in the temperature range (10–50 °C) illustrated.
- After a certain degree of saturation, solids will be formed by the combined contribution of saturated fatty acids and *trans* fatty acids. The example in Fig. 21.5 shows the solid phase lines of soybean oil at 27% saturation, hydrogenated at a low temperature with a fresh catalyst to reduce *trans* formation (the lowest curve of Fig. 21.4). These products are typically used as stable frying oils.
- If hydrogenation continues, more solids will be formed, resulting in higher and steeper solids lines. The steepness of the line depends on the distribution of saturated fatty acids over the triacylglycerol molecules and the level of *trans* fatty acids (C18 *trans* monoene contributes to the solid levels at the lower temperatures (10–20 °C) but does not contribute to solid levels at high

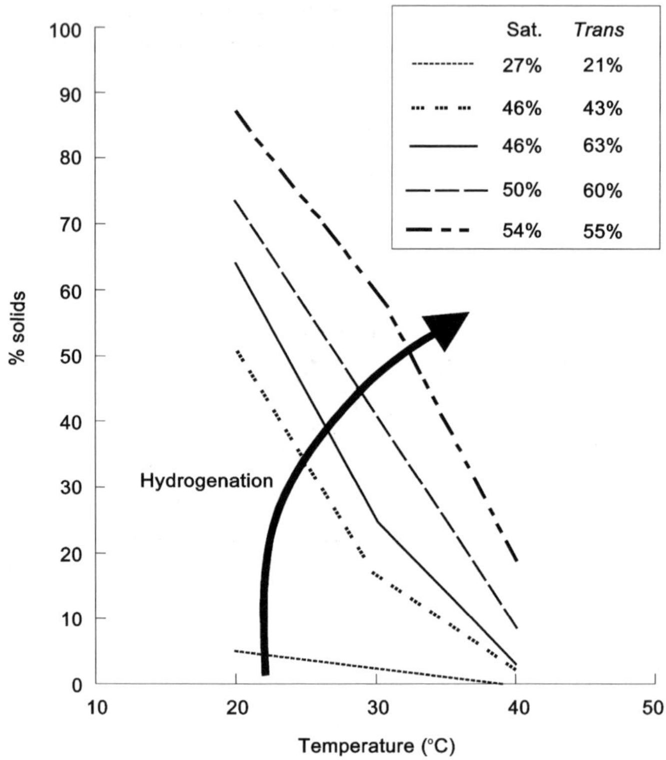

Fig. 21.5 Solid phase lines of hydrogenated soybean oil at different degrees of saturation. The two lines at 46% saturation show a steeper solid line for the product with the higher *trans* level.

temperature (> 40 °C)). This is illustrated in Fig. 21.5 by the two solid phase lines at 46% saturation; the solid phase line of the product with the higher *trans* level is steeper.

- Further saturation will further increase the solid fat content until the optimal solid phase line is obtained (in Fig. 21.5 lines at 50 and 54% saturation and high *trans* levels are also shown).
- At full saturation, the solid fat content will be close to 100% for the full temperature range below the melting point and will drop to zero just above the melting point (the melting point of fully hydrogenated soybean oil is 69 °C).

The above example illustrates that products with a wide range of solid phase lines can be produced by partial hydrogenation of soybean oil. Similar results can be obtained using different liquid oils and tropical oils as feedstocks.

In summary, the desired characteristics of partially hydrogenated hardstocks can be obtained by controlling the degree of saturation and *cis–trans* isomerisation (by optimising the process conditions such as hydrogen pressure, oil temperature and the quality of the catalyst) in combination with the selection of the feedstock. This makes partial hydrogenation a very flexible tool to produce optimal cost-effective margarine hardstocks choosing from a range of available feedstocks.

21.3 Oil modification techniques to produce virtually *trans*-free hardstocks

21.3.1 Virtually *trans*-free margarines

In response to the findings of adverse effect of *trans* fatty acids on blood lipids and CHD risk in the early 1990s, the European margarine industry decided to practically eliminate *trans*-containing components from their fat phase compositions (van Duijn, 2000). In 1995, the International Margarine Association of the Countries of Europe (IMACE) adopted a code of practice to reduce *trans* fatty acid levels in all margarines (retail margarines and margarines used as ingredients in processed foodstuffs) to achieve a *trans* level of 5%. Later in 2003, the target for virtually *trans*-free margarines (retail margarines and fat spreads) was set by IMACE at a maximum of 1% *trans* fatty acids on a product basis. Furthermore, the positive health effects accomplished by the reduction in the *trans* fatty acid content should not be counteracted by an increase in the saturated fatty acids level. This is achieved by:

- optimal combination of hardstock characteristics and margarine processing to produce fat crystal structures that can stabilise a maximum of water-in-oil emulsion with a minimum of solid fat phase;
- the production of *trans*-free hardstocks by combination of full hydrogenation and/or interesterification and/or fractionation. These *trans*-free hardstock production techniques will be introduced in the following sections.

21.3.2 Full hydrogenation

Reduction of the *trans* level to a maximum of 1% in an 80% fat margarine means a maximum of 1.25% *trans* in the margarine fat phase. The liquid oil part of this fat phase may also contain *trans* fatty acids as a result of high-temperature deodorisation (1–1.5% depending on the oil type, see Section 21.4). Hence, the maximum *trans* level in the margarine hardstock should also be around 1.25% to meet the product target. This very low maximum *trans* level can be achieved only by either no hydrogenation or full hydrogenation (as clearly shown in Fig. 21.4). Also hydrogenation with alternative systems such as noble catalysts will not meet this target.

Tropical oils and fats are, in their natural state, relatively saturated and therefore high in solids. Hardstocks can be produced by a combination of interesterification and fractionation of non-hydrogenated tropical oils and fats. Liquid oils contain hardly any solids. Therefore use of interesterification and/or fractionation alone as a means of reducing *trans* in liquid oils used for hardstock production is not an option. Use of full hydrogenation is now necessary to generate the saturated fatty acids, which can subsequently be redistributed by the other modification techniques.

With a factory-scale hydrogenation process, complete saturation of all double bonds is practically not achievable, the residual iodine value (IV) of a fully hydrogenated product will be around 1–2. (The IV is the measure for the degree of unsaturation of an oil or fat. It gives the amount of iodine (in grams) that reacts with 100 g of oil or fat.) A residual IV of 1 corresponds with 1.15% remaining monounsaturated fatty acids in the product. For almost fully hydrogenated fat, the thermodynamic equilibrium ratio between *cis* and *trans* (28/72) is reached. With this ratio, each IV point corresponds with 0.85% *trans* fatty acids. To obtain a product with a *trans* level below 1.25%, the hydrogenation should be continued until an IV below 1.5 is reached (the 'practical' specification of a fully hydrogenated product).

21.3.3 Interesterification

Interesterification permits a rearrangement or redistribution of the fatty acids on the glycerol fragment of the triacylglycerol molecule. Interesterification is promoted by an alkaline catalyst or by lipase (Rozendaal and Macrae, 1997). The most commonly used alkaline catalysts are sodium methylate and sodium ethylate. The mechanism of interesterification is described in detail in the literature (Rozendaal, 1997). Alkaline-catalysed reactions produce a mixture of triacylglycerols where the fatty acids are distributed randomly among the triacylglycerol molecules and among the three available positions within each molecule. Lipases mainly catalyse rearrangements at the 1 and 3 positions of the glycerol, leaving the ester link at the 2 position intact.

The alkaline (sodium (m)ethylate) catalysed reaction takes place in pre-refined oil (low in water and in free fatty acids) at elevated temperatures (100–110 °C). The reaction is very fast; full randomisation is reached within a few minutes even in factory-scale vessels (10–40 tonnes oil content). After the reaction, the catalyst is deactivated by water addition; sodium hydroxide and (m)ethyl esters will be formed. Sodium hydroxide will react with fatty acids and oil into soap, which is removed by water washing and decanting. (M)ethyl esters are more volatile than triacylglycerol molecules and are removed during high-temperature deodorisation.

The modification of the fatty acid distribution of the triacylglycerol molecules by interesterification will in general lead to a modification of the solid phase line resulting in a change of the crystallisation behaviour. This is illustrated by two examples:

- Random interesterification of a mixture of 50% tristearate and 50% trioleate will result in a mixture of six triacylglycerols (see Fig. 21.6). The original binary mixture has a melting point of 65 °C and a solids level of 46% at 60 °C. The melting point of the interesterified mixture with six components has decreased to 50 °C while the solids level at 60 °C dropped to only 5.5%.

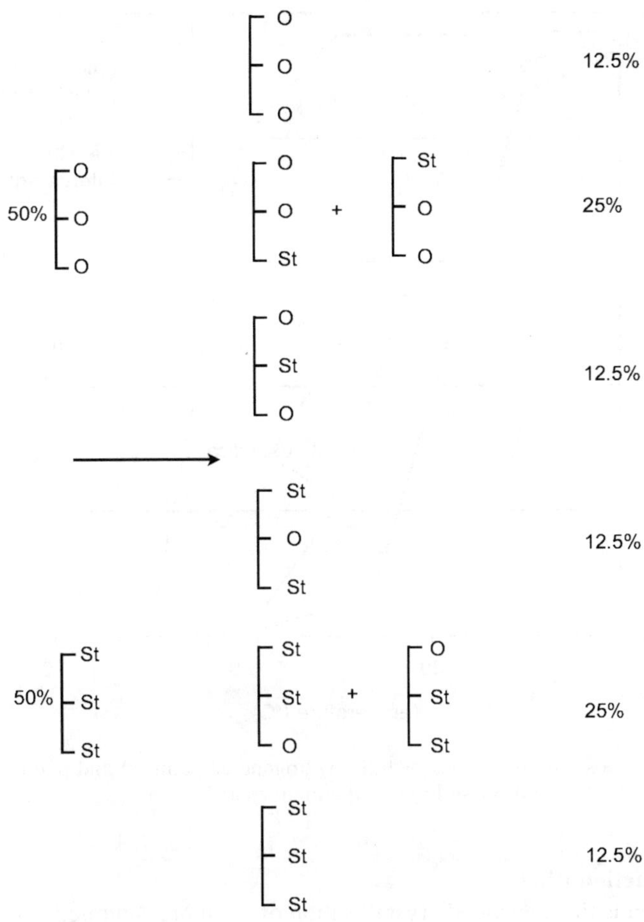

	Trioleate/tristearate mixture	Interesterified mixture
Melting point N60	65°C 46%	50°C 5.5%

Fig. 21.6 Triacylglycerols resulting from the random interesterification of a mixture of 50% tristearate and 50% trioleate.

- Random interesterification of a mixture of two fully hydrogenated components (fully hydrogenated palm oil and fully hydrogenated palm kernel oil). Figure 21.7 shows the solid phase lines of the two separate components, the mixture of the two components and of the interesterified mixture. The solids levels at high temperature (> 50 °C) are clearly reduced by interesterification: this makes the interesterified mixture better suited as margarine hardstock than the mixture before interesterification.

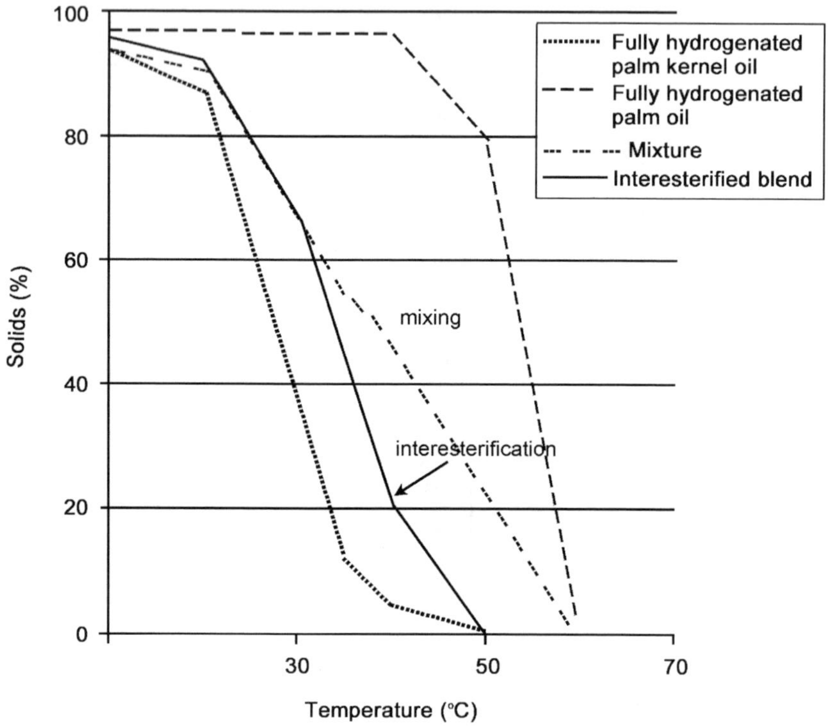

Fig. 21.7 The solid phase lines of fully hydrogenated palm oil and palm kernel oil together with the solid phase lines of the mixture and the interesterified mixture.

21.3.4 Fractionation

Fractionation is the controlled crystallisation of the more saturated and/or longer chain triacylglycerols, followed by separation of the solid phase (named stearin) and liquid phase (named olein). By far the most important oil, fractionated worldwide, is palm oil, the main reason being the demand for clear liquid oil (palm olein). More recently there has been a growing interest in the solid product of palm oil fractionation (palm stearin), for production of cocoa butter equivalents, cocoa butter replacers and margarine hardstocks. Besides palm oil, also palm kernel oil, partly hydrogenated liquid oils, cottonseed oil and milk fat are fractionated.

The fractionation process consists of the following steps:

- crystal nucleation;
- crystal growth;
- crystal slurry filtration;
- filter cake squeezing/pressing.

There are two defined forms of nucleation: primary and secondary. Primary nuclei are formed when oil is supersaturated or under-cooled; this is the driving force of the fractionation process. Secondary nucleation is the result of 'mechanical' attrition of existing crystals. The presence or addition of secondary crystals shortens the induction time necessary for primary nucleation and can initiate a better-controlled crystal growth regime. The aim for fractionation is to grow large, dense crystal agglomerates that can easily be separated from the liquid oil. The level of supersaturation and the presence of growth nuclei essentially drive crystal growth.

Crystal slurry is made up of potentially fragile crystal agglomerates. This slurry must not experience high shear stresses during the transfer to the filter and inside the filter. The filtration characteristics of the slurry depend on size of the crystal agglomerates, the separation efficiency of the slurry and the solid phase content. Most modern fractionation plants use membrane filter presses. These enable the filter cake, produced by simple filtration, to be squeezed to both increase the yield of olein and produce a harder stearin.

The combination of process conditions influencing these fractionation steps determines the characteristics and yield of both the olein and stearin. The most important parameters for solid fat production are:

- the type and quality of the feedstock;
- the crystallisation temperature;
- the type and size of the crystals;
- the efficiency of the separation process.

21.3.5 Virtually *trans*-free hardstock production

The combination of these *trans*-free modification techniques (full hydrogenation, interesterification and fractionation) and the availability of a variety of different feedstocks can be used to produce virtually *trans*-free hardstocks with a range of physical properties such as solid phase lines determining melting performances.

Liquid seed oils, low in solids, are first fully hydrogenated to generate solids combined with a very low *trans* level (< 1.25%). These fully hydrogenated oils may subsequently be interesterified with non-hydrogenated liquid oil to reduce the solid fat content at high temperature (> 40 ºC). This solid fat content can be further reduced by fractionation (see Fig. 21.8). The presence of relatively high solids levels in tropical oils creates more flexibility in oil modification routes. Fractionation alone will produce a relatively soft stearin which is not optimal for structuring margarine. Fractionation followed by interesterification with other (fractionated) components is used to produce 'non-hydrogenated' hardstocks. Full hydrogenation followed by interesterification is an alternative to obtain a hardstock high in solids with a steep melting line, without fractionation (see Fig. 21.8). This combination of techniques creates a tool for optimal hardstock production, which is almost as flexible as partial hydrogenation.

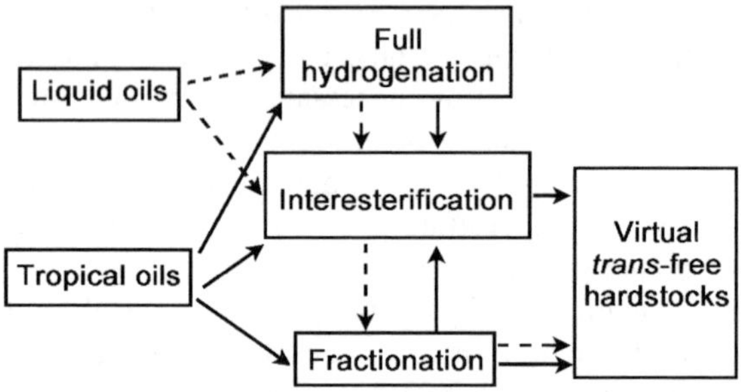

Fig. 21.8 The combination of *trans*-free modification techniques to produce virtual *trans*-free hardstocks.

21.4 The formation of *trans* fatty acids during high-temperature deodorisation

21.4.1 *Trans* formation at high temperature

Trans fatty acid isomers have repeatedly been identified in commercially deodorised oils: total *trans* levels of a few per cent have been observed in linoleic and α-linolenic acid-containing oils. The isomers that have been reported in heated vegetable oils include two *trans* isomers of linoleic acid (C18:2 *cis–trans* and C18:2 *trans–cis*) and six for α-linolenic acid (C18:3 *cis–trans–trans*, C18:3 *trans–cis–trans*, C18:3 *cis–cis–trans*, C18:3 *trans–cis–cis*, C18:3 *cis–trans–cis*, C18:3 *trans–trans–cis*). The full *trans* isomers (C18:2 *trans–trans* and C18:3 *trans–trans–trans*) were not found. The maximum *trans* level found for oleic acid (C18:1 *trans*) is 0.2%.

Within Unilever Research, a kinetic model has been developed to predict the *trans* level. The total concentration of *trans* isomers of a fatty acid (C_{tr}) depends on the original *cis* concentration of that fatty acid (C_0), the temperature (T in kelvin) and the time at this temperature (t_{m} in minutes), according to the following relation:

$$C_{tr} = C_0(1 - e^{-ktm})$$

The rate constant k in this model is temperature dependent. The parameters used to describe this dependency have been determined for linoleic acid and α-linolenic acid from factory scale experiments:

- C18:2, $k = 8 \times 10^8 \times e^{-128/RT}$ $(\mathrm{min})^{-1}$
- C18:3, $k = 6.3 \times 10^{11} \times e^{-145/RT}$ $(\mathrm{min})^{-1}$

Oils high in oleic acid may have an additional contribution to the *trans* level of 0.1–0.2% depending on deodorisation temperature and oleic acid level.

Verification by full-scale deodorisations has shown a good correlation between measured and predicted *trans* values. Lesieur and Cereol (Hénon *et al.*, 1999) have developed a comparable model with similar good prediction.

Table 21.1 Predicted *trans* fatty acid levels (%) in different oils, deodorised at different temperatures and times

Deodorisation temperature	Sunflower oil		Soybean/rapeseed oil	
	30 min	60 min	30 min	60 min
200	0.3	0.3	0.3	0.3
220	0.4	0.4	0.4	0.5
240	0.5	0.7	0.7	1.1
250	0.6	1.0	1.0	1.7
260	0.9	1.4	1.6	2.8

21.4.2 Optimal deodorisation conditions to prevent *trans* formation

The predicted *trans* levels after 30 and 60 minutes of deodorisation at different temperatures (in the range 200–260 °C) for the main liquid seed oils are given in Table 21.1. *Trans* levels higher than 1% will occur in sunflower only at high temperature and long deodorisation time; for soybean and rapeseed oil, a wider range of times and temperatures will result in these *trans* levels. However, high deodorisation temperatures and/or long times may be required for the following reasons:

- The stripping of free fatty acids in physical refining. To reduce a free fatty acid level from more than 1% to below 0.1% often requires deodorisation temperatures above 240 °C combined with a long deodorisation time.
- To ensure removal of pesticides and light polyaromatic hydrocarbons a deodorisation temperature of more than 220 °C is required.
- The higher the temperature, the less stripping steam is needed to obtain a good tasting deodorised product.
- Decomposition of red colour is achieved at high temperature; this is specially applied in palm oil deodorisation where *trans* formation is, however, less important (mainly saturated and monounsaturated fatty acids).

For each deodoriser, the process window of operational parameters should be defined, in which all these requirements (including the maximum *trans* limit) are met. For physical refining of seed oils with a high free fatty acid content and/or high in linolenic acid, this may be a difficult and sometimes impossible task. Relaxation of the free fatty acid specification in the deodorised product, changing to chemical refining or improvement of the deodoriser efficiency will then be required.

21.5 Future trends

The target for virtually *trans*-free margarine production was set at a maximum of 1% on a product basis. Further reduction of this target to a limit of around 0.5% or lower would introduce the following restrictions:

- No hydrogenation, since *trans* levels below 1% in a fully hydrogenated product are not achievable on a production scale.
- Relatively mild deodorisation conditions; reduction of the deodorisation temperature to a maximum of 220 °C.

These restrictions would eliminate all routes using full hydrogenation (see Fig. 21.8). Hardstock production starting from liquid oils only would not be possible, tropical oils would always be needed. For hardstocks with high solid fat contents, special fractions of tropical oils will be required. These can then be interesterified with other tropical oil fractions or liquid oils. An alternative route to eliminate hydrogenation and even reduce the need for interesterification is the development of 'natural' oils and fats with a solid phase line close to the desired one. This can be achieved by developing already existing tropical fruits, containing oils/fats with the desired solid phase line, into an industrial crop. Classical or genetic modification can develop oil seeds containing oils/fats relatively high in solids.

Deodorisation at a relatively low temperature (< 220 °C) requires feedstocks that are low in contaminant levels. These contaminants include 'light' polyaromatic hydrocarbons, some pesticides and other volatile contaminants (e.g. from previous cargoes). At low-temperature deodorisation, the reduction of free fatty acids will also be less. Reduction of deodorisation temperature must therefore be combined with an increase in the crude oil quality by a better control of the crude oil supply chain.

21.6 References

ARO A, ANTOINE JM, PIZZOFERRATO L, REYMER PW, VAN POPPEL G: *Trans* fatty acids in dairy and meat products from 14 European countries: the TransFair Study. *J Food Comp Anal* (1998a) **11** 150–160.

ARO A, VAN AMELSFOORT JMM, BECKER W, VAN ERP-BAART MA, KAFATOS A, STANLEY J, VAN POPPEL G: *Trans* fatty acids in dietary fats and oils from 14 European countries: the TransFair Study. *J Food Comp Anal* (1998b) **11** 137–149.

ARO A, AMARAL E, KESTELOOT H, RIMESTAD AH, THAMM M, VAN POPPEL G: *Trans* fatty acids in French fries, soups and snacks from 14 European countries: the TransFair Study. *J Food Comp Anal* (1998c) **11** 170–177.

HARNACK L, LEE S, SCHAKEL SF, DUVAL S, LUEPKER RV, ARNOLD AH: Trends in the *trans*-fatty acids composition of the diet in a metropolitan area: the Minnesota Heart Survey. *J Am Diet Assoc* (2003) **103** 1160–1166.

HÉNON G, KEMÉNY ZS, ZWOBADA F, KOVARI K: Deodorization of vegetable oils. Part 1: modelling the geometrical isomerization of poly unsaturated fatty acids. *JAOCS* (1999) **76** 1 73–81.

HULSHOF KFAM, VAN ERP-BAART MA, ANNTOLAINEN M *et al.*: Intake of fatty acids in Western Europe with emphasis on *trans* fatty acids: The TRANSFAIR study. *Eur J Clin Nutr* (1999) **53** 143–157.

INSTITUTE OF MEDICINE: *Dietary reference intakes for energy, carbohydrate, fibre, fat, fatty acids, cholesterol, protein, and amino acids*, Nat Acad Press 2003 (website http://www.nap.edu/catalog/10490.html).

IP C, MARSHALL JR: Trans fatty acids and cancer. *Nutr Rev* (1996) **54** 138–145.

JOINT WHO/FAO EXPERT CONSULTATION: *Diet, nutrition and the prevention of chronic diseases*. WHO Tech Report Series 916. WHO, Geneva (2003) (website http://www.who.int/hpr/nutrition/expertconsultationGE.htm accessed March 2003).

LARQUE E, ZAMORA S, GIL A: Dietary *trans* fatty acids in early life: a review. *Early Hum Dev* (2001) **65** S31–S41.

LICHTENSTEIN AH: Trans fatty acids and cardiovascular disease risk. *Curr Opin Lipidol* (2000) **11** 37–42.

MEIJER GW, VAN TOL A, VAN BERKEL THJC, WESTSTRATE JA: Effect of dietary elaidic versus vaccenic acid on blood and liver lipids in the hamster. *Atherosclerosis* (2001) **157** 31–40.

MENSINK RP, ZOCK PL, KESTER ADM, KATAN MB: Effects of dietary fatty acids and carbohydrates on the ratio of serum total to HDL cholesterol and on serum lipids and apoproteins: a meta analysis of 60 controlled trials. *Am J Clin Nutr* (2003) **77** 1146–1155.

PRECHT D, MOLKENTIN J: Recent trends in the fatty acid composition of German sunflower margarines, shortenings and cooking fats with emphasis on individual C16:1, C18:1, C18:2, C18:3 and C20:1 *trans* isomers. *Nahrung* (2000) **44** 222–228.

ROZENDAAL A: New trends in heterogeneously catalyzed hydrogenation of oils and fats. *Proceedings of ISF Congress*, Marseille (1976) 43–70.

ROZENDAAL A, MACRAE AR: Interesterification of oils and fats. *Lipid Technologies and Applications*, Eds F.D. Gunstone and FB. Padley, Marcel Dekker, New York, 1997, 223–263.

SCIENTIFIC PANEL: Opinion of the Scientific Panel on Dietic Products, Nutrition and Allergies on the request from the Commission related to the presence of *trans* fatty acids in foods and the effect on human health of the consumption of *trans* fatty acids. Request No. EFSA-Q-2003-022 (website: http://www.efsa.eu.int/science/nda_ options/catindex_en.html).

STEINHART H, RICKERT R, WINKLER K: *Trans* fatty acids (TFA): analysis, occurrence, intake and clinical relevance. *Eur J Med Res* (2003) **8** 358–362.

VAN DUIJN G: Technical aspects of *trans* reduction in margarines. *Oléagineux Corps Gras Lipides* (2000) **7**95–98.

VAN ERP-BAART M.A, COUET C, CUADRADO C, KAFATOS AG, STANLEY J, VAN POPPEL G: *Trans* fatty acids in bakery products from 14 European countries: the TransFair Study. *J Food Comp Anal* (1998) **11** 161–169.

WEGGEMANS, RM, RUDRUM M, TRAUWTEIN EA: Intake of ruminant versus industrial *trans* fatty acids and risk of coronary heart disease: what is the evidence? *Eur J Lipdi Sci Technol* (2004) **106** 390–397.

ZOCK PL: Dietary fats and cancer. *Curr Opin Lipidol* (2001) **12** 5–10.

22

Novel fats for the future

J. Skorve, K. J. Tronstad, H. V. Wergedahl, K. Berge, Haukeland University Hospital, Norway, J. Songstad, University of Bergen, Norway and R. K. Berge, Haukeland University Hospital, Norway

22.1 Introduction: the concept of modified fatty acids

Disorders of lipid metabolism are intimately connected to many common lifestyle-related diseases, including the Metabolic Syndrome, a serious condition with clustering of risk factors/disorders including overweight, dyslipidaemia, hypertension and insulin resistance/type 2 diabetes.[1,2] Fatty acids and other lipids have multiple roles in the body as they function as structural components, participate in intracellular signalling and serve as metabolic fuel. Long chain omega-3 polyunsaturated fatty acids (PUFAs) from fish and fish oils can protect against coronary heart disease, at least in part due to their beneficial effects on the plasma lipid profile.[3,4] Conversely, there is a strong positive correlation between the dietary intake of saturated fatty acids and *trans*-fatty acids and coronary heart disease.[5]

Owing to such differences in the biological activity of fatty acids, we have used novel fatty acids that have been modified structurally to investigate biochemical mechanisms that control lipid homeostasis. Minor changes in the structure of natural fatty acids, such as insertion of heteroatoms like sulphur, selenium or oxygen in the carbon chain, create modified fatty acids with new regulatory and metabolic properties. Although these modified fatty acids in many respects have properties similar to natural fatty acids, they also have additional biological effects which give them a unique impact on lipid metabolism. A considerable amount of research has been conducted to investigate the effects of heteroatomic modified fatty acids on lipid transport and metabolism in the body, and this work has documented that such compounds may have potential in prevention or treatment of lipid-related disorders.

22.2 Short historical background

A sulphur-containing fatty acid was probably first synthesised in 1948 as a precursor substance in the preparation of new penicillins.[6] Since 1990, various forms of sulphur substituted fatty acids, or thia fatty acids, have been extensively investigated for their effects on cells and tissues. The idea for the synthesis of sulphur-substituted fatty acids evolved from studies using the hypolipidaemic peroxisome proliferator tiadenol (bis(carboxyethylthio)-1,10-decane).[7] Berge *et al.* synthesised various thia fatty acids in order to investigate the structural requirements for peroxisome proliferation.[8] One of them, tetradecylthioacetic acid (TTA, Fig. 22.1) is by far the most studied owing to its diverse and beneficial effects in animal models, including lowering of plasma lipids, improving insulin action, antioxidant effects, anti-inflammatory action and modification of cell proliferation and apoptosis. TTA has a sulphur atom inserted in the 3-position from the carboxylic end, which prevents normal β-oxidation. Indeed, this modified fatty acid can be classified as a hypolipidaemic peroxisome proliferator. However, the plasma lipid-lowering effect seems to be mediated through the mitochondria rather than the peroxisomes (reviewed in ref. 9).

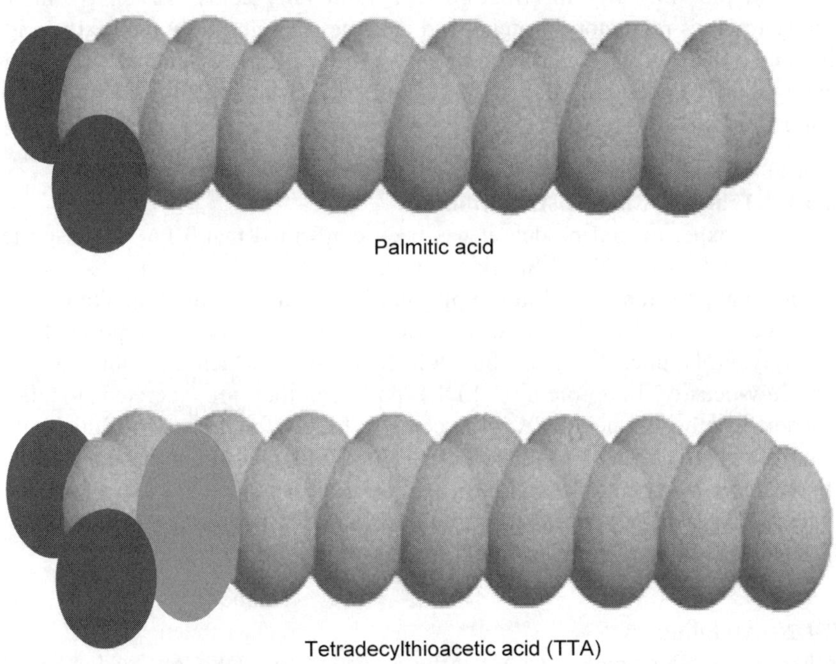

Fig. 22.1 The molecular structure of palmitic acid and TTA.

22.3 Structure and properties of tetradecylthioacetic acid (TTA)

When a sulphur atom is inserted in the carbon chain of a saturated fatty acid, as in TTA, the geometrical structure of the molecule is only slightly altered.[10] A slight torsion of the molecule around the sulphur atom of approximately 60º is to be expected. The sulphur atom is more electronegative than carbon. Hence, thia fatty acids are slightly more acidic than the corresponding fatty acid. Thia fatty acids are also more polar and slightly more soluble in water than fatty acids of corresponding chain length.

The synthesis of TTA and similar thia fatty acids is relatively simple and the most convenient method is by a condensation reaction (nucleophilic attack) between a thiodianion and an alkylbromide.[11] For TTA, the purified product has a melting point of 65–67 °C, and mass spectrometry of this product contains a major peak at 288 as expected. TTA is a colourless, crystalline substance with no odour or taste, and is non-hygroscopic. TTA is nearly indefinitely stable when stored in darkness, preferably at 0 °C. In aqueous solution it is oxidised very slowly by molecular oxygen to a sulphoxide.

22.4 Properties of 3-thia fatty acids

Owing to the similarity in structure to natural fatty acids, TTA has binding affinity towards regulatory proteins and enzymes that normally bind fatty acids. The metabolism of TTA is therefore very similar to that of dietary fatty acids, although differences are seen with respect to its catabolism and distribution within lipid classes.

22.4.1 Transport and distribution

In various experimental models it has been confirmed that TTA is transported into cells and tissues.[9,12–14] Similar to normal fatty acids, TTA is absorbed by the intestine and transported in the plasma, followed by a rapid uptake (plasma clearance) in the liver.[15] In hepatocytes, fatty acids are incorporated into triacylglycerols, phospholipids and cholesteryl esters, which are components of very low-density lipoprotein (VLDL) particles that are secreted for lipid transport to other tissues. TTA also seems to follow this transport route as it is found in the liver and VLDL particles,[16] and in tissues such as the kidneys, adipose tissue and heart.[17] After intravenous injection of [^{14}C]-TTA in rats, most of the radioactivity was detected in the liver within 1 min of administration, but significant amounts were also found in heart and adipose tissue.[18]

22.4.2 Metabolism

Following cellular uptake, TTA can be activated to TTA-CoA by long chain acyl-CoA synthetase, which occurs at a rate approximately half that of palmitic acid in rat liver preparations.[19] As for normal long chain acyl-CoAs, the TTA-

CoA ester can be used as substrate for biosynthesis of complex lipid classes. The acyl-chain of TTA is primarily found in the phospholipid fraction of rat liver, but there is clearly also some incorporation into triacylglycerols and cholesteryl esters.[15–17,20] TTA is a substrate for acyl-chain desaturation and the Δ9-desaturated product appears as a component of phospholipids and cholesteryl esters in rat liver.[16] Small amounts of the elongated product of TTA have also been found in liver after TTA administration to rats (unpublished data). Alternatively to the incorporation into esterified lipids, TTA-CoA may follow the normal transport route of long chain fatty acids into the oxidation pathway in the mitochondria. As with conventional fatty acids, the acyl-CoAs are then converted into acyl-carnitines by carnitine palmitoyltransferase (CPT) I, an enzyme of the outer mitochondrial membrane,[21] before they are carried across the inner mitochondrial membrane by carnitine: acylcarnitine translocase.[22]

CPT II is located in the inner mitochondrial membrane and catalyses the transfer of fatty acyl residues from carnitine to CoA, producing long-chain acyl-CoAs,[23] which subsequently enter the β-oxidation spiral in the mitochondrial matrix. TTA-CoA is a substrate for CPT I, and TTA-carnitine can be detected in liver (unpublished data), but it is clearly a poor substrate compared with palmitoyl-CoA.[24] Furthermore, in contrast to conventional acyl-CoAs in the mitochondrial matrix, TTA-CoA cannot be β-oxidised in the mitochondria due to the sulphur atom in the 3-position. TTA is, however, found as a component of structural mitochondrial lipids.[25] After *in vivo* injection of [1-^{14}C]-labelled 3-thia fatty acids, only trace amounts are converted to [^{14}C]-CO_2,[26] demonstrating that β-oxidation, as well as α-oxidation, is of little importance in the breakdown of these fatty acids. In rats, 3-thia fatty acids appear to be catabolized by ω-oxidation and sulphur oxidation in endoplasmic reticulum and peroxisomes,[26,27] leading to secretion of short sulphoxy dicarboxylic acids via urine.[10]

22.4.3 Kinetics of TTA in plasma

Kinetic studies of plasma TTA concentrations in rats and dogs have shown that systemic accumulation of TTA, and more markedly the desaturated form of TTA, was increased with repeated daily administration. Non-compartmental analysis of the plasma concentration data found a dose-independent terminal elimination half-life of 9 h following a single dose of TTA, and this was slightly increased with daily dosing. A dose-dependent increase in peak plasma concentrations of TTA was observed. The compound was extensively distributed in the extravascular space as indicated by a high volume of distribution. Plasma kinetic data in the dog are largely similar to the rat.

22.5 Modified fatty acids and the metabolic syndrome

Studies on modified fatty acids have revealed that such compounds may have a promising potential in the treatment of disorders that are tightly connected to development of cardiovascular disease, including common lipid disorders and insulin resistance. TTA is of particular interest due to its beneficial effects on lipid transport and utilization.[9] 3-Thia fatty acids affect the activities of various regulatory factors and enzymes via direct physical interaction, transcriptional regulation and by influencing the levels and composition of metabolites such as fatty acids in the cells. In the following, a survey is presented of the effects of TTA on individual risk factors of the metabolic syndrome, and the possible mechanisms involved in the biological responses.

22.5.1 Hypolipidaemic effects, mitochondrial function and PPAR activation

High plasma levels of lipid-rich lipoproteins and their remnants are important risk factors for coronary artery disease. The beneficial effects of hypolipidaemic agents are due to the reduction of plasma cholesterol, plasma triacylglycerols or both. Omega-3 fatty acids of fish origin, especially eicosapentaenoic acid (EPA), reduce plasma triacylglycerols and cholesterol in rodents,[28,29] but a high fish diet predominantly affects the plasma triacylglycerol level in humans. The hypolipidaemic effects are more dominant with 3-thia fatty acids and moderate doses of TTA decreased both plasma cholesterol and triacylglycerol levels in animals like rats, mice, rabbits and dogs within 2–3 days of treatment.[17,30–32]

Results from *in vivo* and *in vitro* experiments indicate that reduced triacylglycerol synthesis and secretion from the liver contribute to the hypolipidaemic effect of omega-3 fatty acids, and is due to increased fatty acid oxidation.[33–35] Similarly, feeding TTA to rats modulates hepatic gene expression and enzyme activities and causes a significantly increased mitochondrial and peroxisomal fatty acid oxidation.[36–38] TTA itself is unable to undergo β-oxidation and the stimulated fatty acid catabolism therefore leads to increased usage of endogenous fatty acids.

The increased expression of proteins involved in fatty acid transport and catabolism seems at least in part to be due to activation of peroxisome proliferator-activated receptors (PPARs), which are pleiotropic regulators of cellular proliferation, differentiation and lipid homeostasis. The PPAR family comprises the three subtypes PPARα, PPARγ and PPARδ, with different tissue distribution patterns and expression levels.[39] PPARs are activated by a number of pharmacological compounds, as well as by fatty acids and fatty acid-derived molecules. These ligands include fibrates, non-steroidal anti-inflammatory drugs and the antidiabetic glitazones, as well as natural ligands such as PUFAs, arachidonic acid metabolites and fatty acid-derived components of oxidised LDL.[40–42] Now, it is established that TTA acts as a ligand and activator of all three PPAR subtypes.[34,41,43,44] Transient transfection experiments have revealed that the activation potency depends on both the cell type and the species examined.[45,46]

A contribution of PPARα in mediating the effects of TTA has been demonstrated,[44] but experiments in PPARα-deficient mice indicate that PPARα-

independent mechanisms also seem to be involved.[25] Both fish oil and conjugated linoleic acid (CLA) decrease plasma triacylglycerols in PPARα-deficient mice.[47,48] In accordance, the gene expression of mitochondrial fatty acid oxidation enzymes were upregulated in PPARα-null mice given CLA,[48] whereas no induction was observed after treatment with the peroxisome proliferator Wy 14,643.[49] Similar effects have been observed in PPARα-deficient mice treated with TTA, in contrast to the PPARα ligand fenofibrate, which neither increased fatty acid oxidation nor decreased plasma triacylglycerols (unpublished data). The divergent regulation of lipid metabolism by peroxisome proliferators, fish oil, TTA and CLA, which all activate PPARα, argues that additional control mechanisms, besides activation of PPARα, are involved.

PPARδ has emerged as an important player in the regulation of lipid metabolism, and this transcription factor and certain nuclear receptor coregulators have been linked to the control of energy homeostasis and fat accumulation. Agonists specific to PPARδ decrease plasma lipids and insulinaemia in obese animals and recent data indicate that this receptor plays a central role in the regulation of fatty acid oxidation in several tissues, such as skeletal muscle and adipose tissue.[50,51] It has been demonstrated that TTA activates PPARδ in transfected skeletal muscle cells (unpublished data).

Rat experiments have further demonstrated that TTA affects mitochondrial function and energy state parameters.[25] Increased β-oxidation rate in liver of TTA-treated rats was associated with a lowered energy state, a lowered mitochondrial proton electrochemical potential (Δp) and altered mitochondrial fatty acid composition. Under these conditions, uncoupling of mitochondria involved depletion of the electrical potential difference ($\Delta\Psi$ component), but not the pH gradient, indicating a possible stimulation of electrogenic ion transport systems. Putative candidates in this regard are the ADP/ATP antiporter and the uncoupling proteins (UCPs). UCP homologues form a family of mitochondrial carriers that are capable of depleting the proton gradient. Accordingly, the demonstration of increased expression of hepatic UCP-2 by TTA may indicate that this transporter is of importance for the moderate uncoupling caused by TTA.[25] UCP-2 is under PPARα regulation, and the PPARα selective drug fenofibrate significantly induced the hepatic UCP-2 expression in wild type mice, but not in PPARα-deficient mice. However, UCP-2 expression could also be induced via a PPARα-independent mechanism as demonstrated by the equal level of induction in wild-type and PPARα-deficient mice after TTA treatment.[25]

22.5.2 Reduced obesity and improved insulin sensitivity

Since hypertriglyceridaemia is associated with the metabolic syndrome, triglyceride-derived fatty acids are thought to play a key role in the development and progression of this metabolic disorder. Normally, the level of free fatty acids in the blood is determined by the relative rates of fatty acid release (lipolysis) and accumulation (esterification) in adipose tissue, and the uptake in muscles. In muscle tissue, free fatty acids inhibit glucose uptake and oxidation. Thus, increased availability of fatty acids and triacylglycerols in blood and muscles correlates with obesity and insulin resistance, and a reduced ability to metabolise glucose.[52,53] Stimulation of fatty acid oxidation and ketogenesis in the liver, and decreased fatty acid concentration in the plasma, may reduce the fatty acid load reaching skeletal muscle tissue and thereby maintain glucose uptake and utilisation in skeletal muscle.

TTA prevents high-fat diet-induced insulin resistance and adiposity in rats. In obese Zucker (fa/fa) rats, TTA reduced adiposity and hyperglycaemia, and markedly improved insulin sensitivity as determined by the intravenous glucose tolerance test.[54] Similarly, experiments with male Wistar rats fed a high-fat diet for 7 weeks clearly showed the antiadipogeneic properties of TTA. TTA supplementation substantially decreased body weight gain and significantly improved the catabolic efficiency (body weight gain/food intake), compared with control and omega-3 fatty acid supplementation. TTA decreased the mass of different adipose depots during high-fat feeding, as determined with nuclear magnetic resonance (NMR) (unpublished data).

Hormone-sensitive lipase is responsible for mobilisation of fatty acids from adipose tissue to the bloodstream, and is therefore important in the regulation of free fatty acids in blood. Interestingly, reduced adiposity in TTA-treated rats is not associated with stimulation of hormone-sensitive lipase.[55] This suggests that TTA does not stimulate mobilisation of free fatty acids from white adipose tissue, which is further supported by reduction in the level of free fatty acids in plasma.

It has been shown that modulation of triacylglycerol-derived fatty acid disposal from lipoproteins can directly affect the development of obesity and insulin resistance. Thus, the importance of apo C-III in modulating triglyceride-derived fatty acid fluxes should be considered.[56] One function of apo C-III is to inhibit lipoprotein lipase (LPL) and prevent a direct uptake of VLDL in the liver. TTA reduced the expression of hepatic apo C-III mRNA.[44] Hence, the uptake of VLDL and chylomicrons by the liver might be stimulated, establishing a direct route of fatty acid transport from the intestine to the liver and/or re-uptake of VLDL formed in the liver itself. The level of free fatty acids in the blood is determined by the relative rates of lipolysis and esterification in the adipose tissue and the uptake of free fatty acids in the muscles. As the transport of free fatty acids to the liver is relatively minor (a few per cent) in relation to the total turnover (lipolysis, re-esterification), the liver has little immediate influence on the plasma levels of free fatty acids. However, over time, free fatty acids may be drained from the blood because of a stimulated fatty acid oxidation and ketogenesis in the liver. Indeed, the plasma concentrations of free fatty acids and ketone bodies were decreased and increased, respectively, after TTA treatment. Additionally, the gene expression of LPL was increased in liver but not in adipose tissue (data to be published), further indicating a specific enhancement of fatty acid import into the liver.

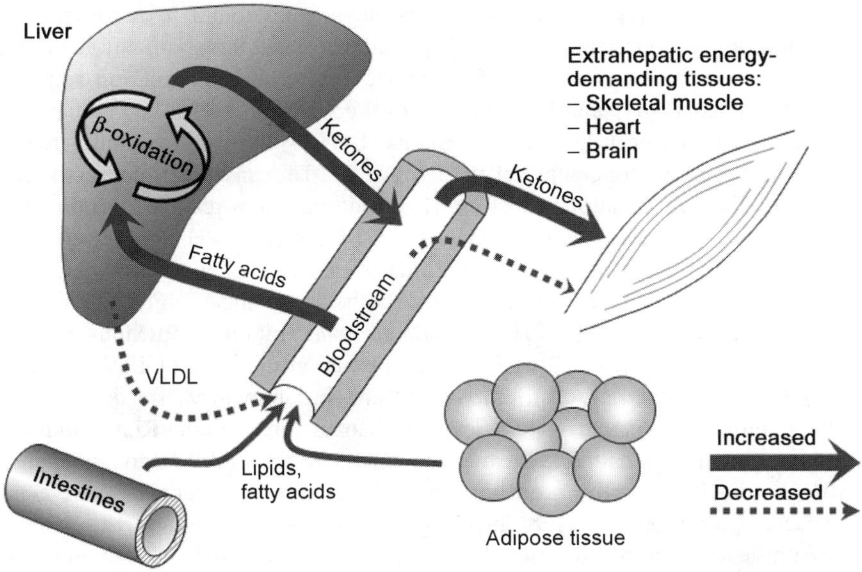

Fig. 22.2 The hepatic fatty acid drainage hypothesis, depicting the relationship between increased hepatic fatty acid oxidation and reduced fatty acid load in peripheral tissue.

Therefore, the hypolipidaemic and antiadipogenic effects of TTA are most likely explained by an increased fatty acid uptake and oxidation in other tissues, particularly in liver. This constitutes the basis of 'the hepatic fatty acid drainage hypothesis'[55] in which it is suggested that under the circumstances of TTA treatment, fatty acids are transported into hepatocytes and oxidised within the mitochondria, accompanied by an increased production of ketone bodies (Fig. 22.2). This hypothesis is supported by an induction of mitochondrial proliferation and a significant stimulation of β-oxidation and ketogenesis. The molecular mechanisms underlying this metabolic shift seem to involve *in vivo* activation of PPARα and the regulation of PPARα target genes in the liver.[9,55,57,58] Whether other PPAR subtypes are involved in this draining of fatty acids to the liver is under investigation. Thus, stimulated hepatic fatty acid oxidation and reduced VLDL formation could explain the anti-adiposity effect and improved insulin sensitivity after TTA administration. Another mechanism for removal of fatty acids from plasma may be an increased oxidation in adipose tissue and/or skeletal muscle. For instance, PPARα agonists reduce mRNA levels of adipocyte differentiation markers and increases fatty acid oxidation in adipocytes.[59]

22.5.3 Attenuation of atherosclerosis and vascular inflammation

Key features of the metabolic syndrome, including obesity, hypertension and dyslipidaemia, individually and interdependently lead to a substantially increased risk for cardiovascular disease morbidity and mortality. Inflammatory and immunological mediators may play important roles in cardiovascular pathogenesis. A range of lipid mediators have been found to modulate the inflammatory response including PUFAs and various agonists of the different PPAR subtypes.[60] In addition, PPARs interfere with chemo-attraction and cell adhesion of monocytes and lymphocytes in the vascular wall.

The modulation of inflammatory response by TTA has been demonstrated in peripheral blood mononuclear cells (PBMC).[61,62] TTA markedly depressed the release of the inflammatory cytokine IL-2, without significantly affecting the release of IL-1β or TNFα when PBMC were stimulated by PHA or LPS. On the other hand, the release of the anti-inflammatory IL-10 was enhanced nearly 10-fold when PBMC were stimulated by both PHA and TNFα. TTA also significantly suppressed the PHA stimulated proliferation of PBMC, and this suppression was not affected by blocking the action of IL-10 or IL-2. Thus, it seems likely that the anti-proliferative and anti-inflammatory effects represent distinct biological mechanisms. The mechanism by which TTA modifies cytokine production and release may be mediated by PPAR, through altered prostaglandin levels or by modification of lipid mediated signal transduction, which has been proposed as the mechanism of action of PUFAs.

Reactive oxygen species (ROS) are involved in a variety of pathological events, including atherosclerosis and inflammation. ROS-mediated oxidation of LDL and cholesterol accumulation in the arterial wall are two of the initial steps in atherosclerotic plaque formation. Studies in different animal models indicate that antioxidants may decrease the oxidative modification of LDL cholesterol and reduce plaque formation. TTA has antioxidant properties in biological systems, which may be explained both by the reducing power of sulphur and by biochemical changes affecting metabolites and enzymes involved in ROS generation and detoxification. The Cu^{2+}-induced oxidation of LDL particles is significantly reduced by TTA.[63,64] The antioxidant properties of TTA have also been demonstrated *in vivo*.[65] Triacylglycerol-rich lipoproteins isolated from rats fed TTA for 1 week altered fatty acid composition and significantly reduced the level of lipid peroxides. They were also much less susceptible to Cu^{2+}-induced lipid oxidation *in vitro*. The potent *in vivo* antioxidant capability of TTA, beside its hypolipidaemic effect, might therefore be of importance in relation to the development of atherosclerosis. Other redox-connected parameters that are affected in rats include reduction in plasma lipid peroxides and increase in liver glutathione content.[66,67]

22.5.4 Modulation of fatty acid composition

Owing to regulation of several enzymes involved in lipid metabolism, TTA alters the fatty acid composition in hepatic as well as plasma lipids. TTA has distinct effects on the cellular fatty acid desaturation and elongation system that are different from the action of unsaturated fatty acids. Twelve weeks of TTA administration nearly doubled the hepatic content of monounsaturated fatty acids (mainly oleic acid), probably because of increased activity of the $\Delta 9$ desaturase.[16] This is an interesting feature as an increased level of oleic acid may have a cardioprotective effect. Enrichment of LDL particles with oleic acid seems to make them more resistant to oxidative modifications. The content of PUFAs (mainly linoleic acid and docosahexaenoic acid) was decreased. This decrease was, however, not observed in the heart.[16,17,31]

22.5.5 Antihypertensive effects

Hypertension, dyslipidaemia and diabetes frequently cluster and share common pathogenic mechanisms, resulting in a complex interplay between these apparently disparate risk factors. Obesity is associated with activation of the renin–angiotensin system and hyperinsulinaemia, which may contribute to renal hypertension via sodium reabsorption and associated fluid retention.[68] Other risk factors such as hyperlipidaemia and hyperglycaemia may provoke additional potentially nephrotoxic mechanisms such as hyperfiltration and increased blood pressure. Obese individuals tend to have glomerular hyperfiltration and these increased filtration rates correlate well with fasting insulin levels. High levels of free fatty acids are thought to raise blood pressure, and these levels are increased in obese subjects.

Thiazolidinediones represent a class of drugs that act as PPARγ agonists and insulin sensitisers. These agents have been shown to have antihypertensive properties in rats and humans, and this is likely to be caused by modulation of lipid metabolism and a decrease in the level of free fatty acids in the plasma.[69] High intake of fish oil may lower blood pressure, especially in older and hypertensive subjects.[70] Studies in rats with renal hypertension have shown that TTA administration normalised blood pressure, accompanied by a normalisation of the renin production. The data suggest that TTA interfere with the activity of the renin–angiotensin system. Hypertension is probably reduced through down-regulation of COX-2 followed by inhibition of renin release and normalisation of the vascular response to angiotensin II, a peptide with strong vasoactive actions (data to be published). TTA had only minor effect on the blood pressure in normotensive rats and in rats with genetic hypertension. Since TTA lowered both plasma triacylglycerols and cholesterol in rats with renal hypertension as well as in genetically hypertensive rats, the lowering of blood pressure in the high-renin hypertensive rats cannot be explained by the lipid-lowering effect of TTA. Further studies will be needed to obtain a more comprehensive understanding of the mechanisms involved.

22.6 Health benefits for humans

As outlined in the preceding sections, the pleiotropic effects of TTA in animal models suggest that modified fatty acids could potentially provide great benefits in the prevention or treatment of the metabolic syndrome in humans. TTA has recently been evaluated in human studies. Small trials have been conducted with selected groups of patients, including diabetic and moderately dyslipidaemic patients. In these studies the subjects received 1 g TTA (approx. 15 mg/kg body weight) daily for 4 weeks.[71] These studies have been conducted to evaluate how TTA affects lipid metabolism, insulin action and vascular inflammation, in addition to an assessment of the antioxidant properties of TTA in humans. TTA administration was generally well tolerated in these studies, and no clinically adverse events were observed.

These human studies have documented for the first time that TTA affects lipid metabolism and that it decreases plasma lipids in humans. A significant reduction in plasma LDL cholesterol and in plasma triacylglycerols was observed, and after 4 weeks of treatment the decrease in plasma lipids was in the order of 15–20%. Such short-term treatment with TTA did not influence blood glucose control, but an indication was obtained that TTA may reduce the oxidisability of plasma LDL. TTA also influenced parameters related to vascular inflammation and lipoprotein metabolism. The plasma level of the adhesion molecule VCAM-1, involved in the process of atherosclerosis, was shown to be decreased by approximately 30% in subjects receiving TTA compared with placebo.[72] Slightly reduced plasma levels of apolipoprotein B and apolipoprotein A have also been observed in these studies. Additionally, blood pressure was affected, with a significant decrease in diastolic blood pressure.

The human studies have confirmed the large distribution volume of TTA, as demonstrated by rat plasma kinetic data. The plasma half-life of TTA, in the order of 12 h, as well as the plasma TTA levels, were comparable to the data obtained in plasma of rats. For a more extensive evaluation of the modulation of human metabolism by TTA, trials with larger cohorts of subjects will have to be conducted for at least 3 months.

22.7 Future trends

The use of modified fatty acids in food products will depend both on the documented biological effects and on identifying molecular entities and formulations that have satisfactory technological characteristics and show the highest bioavailability. Thia fatty acids appear most biologically active if the total number of carbon atoms in the carbon chain is between 14 and 18, and the sulphur atoms are inserted in uneven numbered positions such as 3, 5 and 7.[71] The metabolism and biological effects have not yet been studied in detail for all these molecular species and their tissue distribution and biological half-life may be different. It is a matter of concern and an important future research topic to determine the extent to which modified fatty acids may accumulate in specific tissues in the body.

The bioavailability of modified fatty acids may depend on the actual molecular species employed. As discussed in the section on the metabolism of 3-thia fatty acids, TTA is extensively incorporated into esterified lipids, especially phospholipids. Phospholipids and triacylglycerols with TTA as the fatty acid component have been synthesised. Studies with these compounds have demonstrated a high recovery of TTA in plasma and liver in rodents fed these esterified compounds, and especially with TTA in a phospholipid, as compared to feeding TTA as a free fatty acid (unpublished data). This is indicative of an increased intestinal absorption of TTA when esterified in phospholipids.

The esterification of TTA has been observed in rodents, and by including TTA in fish feed, similar observations have been made in salmon. TTA has been recovered from salmon muscle in esterified form, with a high preponderance for the phospholipid fraction.[73] The same will probably be true also for domestic animals. Thus, it should be entirely feasible to incorporate thia fatty acids in functional food products through inclusion as a feed component. Future research will have to focus on the level attainable and on the bioavailability of modified fatty acids when incorporated especially into the skeletal muscle of domestic animals. Research should also be directed towards alternative ways of incorporating modified fatty acids in functional food products, including liquid and solid emulsions such as fruit drinks, yoghurts and spreads.

Of further interest is the possible change in fatty acid composition as a result of thia fatty acid feeding. As discussed previously it is reasonable to assume that TTA feeding should result in a more beneficial fatty acid composition in the animal, in particular by increasing the content of monounsaturated fatty acids.

Another important topic to be addressed is the potential for additive or synergistic effects when combining various bioactive lipids. Differences in mode of action with respect to gene expression and metabolic fate suggest that a broader and more optimal range of biological effects may be attainable by combining modified fatty acids and other bioactive fatty acids such as monounsaturates and polyunsaturates. Evidence has been provided that TTA fed in combination with fish oil will have additive effects with respect to plasma lipids. Future research will have to identify optimal combinations of such bioactive lipids for enhanced biological effects, in much the same way as optimal ratios of unsaturated fatty acids have been identified.

22.8 References

1. GRUNDY, S.M., BREWER, H.B., JR., CLEEMAN, J.I., SMITH, S.C., JR., and LENFANT, C. (2004). Definition of metabolic syndrome: Report of the National Heart, Lung, and Blood Institute/American Heart Association conference on scientific issues related to definition. *Circulation* **109**, 433–438.
2. HUNT, K.J., RESENDEZ, R.G., WILLIAMS, K., HAFFNER, S.M., and STERN, M.P. (2004). National Cholesterol Education Program versus World Health Organization metabolic syndrome in relation to all-cause and cardiovascular mortality in the San Antonio Heart Study. *Circulation* **110**, 1251–1257.
3. CONNOR, W.E. (2000). Importance of n-3 fatty acids in health and disease. *Am J Clin Nutr* **71**, 171S–175S.
4. DIN, J.N., NEWBY, D.E., and FLAPAN, A.D. (2004). Omega 3 fatty acids and cardiovascular disease – fishing for a natural treatment. *BMJ* **328**, 30–35.
5. HU, F.B., MANSON, J.E., and WILLETT, W.C. (2001). Types of dietary fat and risk of

coronary heart disease: a critical review. *J Am Coll Nutr* **20**, 5–19.

6. SOPER, Q.F., WHITEHEAD, C.W., BEHRENS, O.K., CORSE, J.J., and JONES, R.G. (1948). Biosynthesis of penicillins. VII. Oxy- and mercaptoacetic acids. *J Am Chem Soc* **70**, 2849–2855.
7. BERGE, R.K., and BAKKE, O.M. (1981). Changes in lipid metabolizing enzymes of hepatic subcellular fractions from rats treated with tiadenol and clofibrate. *Biochem Pharmacol* **30**, 2251–2256.
8. BERGE, R.K., AARSLAND, A., KRYVI, H., BREMER, J., and AARSAETHER, N. (1989). Alkylthio acetic acids (3-thia fatty acids) – a new group of non-beta-oxidizable peroxisome-inducing fatty acid analogues – II. Dose–response studies on hepatic peroxisomal- and mitochondrial changes and long-chain fatty acid metabolizing enzymes in rats. *Biochem Pharmacol* **38**, 3969–3979.
9. BERGE, R.K., SKORVE, J., TRONSTAD, K.J., BERGE, K., GUDBRANDSEN, O.A., and GRAV, H. (2002). Metabolic effects of thia fatty acids. *Curr Opin Lipidol* **13**, 295–304.
10. SKREDE, S., SORENSEN, H.N., LARSEN, L.N., STEINEGER, H.H., HOVIK, K., SPYDEVOLD, O.S., HORN, R., and BREMER, J. (1997). Thia fatty acids, metabolism and metabolic effects. *Biochim Biophys Acta* **1344**, 115–131.
11. SPYDEVOLD, O., and BREMER, J. (1989). Induction of peroxisomal beta-oxidation in 7800 C1 Morris hepatoma cells in steady state by fatty acids and fatty acid analogues. *Biochim Biophys Acta* **1003**, 72–79.
12. SKREDE, S., NARCE, M., BERGSETH, S., and BREMER, J. (1989). The effects of alkylthioacetic acids (3-thia fatty acids) on fatty acid metabolism in isolated hepatocytes. *Biochim Biophys Acta* **1005**, 296–302.
13. BREMER, J. (2001). The biochemistry of hypo- and hyperlipidemic fatty acid derivatives: metabolism and metabolic effects. *Prog Lipid Res* **40**, 231–268.
14. PETTERSEN, R.J., KUIPER, K.K., FROYLAND, L., BERGE, R.K., and NORDREHAUG, J.E. (2001). Long-term retention of a novel antioxidant sulphur-substituted fatty acid analogue after local delivery in porcine coronary arteries. *Scand Cardiovasc J* **35**, 101–106.
15. GRAV, H.J., ASIEDU, D.K., and BERGE, R.K. (1994). Gas chromatographic measurement of 3- and 4-thia fatty acids incorporated into various classes of rat liver lipids during feeding experiments. *J Chromatogr B Biomed Appl* **658**, 1–10.
16. MADSEN, L., FROYLAND, L., GRAV, H.J., and BERGE, R.K. (1997). Up-regulated delta 9-desaturase gene expression by hypolipidemic peroxisome-proliferating fatty acids results in increased oleic acid content in liver and VLDL: accumulation of a delta 9-desaturated metabolite of tetradecylthioacetic acid. *J Lipid Res* **38**, 554–563.
17. ASIEDU, D.K., FROYLAND, L., VAAGENES, H., LIE, O., DEMOZ, A., and BERGE, R.K. (1996). Long-term effect of tetradecylthioacetic acid: a study on plasma lipid profile and fatty acid composition and oxidation in different rat organs. *Biochim Biophys Acta* **1300**, 86–96.
18. ELHOLM, M., GARRAS, A., NEVE, S., TORNEHAVE, D., LUND, T.B., SKORVE, J., FLATMARK, T., KRISTIANSEN, K., and BERGE, R.K. (2000). Long-chain acyl-CoA esters and acyl-CoA binding protein are present in the nucleus of rat liver cells. *J Lipid Res* **41**, 538–545.
19. AARSLAND, A., and BERGE, R.K. (1991). Peroxisome proliferating sulphur- and oxy-substituted fatty acid analogues are activated to acyl coenzyme A thioesters. *Biochem Pharmacol* **41**, 53–61.
20. WU, P., GRAV, H.J., HORN, R., and BREMER, J. (1996). Effects of chain length and sulphur position of thia fatty acids on their incorporation into phospholipids in 7800 C1 hepatoma cells and isolated rat hepatocytes, and their effects on fatty acid composition of phospholipids. *Biochem Pharmacol* **51**, 751–758.

21. MURTHY, M.S., and PANDE, S.V. (1990). Characterization of a solubilized malonyl-CoA-sensitive carnitine palmitoyltransferase from the mitochondrial outer membrane as a protein distinct from the malonyl-CoA-insensitive carnitine palmitoyltransferase of the inner membrane. *Biochem J* **268**, 599–604.
22. PANDE, S.V. (1975). A mitochondrial carnitine acylcarnitine translocase system. *Proc Natl Acad Sci USA* **72**, 883–887.
23. MURTHY, M.S., and PANDE, S.V. (1987). Some differences in the properties of carnitine palmitoyltransferase activities of the mitochondrial outer and inner membranes. *Biochem J* **248**, 727–733.
24. MADSEN, L., GARRAS, A., ASINS, G., SERRA, D., HEGARDT, F.G., and BERGE, R.K. (1999). Mitochondrial 3-hydroxy-3-methylglutaryl CoA synthase and carnitine palmitoyltransferase II are potential control sites of hepatic ketogenesis under conditions of peroxisome proliferation. *Biochem Pharmacol* **57**, 1011–1019.
25. GRAV, H.J., TRONSTAD, K.J., GUDBRANDSEN, O.A., BERGE, K., FLADMARK, K.E., MARTINSEN, T.C., WALDUM, H., WERGEDAHL, H., and BERGE, R.K. (2003). Changed energy state and increased mitochondrial beta-oxidation rate in liver of rats associated with lowered proton electrochemical potential and stimulated uncoupling protein 2 (UCP-2) expression: evidence for peroxisome proliferator-activated receptor-alpha independent induction of UCP-2 expression. *J Biol Chem* **278**, 30525–30533.
26. BERGSETH, S., and BREMER, J. (1990). Alkylthioacetic acids (3-thia fatty acids) are metabolized and excreted as shortened dicarboxylic acids *in vivo*. *Biochim Biophys Acta* **1044**, 237–242.
27. HVATTUM, E., BERGSETH, S., PEDERSEN, C.N., BREMER, J., AARSLAND, A., and BERGE, R.K. (1991). Microsomal oxidation of dodecylthioacetic acid (a 3-thia fatty acid) in rat liver. *Biochem Pharmacol* **41**, 945–953.
28. WILLUMSEN, N., SKORVE, J., HEXEBERG, S., RUSTAN, A.C., and BERGE, R.K. (1993). The hypotriglyceridemic effect of eicosapentaenoic acid in rats is reflected in increased mitochondrial fatty acid oxidation followed by diminished lipogenesis. *Lipids* **28**, 683–689.
29. FROYLAND, L., VAAGENES, H., ASIEDU, D.K., GARRAS, A., LIE, O., and BERGE, R.K. (1996). Chronic administration of eicosapentaenoic acid and docosahexaenoic acid as ethyl esters reduced plasma cholesterol and changed the fatty acid composition in rat blood and organs. *Lipids* **31**, 169–178.
30. ASIEDU, D.K., AL-SHURBAJI, A., RUSTAN, A.C., BJORKHEM, I., BERGLUND, L., and BERGE, R.K. (1995). Hepatic fatty acid metabolism as a determinant of plasma and liver triacylglycerol levels. Studies on tetradecylthioacetic and tetradecylthiopropionic acids. *Eur J Biochem* **227**, 715–722.
31. FROYLAND, L., MADSEN, L., SJURSEN, W., GARRAS, A., LIE, O., SONGSTAD, J., RUSTAN, A.C., and BERGE, R.K. (1997). Effect of 3-thia fatty acids on the lipid composition of rat liver, lipoproteins, and heart. *J Lipid Res* **38**, 1522–1534.
32. FROYLAND, L., ASIEDU, D.K., VAAGENES, H., GARRAS, A., LIE, O., TOTLAND, G.K., and BERGE, R.K. (1995). Tetradecylthioacetic acid incorporated into very low density lipoprotein: changes in the fatty acid composition and reduced plasma lipids in cholesterol-fed hamsters. *J Lipid Res* **36**, 2529–2540.
33. WONG, S.H., NESTEL, P.J., TRIMBLE, R.P., STORER, G.B., ILLMAN, R.J., and TOPPING, D.L. (1984). The adaptive effects of dietary fish and safflower oil on lipid and lipoprotein metabolism in perfused rat liver. *Biochim Biophys Acta* **792**, 103–109.
34. BERGE, R.K., MADSEN, L., VAAGENES, H., TRONSTAD, K.J., GOTTLICHER, M., and RUSTAN, A.C. (1999). In contrast with docosahexaenoic acid, eicosapentaenoic acid and

hypolipidaemic derivatives decrease hepatic synthesis and secretion of triacylglycerol by decreased diacylglycerol acyltransferase activity and stimulation of fatty acid oxidation. *Biochem J* **343**, 191–197.

35. WILLUMSEN, N., VAAGENES, H., LIE, O., RUSTAN, A.C., and BERGE, R.K. (1996). Eicosapentaenoic acid, but not docosahexaenoic acid, increases mitochondrial fatty acid oxidation and upregulates 2,4-dienoyl-CoA reductase gene expression in rats. *Lipids* **31**, 579–592.
36. ASIEDU, D.K., SKORVE, J., WILLUMSEN, N., DEMOZ, A., and BERGE, R.K. (1993). Early effects on mitochondrial and peroxisomal beta-oxidation by the hypolipidemic 3-thia-fatty acids in rat livers. *Biochim Biophys Acta* **1166**, 73–76.
37. FROYLAND, L., MADSEN, L., VAAGENES, H., TOTLAND, G.K., AUWERX, J., KRYVI, H., STAELS, B., and BERGE, R.K. (1997). Mitochondrion is the principal target for nutritional and pharmacological control of triglyceride metabolism. *J Lipid Res* **38**, 1851–1858.
38. VAAGENES, H., MADSEN, L., ASIEDU, D.K., LILLEHAUG, J.R., and BERGE, R.K. (1998). Early modulation of genes encoding peroxisomal and mitochondrial beta-oxidation enzymes by 3-thia fatty acids. *Biochem Pharmacol* **56**, 1571–1582.
39. TORRA, I.P., CHINETTI, G., DUVAL, C., FRUCHART, J.C., and STAELS, B. (2001). Peroxisome proliferator-activated receptors: from transcriptional control to clinical practice. *Curr Opin Lipidol* **12**, 245–254.
40. DELERIVE, P., FURMAN, C., TEISSIER, E., FRUCHART, J., DURIEZ, P., and STAELS, B. (2000). Oxidized phospholipids activate PPARalpha in a phospholipase A2-dependent manner. *FEBS Lett* **471**, 34–38.
41. FORMAN, B.M., CHEN, J., and EVANS, R.M. (1997). Hypolipidemic drugs, polyunsaturated fatty acids, and eicosanoids are ligands for peroxisome proliferator-activated receptors alpha and delta. *Proc Natl Acad Sci USA* **94**, 4312–4317.
42. LEHMANN, J.M., LENHARD, J.M., OLIVER, B.B., RINGOLD, G.M., and KLIEWER, S.A. (1997). Peroxisome proliferator-activated receptors alpha and gamma are activated by indomethacin and other non-steroidal anti-inflammatory drugs. *J Biol Chem* **272**, 3406–3410.
43. GOTTLICHER, M., DEMOZ, A., SVENSSON, D., TOLLET, P., BERGE, R.K., and GUSTAFSSON, J.A. (1993). Structural and metabolic requirements for activators of the peroxisome proliferator-activated receptor. *Biochem Pharmacol* **46**, 2177–2184.
44. RASPE, E., MADSEN, L., LEFEBVRE, A.M., LEITERSDORF, I., GELMAN, L., PEINADO-ONSURBE, J., DALLONGEVILLE, J., FRUCHART, J.C., BERGE, R., and STAELS, B. (1999). Modulation of rat liver apolipoprotein gene expression and serum lipid levels by tetradecylthioacetic acid (TTA) via PPARalpha activation. *J Lipid Res* **40**, 2099–2110.
45. BERGE, K., TRONSTAD, K.J., FLINDT, E.N., RASMUSSEN, T.H., MADSEN, L., KRISTIANSEN, K., and BERGE, R.K. (2001). Tetradecylthioacetic acid inhibits growth of rat glioma cells *ex vivo* and *in vivo* via PPAR-dependent and PPAR-independent pathways. *Carcinogenesis* **22**, 1747–1755.
46. WESTERGAARD, M., HENNINGSEN, J., SVENDSEN, M.L., JOHANSEN, C., JENSEN, U.B., SCHRODER, H.D., KRATCHMAROVA, I., BERGE, R.K., IVERSEN, L., BOLUND, L., KRAGBALLE, K., and KRISTIANSEN, K. (2001). Modulation of keratinocyte gene expression and differentiation by PPAR-selective ligands and tetradecylthioacetic acid. *J Invest Dermatol* **116**, 702–712.
47. DALLONGEVILLE, J., BAUGE, E., TAILLEUX, A., PETERS, J.M., GONZALEZ, F.J., FRUCHART, J.C., and STAELS, B. (2001). Peroxisome proliferator-activated receptor alpha is not rate-limiting for the lipoprotein-lowering action of fish oil. *J Biol Chem* **276**, 4634–4639.

48. PETERS, J.M., PARK, Y., GONZALEZ, F.J., and PARIZA, M.W. (2001). Influence of conjugated linoleic acid on body composition and target gene expression in peroxisome proliferator-activated receptor alpha-null mice. *Biochim Biophys Acta* **1533**, 233–242.
49. AOYAMA, T., PETERS, J.M., IRITANI, N., NAKAJIMA, T., FURIHATA, K., HASHIMOTO, T., and GONZALEZ, F.J. (1998). Altered constitutive expression of fatty acid-metabolizing enzymes in mice lacking the peroxisome proliferator-activated receptor alpha (PPARalpha). *J Biol Chem* **273**, 5678–5684.
50. FREDENRICH, A., and GRIMALDI, P.A. (2004). Roles of peroxisome proliferator-activated receptor delta in skeletal muscle function and adaptation. *Curr Opin Clin Nutr Metab Care* **7**, 377–381.
51. WANG, Y.X., LEE, C.H., TIEP, S., YU, R.T., HAM, J., KANG, H., and EVANS, R.M. (2003). Peroxisome-proliferator-activated receptor delta activates fat metabolism to prevent obesity. *Cell* **113**, 159–170.
52. OLEFSKY, J.M. (2000). Treatment of insulin resistance with peroxisome proliferator-activated receptor gamma agonists. *J Clin Invest* **106**, 467–472.
53. GUERRE-MILLO, M., GERVOIS, P., RASPE, E., MADSEN, L., POULAIN, P., DERUDAS, B., HERBERT, J.M., WINEGAR, D.A., WILLSON, T.M., FRUCHART, J.C., BERGE, R.K., and STAELS, B. (2000). Peroxisome proliferator-activated receptor alpha activators improve insulin sensitivity and reduce adiposity. *J Biol Chem* **275**, 16638–16642.
54. MADSEN, L., GUERRE-MILLO, M., FLINDT, E.N., BERGE, K., TRONSTAD, K.J., BERGENE, E., SEBOKOVA, E., RUSTAN, A.C., JENSEN, J., MANDRUP, S., KRISTIANSEN, K., KLIMES, I., STAELS, B., and BERGE, R.K. (2002). Tetradecylthioacetic acid prevents high fat diet induced adiposity and insulin resistance. *J Lipid Res* **43**, 742–750.
55. BERGE, R.K., TRONSTAD, K.J., BERGE, K., ROST, T.H., WERGEDAHL, H., GUDBRANDSEN, O.A., and SKORVE, J. (2005). The metabolic syndrome and the hepatic fatty acid drainage hypothesis. *Biochimie* **87**, 15–20.
56. VAN DIJK, K.W., RENSEN, P.C., VOSHOL, P.J., and HAVEKES, L.M. (2004). The role and mode of action of apolipoproteins CIII and AV: synergistic actors in triglyceride metabolism? *Curr Opin Lipidol* **15**, 239–246.
57. BERGE, R.K., STENSLAND, E., AARSLAND, A., TSEGAI, G., OSMUNDSEN, H., AARSAETHER, N., and GJELLESVIK, D.R. (1987). Induction of cytosolic clofibroyl-CoA hydrolase activity in liver of rats treated with clofibrate. *Biochim Biophys Acta* **918**, 60–66.
58. GUDBRANDSEN, O.A., DYRØY, E., BOHOV, P., SKORVE, J., and BERGE, R.K. (2005). The metabolic effects of thia fatty acids in rat liver depend on the position of the sulfur atom. *Chem Biol Interact* **155**, 71–81.
59. CABRERO, A., ALEGRET, M., SANCHEZ, R.M., ADZET, T., LAGUNA, J.C., and VAZQUEZ, M. (2001). Bezafibrate reduces mRNA levels of adipocyte markers and increases fatty acid oxidation in primary culture of adipocytes. *Diabetes* **50**, 1883–1890.
60. DELERIVE, P., FRUCHART, J.C., and STAELS, B. (2001). Peroxisome proliferator-activated receptors in inflammation control. *J Endocrinol* **169**, 453–459.
61. AUKRUST, P., WERGEDAHL, H., MULLER, F., UELAND, T., DYROY, E., DAMAS, J.K., FROLAND, S.S., and BERGE, R.K. (2003). Immunomodulating effects of 3-thia fatty acids in activated peripheral blood mononuclear cells. *Eur J Clin Invest* **33**, 426–433.
62. TRONSTAD, K.J., BRUSERUD, O., BERGE, K., and BERGE, R.K. (2002). Antiproliferative effects of a non-beta-oxidizable fatty acid, tetradecylthioacetic acid, in native human acute myelogenous leukemia blast cultures. *Leukemia* **16**, 2292–2301.
63. MUNA, Z.A., BOLANN, B.J., CHEN, X., SONGSTAD, J., and BERGE, R.K. (2000). Tetradecylthioacetic acid and tetradecylselenoacetic acid inhibit lipid peroxidation and

interact with superoxide radical [In Process Citation]. *Free Radic Biol Med* **28**, 1068–1078.

64. MUNA, Z.A., DOUDIN, K., SONGSTAD, J., ULVIK, R.J., and BERGE, R.K. (1997). Tetradecylthioacetic acid inhibits the oxidative modification of low density lipoprotein and 8-hydroxydeoxyguanosine formation *in vitro*. *Arterioscler Thromb Vasc Biol* **17**, 3255–3262.
65. MUNA, Z.A., GUDBRANDSEN, O.A., WERGEDAHL, H., BOHOV, P., SKORVE, J., and BERGE, R.K. (2002). Inhibition of rat lipoprotein oxidation after tetradecylthioacetic acid feeding. *Biochem Pharmacol* **63**, 1127–1135.
66. DEMOZ, A., SVARDAL, A., and BERGE, R.K. (1993). Relationship between peroxisome-proliferating sulfur-substituted fatty acid analogs, hepatic lipid peroxidation and hydrogen peroxide metabolism. *Biochem Pharmacol* **45**, 257–259.
67. DEMOZ, A., ASIEDU, D.K., LIE, O., and BERGE, R.K. (1994). Modulation of plasma and hepatic oxidative status and changes in plasma lipid profile by n-3 (EPA and DHA), n-6 (corn oil) and a 3-thia fatty acid in rats. *Biochim Biophys Acta* **1199**, 238–244.
68. ANEJA, A., EL-ATAT, F., MCFARLANE, S.I., and SOWERS, J.R. (2004). Hypertension and obesity. *Recent Prog Horm Res* **59**, 169–205.
69. MIYAZAKI, Y., MAHANKALI, A., WAJCBERG, E., BAJAJ, M., MANDARINO, L.J., and DEFRONZO, R.A. (2004). Effect of pioglitazone on circulating adipocytokine levels and insulin sensitivity in type 2 diabetic patients. *J Clin Endocrinol Metab* **89**, 4312–4319.
70. GELEIJNSE, J.M., GILTAY, E.J., GROBBEE, D.E., DONDERS, A.R., and KOK, F.J. (2002). Blood pressure response to fish oil supplementation: metaregression analysis of randomized trials. *J Hypertens* **20**, 1493–1499.
71. FREDRIKSEN, J., UELAND, T., DYROY, E., HALVORSEN, B., MELBY, K., MELBYE, L., SKALHEGG, B.S., BOHOV, P., SKORVE, J., BERGE, R.K., AUKRUST, P., and FROLAND, S.S. (2004). Lipid-lowering and anti-inflammatory effects of tetradecylthioacetic acid in HIV-infected patients on highly active antiretroviral therapy. *Eur J Clin Invest* **34**, 709–715.
72. DYRØY, E., YNDESTAD, A., UELAND, T., AUKRUST, P., and BERGE, R.K. (2005). Anti-inflammatory effects of tetradecylthioacetic acid involve both peroxisome proliferator-activated receptor alpha-dependent and -independent pathways. *Arterioscler Thromb Vasc Biol* **25**, 1364–1369.
73. MOYA-FALCON, C., HVATTUM, E., DYROY, E., SKORVE, J., STEFANSSON, S.O., THOMASSEN, M.S., JAKOBSEN, J.V., BERGE, R.K., and RUYTER, B. (2004). Effects of 3-thia fatty acids on feed intake, growth, tissue fatty acid composition, beta-oxidation and Na^+,K^+-ATPase activity in Atlantic salmon. *Comp Biochem Physiol B Biochem Mol Biol* **139**, 657–668.

Index